ADVANCED SKILLS
for
HEALTH CARE
PROVIDERS
SECOND EDITION

ADVANCED SKILLS
for
HEALTH CARE
PROVIDERS

SECOND EDITION

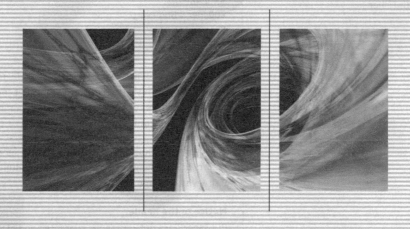

Barbara Acello, MS, RN

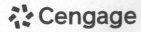
Cengage

Australia • Brazil • Canada • Mexico • Singapore • United Kingdom • United States

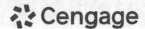

Advanced Skills for Health Care Providers,
Second Edition
Barbara Acello

Vice President, Health Care Business Unit:
William Brottmiller

Director of Learning Solutions: Mathew Kane

Managing Editor: Marah Bellegarde

Associate Acquisitions Editor: Matthew Seeley

Editorial Assistant: Jadin Babin-Kavanaugh

Marketing Director: Jennifer McAvey

Marketing Manager: Michele Gleason

Technology Director: Laurie Davis

Production Director: Carolyn Miller

Production Manager: Barbara A. Bullock

Art and Design Specialist: Alexandros Vasilakos

Content Project Manager: Thomas Heffernan

Project Editor: Ruth Fisher

For product information and technology assistance, contact us at
Cengage Customer & Sales Support, 1-800-354-9706
or support.cengage.com.

For permission to use material from this text or product, submit all
requests online at **www.copyright.com**.

Library of Congress Control Number: 2005037322

ISBN-13: 978-1-4180-0133-9
ISBN-10: 1-4180-0133-3

Cengage
200 Pier 4 Boulevard
Boston, MA 02210
USA

Cengage is a leading provider of customized learning solutions
with employees residing in nearly 40 different countries and sales in more
than 125 countries around the world. Find your local representative at:
www.cengage.com.

To learn more about Cengage platforms and services, register or access
your online learning solution, or purchase materials for your course,
visit **www.cengage.com**.

Notice to the Reader
Publisher does not warrant or guarantee any of the products described
herein or perform any independent analysis in connection with any of
the product information contained herein. Publisher does not assume,
and expressly disclaims, any obligation to obtain and include information
other than that provided to it by the manufacturer. The reader is expressly
warned to consider and adopt all safety precautions that might be indicated
by the activities described herein and to avoid all potential hazards. By
following the instructions contained herein, the reader willingly assumes
all risks in connection with such instructions. The publisher makes no
representations or warranties of any kind, including but not limited to, the
warranties of fitness for particular purpose or merchantability, nor are any
such representations implied with respect to the material set forth herein,
and the publisher takes no responsibility with respect to such material. The
publisher shall not be liable for any special, consequential, or exemplary
damages resulting, in whole or part, from the readers' use of, or reliance
upon, this material.

Printed in the United States of America
Print Number: 15   Print Year: 2022

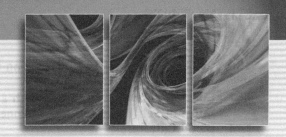

Contents

xiii | Preface

CHAPTER 1
Health Care Delivery for the 21st Century 1

1 | Health Care Delivery from 1980 to the Present
2 | Quality Assurance
6 | Patient-Focused Care
10 | Delegation
12 | Teamwork
13 | Desirable Qualities of the PCT
15 | Professional Boundaries
16 | Communication
19 | Developmental Tasks
19 | Age-Appropriate Care
32 | Restorative Nursing Care

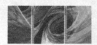

CHAPTER 2
Observation, Documentation, and Reporting to the RN 38

38 | Communicating with Other Members of the Health Care Team
39 | Observing the Patient
45 | Pain
47 | Reporting Observations
47 | Recording Observations on the Medical Record
49 | Legal Considerations
50 | Guidelines for Charting
50 | Computers in Health Care Facilities
53 | Guidelines for Documentation on the Computerized Medical Record

CHAPTER 3
Infection Control 57

57 | Spread of Infection
58 | Handwashing
62 | Guidelines for Times When Handwashing Should Be Done

63 | Waterless Hand Cleaners
64 | Standard Precautions
73 | Isolation Measures
78 | Guidelines for Putting on Personal Protective Equipment
80 | Guidelines for Removing Personal Protective Equipment
80 | Beginning and Ending Procedure Actions
80 | Bioterrorism

CHAPTER 4
Surgical Asepsis 88

88 | Sterile Technique
89 | Guidelines for Sterile Procedures
91 | Setting Up a Sterile Field
94 | Sterile Gloves
96 | Sterilization

CHAPTER 5
Wound Care 100

100 | The Skin
102 | Factors Affecting Wound Healing
104 | Removing a Dressing
105 | Cleansing the Wound
106 | Guidelines for Wound Irrigation
106 | Dressings and Bandages
107 | Sterile Technique and Clean Technique
108 | Applying a Dressing
112 | Managing Wounds with Drains
113 | Wet–to–Dry Dressings
114 | Transparent Film and Hydrocolloid Dressings
116 | Pin Care
117 | Removing Sutures and Staples

CHAPTER 6
Phlebotomy 123

123 | Phlebotomy
125 | Standard Precautions
125 | Methods of Drawing Blood
129 | Selecting a Vein and Performing the Venipuncture

136 | Collecting a Blood Specimen Using the Vacuum-Tube System
141 | Collecting a Blood Specimen with a Winged Infusion Set (Butterfly) and Syringe
144 | Blood Cultures
146 | Drawing Blood Using a Lancet for a Microdraw or Infant Heel Stick
150 | Measuring Bleeding Time
152 | Transporting Specimens to the Laboratory
152 | The Centrifuge

CHAPTER 7
Intravenous Therapy   157

157 | Intravenous Therapy
161 | Inserting a Peripheral IV in an Adult
168 | Heparin Locks
169 | Inserting an IV Using a Butterfly Needle
170 | Inserting a Peripheral IV in a Child
171 | Monitoring Intravenous Flow Rate
173 | Using IV Pumps and Controllers
173 | Complications of IV Therapy
177 | Changing a Peripheral IV Dressing
179 | Discontinuing a Peripheral IV
179 | Assisting the RN with a Central Intravenous Catheter Change
182 | Blood Administration

CHAPTER 8
Urinary and Bowel Elimination   189

189 | Role of the PCT in Assisting Patients with Elimination Procedures
190 | Testing Urine
196 | Catheters
207 | Guidelines for Opening a Closed Drainage System
208 | Guidelines for Applying a Urinary Leg Bag
209 | Guidelines for Drainage Bag Disinfection
209 | Suprapubic Catheters
210 | Nephrostomy Tubes
213 | Bladder Irrigation
216 | Removing an Indwelling Catheter
217 | Care of the Patient Who Is Receiving Dialysis
219 | Bowel Elimination
223 | Guidelines for Enema Administration
229 | Caring for Patients with Ostomies
230 | Guidelines for Caring for an Ostomy

CHAPTER 9
Enteral Nutrition   239

239 | Tube Feeding
240 | Nasogastric Tube Insertion and Care
243 | Checking Nasogastric Tube Placement

245 | Determining Residual Stomach Contents
246 | Irrigating a Nasogastric Tube
247 | Removing a Nasogastric Tube
248 | Caring for a Patient with a Gastrostomy
251 | Feeding Patients with an Enteral Tube
261 | Equipment Alarms

CHAPTER 10
Specimen Collection   266

266 | Specimen Collection
267 | Guidelines for Collecting a Specimen
267 | Culture and Sensitivity Testing
268 | Guidelines for Collecting Culture and Sensitivity Specimens
269 | Throat Culture
270 | Testing for Group A Streptococcus Antigen
271 | Wound Infection
273 | Sputum Culture
274 | Gastric Specimen
274 | Urine Specimen Collection
282 | Stool Specimen
286 | Measuring Blood Glucose
290 | Measuring Glycated Hemoglobin

CHAPTER 11
Perioperative Care   298

298 | Perioperative Nursing Care
300 | Advances in Caring for Surgical Patients
300 | Preoperative Skin Care
302 | During the Operative Period
303 | Postoperative Care
308 | Guidelines for Leg Exercises
310 | Respiratory Exercises
312 | Support Hosiery
314 | Guidelines for Applying Antiembolism Stockings
316 | Pneumatic Cuffs
318 | Caring for Patients Who Have Orthopedic Disorders

CHAPTER 12
Heat and Cold Applications   338

338 | Heat and Cold Treatments
339 | Guidelines for Using Heat and Cold Applications
340 | Heat Treatments
350 | Hydrotherapy
351 | Guidelines for Giving a Whirlpool Bath
352 | Guidelines for Monitoring Hydrotherapy Equipment
358 | Cold Applications
362 | Warm and Cool Eye Compresses

363 | Hypothermia
365 | Heat-Related Illness
366 | The Hypothermia-Hyperthermia Blanket

CHAPTER 13
Caring for Patients with Special Needs 373

373 | Special-Needs Patients
374 | Working with Interpreters
374 | Guidelines for Working with Interpreters in the Health Care Facility
376 | Domestic Violence
382 | Delirium
383 | Caring for Patients with Seizure Disorders
388 | Spinal Cord Injuries
392 | Caring for Patients Who Are Receiving Chemotherapy
394 | Caring for the Patient Who Is Receiving Radiation Therapy
395 | Guidelines for Working with Radiation Therapy and Brachytherapy Patients
397 | Caring for the Patient Who Is Receiving Immunotherapy
397 | The Rehabilitation Services Team
401 | The Pain Problem
402 | Pain Management Procedures

CHAPTER 14
Respiratory Procedures 415

415 | Structure and Function of the Respiratory System
417 | Caring for Patients Who Have Respiratory Conditions
418 | Capillary Refill
418 | The Pulse Oximeter
421 | Oxygen Therapy
424 | Guidelines for Oxygen Safety
431 | Oropharyngeal Airway
433 | Nasopharyngeal Airway
434 | Suction
438 | Small-Volume Nebulizer Treatment
440 | Noninvasive Mechanical Ventilation
441 | Postural Drainage

CHAPTER 15
Advanced Respiratory Procedures 448

448 | Endotracheal Intubation
453 | Patients Who Breathe Through the Neck
462 | Chest Tubes
464 | Caring for a Patient Who Is Mechanically Ventilated

CHAPTER 16
Cardiac Care Skills 470

470 | Electrical Conduction of the Heart
472 | Monitoring the Heartbeat
475 | Identifying Cardiac Rhythms
488 | Performing an ECG
495 | Continuous Cardiac Monitoring
498 | Monitoring the Pulse to Evaluate Circulation
502 | Blood Pressure
504 | Guidelines for Electronic Blood Pressure Monitoring
505 | Caring for a Patient Following an Angiogram or Arteriogram
505 | Guidelines for Caring for a Patient Post-Arteriogram (or Angiogram)
506 | Cardiac Catheterization

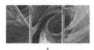

CHAPTER 17
Emergency Procedures 511

511 | Resuscitation
512 | The ABCs of Emergency Care
513 | Protecting the Airway
513 | Maintaining the Patient's Breathing
519 | Cardiopulmonary Resuscitation
522 | The Recovery Position
523 | Introduction to the Crash Cart
523 | Defibrillation
527 | Postresuscitation Care

APPENDIX A
Guidelines for Hand Hygiene 531

531 | Introduction
533 | Latex Allergy
536 | Mercury
537 | Mercury Spills

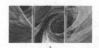

APPENDIX B
Abbreviations and Medical Terminology 538

538 | Abbreviation Problems
542 | General Abbreviations
556 | Medical Terminology

APPENDIX C
Electronic Communication 560

563 | Medication and Treatment Orders

APPENDIX D
Procedures and Other Useful Information 566

566 | Caring for a Patient with a T–Tube
568 | Using a Closed Wound Drainage System
570 | Additional Methods for Versatile Cardiac Monitoring

573 | Heart and Electrocardiogram Study Guide
575 | Calculating Intravenous Drip Rates

GLOSSARY 579

INDEX 592

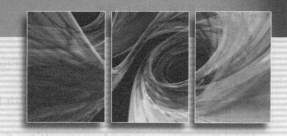

Procedure List

62 | Procedure 1 Handwashing

67 | Procedure 2 Applying Disposable Gloves

68 | Procedure 3 Removing Disposable Gloves

68 | Procedure 4 Applying a Gown

70 | Procedure 5 Removing a Gown

71 | Procedure 6 Applying a Surgical Mask

72 | Procedure 7 Removing a Surgical Mask

72 | Procedure 8 Applying Protective Eyewear

72 | Procedure 9 Removing Protective Eyewear

75 | Procedure 10 Applying a NIOSH-Approved Respirator

76 | Procedure 11 Removing a NIOSH-Approved Respirator

90 | Procedure 12 Opening a Sterile Tray

91 | Procedure 13 Opening a Sterile Package

92 | Procedure 14 Setting Up a Sterile Field Using a Sterile Drape

93 | Procedure 15 Adding an Item to a Sterile Field

93 | Procedure 16 Adding Liquids to a Sterile Field

94 | Procedure 17 Applying and Removing Sterile Gloves

96 | Procedure 18 Using Transfer Forceps

108 | Procedure 19 Changing a Clean Dressing

109 | Procedure 20 Applying a Bandage

111 | Procedure 21 Applying a Sterile Dressing

112 | Procedure 22 Applying a Dressing Around a Drain

113 | Procedure 23 Changing Wet-to-Dry Dressings

115 | Procedure 24 Applying a Transparent Film Dressing

116 | Procedure 25 Applying a Hydrocolloid Dressing

117 | Procedure 26 Pin Care

118 | Procedure 27 Removing Sutures

119 | Procedure 28 Removing Staples

133 | Procedure 29 Performing a Venipuncture

140 | Procedure 30 Collecting a Blood Specimen Using the Vacuum-Tube System

143 | Procedure 31 Collecting a Blood Specimen Using a Butterfly Needle and Syringe

144 | Procedure 32 Using the Blood Transfer Device

145 | Procedure 33 Collecting a Blood Culture

149 | Procedure 34 Drawing Blood Using a Lancet for a Microdraw or Infant Heel Stick

150 | Procedure 35 Measuring Bleeding Time

160 | Procedure 36 Assembling and Priming a Basic Administration Set

166 | Procedure 37 Inserting a Peripheral IV in an Adult

168 | Procedure 38 Inserting a Heparin Lock

169 | Procedure 39 Inserting an IV with a Butterfly Needle

171 | Procedure 40 Inserting a Peripheral IV in a Child

172 | Procedure 41 Monitoring the Intravenous Flow Rate

178 | Procedure 42 Applying a Transparent Film Dressing to an Intravenous Infusion Site

179 | Procedure 43 Discontinuing a Peripheral IV

181 | Procedure 44 Assisting the RN with a Central IV Dressing Change

183 | Procedure 45 Obtaining and Checking Blood from the Blood Bank

183 | Procedure 46 Checking Blood Products on the Nursing Unit

192 | Procedure 47 Testing Urine with Reagent Strips

194 | Procedure 48 Measuring Urine Specific Gravity with a Urinometer

195 | Procedure 49 Measuring Urine Specific Gravity with a Refractometer

195 | Procedure 50 Multistix Urine Testing

199 | Procedure 51 Inserting a Straight Catheter

202 | Procedure 52 Inserting an Indwelling Catheter

212 | Procedure 53 Changing a Nephrostomy Tube Dressing

213 | Procedure 54 Open Bladder Irrigation

215 | Procedure 55 Closed Bladder Irrigation

215 | Procedure 56 Continuous Bladder Irrigation

216 | Procedure 57 Removing an Indwelling Catheter

220 | Procedure 58 Inserting a Rectal Tube and Flatus Bag

221 | Procedure 59 Inserting a Rectal Suppository

224 | Procedure 60 Administering a Cleansing Enema

226 | Procedure 61 Administering a Commercially Prepared Enema

228 | Procedure 62 Breaking Up and Removing a Fecal Impaction

231 | Procedure 63 Changing an Ostomy Appliance

232 | Procedure 64 Irrigating a Colostomy

241 | Procedure 65 Inserting a Nasogastric Tube

245 | Procedure 66 Checking Nasogastric Tube Placement

246 | Procedure 67 Aspirating for Residual Stomach Contents

247 | Procedure 68 Irrigating a Nasogastric Tube

247 | Procedure 69 Removing a Nasogastric Tube

249 | Procedure 70 Gastrostomy Tube Care

250 | Procedure 71 Inserting a Gastrostomy Tube into an Established Tract

259 | Procedure 72 Bolus Enteral Feeding

260 | Procedure 73 Continuous Enteral Feeding with a Pump

270 | Procedure 74 Collecting a Throat Culture

272 | Procedure 75 Obtaining a Swab Culture from a Wound

273 | Procedure 76 Collecting a Sputum Specimen

274 | Procedure 77 Collecting a Specimen for Gastric Analysis

275 | Procedure 78 Collecting a Midstream Urine Sample

276 | Procedure 79 Collecting a 24-Hour Urine Specimen

277 | Procedure 80 Collecting a Sterile Urine Specimen from an Indwelling Catheter

278 | Procedure 81 Obtaining a Urine Specimen Using the Speci-Cath Collection Device

281 | Procedure 82 Straining the Urine for Renal Calculi

282 | Procedure 83 Collecting a Pediatric Urine Specimen

283 | Procedure 84 Collecting a Stool Specimen

284 | Procedure 85 Collecting a Rectal Swab Specimen for Culture and Sensitivity

285 | Procedure 86 Collecting and Testing a Stool Specimen for Occult Blood

290 | Procedure 87 Obtaining a Fingerstick Blood Sugar

302 | Procedure 88 Shaving the Operative Site

310 | Procedure 89 Coughing and Deep Breathing Exercises

312 | Procedure 90 Incentive Spirometry

314 | Procedure 91 Applying Antiembolism Stockings (Graduated Compression Hosiery)

317 | Procedure 92 Applying the Pneumatic Compression Device

320 | Procedure 93 Applying an Arm Sling

325 | Procedure 94 Continuous Passive Motion Therapy

330 | Procedure 95 Setting Up Traction (Claw-Type Basic Frame)

341 | Procedure 96 Applying a Hot Water Bottle, Gel Pack, or Chemical Hot Pack

343 | Procedure 97 Performing a Warm Soak

344 | Procedure 98 Applying Warm, Moist Compresses

346 | Procedure 99 Applying an Aquathermia Pad (K-Pad)

349 | Procedure 100 Applying Moist Hot Packs (Hydrocollator Tank)

354 | Procedure 101 Giving a Tepid Sponge Bath to an Adult

355 | Procedure 102 Giving a Tepid Bath to a Child

357 | Procedure 103 Giving a Sitz Bath

359 | Procedure 104 Applying an Ice Bag, Ice Collar, Gel Pack, or Chemical Cold Pack

361 | Procedure 105 Applying Cool, Moist Compresses

361 | Procedure 106 Performing a Cool Soak

363 | Procedure 107 Applying Warm or Cool Eye Compresses

367 | Procedure 108 Applying the Hypothermia-Hyperthermia Blanket

387 | Procedure 109 Caring for the Patient Who Is Having a Seizure

418 | Procedure 110 Checking Capillary Refill

420 | Procedure 111 Using a Pulse Oximeter

425 | Procedure 112 Preparing Wall-Outlet Oxygen

426 | Procedure 113 Preparing the Oxygen Cylinder

428 | Procedure 114 Attaching the Humidifier to the Oxygen Flow Meter or Regulator

429 | Procedure 115 Administering Oxygen Through a Nasal Cannula

430 | Procedure 116 Administering Oxygen Through a Mask

432 | Procedure 117 Inserting the Oropharyngeal Airway

434 | Procedure 118 Inserting the Nasopharyngeal Airway

436 | Procedure 119 Oropharyngeal Suctioning

437 | Procedure 120 Nasopharyngeal Suctioning

439 | Procedure 121 Administering a Small-Volume Nebulizer Treatment

443 | Procedure 122 Assisting with Postural Drainage

452 | Procedure 123 Assisting with Endotracheal Intubation

453 | Procedure 124 Ventilating an Endotracheal Tube Using a Bag-Valve Device

456 | Procedure 125 Ventilating a Tracheostomy Using a Bag-Valve Device

457 | Procedure 126 Suctioning a Tracheostomy

458 | Procedure 127 Giving Tracheostomy/Stoma Care Using a Nondisposable Inner Cannula

460 | Procedure 128 Giving Tracheostomy/Stoma Care Using a Disposable Inner Cannula

462 | Procedure 129 Applying a Tracheostomy Dressing and Ties

493 | Procedure 130 Performing a 12-Lead ECG

498 | Procedure 131 Setting Up for Continuous Cardiac Monitoring

499 | Procedure 132 Counting the Apical-Radial Pulse

501 | Procedure 133 Checking the Pulses in the Legs and Feet

502 | Procedure 134 Using a Doppler to Hear Pulse Sounds

504 | Procedure 135 Taking Blood Pressure with an Electronic Blood Pressure Apparatus

506 | Procedure 136 Monitoring after Cardiac Catheterization

514 | Procedure 137 Head-Tilt, Chin-Lift Maneuver

515 | Procedure 138 Jaw-Thrust Maneuver

516 | Procedure 139 Obstructed Airway Procedure, Conscious Patient

518 | Procedure 140 Mouth-to-Mask Ventilation

519 | Procedure 141 Bag-Valve Mask Ventilation, Two Rescuers

520 | Procedure 142 One-Rescuer CPR, Adult

521 | Procedure 143 Two-Rescuer CPR, Adult

523 | Procedure 144 Positioning the Patient in the Recovery Position

525 | Procedure 145 Managing Cardiac Arrest Using an AED

567 | Procedure D1 Caring for a T-Tube or Similar Wound Drain

568 | Procedure D2 Caring for a Closed Wound Drainage System

569 | Procedure D3 Discontinuing an IV and Switching to a Heparin Lock

572 | Procedure D4 Applying a Holter Monitor

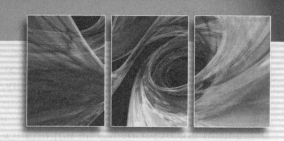

Preface

INTRODUCTION

During the 1990s many changes occurred in health care. Among these, the scope of practice of unlicensed assistive personnel was expanded to include skills that were formerly performed only by nurses or caregivers from other disciplines. New courses of instruction were developed to prepare competent caregivers to practice these advanced skills.

Advanced Skills for Health Care Providers is a comprehensive text that consolidates advanced procedural skills from many sources to make it easier for students and instructors to find and use the information. The book was written for those caregivers or patient care technicians (PCTs) who will perform advanced skills in acute care facilities, clinics, HMOs, home health care agencies, and other facilities.

TEXT DEVELOPMENT

In the United States, there is no standard or formal scope of practice for the PCT. Individual state nurse practice acts vary, and these have a profound effect on the advanced care skills that PCTs are allowed to perform. Similarly, facility and agency policies and practices vary. As a result, some of the procedures in this book may not be used in some facilities, agencies, or states.

This book is written to meet a market need for an all-inclusive source of advanced patient care information. During the initial stages of development, instructors in PCT programs were surveyed for course information and lists of procedures taught in their programs. The content of the book is based largely on the information gained from these surveys. The book was extensively peer-reviewed by instructors, as well as specialists in various health care fields. Consideration was given to procedural scope, procedural accuracy, and the students' reading level.

The user of this book must have some patient care knowledge, such as can be obtained through nursing assistant or basic PCT education. Previous experience in providing basic patient care as a nursing assistant or PCT is invaluable. The information herein will assist the reader in integrating basic information with chapter content, enabling him or her to achieve advanced level skills.

We recognize that the PCT will be supervised by a licensed health professional, but the title and licensure of this individual may vary with the practice setting. In this book, the registered nurse (RN) is the supervisor, although the reporting information is appropriate for other licensed personnel as well. The individual receiving care is called the *patient*. There are many titles for unlicensed individuals providing patient care. We have chosen *patient care technician,* which is commonly used, for use in this book.

Each patient must be admitted to the health care facility with physician approval. The patient's care must be supervised by a licensed physician who has admitting and other privileges. Some facilities and physicians employ other licensed professionals, such as nurse practitioners (NP), clinical nurse specialists (CNS), and physician assistants (PA) to work in collaboration with the physician(s). Today, non-physician practitioners are increasingly assuming primary health care duties that were formerly the exclusive province of physicians. The author and publisher acknowledge the many positive contributions that these non-physician practitioners make to quality patient care. However, for ease of reading and grammar, this book uses the terms "doctor" and "physician" when referring to the primary health care provider. This is not meant to devalue the contributions that nurse practitioners, clinical nurse specialists, or physician assistants make to facility operations and patient care.

CONTENT ORGANIZATION

The book begins with an overview of the changes in the health care industry spanning the past 25 years; this continues into a description of how the PCT role evolved. The role of the PCT is described, as are his or her responsibilities to patients, supervisor, and the facility or agency. Legal issues involving scope of practice, nurse practice acts, and delegation are described. The importance of using good communication skills begins in Chapter 1 and is emphasized throughout the book.

Making observations, reporting these observations to the licensed supervisor, and documentation are covered in Chapter 2. Chapters 3 and 4 describe infection control and sterile technique. The information in the first four chapters establishes the groundwork for the remainder of the book. Chapters 5 through 17 contain procedural content, including wound care, phlebotomy and intravenous therapy, procedures related to urine and bowel elimination, enteral nutrition, specimen collection, perioperative care, respiratory care procedures, cardiac care skills, and emergency care. Each chapter emphasizes the importance of safety, infection control, patient rights, and communication skills.

Appendices were added to this edition to provide additional information on subject matter for which PCT is responsible, but has not necessarily committed to memory. This includes infection control and latex allergies, medical terminology, HIPAA-compliant electronic communication, transcription of physician orders, and advanced procedures for which some PCTs are responsible. This content was identified and requested by a peer review team, the members of which instruct and supervise PCTs in the classroom, skills lab, and clinical environment.

FEATURES

The following features are provided to aid the learner in understanding critical content.

- Objectives appear at the beginning of every chapter, to focus readers on the concepts they will be introduced to in the chapter.
- Key terms are bolded within the text so that they can easily be identified by the reader. Additionally, the definition of the term is given within the paragraph so that the reader is exposed to the term in context.
- The "Chapter Review," found at the end of each chapter tests readers comprehension of the chapter concepts, and allows self-evaluation of the need for review or further study.
- "Key Points" summarize the concepts presented in each chapter.

- "Clinical Applications" exercises ask the readers to apply the concepts they have learned to a scenario and determine the appropriate action.
- The importance of reporting information and observations to the licensed supervisor is emphasized throughout the book. To this end, most chapters contain special "Observe & Report" sections listing observations to be reported and recorded.
- "Guideline" boxes have been added to highlight and summarize important points.
- Alerts have been added with pertinent information on "Infection Control," "OSHA," "Communications," "Age-Appropriate Care," "Legal Implications," "Safety," "Culture," "Difficult Patient Care," and "Health Care."
- Website addresses have been added to each chapter so that readers can find further information.

NEW TO THE SECOND EDITION

Numerous changes were made in the second edition of *Advanced Skills for Health Care Providers*, to better prepare the PCT to meet the needs of the evolving patient base in the changing regulatory climate. New information has been added to reflect the current trends in infection control, disease management, industry trends, and patient care. The following updated and advanced content addresses the changing character of PCT responsibilities.

- HIPAA is introduced, and the documentation section has been explained with a focus on electronic documentation.
- The infection control content has been updated to reflect the use of alcohol-based hand cleaners, the addition of expanded precautions, and the new CDC recommendations.
- A chapter has been added describing heat and cold applications.
- A chapter has been added describing the care of patients with special needs, such as:
  - Patients who need the services of an interpreter
  - Victims of domestic and relationship violence
  - Patients who have signs and symptoms of delirium
  - Patients who have seizures

- Patients with paralysis, including recognition of automatic dysreflexia
- Patients who are receiving chemotherapy, radiation therapy, brachytherapy, and immunotherapy
- Patients with rehabilitation needs
- Patients who have pain
- Patients who have epidural catheters or implanted medication pumps
- Patients who are receiving transcutaneous electrical nerve stimulation

Other new content and procedures include:

- 2003 National Institutes of Health blood pressure guidelines
- Caring for a patient who is on dialysis
- Caring for patients who have suprapubic catheters
- Caring for patients who have nephrostomy tubes
- Caring for the patient who uses a urinary leg bag
- Administering enemas
- Inserting a rectal tube
- Inserting a gastrostomy tube into an established stoma/tract
- Collecting a urine specimen from an infant
- Straining urine
- Collecting a rectal swab and wound culture
- Providing perioperative nursing care
- Appling antiembolism hose
- Identifying compartment syndrome
- Caring for a patient who has a laryngectomy
- Differentiating a tracheostomy from a laryngectomy
- Caring for a patient who is on a ventilator
- Caring for a patient who uses CPAP or BiPap
- Caring for a patient who has a chest tube
- Taking an apical-radial pulse
- Taking a femoral pulse
- Using a Doppler to hear pulse sounds
- Using an electronic blood pressure apparatus
- Caring for a patient after an arteriogram or angiogram
- Operating the automatic external defibrillator
- Giving a small-volume nebulizer treatment
- Irrigating a wound
- Caring for a T-tube or comparable drain
- Applying a Holter monitor
- Caring for patients who have orthopedic disorders or who have had hip surgery

SUPPLEMENTS

Instructor Supplements

New to this edition is an accompanying Electronic Classroom Manager CD-ROM. This includes an Instructor's Manual, Computerized Testbank, and PowerPoint presentation. The **Instructor's Manual** contains teaching methods and strategies, lesson plans, student and instructor resources, quizzes and testing material, crossword puzzles and solutions, performance competency checklists for all procedures, and student handouts. The **Computerized Testbank** supplies approximately 800 questions. The software allows instructors to use questions as is, alter existing questions, or write their own. The Electronic Classroom Manager also includes a **PowerPoint slide presentation** that is designed to enhance classroom instruction. The presentation can be used as is, or altered to meet instructor needs.

Order Number 1-4180-01341.

Student Supplements

A *Workbook to Accompany Advanced Skills for Health Care Providers* has been added to enhance student learning, retention of material, and ability to use critical thinking skills. Use of the workbook will assist students in mastering the material and applying the principles learned to a wide variety of patient care situations.

Order Number 1-4180-0135X

Although the text may be used as a stand-alone item, the various teaching aids will meet the needs of a wide variety of programs. We believe that this comprehensive training package will meet the needs of most agencies.

ABOUT THE AUTHOR

Barbara Acello, MS, RN, is an independent nurse consultant in the Dallas-Fort Worth, Texas, area. She has many years of experience both as a hands-on clinician and as an educator in acute and long-term care, as well as emergency care in the streets. Mrs. Acello is a diploma nursing graduate with a bachelor's degree in health care administration and a master's degree in education.

ACKNOWLEDGMENTS

The author wishes to thank Marah Bellegarde, Acquisitions Editor of Thomson Delmar Learning, for initiating this project. I sincerely appreciate her responsiveness to meeting current industry needs. Jadin Babin-Kavanaugh, Editorial Assistant, has done a magnificent job of coordinating many facets and minuscule but important details of manuscript production, copying, and shipping. Many unnamed individuals at Delmar Learning provided their talents and abilities to move this project from idea to finish, ensuring that you receive a high-quality product. The book was designed and assembled by Carlisle Publishing Services in Dubuque, IA. Angela Kearney, the project editor has done an awesome job in taking several thousand pages of raw manuscript and turning it into the attractive, legible book that you hold in your hands. Layout, design, and legibility are key to student mastery of the content, and Carlisle has done a tremendous job in ensuring a high quality finished product. I am grateful for their effort, assistance, and commitment to quality. Brooke Graves, the copy editor, is always a joy to work with. Her attention to grammatical and organizational detail helps ensure a quality book. I am always delighted when Brooke works on my projects!

My books often turn into a community effort in our self-employed household. I could not do what I do without the assistance of my husband Fran, daughter Laura, and son Jon. Laura made herself invaluable by taking over many of my other responsibilities so I could devote time to this book. She also lent her many talents and abilities to assembly of the art manuscript. My middle grandson, Chris, who generally hates art, glued most of the figure tags to the hundreds of loose art manuscript pages. This tedious, messy job is essential to ensuring proper figure placement. I sincerely appreciate the love and support that you all freely give.

Many individuals and organizations contributed to the photographs, drawings, and forms in this text. I sincerely appreciate your assistance. Writing is the easy part! Gathering the art manuscript is difficult for me, and your cooperation made this task relatively painless.

A team of peer reviewers dedicated many hours to reviewing this manuscript and providing helpful comments throughout development of the text. This book is especially difficult to review because there is no standardized curriculum for the PCT caregiver, and the skills taught vary from state to state and from one facility to the next. Colleges and facilities teaching this content do so because of an expressed community need for the caregivers; the instructor designs a class and the skills to be taught to meet this need. Thus, classes and content vary widely. Hence, reviewers for this subject matter must avoid tunnel vision and look beyond the walls of their own institutions.

Elizabeth Patterson, RT (R), RDMS, RDCS
    Health Programs Coordinator
    Edmonds Community College
    Lynnwood, WA
Ann Simms, RN
    Program Director, Nursing Assistant Programs
    Albuquerque Technical Vocational Institute
    Albuquerque, NM
Lois Stotter, BSN, RNC, MSN (c)
    Clinical Nurse Educator
    Borgess Medical Center
    Kalamazoo, MI
Judith E. Wilcock, RN, BSN
    Health Services Instructor
    West Central Technical College
    Newnan, GA

FEEDBACK

I welcome your comments and feedback about this book. Please feel free to contact me through Delmar Thomson Learning or at bacello@spamcop.net.

Barbara Acello, MS, RN

CHAPTER 1

Health Care Delivery for the 21st Century

OBJECTIVES:

After reading this chapter, you should be able to:

- Spell and define key terms.
- Define *workplace redesign* and describe changes in the nursing department that have occurred because of restructuring.
- Describe the role, responsibilities, and scope of practice of the patient care technician, and explain why standards of care are important.
- List the five rights of delegation and give examples of situations in which delegating a procedure to a PCT is not appropriate.
- Differentiate an intradisciplinary team from an interdisciplinary team and list some general responsibilities of teams.
- List at least 10 desirable qualities of the PCT.
- Identify professional boundaries in relationships with patients and families.
- List five methods of communicating with others and demonstrate how to communicate with patients.
- List at least one developmental task for each age group.
- Describe three aspects of care that must be adjusted to the patient's age.
- List the principles of restorative nursing care.
- State the purpose of process improvement, and list some benefits.

HEALTH CARE DELIVERY FROM 1980 TO THE PRESENT

Health care is provided in many settings. Many professional and nonprofessional workers provide patient care. The type of care given is determined by the types of services the agency delivers. Health care workplace organization remained largely the same for many years.

Before the mid-1980s, health care facilities were set up so that many departments provided services to the patients. Each department provided a distinct service. Workers were specially trained to provide that service. In a large acute care hospital, each patient would receive services from an average of 40 to 60 different health care workers. This was confusing for the patients. Providing services in this manner was not cost-effective for the health care facility. A great deal of time was wasted coordinating and scheduling services between departments. Long delays waiting for services to be delivered were common.

Changes in Reimbursement

Changes in reimbursement for health care services began with the federal government in the late 1970s. This was done to save Medicare money. The method of reimbursement for private insurers also changed. In the mid-1980s, changes began to have a profound effect on the health care industry. These changes caused modifications in the operation of physicians' offices, clinics, laboratories, hospitals, and long-term care facilities. The face of health care delivery changed extensively in the

1990s, affecting reimbursement in all practice settings. Changes in reimbursement are expected to continue. These changes affect health care delivery methods and practices.

Workplace Reorganization

Most health care facilities studied their operations to see how they could become more efficient. This was necessary because reimbursement for services was less than it had been previously. Organizations had to figure out how to provide the same services at a lower cost. Saving money was necessary for survival. Some hospitals closed because they could not operate on lower revenues.

Efficiency studies were done and many agencies learned that they could save money if they combined the services that departments and workers deliver. Small departments merged, becoming parts of larger departments. The workers were taught to perform new patient care procedures. As staff within larger departments, workers provide more services to patients than they did previously. Many workers from various departments used to care for each patient. Now fewer workers provide a broader spectrum of care. Each worker provides services that other departments used to be responsible for. Collectively, these changes in health care delivery are called **workplace redesign.** They may also be called **restructuring** or **re-engineering.**

Effect of Workplace Redesign

All health care workers have been affected in some way by workplace redesign. In most health care agencies, the nursing department's responsibilities have been expanded. Staff is given additional training in procedures that nursing was not responsible for previously. In some agencies, nursing assistants and other unlicensed care providers are taught to provide advanced technical skills. Training of this type is called **multiskilling** or **cross-training.** The multiskilled worker has completed a basic nursing assistant or other educational program to learn to provide personal care and basic comfort measures to patients. The assistant attends classes to learn additional technical skills. Some of these may be procedures previously performed by other departments. Some are activities that nurses historically performed. Many agencies have changed the assistant's title to reflect these changes in responsibilities. Common titles being used by health care agencies to describe this new position are listed in **Figure 1-1.** In this book, we call the multiskilled

Care Partner	Patient Care Technician
Clinical Associate	Patient Service Associate
Clinical Care Associate	Patient Support Associate
Clinical Care Technician	Patient Support Partner
Clinical Support Associate	Personal Care Aide
Clinical Technician	Personal Care Assistant
Direct Caregiver	Personal Care Attendant
Health Care Associate	Primary Caregiver
Health Care Technician	Support Aide
Nurse Extender	Support Partner
Nursing Associate	Team Care Member
Nursing Attendant	Unit Representative
Nursing Technician	Unit Support Associate
Patient Care Associate	Unit Support Technician
Patient Care Attendant	Zone Service Worker
Patient Care Specialist	
(This list was compiled with the assistance of the nurses on the Nursenet listserv.)	

FIGURE 1-1 Titles for multiskilled workers

worker a *patient care technician* (PCT) and the person who receives care the *patient.*

QUALITY ASSURANCE

All health care facilities have an internal program for **process improvement.** This is commonly called **quality improvement (QI),** but may also be called **quality assurance (QA)** or **continuous quality improvement (CQI).** You may be asked to participate on the quality assurance committee. The purpose of quality assurance is to identify problems or potential problems and find solutions for improvement. The quality assurance committee meets to conduct internal reviews and evaluate care provided and practices used in the facility. Restraint use, infections, pressure ulcers, and infection control are some areas that may be reviewed. Committee members will audit practices on each unit and make recommendations to improve care.

The facility should continuously reevaluate and adjust care to meet the needs of the patients who receive services. The quality assurance program performs this important function. Accreditation standards state that *all personnel must be competent in their responsibilities.* The facility must evaluate staff competence periodically, and maintain a record of these checks. In some facilities, the quality assurance committee also evaluates staff competence.

The quality assurance committee is very important to the operation of the facility and its successful performance on facility surveys. The committee identifies and corrects problems. This improves the quality of care.

A Process Improvement Study: Emphasis on Noise

As a PCT, you know that comfort, rest, and sleep are important for patient well-being. Excessive noise delays healing, impairs immune function, causes stress, and increases heart rate and blood pressure. Patients who do not sleep well at night may be unhappy with their care and unable to stay awake during the day for meals and therapy. Some patients become confused and agitated when sleep-deprived. A process improvement study done by the staff of one hospital unit has direct implications for PCTs.[1] The staff measured noise levels with special instruments during the night. The workers who were on duty were not aware that noise was being measured.

The Occupational Safety and Health Administration (OSHA) has established noise standards for employee safety. Under these standards, workers should not be exposed to 90 decibels of sound for more than eight hours. Average noise levels are listed in **Table 1-1**. The Environmental Protection Agency (EPA) recommends that hospital noise levels not exceed 45 decibels during the day. Examples of various types of noise are pictured in **Figure 1-2**. During the study, decibel levels as high as 113 were recorded at night. The noisiest time was at shift change, when more visitors, physicians, and nursing staff were entering or leaving the unit. Two nurses who acted as patients noted that this noise prevented them from falling asleep. They noted that, once asleep, noise from equipment alarms, telephones, carts, X-ray machines, opening and closing doors, the paging and intercom system, roommates, and nursing personnel

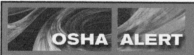
OSHA ALERT

The Occupational Safety and Health Administration is a governmental agency that protects the health and safety of employees and surveys health care facilities. The inspectors review infection control, isolation practices, tuberculin testing, material safety data sheets (MSDS), and other policies and facility practices. The OSHA surveyor interviews employees, tours the facility, and asks questions about health and safety practices. If unsafe conditions are found, the inspector will make recommendations for correction. The facility may receive a citation or fine. A citation is a written notice that informs the facility of the violations. The employer must post the report of each citation at or near the place the violation occurred for three days, or until the unsafe condition is corrected.

[1]Cmiel, C. A., et al. (2004). Noise control: A nursing team's approach to sleep promotion. *American Journal of Nursing 104*(2), 40–48.

Table 1-1	
Noise in Decibels (dB)	Source (range in dB)
194	loudest tone possible
180	rocket launch
165	12-gauge shotgun
140	jet engine at takeoff
120	ambulance siren
119	pneumatic percussion drill
110	chainsaw
108	continuous miner
105	bulldozer, spray painter
98	hand drill
96	tractor
93	belt sander
90	hair dryer, power lawn mower
80	ringing telephone
60	normal conversation
30	whisper
0	weakest sound heard by the average human ear

(Modified from National Institute for Occupational Safety and Health (NIOSH). (2001). General estimates of work-related noises. Accessed November 15, 2004, from http://www.cdc.gov/niosh/01-104.html)

interrupted their sleep. Noises that were tolerable during the day were more disruptive at night.

The effects of noise and sleep in the hospital are areas of ongoing study. Because the nurses who conducted this study published their findings, we have a good example of how the process improvement activities in one hospital can benefit many facilities, and open areas of ongoing research. It is safe to say that the study proves that nighttime noise is disruptive to hospital patients. Follow your facility policies and do all you can to reduce noise when you are on duty!

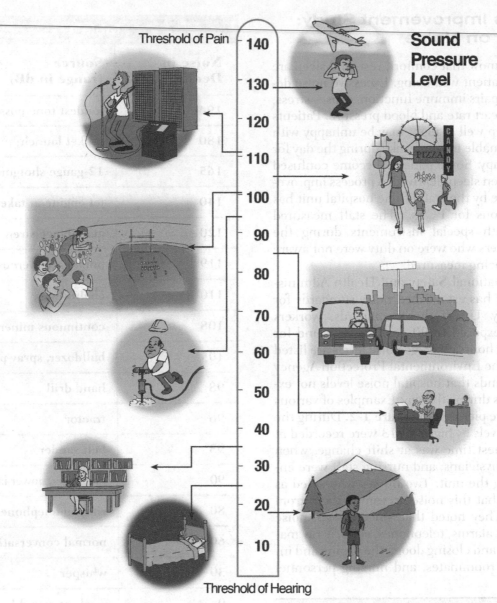

FIGURE 1-2 Sound intensity generated by various activities. In one study, hospital noises during the night approached the levels of chainsaws or jackhammers, making it difficult for patients to sleep. The nurses found that simple steps, such as closing the doors to patients' rooms and muffling the clatter of clipboards, can help.

Benchmarking

Benchmarking is an important part of the quality improvement process. Any aspect of the organization can be benchmarked. Benchmarking is essential to identifying the standard of care. You must be able to identify and define the standard before you can compare your organization with it. The **benchmark** is a standard reference point against which performance is measured. **Benchmarking** is an activity in which an organization establishes best practices by comparing what it is doing with what other, similar organizations are doing. By benchmarking with other organiza-

tions, the facility can improve its processes and achieve excellence.

Critical thinking describes clear, precise, and purposeful mental activities. This skill is essential to solving complex problems, identifying solutions, drawing conclusions, combining information, separating fact from opinion, and estimating potential outcomes. Benchmarking does not involve copying what other facilities are doing. Rather, it uses critical thinking (problem solving) to identify and correct problems. Hospitals will identify new ways of solving a problem that work best in their facility. The supply of data that can be benchmarked in every health care facility is limitless.

Quality Indicators

Monitoring quality indicators has become popular in health care. **Quality indicators** are decision-making and research tools that are used for tracking changes, recognizing potential quality problems, and identifying areas that warrant further study and research. Indicators that reflect the type of services a facility provides can be measured. If the facility is not happy with its performance, it can change. Quality indicators are also a type of benchmark. They reveal how patients in other facilities are similar, and how they are different. They provide information about patient outcomes, access to care, utilization, and costs.

Serious Events

The quality assurance team reviews incidents in which injury or the potential for injury exists. These fall into four main categories:

1. **Adverse events**—incidents, accidents, events, and injuries associated with patient care and services. An adverse event may result from commission or omission. In other words, the staff did something they should not have done, or failed to do something they should have done. Examples of adverse events are falls and medication errors.

2. **Close calls**—situations that could have resulted in an adverse event but did not, either by chance or through timely action of the staff. These incidents may also be called *near misses*. An example is preparing to perform a procedure on the wrong patient, but catching the mistake at the last minute. Close calls always present opportunities for learning and further study. They are given as much attention as events that result in injury.

3. **Intentionally unsafe acts**—result from criminal acts, purposefully unsafe actions, acts related to alcohol or substance abuse by workers, or patient abuse or neglect.

4. **Sentinel events**—a type of adverse event. These are serious incidents that result in patient death or serious physical or psychological injury. Some sentinel events create a risk of death or serious injury, such as medication errors and wrong-site surgery. Sentinel events are always reported and tracked.

Root Cause Analysis

Most progressive hospitals are taking an innovative approach to incident reporting. Rather than blam-

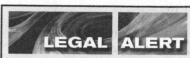

ing a staff person for the occurrence of an incident, they evaluate the organization to learn if a system breakdown or policy caused or contributed to the event. If so, they use critical thinking to identify ways of correcting the problem. **Root cause analysis (RCA)** is a process for identifying the cause or contributing factors associated with untoward events. An RCA is a review of unsafe acts, adverse events, close calls, or sentinel events. Your facility will have guidelines for conducting a root cause analysis investigation. Root cause analyses:

- Are interdisciplinary, involving personnel who are knowledgeable about the processes involved.
- Focus mainly on systems and processes rather than individual performance.
- Ask "what" and "why" until all aspects of the process have been reviewed and contributing factors identified.
- Identify potential procedural changes to reduce the risk of adverse events or close calls.

Root cause statements:

- Identify the cause and effect of the event
- Recognize that most incidents have many underlying causes; there is seldom only one cause of an adverse event
- Use positive terms
- Recognize that each human error has a cause. Procedure violations are not considered root causes. They must have a preceding cause. Failure to act is a root cause only if the staff member involved has a duty to act
- Review potential work system redesign to reduce the risk of recurrence
- Should be consistent and not contradictory. All obvious questions should be answered

- Consider relevant literature
- Include corrective actions, outcome measures, and management approval
- Meet facility and accrediting body requirements

Root cause analysis does not involve placing blame. Instead, it focuses on learning how an incident occurred, and applies the learning to develop preventive measures and solutions. **Transparency** is the part of the investigative process that involves keeping people informed. Having transparency is critical to improving patient safety. The results of an investigation do no good unless they are accessible and understandable. Therefore, everyone should know how (and where) to access the information and understand the findings. People do not usually trust information they cannot see or understand. Because of this, readers of the RCA data should be able to:

- Find all the information of concern.
- See what questions were asked during the investigation.
- See what evidence confirms each fact.
- See what theories were explored, ruled out, and why.

Transparency promotes learning and understanding, and enhances trust in the RCA process. It gives employees, patients, and others greater confidence in our knowledge of the problem, and whether the proposed solutions will meet the need.

The goals of the quality assurance program are many. Root cause analysis is a critical part of the process. Some of the most important goals involve prevention of injury to patients, visitors, and employees. As you can see, everyone benefits. Cooperating with and participating in your facility quality assurance program promotes patient and employee safety and satisfaction.

Customer Satisfaction and Service

In addition to performance review programs that improve quality of care, many health care facilities have adapted programs first used in the retail industry to ensure that the customer is happy and returns again. These programs are used with patients, visitors, and employees to retain and expand facility business and prevent financial losses. In some facilities, the program involves simple measures, such as asking each patient if he or she needs anything else before leaving the room. Some provide a flower for each patient. Employees may receive

bonuses for certain activities, such as implementing quality improvements or meeting patient care and safety goals. Some facilities have added specialized services, and others have remodeled and expanded to enable them to change from the traditional two-bed rooms to all private rooms. A few have added Internet access to all patient rooms. Some have touch-screen televisions that enable patients to check their e-mail, play games, watch videos or television programs, or learn about hospital services. You can expect customer service to be an important focus in years to come, and hospitals will be adding new electronic services to meet patient demands for new technology.

This is a time of great change. As a PCT, you have a key role in ensuring patient satisfaction. Cooperate as changes occur, and learn all you can about the new systems and information processes used by your facility.

Institute for Healthcare Improvement

The **Institute for Healthcare Improvement (IHI)** is a not-for-profit organization that has become a very important part of hospital-based health care. Membership is voluntary. Many of the IHI's initiatives affect how care is delivered in hospitals today. The IHI promotes timely, safe, effective, efficient, patient-centered care. Its mission is to improve health care by turning promising concepts for improving care into action. The goals are to deliver health care with no:

- needless deaths
- unnecessary pain or suffering
- helplessness in those served or serving
- unwanted waiting
- waste

Health care facilities need support to effect positive change. IHI helps facilities find solutions for action, teaches about quality improvement, and provides information about health care quality.

PATIENT-FOCUSED CARE

Along with workplace redesign came a movement toward **patient-focused care.** The purpose of patient-focused care is to bring services to patients, instead of bringing patients to services. This care model is more flexible in meeting patient needs and puts more responsibility for decision making into the hands of health care workers. Fewer workers are needed to provide services to each patient under this model of care. Workers are members of teams that meet the needs of patients as efficiently as possible.

Unlicensed Assistive Personnel

Some health care agencies refer to unlicensed health care workers as **unlicensed assistive personnel (UAPs).** UAPs are defined by the National Council of State Boards of Nursing as "individuals who assist the licensed nurse in the role of providing direct nursing care to health care consumers as delegated by, and under the supervision of, the licensed nurse." According to this definition, any direct care provider without a license is a UAP. Nursing assistants who complete a state-approved program are not licensed in most states. A few do issue licenses to CNAs. Upon successful completion of a prescribed education and competency evaluation program, these important workers are listed with the state nursing assistant reg-

istry. Listing an assistant on the registry is different from licensure. Some nursing assistant programs are not state-approved, so their graduates are not listed on the registry.

Role and Responsibilities of the Patient Care Technician

Patient care technicians work in physicians' offices; clinics; surgical centers; hospitals; subacute, rehabilitative, and long-term care facilities; hospices; and other community agencies. The role and responsibilities of the PCT vary from one agency to the next. Understanding what you can and cannot do is very important. Your employer will give you a job description, listing your responsibilities. A sample job description is given in **Figure 1-3**. The job description is developed by your employer based on your state laws and facility policies.

Title: Patient Care Technician

Department: Nursing Service

Overview: Functions as a direct caregiver and member of the patient care team. Provides age-appropriate patient care. This includes assisting patients with activities of daily living, taking vital signs, phlebotomy, EKGs, catheterization, wound care and dressing changes, obtaining specimens, providing intravenous therapy, administering enteral feedings, pre- and postoperative care, caring for patients with tracheostomies, basic airway management, and assisting with life-sustaining procedures, including CPR. Provides physical and emotional support to patients. Reports changes in patient condition to RN supervisor in a timely manner. Records patient information in the medical record. Communicates effectively, and cooperates with other team members to ensure continuity of care. Responsibilities may vary slightly depending on assigned unit and shift.

A. Duties and Responsibilities
1. Takes and records vital signs. Reports abnormal values to RN.
2. Assists patients with ADLs, grooming, elimination, fluid balance, personal hygiene, mobility, exercise, ambulation, feeding, comfort, and preventive measures. Follows infection control policies and procedures.
3. Avoids using restraints whenever possible. Monitors and reports changes in patients' behavior. Follows the care plan for behavior management.
4. Monitors and observes patients' condition and reports changes to RN manager.
5. Performs technical procedures including:
   a. Standard precautions, personal protective equipment, medical and surgical asepsis, isolation and good handwashing.

b. Sterile procedures.
c. Clean and sterile dressing change.
d. Other wound care, including wet to dry dressings, transparent film, and hydrocolloid dressings.
e. Pin care; suture and staple removal.
f. Phlebotomy, specimen collection, and limited specimen testing.
g. Intravenous therapy initiation, monitoring, site care, and removal.
h. Catheter insertion, removal, irrigation, and maintenance.
i. Assisting with fecal elimination, including enemas, removal of fecal impaction, ostomy care, maintenance, and irrigation.
j. Nasogastric tube insertion and removal, maintenance, and feeding; care and feeding through enteral tubes.
k. Pre- and postoperative care, including shaving, assisting patients with coughing and deep breathing, incentive spirometer, pneumatic hose, traction, hypo- and hyperthermia blanket.
l. Insertion and maintenance care for oropharyngeal and nasopharyngeal airways; oropharyngeal and nasopharyngeal suctioning; pulse oximetry; oxygen administration, monitoring, and care; and assisting with emergency procedures.
m. Assisting with intubation; caring for the endotracheal tube.
n. Providing tracheostomy and stoma care, including suctioning.
o. ECG monitoring.
p. Performing postcardiac catheterization check.
6. Works as a team member, assisting and providing support as needed.

FIGURE 1-3 Sample PCT job description

(continues)

7. Answers call signals and meets patient needs or reports to the appropriate team member.
8. Applies principles of infection control in daily practice.
9. Maintains an orderly, tidy unit by following all infection control precautions, emptying trash, and cleaning equipment, supplies, and work areas as assigned.
10. Restocks supplies, equipment, and linen as needed.
11. Follows all safety policies and procedures; teaches patient safety.
12. Employs the principles of good body mechanics for lifting and moving patients and heavy objects.
13. Assists licensed nurses and physicians with procedures, as directed.
14. Maintains a positive relationship with patients, visitors, physicians, and staff.
15. Attends educational programs and meetings.
16. Participates in committees as requested. Cooperates with and follows safety committee, infection control committee, ergonomics committee, and quality assurance committee policies and procedures.

B. Education
1. High school graduate or equivalent.
2. Successful completion of basic nursing assistant program.
3. Successful completion of PCT program.

C. Knowledge, Skills, and Abilities
1. Sincerely likes and believes in people.
2. Is considerate and understanding to patients, visitors, and other staff members.
3. Follows directions and functions according to expectations with minimal supervision.
4. Provides quality care according to RN directions and the patient's care plan.
5. Proficient in documentation for assigned procedures.

D. Physical Requirements
1. Ability to lift 50 pounds.
2. Ability to carry objects weighing 15 pounds.
3. Ability to stand for at least three hours at a time.
4. Able to stoop, bend, reach, and grasp. Able to use hands and arms to push and pull wheelchairs, stretchers, beds, and carts as necessary.
5. Able to use the principles of good body mechanics for lifting, moving, and positioning patients and heavy objects at least hourly.

E. Reporting Responsibilities
1. Assigned to a team by the nurse manager. Works under the general supervision of a registered nurse (RN).
2. Functions as a member of a self-directed work team; assists and supports other team members with patient care, support services, and clerical functions as necessary.

F. Working Conditions
1. Works on a unit with exposure to infectious disease. Risk for harm is limited if employee follows all infection control procedures and agency policies.

G. Ethics
1. Honesty demands that time paid by the employer be used profitably. If the work assigned is insufficient to occupy the time, report to the RN or nurse manager for additional duties.
2. Employees must not sleep, smoke, or eat in public areas or on patient care units.
3. Meals and break time will be assigned. Report to the RN before leaving the unit, and again upon your return.
4. Conserve supplies, electricity, and other commodities at all times.

This job description provides an overview of the requirements for the patient care technician. It is not an exhaustive, comprehensive, or all-inclusive description of job duties, requirements, or responsibilities.

FIGURE 1-3 Sample PCT job description—Continued

Please keep in mind that this job description is only an example. In some states, this sample job description might be too broad in scope, because state laws prohibit the PCT from performing all the procedures listed. The description will be appropriate in other states. As you will see, the role and responsibilities of the PCT vary widely from employer to employer and state to state. There are no uniform job descriptions or responsibilities. Your instructor will guide you in procedures that are legal and appropriate for your state and are permitted by your employer.

You will be supervised by a registered nurse (RN) or other licensed health care provider. In this text, we will call the RN your supervisor. He or she is accountable for the patient's well-being. You must report changes in patient condition to your supervisor promptly.

Sometimes the RN will perform tasks that you have been taught to provide. Do not be offended if this happens. A nurse can legally assign tasks to an unlicensed assistant in certain situations. The RN must believe that delegating the activity will be safe for the patient. If the nurse believes that the patient is not stable, or if further assessment is necessary during the procedure, he or she will perform the task.

Nurse Practice Acts

Nursing practice is regulated by a board of nursing or other governing body in each state. This agency governs nursing practice by providing a **nurse practice act.** The nurse practice act describes the nurses' scope of practice in your state. In some states, unlicensed assistants cannot perform nursing functions unless they meet the education and licensure requirements stated in the nurse practice act. This means that, indirectly, in these states, the state nurse practice act also governs the scope of your practice. The act is used as a guide when facilities develop job descriptions and determine which skills you can perform. The act may also describe circumstances under which an unlicensed assistant can or cannot perform these skills.

Scope of PCT Practice

The procedures in this book are all performed by unlicensed assistive personnel in some health care facilities. Some procedures are simple, but some are more advanced. Your ability to perform them will be determined by your state nurse practice act, state laws, facility policies, and your job description. In addition, you must be taught to perform these procedures, and you must be properly supervised in your work. Never perform procedures that you have not been taught to provide, or that are illegal for patient care technicians in your state. Follow the directions of the RN for providing care, and perform procedures as assigned.

Standards of Care

Although health care is delivered in many different settings, the legal requirements for PCTs are similar in all settings. **Standards of care** are common health care practices based on:

- laws
- facility policies and procedures
- information learned in class
- your job description
- published information

Standards may be defined by community, state, and national practices. Applying standards of care means using the degree of care or skill that is expected in a particular circumstance or role. Standards are used to measure workers' efficiency. They enable you to be evaluated based on what is expected of a worker with your education and experience. All facilities have *standards of performance* that their workers must follow. Applying the standard of care involves doing what the reasonable, prudent worker would do based on his or her education and experience. Adhering to *standards of practice* or standards of care is very important. Many standards apply to each patient, each profession, and each situation. No single standard encompasses all workers who care for patients.

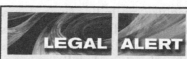

LEGAL ALERT

From a legal standpoint, you will be held to the same standard of care as the average worker in your position. You are not expected to do what the best worker would do, but rather what any reasonable worker would do in the same or similar situation. If a worker holds certifications or advanced education, he or she is held to the same standard as other workers with similar qualifications.

Negligence is failure to exercise the degree of care considered reasonable in a situation. It is the failure to act with the care that a person with equal qualifications would exercise in the same situation. In other words, it is failure to meet the standard of care. A negligent act may be accidental or deliberate. It may involve a commission or omission. For example, forgetting to serve a confused patient's meal tray is an omission. The patient cannot tell anyone he missed a meal. This is accidental. Intentionally not serving the same patient's meal tray because he takes too long to feed is deliberate negligence. **Malpractice** is the failure to act according to the acceptable course of conduct, resulting in harm or injury to the patient. It may also be accidental or deliberate. As you can see, deviating from the standards of care can be risky for both patients and health care workers.

Becoming familiar with the location and contents of facility policy and procedure manuals will help you do your job and remain within your scope of practice. However, technology and research frequently drive changes in practices, so you should attend inservices and review current journals to ensure that you are using the most up-to-date information.

Continuing Your Education

The golden rule implies your intent to provide adequate care. However, your intentions are effective only when you act on them. You have the ethical responsibility to maintain competence in your practice.

The Joint Commission on Accreditation of Healthcare Organizations (JCAHO) accredits many different types of health care agencies. The JCAHO requires health care facilities to ensure that workers are **competent** in their responsibilities. This means that you must know how to perform correctly the procedures that you are responsible for. Your employer will evaluate your skills each year. It may do this by observing you or by giving a written test. This is a JCAHO requirement for accredited facilities. The federal laws governing the long-term care industry also require periodic competency evaluation. This is managed differently in various states and facilities. Many long-term care facilities also require an annual evaluation of skills.

Health care is always changing, so you must attend educational classes to stay abreast of current information. Look forward to taking classes to learn new things that will benefit both you and the patients. New procedures and equipment are introduced frequently. When your unit begins using a new procedure or piece of equipment, you will be taught how to use it correctly. You will be expected to show that you are competent in the new procedure before you perform it on a patient.

Health care workers have a broad knowledge of many subjects. All have specific, specialized knowledge in their selected areas of expertise and practice. Knowing all you need to know about every subject is impossible. For the most part, your general knowledge will sustain you, but there will be times when you must learn more about current standards in areas in which you work infrequently, or those outside your specialty area. Even then, there will be times when you must research and review the standards, even if you know them well.

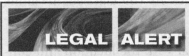

LEGAL ALERT

Becoming familiar with and following the standards of care for PCTs is essential. "Scope of practice" is a very important legal concept. Your scope of practice is defined by your job description. Functioning within this scope of practice protects you and the facility.

Education in some subjects is mandatory in health care facilities. These subjects will be presented to you upon orientation and periodically after that. Review or updates on things such as fire and disaster preparedness, infection control (Figure 1-4) and patient or resident rights may be required each year.

You must be competent in your work to protect patient safety. You can keep your skills and knowledge current by:

- reading health care books and journals
- taking classes and studying
- practicing procedures
- observing nurses
- asking questions

The federal laws specify education and competency requirements for nursing assistants who care

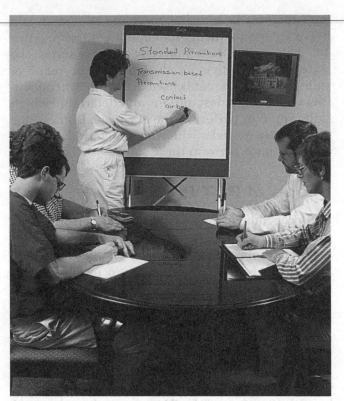

FIGURE 1-4 Health care is always changing, and you will be attending classes regularly, which will enable you to learn new information, practices, and techniques.

for the elderly in long-term care facilities. As you can see, there is no uniform code of practice for PCTs or other unlicensed health care providers in the United States. Nursing assistants working in long-term care are the only group of unlicensed assistants with a defined scope of practice. The scope of practice varies slightly from state to state in long-term care.

DELEGATION

Delegation is the transfer of responsibility for a nursing activity from a licensed nurse who is authorized to perform the activity to someone who does not already possess such authority. After the task has been **delegated,** only the person given the authority may perform the task. In other words, this person cannot delegate the assignment to someone else. The licensed nurse is accountable for the task and its outcome. Because the nurse is accountable, he or she must be confident that the unlicensed person can complete the assignment correctly.

In some states, the nurse practice act describes how nurses **assign** or delegate duties to unlicensed assistants. The practice act specifies what qualifications you must have before the nurse may assign certain duties to you. In other states, the nurse practice act does not discuss delegation of specific duties. In these states, laws governing health care facilities, rules of accrediting organizations, and facility policies may describe tasks that can be delegated by the nurse. Some states have passed laws that specifically prohibit unlicensed assistants from performing certain activities.

Some states further define the terms *assign* and *delegate*. In these states, an RN assigns tasks to unlicensed workers. In this context, *assigning* means advising, instructing, or directing another person to complete a task. The person assigning the task must possess the authority to make the assignment. Tasks are delegated only to other licensed nurses, including RNs, LPNs, and LVNs. In these states, the term *delegation* means to authorize or entrust another person to do a job. In delegating a task, the RN is authorizing another nurse to do the job and entrusting him or her with the responsibility for completing the task. Your instructor will clarify the definitions used by your state.

Five Rights of Delegation

Before delegating a task to a PCT, the nurse must decide if delegation is appropriate. Appropriate delegation ensures that:

- The PCT has been taught to perform the procedure. If asked, he or she can demonstrate the procedure safely and correctly.
- The patient does not need frequent, repeated assessments during the procedure.
- The patient's response to the procedure is reasonably predictable.
- In the nurse's opinion, the PCT will obtain the same or similar results as an RN in performing the procedure.
- The nurse is certain that delegating the activity to a PCT is not against the law.

The National Council of State Boards of Nursing has developed a guide called the Five Rights of Delegation. Nurses use this list to help them delegate correctly. Reading this list will help you learn if a delegation is appropriate. The rights are listed in Figure 1-5.

Not all nursing procedures can be delegated at all times. In certain situations, delegating even simple activities is inappropriate. For example, the PCT can safely take the vital signs of a stable patient. However, assigning a PCT to take the vital

- Right Task—one that can legally be delegated to a PCT who is trained and competent in performing the procedure
- Right Circumstances—the PCT understands the purpose of the procedure, can perform it safely in an appropriate setting, and has the right supplies or equipment to perform the procedure
- Right Person—the right person delegates the right task to the right PCT, to be performed on the right patient
- Right Direction/Communication—the person delegating the activity has described it clearly, including directions, limits, and the expected outcome
- Right Supervision—the nurse delegating the activity answers the PCT's questions and is available to handle problems if the patient's condition changes. The PCT who performed the activity reports its completion and the patient's response to the nurse who delegated the activity.

FIGURE 1-5 Five rights of delegation. (Modified from the National Council of State Boards of Nursing Guidelines.)

signs of an unstable patient who is in shock is probably inappropriate. This patient needs the assessment skills of a licensed nurse. By law, only an RN can assess patients. Assessment cannot be delegated. However, the LPN or LVN, PCT, and others may assist the RN with data collection necessary for the assessment. For example, taking routine vital signs is part of some assessments. The PCT also makes observations and reports them to the RN. These examples of data collection are part of the assessment that are well within the scope of PCT practice.

Part of the assessment process consists of organizing, analyzing, prioritizing, evaluating, and synthesizing the data collected. Based on this information, the RN identifies actual and potential health problems. Only the RN can perform these functions and develop a plan for using the information. The plan will list goals and nursing interventions to assist the patient in meeting these goals. However, others may contribute to the development of goals and interventions by providing information about the patient and sharing observations.

Performing Delegated Activities

As you can see, delegating activities to a PCT is a serious matter for nurses. When you accept the responsibility for a delegated task, you are responsible for your own actions. Never perform a procedure if

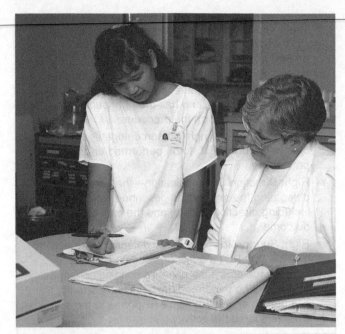

FIGURE 1-6 The RN will give you your assignment. Check with him or her if you have questions or need clarification.

you have not been taught, or are not allowed to do it according to your state law or facility policy. Make sure that the proper supplies are available to complete the procedure safely. Always ask for directions if you do not understand your assignment (**Figure 1-6**). If you think that performing a procedure is unsafe for the patient, discuss your feelings with the RN. Report any applicable observations about the patient's condition. Ask for help, if necessary. Notify the RN immediately if the patient's condition changes.

Refusing Delegation

If you believe that a procedure is not within your legal scope of practice, if you have not been taught to perform that procedure, or if you believe that the activity will harm the patient, you may refuse the delegation. Likewise, if you do not understand the directions, or do not have the proper supplies, you may also refuse. However, you must explain the reason for your refusal to the RN. He or she can probably resolve your concerns, enabling you to complete the activity. Do not refuse because you do not have time or because the procedure is unpleasant. The RN can show you how to perform the procedure, or help you if you are not comfortable with it. He or she can help you adjust your schedule to make the time. Be honest with the RN.

Good communication is the key to successful delegation and patient safety. Be tactful. This is a sensitive issue. If honest communications are inef-

fective, you can use the chain of command to address the problem with the next person in line.

Protecting the patient is always a top priority. If you are assigned to a task, your supervisor assumes that you will do it. Never ignore an assignment. If you cannot complete the activity, discuss the situation with your supervisor.

Completing an Assignment

Report the completion of the task and the patient's response to the RN. Reporting even simple tasks may be important. Verbally informing the nurse of the outcome is an important step in the procedure. You may be tempted to skip reporting if you are responsible for documenting the activity. Do not neglect reporting! After informing the nurse, document according to facility policy.

TEAMWORK

As health care facilities restructure, many have assigned their employees to permanent work teams. These teams must function as harmoniously as possible, and are important for patient well-being. Nursing teams are responsible for many patient services, such as phlebotomy (**Figure 1-7**) and EKG, that were formerly provided by other departments. **Intradisciplinary teams** are composed of workers from the same discipline. They have similar education, scopes of responsibility, and levels of expertise. **Interdisciplinary teams** are made up of workers from different disciplines. Team members have different qualifications, scopes of responsibility, and levels of expertise. **Intradepartmental teams** consist of workers from

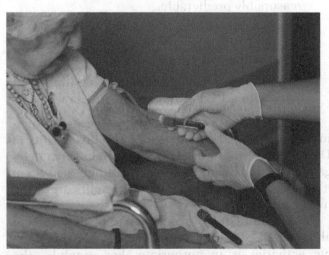

FIGURE 1-7 Phlebotomy is the task of drawing blood. Previously, another department was responsible for this function.

> **Responsibilities of Team Members**
> - Work together to perform job duties and provide patient care
> - Coordinate work assignments
> - Cooperate with others
> - Share resources and information
> - Organize special projects
> - Set standards and monitor outcomes
> - Recommend quality improvements
> - Participate in the development of policies and procedures
> - Test and evaluate new technology
> - Identify training needs
> - Participate in special work groups and committees

FIGURE 1-8 Responsibilities of team members

the same department. **Interdepartmental teams** are composed of workers from two or more different departments.

Teams assigned to care for specific patients learn the patients' needs very quickly. The patients also get to know their caregivers well. This decreases the patients' stress and increases satisfaction. Team members also like the close patient contact. Most also like the increased responsibility that comes with being a team member. Some responsibilities of team members are listed in **Figure 1-8**.

Team Success

Expect to make changes and to learn new things when working as a member of a team. Also, expect your team responsibilities to change from time to time. Be willing to change. Health care is always changing, and you must change with it. Cooperate with others. The success of the team begins with each member. All members must carry their share of the load for the team to function well. Treat others as you would like to be treated. If another worker needs help, be there to assist. Remember, the team will only be as successful as its weakest member.

DESIRABLE QUALITIES OF THE PCT

The PCT is a special person. The successful PCT likes people, takes responsibility seriously, and believes in the importance of the position. A pleasant personality is an important quality. Being pleasant and polite, treating others with respect and dignity, and showing a genuine concern for your patients and coworkers are positive traits. Be available to help others and accept help if you need it. Respect others' opinions and beliefs and avoid judging people's feelings. You will gain skill in helping patients with their feelings and emotional needs as you gain experience. Many things, including culture, personality, illness, and emotional health, influence behavior. Understanding why others respond as they do will help you accept and deal with people's behavior.

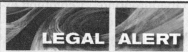

LEGAL ALERT

At some point in your life, you learned the Golden Rule, "Do unto others as you would have them do unto you." An alternative to the Golden Rule is the Platinum Rule: "Treat others the way they want to be treated." Think about how this affects feelings and relationships. The Platinum Rule shifts the focus from treating everyone alike to providing highly individualized care. Find out what the patients want, and give it to them, as much as possible, and in keeping with their plans of care. Use both principles to guide your practice. You will find many instances in which personal comfort and convenience potentially interfere with the care you give. By placing the patients' interests ahead of your own, you are fulfilling the ethical and legal obligations of your practice, protecting patient safety, enhancing patient comfort and satisfaction with care, and reducing your personal risk of legal exposure.

Learn to work as a team player. This involves depending on others to help care for the patients. It also means that others can depend on you. One person or department cannot accomplish good patient care. It takes many people and departments working together to meet each patient's needs. The expression, "It takes a village to raise a child," has an analogy in health care. In this case, it takes the expertise of an entire interdisciplinary team of professionals and **paraprofessionals** to care for each patient. In health care, paraprofessional workers are qualified, educated assistants to licensed workers. For effective, interdisciplinary care, lines of communication must be open and precise. Documentation must be accurate. Team members must communicate with each other regularly. Team members use the nursing process in the care of patients.

Practice tact. **Tact** involves the ability to say and do things at the right time. Being tactful means you are considerate, polite, and thoughtful. Be sensitive to the problems and needs of others. Do not judge others or give advice. Treat patients and coworkers with courtesy, respect, and consideration.

Do not argue, gossip, criticize your employer or others, or use abusive language.

Ethics are principles of conduct and moral values. Discussing facility business with patients, family members, and others outside the facility is not ethical. Be tactful and professional in revealing information. For example, telling patients or family members that you are "short of staff," or discussing working conditions, salary, benefits, or other information about facility operations, is not ethical. Discussing this information or complaining to others in the community is also inappropriate. A common expression in the field is: "The employees are the facility's worst enemies." When employees make negative comments and reveal private information, it sends a negative message about all parties involved. You have a moral and ethical obligation to your employer.

Complaining to others does not solve problems. In fact, it often makes problems worse. If you have concerns about staffing, working conditions, or other situations, use the chain of command within the facility to resolve them. Be proud of what you do and feel good about yourself. It takes a special person to provide personal care to other people! The role of the PCT is very important to the operation of the facility. Do the best job you can. Others will follow your example.

Organizing Your Work

Practice organizing your work. Organization is not something that can be taught in the classroom. Your instructor will teach you the principles of organization, but it is up to you to learn, practice, and master them. Organizing your work means learning how to set **priorities.** This means performing tasks in order of importance. It also means that you anticipate your own supply needs and patients' personal needs. Bring needed items to the room before you begin care. This saves time and steps. If you plan and prepare to meet these needs in advance, the quality of care you give will be better and the job will be much easier for you.

Good organization also reduces stress. Set priorities at the beginning of your shift to make the most of your day. When organizing your work, rate each task in order of importance. Priorities are constantly changing in health care because of patient illness, admissions, discharges, and emergencies. Do not become frustrated if your priorities change or must be adjusted partway through the shift. Readjust your plan and continue.

After you have set your priorities, plan your work for the most efficient use of your time. Identify tasks that can be grouped together. For example, you can make the bed while the patient is sitting in a chair or washing at the sink. Plan your schedule around mealtimes, activities, appointments, and the patients' therapy schedule. Plan for tasks that will require someone else to help you or for which you will need special equipment. If organization or time management is a problem for you, ask other workers for tips and techniques to use.

Check on all your patients before beginning your assignment. Take care of immediate needs. List special procedures that must be done and the time. Check to see if patients are scheduled for tests, appointments, or other activities during your shift. Follow your assignment sheet and each patient's care plan.

Remember that while you are at work, you are on duty. You are being paid to work the whole time. If you run out of things to do, help your coworkers or do things that have to be done on your unit. Do these things without being told.

Responsible Behavior

Responsible behavior is essential for workers in health care professions. Responsible workers are dependable and trustworthy. They follow the rules even if they do not agree with them. They take initiative to do things without being asked. Everyone suffers if team members are not responsible. Because you care for the health and welfare of human beings, you must take your job duties very seriously. Think how you would feel if a family member was a patient in a health care facility: you would want the best care possible for your loved one. To deliver the best care, all team members must demonstrate responsible behavior. This includes:

- Reporting to work on time and using your time well while at work.

- Keeping absences to a minimum. If you must be absent, follow your facility policy for reporting your absence. Notify the facility as early as possible so they can call in a replacement. If the facility does not know you will be absent, care will suffer and your coworkers will work much harder than usual.

- Keeping your promises to patients and other staff members.

- Following each patient's care plan and giving personalized care that meets each patient's needs.

- Doing assigned tasks quickly and accurately.

- Doing things the right way and avoiding shortcuts that can be dangerous.
- Treating each patient with respect and dignity.
- Keeping patient information confidential.
- Cooperating with other staff in all departments.
- Reporting safety and infection control problems.
- Practicing according to your job description and scope of practice.
- Reporting mistakes if you make them.
- Giving proper notice of resignation if it becomes necessary to resign from your position. The length of time varies with facility policy, but it is usually equal to one pay period, or a minimum of two weeks' notification.

PROFESSIONAL BOUNDARIES

As a PCT, you must stay within certain **professional boundaries** in the care of each patient. You may cross these boundaries accidentally or deliberately, thinking you are meeting a patient's needs. Respecting boundaries is one way of showing job responsibility. Boundaries limit and define how workers act with patients. You cannot see a boundary. You must use good judgment and experience to identify boundaries and keep from crossing them. When driving the car, you do not see the boundaries when you cross from one city to the next. Professional boundaries are similar: they exist, but you cannot see them. Being aware of them and using your best behavior, ethical practices, good judgment, and common sense will help you avoid crossing them. This is very important when caring for patients who are under emotional stress. Patients who are at risk of inappropriate relationships with health care workers usually have one or more of these risk factors:

- mental or emotional problems
- poor impulse control
- marital problems
- low self-esteem
- loneliness

Health care workers who are at greatest risk for boundary problems usually have one or more of these risk factors:

- family or marital problems
- naïveté

- low self-esteem
- loneliness, feelings of isolation
- addiction (chemical or sexual)
- financial problems
- stress, burnout

To avoid boundary violations, avoid putting yourself in a position in which you think and act as a family member or friend. Determine how much contact and assistance are right for each patient. Consult the RN if you are unsure. Too much or too little contact can be unhealthy. Treat all patients professionally.

As a PCT, patients expect you to act in their best interests and treat them with dignity. You do this by not taking advantage of a patient's situation and avoiding inappropriate involvement in the patient's personal and family relationships. Some relationships with patients and families are not healthy for the patient or the PCT. Once you have crossed over a boundary line, turning back may be difficult. Recognizing unhealthy relationships is not always easy until it is too late. Because of this, strive to keep your relationships professional. If any of the following occur, you are probably entering a relationship danger zone:

- Discussing your personal problems with the patient or family members
- Being flirtatious with a patient, including sexual innuendos, jokes that are sexual in nature, or using offensive language
- Discussing your feelings of sexual attraction with a patient
- Feeling that you may become involved in a sexual relationship with a patient
- Keeping secrets with a patient
- Becoming defensive when someone questions your relationship or involvement with the patient's personal life
- Thinking that you are immune from having an unhealthy relationship with a patient
- Believing that you are the only worker who can meet the patient's needs
- Spending an inappropriate amount of time with the patient, including making off-duty visits or trading assignments with others so you can be with the patient
- Reporting only partial information about the patient because you fear mentioning

unfavorable information or secrets the patient has told you

- Feeling that you must protect the patient from other health care workers and always siding with the patient

Consequences of Boundary Violations

Boundary violations lead to inappropriate relationships with patients or families. These violations cloud your clinical judgment and may lead to serious consequences, such as inappropriate sexual relationships. They often carry over into your personal life. The improper relationship may cause you to do things that you would not ordinarily do (such as stealing or using drugs). There are many serious personal, legal, and professional consequences of inappropriate relationships. For your own well-being, be aware that professional boundaries exist, and actively take steps to keep from crossing them.

COMMUNICATION

Communication involves sending and receiving messages to exchange information with others. You will communicate verbally, in writing, through gestures, and by using your body. To be successful, you must understand and practice effective techniques. You will exchange messages with patients, families, visitors, coworkers, and managers. Your messages must be adjusted to fit the age and condition of the patient. The messages must be interpreted accurately. Communication is more than saying words. It is showing honest concern and caring for other people.

Communication is important to the operation of the health care facility. Misinterpreted messages create many problems. Listening is also part of communication. Be a good listener. Gestures, posture, body language, and touch are also part of the message. Making eye contact is important. The eyes are very powerful messengers. A great deal can be learned about how a person is feeling or thinking by looking at the eyes, even if the body is still (**Figure 1-9**). Make sure your eyes and body send the same message that you are speaking. Be open-minded and try to understand others' opinions and feelings.

Most communication is verbal. Although the words that you speak are important, your tone of voice also affects your message. The tone and pitch of your voice and your body language can change the message you are sending. When speaking with others, always remember the effect of nonverbal communication. Your words represent only 7 percent of your message. The remainder is communicated through facial ex-

Messengers

They express anger; That is easily detected. They express hopelessness; When we feel dejected.

They express delight; When we achieve. They express sorrow; When we grieve.

They express victory; When we win. They express forgiveness; For an imagined sin.

They express confusion; When we don't perceive. They express appreciation; For what we receive.

They express happiness; For all we hold dear. They express fright; When we encounter a fear.

They express disappointment; When we lose. They express indecision; When we must choose.

They express patience; For a child. They express excitement; When our imagination runs wild

They express love; It's perfectly clear. They speak a language; For all to hear.

In one fluid motion; As they part. The hands become Messengers of the heart.

To really know a person; If this is your goal. Look deep into their eyes; The Messengers of the soul.

FIGURE 1-9 An original poem by Marilyn Sossaman, LPN. Used with permission.

> Your verbal message is interpreted like this:
> 7% words
> + 38% tone of voice
> + 55% facial expression, body language, gestures
> ——————————————————————
> = 100% total communication

FIGURE 1-10 Be aware of the effects that body language and the tone, pitch, and quality of voice have on the way your message is interpreted. If the tone and pitch of your voice contradict your spoken words, the tone and pitch will overshadow the message.

pressions, gestures, and overall body language (Figure 1-10). Choose your words carefully. Avoid using slang or words with more than one meaning. Use words with which the receiver is familiar. Speak slowly and clearly. Look at the receiver when speaking.

A positive attitude is an important characteristic to bring to your job. Your attitude is the outer reflection of the way you feel. Your attitude shows in your behavior, including your speech and body language. Your attitude will be reflected in your work. It affects the patients' motivation. Believe in what you are doing and in the benefits to the patients. Be positive about your job and your contribution to patient care.

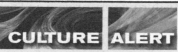

COMMUNICATION ALERT

Remember that one of the most important and powerful messages you send to patients is that you care about them. You do this in many ways, including your demeanor when you enter the room, your body language, your tone of voice, and your touch. With some patients, verbal communication will be very limited. Use your nonverbal communication skills to send the message that you care to all patients.

Review the communication guidelines from your basic patient care or nursing assistant program. Excellent skills are necessary for proper team functioning. Developing effective skills is a challenging, ongoing process. Work on your communication skills to make sure they contribute to the success of your unit or team. Cultural influences on communication are listed in the Culture Alert box.

CULTURE ALERT

Factors That Influence Communication with Patients
Sickness, medication, anesthesia, pain, aging, culture, and disease can affect the ability to communicate. Some patients have trouble seeing, hearing, or speaking. Some have language barriers and do not speak English. Be empathetic with patients who have difficulty. This involves understanding how the patient feels. Tell the patient that you understand by making statements such as, "I know this is very frustrating for you." Imagine how frustrating it would be if you were unable to make your needs known! Be tolerant and patient when speaking with patients who have physical or mental impairments. Do not assume that patients who cannot speak are mentally confused. They may understand what you are saying. Explain who you are and what you are doing when you enter the room. Speak when giving care. Treat all patients with dignity and respect.
Physical Distance
Physical distance is important for effective communication. In the United States, a comfortable physical distance from others is about 18 to 36 inches. If you are closer than this, others may be uncomfortable. If you are farther away, the receiver may be offended, or the message may be misinterpreted because the receiver could not see or hear you correctly. Establish a comfortable physical distance depending on the cultures of the patient and PCT.

Sympathy and Empathy

Sympathy means feeling sorry for patients, and taking on their feelings as your own. Feeling sorry will not help the patients. **Empathy** is understanding how the patient feels. It involves connecting with and supporting a patient when he or she works through difficult times. Try to understand patients' feelings of frustration and assist if you can. Spending a few minutes with the patient just to listen and provide support can be very helpful. This often allows the patient to release an emotional burden and brings a great sense of inner peace.

DIFFICULT PATIENT ALERT

Health care personnel are privileged to have a presence in very personal times of stress and turmoil in patients' lives. Pay attention to what patients are saying. Your role is to listen, to reflect, and to clarify information. This will help the patient work through the problem and express his or her feelings. Avoid giving advice or imposing your beliefs on the patient. Avoid pat, uncaring answers to questions. Never give patients false hope. Admitting that you do not know an answer is all right.

Caring for patients during very private and personal moments is a privilege. Do not be so distracted with your work or the environment that you fail to show sensitivity when patients express concerns. Provide privacy and support while they work through challenges to their health and well-being. Inform the RN of the patients' concerns. The RN may be able to provide assistance, intervention, or referrals to other sources of help.

Communicating with the Patients' Family, Friends, and Visitors

You are a representative of the health care facility. Speak and smile at visitors in the hallway. If someone looks lost, ask if you can help. Maintain an open, friendly, and supportive attitude. Show visitors where the lounges, vending machines, cafeteria, and restrooms are. Answer questions about your facility's policies and procedures. However, you must protect patient confidentiality, even with family members. If they ask you questions about the patient's condition, refer them to the RN. You may tell them something about the patient's activities, such as "He ate a good lunch."

The family is an extension of the patient. Families must make many adjustments when a loved one is admitted to a health care facility. This may be a very emotional time. Emotions range from relief in getting help, to guilt for being unable to care for the loved one, to anxiety about outcome or cost. Other common emotions family members experience are:

- *Fear*—Some family members feel fearful about leaving their relative. They may have preconceived notions about the care based on news reports, rumors, or other sources.
- *Anger*—Some families become angry about the admission. They feel as if they are losing control. They may take their anger out on the staff.
- *Uncertainty*—The family may feel uncertain and fear the outcome of the patient's illness. They may seem afraid, nervous, and tense.
- *Sadness*—Family members may have difficulty coping with being separated from the patient.
- *Guilt*—The family may feel guilty for turning the care of the patient over to complete strangers, for insisting that the patient go to the hospital, or for not seeking help sooner. They may find many things to feel guilty about.
- *Helplessness*—Family members may feel helpless because the patient's physical and/or mental condition has worsened and, despite their best efforts, they cannot change the situation.
- *Worry*—Family members may worry about their loved one's well-being. They may worry about how to pay the bills, or what to do with the patient's pets. They may feel overwhelmed with decisions and responsibilities.

Understanding the emotions that families experience should give you an appreciation of why good communication and making a good first impression are important. Greet each family member with warmth, courtesy, kindness, and respect. Be empathetic. Introduce yourself and explain your responsibilities as a nursing assistant in the care of their loved one. Introduce the patient and family to roommates and other staff members. Make them feel welcome, and show that you are sincerely interested in the patient's well-being. If appropriate, make comments such as, "I know this must be very difficult for you." Avoid arguing with family members. If they have complaints or if you believe they are upsetting the patient, notify the RN.

Knowing when to ask a visitor to leave the room takes tact and diplomacy. Try to schedule your care when the patient is alone, if possible. If not, ask visitors to leave any time the patient's body will be exposed or a procedure will be performed. Just ask them to step out until you have finished, and show them where they can wait. When you are done, inform them that they can return. If the patient requests that a visitor be allowed to stay, honor the request. However, do not ask the patient if he or she would like the visitor to stay in the presence of others. Consult the nurse if you are unsure of how to handle a visitor situation.

Answering the Telephone

You may be required to answer the telephone on your unit. If this is your responsibility, answer the phone by stating the name of your unit, then identify yourself by name and title. Be courteous and polite. If a physician calls to give orders, you must get a nurse to take the call. Unlicensed personnel cannot legally take orders from the physician. If the caller is not a physician, provide the requested information, if possible. However, avoid giving out personal information about patients. If the caller is not a physician, obtain the information, or transfer the call to the proper person. If the person being called cannot come to the telephone, take a message. Write down the date, time, the name of the caller, and a brief message. Sign your name and title. Inform the caller that you will deliver the message. Thank the person for calling.

DEVELOPMENTAL TASKS

All humans have **developmental tasks** that must be completed during each stage of life. These are intellectual, social, and emotional skills that a person must accomplish at a certain age. Tasks seem simple in early childhood, becoming more complex as a person grows and ages. Developmental tasks are described in **Table 1-2.** Depending on the diagnosis, length of stay, and condition, some patients will complete developmental tasks during their stay in the facility.

AGE-APPROPRIATE CARE

Age is an important consideration in patient care. You must approach and respond to patients in a way that is appropriate to their age (Figure 1-11). For example, an infant will not understand a complex explanation of a procedure. Likewise, an alert, elderly patient would be offended if you used baby talk. The three main areas of care that must be adjusted according to the patients' age are:

- Communication
- Safety and security
- Personal care and comfort

Adjust your communications and care to the patient's age and needs.

Table 1-2 Developmental Tasks		
Age	**Stage of Development**	**Developmental Tasks**
Birth to 1 year	Infant	Learns to trust self and others
Toddler	1–3 years	Learns to differentiate self from other people
Preschool	3–5 years	Develops initiative and is able to plan and initiate tasks; recognizes self as a member of a family unit
School Age	6–11 years	Develops physical and mental ability; develops relationships with others
Adolescence	12–18 years	Develops a sense of identity and sexuality
Young Adulthood	19–25 years	Establishes intimate relationships with a mate, spouse, significant other, or life partner
Middle Adulthood	26–50 years	Self-realization in marriage and family; establishes a career, works to create a satisfying and productive life
Late Adulthood	51–65 years	Adjusts to the effects of the aging process and chronic disease; helps adult children
Old Age	65 + years	Critical review of the events and circumstances of life; develops feelings of fulfillment, acceptance, and self-worth; copes with losses of friends and family; resolves remaining life conflicts, completes unfinished business

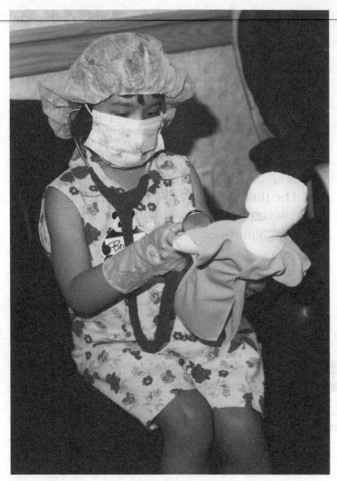

FIGURE 1-11 The child is playing with equipment before beginning a procedure. Allowing children to play with equipment reduces fear.

An overview of age-appropriate strategies is listed in **Table 1-3.** Treat each patient as an individual. Treat all patients with dignity and respect. Honor patients' rights. Remember that illness, injury, and culture may affect behavior. Adjust your approach to the patient's problem, needs, and culture. Be supportive, empathetic, and reassuring.

Special Situations

You have learned that age-appropriate communication is essential to your ability to provide care. A **barrier** is something that interferes with communication. It can be physical, such as trying to speak with a patient whose ears are bandaged. Eliminate barriers whenever possible. If this is not possible, find other means of communicating, such as writing. Barriers can also be mental. Mental barriers arise when you have formed a negative opinion about another person or culture. Avoid forming opinions about others based on appearances. Enter

each communication and greet each person with an open mind.

Other barriers may be present, such as patients with mental confusion, speech and hearing disorders, or those who do not speak English. If you are not sure of the patient's ability to communicate, ask the patient's name and speak with him or her about the weather. Provide orienting information if necessary and evaluate the patient's response. Keep your questions simple and ask only one question at a time. If the patient does not understand, rephrase the question. Never make fun of the patient's lack of understanding. Laugh with the patient, if appropriate. Use the information you have obtained from your evaluation of the patient's understanding to plan your care.

COMMUNICATION ALERT

Try to develop a rapport with the patient on your first contact. At times, this is difficult because some conditions, such as a stroke, may cause changes in mental status, mood, or behavior. Be consistent and avoid becoming discouraged. Try to remember that the illness is causing the problem. Find the most effective means of communicating. Ask yes or no questions whenever possible. Avoid treating the patient like a child. Do not correct the patient's speech. If you must repeat yourself, do so quietly and calmly. Use gestures, if necessary.

The suggestions in **Figure 1-12** will help you communicate effectively with patients who have special needs.

Safety and Security

Keep safety in mind at all times. Age, injury, and certain diseases may affect safety awareness. Teach patients about safety, whenever possible. However, do it in a way that does not insult their intelligence. Some adults, particularly those who are elderly, do not like to be reminded that their activities are not safe. Some patients may not be aware that their activities can be harmful to them. Some may resent the staff's efforts to protect them. They feel that they can protect themselves. Patients may also be in **denial.** When a person is in denial, he or she is afraid to admit that something is the truth. Patients may be afraid that if they admit to having a safety need, they will no longer be independent. Explain what you are doing to keep the environment safe. Explain safety to patients in procedures that you do. Always be alert to safety factors when you enter and leave a room.

Table 1-3 Age-Appropriate Care

Age	Communication	Safety and Security	Personal Care and Comfort
Newborn to 12 months	• Smile	• Keep bed rails up when not at the bedside	• Cuddle, rock, and hold infant
	• Be gentle; responds to faces, voices, and touch as means of communication	• Avoid leaving small or sharp objects within infant's grasp	• Keep infant warm
			• Check and change diapers regularly
	• Speak softly and slowly, or sing during care	• Keep patient safe when out of bed by using safety straps, infant seats, etc.	• Provide food or offer a bottle regularly; do not make infant wait for food
	• Introduce yourself to parents	• Cuddle, rock, and hold infant to make infant feel safe and secure	• Allow parents to remain nearby when providing care; avoid separating child from parent, if possible
	• Explain procedures to parents	• Provide safe toys with large parts that cannot be swallowed	
			• Avoid loud noise and bright lights
		• Monitor rate of IV infusion, oxygen flow rate, equipment alarm status, and other safety precautions each time you are in the room	• Provide comfort object, such as pacifier, if used
		• Check for safety factors upon entering the room and before leaving the room	
1–3 years	• Tell child who you are	• Keep bed rails up when not at the bedside	• Check and change diapers regularly, or toilet according to child's routine; avoid scolding for accidents
	• Call child by name		
	• Introduce yourself to parents	• Avoid leaving small or sharp objects within child's grasp	
	• Explain procedures to parents; ask them to explain to child	• Keep chemicals and other potentially toxic liquids locked up, or under visual control when in use (such as housekeeping chemicals)	• Provide food or fluid according to regular schedule
	• Allow child to handle equipment under supervision		• Allow parents to remain nearby when providing care; avoid separating child from parent for prolonged periods of time, if possible

(continues)

Table 1-3 Age-Appropriate Care (Continued)

Age	Communication	Safety and Security	Personal Care and Comfort
1–3 years, *continued*	• Use simple words and commands to communicate • Allow time for child to respond to you • Smile • Be gentle • Speak to child during care • Stress that the illness is not child's fault • Provide reassurance • Be honest with child • Avoid preparing child for a procedure in advance; children have no concept of time and advance warnings may increase anxiety	• Keep patient safe when out of bed by using safety straps during transport, in high chair, etc.; anticipate child's ability to climb • Provide safe toys with large parts that cannot be swallowed • Avoid toys with sharp edges, long strings, or small, removable parts • Avoid balloons unless child is supervised • Monitor rate of IV infusion, oxygen flow rate, equipment alarm status, and other safety precautions each time you are in the room • Check for safety factors upon entering the room and before leaving the room	• Allow child to be as independent as possible; provide opportunities for making choices
3–5 years	• Tell child who you are • Call child by name • Introduce yourself to parents • Explain procedures to parents • Explain procedures to child in simple language; be honest • Tell child what you will do each time; don't assume that child will remember	• Keep bed rails up when not at the bedside • Keep bed in low position • Allow child to have comfort object, if desired; avoid negative comments about using it • Never leave child unattended in the tub • Avoid leaving small or sharp objects within child's grasp	• Toilet regularly, or on demand, according to routine; use the same words for elimination that child uses at home • Can tolerate separation from parents for short time • Talk to and reassure child • Allow child to be as independent as possible; provide opportunities for making choices

Table 1-3 Age-Appropriate Care (Continued)

Age	Communication	Safety and Security	Personal Care and Comfort
3–5 years, *continued*	• Demonstrate procedures on doll, teddy bear, or other object	• Provide safe toys appropriate to child's age that cannot cause injury	• Give child as much control as possible
	• Allow child to explore equipment under supervision	• May fear the dark; leave a nightlight on	
	• Use simple words and short sentences to communicate	• Maintain a consistent schedule	
	• Smile	• Avoid allowing child to play or run with objects in the mouth	
	• Be gentle		
	• Speak to child during care	• Keep doors to storage areas closed	
	• Stress that the illness is not child's fault	• Monitor rate of IV infusion, oxygen flow rate, equipment alarm status, and other safety precautions each time you are in the room	
	• Teach child to use call signal		
	• Children have a limited concept of time; use familiar time references such as before lunch, or after nap time	• Check for safety factors upon entering the room and before leaving the room	
	• Set limits; reward positive behavior		
	• Encourage/allow child to talk about fears		
6–12 years	• Tell child who you are	• Remind and teach safety procedures	• Talk to and reassure child
	• Call child by name	• Keep bed in low position	• Allow child to be as independent as possible; provide opportunities for making choices
	• Explain procedures to child in simple terms; however, use proper names of body parts	• Allow child to have comfort object, if desired; avoid negative comments about using it	
	• Encourage/allow child to ask questions		• Give child as much control as possible

(continues)

Table 1-3 Age-Appropriate Care (Continued)

Age	Communication	Safety and Security	Personal Care and Comfort
6–12 years, *continued*	• Set limits, if necessary • Allow child to make decisions • Reason with child, if necessary • Smile • Speak to child during care • Teach child to use call signal • Allow child to call schoolmates on phone, or assist to write letters	• May fear the dark; leave a nightlight on • May fear he or she caused the illness; listen for subtle clues and be reassuring • Maintain a consistent schedule • Avoid allowing child to play or run with objects in the mouth • Keep doors to storage areas closed • Monitor rate of IV infusion, oxygen flow rate, equipment alarm status, and other safety precautions each time you are in the room • Check for safety factors upon entering the room and before leaving the room	• Provide privacy during care • Be aware that child will try to delay uncomfortable procedures; may need to set limits on this behavior • Responds well to distraction during painful procedures • Stay with child during painful procedures; speak with, reassure, and comfort child during the procedure
13–18 years	• Introduce yourself • Explain procedures in adult terms; avoid talking down to child • Encourage questions • Spend time talking with child • Avoid using an authoritarian approach; maintain a nonthreatening demeanor • Avoid power struggles with child	• May fear body image changes; listen for subtle clues and be reassuring • Remind and teach safety procedures • Be aware that emotional problems related to weight are common, particularly with girls; report failure to eat/other signs of eating disorders to nurse	• Allow to be as independent as possible • Give child as much control as possible; allow him/her to make choices and decisions • Allow child to set his/her own routine, as much as possible • Provide privacy during care and procedures

Table 1-3 Age-Appropriate Care (Continued)

Age	Communication	Safety and Security	Personal Care and Comfort
13–18 years, *continued*	• Advise of policies and routines upon admission; however, be as flexible as possible • Set limits, if necessary • Speak to child honestly • Assist/allow child to make phone calls to friends • Introduce to others of the same age; encourage socialization • Ensure that child keeps you informed of his/her whereabouts if leaving the room • Teenagers are sensitive to caregivers' body language; make sure yours is appropriate	• Follow agency policy for checking electrical equipment such as hair dryers, radios, etc., to ensure safety • Review smoking policies with adolescent • Reinforce that illicit drugs and alcohol are not permitted • Ensure that child wears shoes/slippers when out of bed, to prevent injury • Assist with bathing, if necessary; child may not ask for help • Monitor rate of IV infusion, oxygen flow rate, equipment alarm status, and other safety precautions each time you are in the room • Check for safety factors upon entering the room and before leaving the room	• Encourage child in his/her normal grooming routine; body image is very important and can be disrupted by illness • Allow child to wear own pajamas, if possible • Be as flexible as possible • Teach personal hygiene, if hygienic practices are poor
18–65 years	• Introduce yourself • Address by title and last name, unless patient instructs you otherwise; avoid pet or demeaning names such as "honey" • Explain procedures; allow/encourage questions • Treat with respect	• Be aware that illness or injury may increase safety risk; take precautions appropriate to the condition • Teach safety precautions appropriate to illness or condition • Keep bed in lowest horizontal position when not performing bedside care	• Provide privacy • Adjust room temperature according to patient's preference • Allow to be as independent as possible • Assist with personal hygiene and grooming as needed

(continues)

Table 1-3 Age-Appropriate Care (Continued)

Age	Communication	Safety and Security	Personal Care and Comfort
18–65 years, *continued*	• Adults are sensitive to caregivers' body language; make sure yours is appropriate	• Wipe spills immediately	• Give as much control as possible; allow to make choices and decisions
	• Inform about available services, policies, and routines upon admission	• Maintain a well-lit environment	• Allow patient to set his/her own routine, as much as possible
	• Be sensitive to patient's need to communicate	• Warn of hazards in the environment	• Provide privacy during care and procedures
	• Be a good listener	• Avoid obstacles in the environment	
		• Observe for unsteady gait	• Be as flexible as possible
		• Transport in wheelchair or use assistive device, if necessary	• Teach personal hygiene, if hygienic practices are poor
		• Monitor rate of IV infusion, oxygen flow rate, equipment alarm status, and other safety precautions each time you are in the room	• Control environmental noise as much as possible
		• Check for safety factors upon entering the room and before leaving the room	
Over age 65	• Introduce yourself	• Be aware that illness or injury may increase safety risk; take precautions appropriate to the condition	• Provide privacy
	• Address by title and last name, unless patient instructs you otherwise; avoid pet or demeaning names such as "honey"	• Teach safety precautions appropriate to illness or condition	• Adjust room temperature according to patient's preference
	• Speak slowly and clearly; make eye contact		• Allow to be as independent as possible
		• Protect patients who are cognitively impaired	• Assist with personal hygiene and grooming as needed

Table 1-3 Age-Appropriate Care (Continued)

Age	Communication	Safety and Security	Personal Care and Comfort
Over age 65, *continued*	• Inform about available services, policies, and routines upon admission	• Keep bed in lowest horizontal position when not performing bedside care	• Give as much control as possible; allow to make choices and decisions
	• Explain procedures; allow and encourage questions	• Wipe spills immediately	• Allow patient to set his/her own routine, as much as possible
	• Be alert to problems with vision and hearing; do not assume that patient is mentally impaired	• Avoid changing position too rapidly	• Provide privacy during care and procedures
		• Allow to dangle before transfers and ambulation	
	• Make adaptations as necessary for vision/hearing impairments	• Warn of hazards in the environment	• Be as flexible as possible
			• Teach personal hygiene, if hygienic practices are poor
		• Maintain a well-lit environment	
	• Allow adequate time for patient to respond to you	• Avoid obstacles in the environment	• Control environmental noise as much as possible
	• Treat with respect	• Observe for unsteady gait	
	• Adults are sensitive to caregivers' body language; make sure yours is appropriate	• Transport in wheelchair or use assistive device, if necessary	
	• Be sensitive to patient's need to communicate	• Monitor rate of IV infusion, oxygen flow rate, equipment alarm status, and other safety precautions each time you are in the room	
	• Be a good listener		
		• Check for safety factors upon entering the room and before leaving the room	

Techniques to Use with Patients Who Have Vision Impairment

- Knock on the door and identify yourself by name and title before entering the room.
- Call the patient by the preferred name.
- Assist patients to clean their glasses and encourage patients to wear them.
- When speaking, sit with the light in your face. The light source should not be behind your back, as it will shine in the patient's eyes from this position.
- Speak clearly and directly in a normal tone of voice. Vision problems do not interfere with the ability to hear.
- Use touch to communicate, if appropriate; move slowly and gently to avoid startling the patient.
- When working in the room, tell the patient what you are doing. Talk to the patient about things you see, interesting changes, and what various people are doing. This is not offensive. You are the patient's eyes!
- Ask patients what they want to wear. Describe the color and style of the clothes.
- Tell the patient when you are finished.
- Replace everything in its original location.
- Tell the patient when you are leaving the room. Make sure the patient is comfortable and safe, with the call signal and needed personal items within reach.

- When assisting patients who have visual impairments with walking, have the patient hold your upper arm. Walk alongside and slightly ahead of the patient. The patient can tell a great deal from feeling your body movement. Walk naturally at the patient's pace. Tell the patient when there are steps, obstacles, when to turn left or right, if you must go through a door, and so forth. Be specific when giving directions. Pause slightly before stairs or when making a turn. Avoid revolving doors and escalators if you are in a public place. If you are walking and are interrupted by someone, let the patient know you will be stopping.
- When using stairs, guide the patient's hand to the railing. Stop on each step before proceeding to the next.
- When seating the patient, place his or her hand on the back or arm of the chair.
- Don't leave a patient who is visually impaired or blind in an open area. Lead him or her to the side of a room, chair, or landmark from which he can obtain a direction for travel.

Techniques to Use with Patients Who Have Hearing Impairment

- Approach the patient from the front or side. Lightly touch the patient's arm or shoulder without startling the patient.
- Eliminate as much background noise and activity as possible.
- Assist the patient to use a hearing aid, if applicable.
- If the patient hears better in one ear, position yourself on that side when speaking.
- Sit in a good light where the patient can see your face. The light source should not be behind your back. Avoid standing in shadows or silhouette.
- Avoid chewing gum, eating, or putting your hands in front of your mouth when speaking.
- Be considerate and try to make the patient feel confident in you.
- Look directly at the patient when speaking.
- Speak slowly, clearly, and distinctly. Use your lips to emphasize words. Make sure the patient can see your lips.
- Choose short, simple words. Use short sentences.
- If it is difficult for a person to understand, find another way to say the same thing, rather than repeating the original words again and again; try moving to a quieter location.
- Recognize that hard-of-hearing people hear and understand less well when they are tired or ill.
- Never talk from another room. Get the attention of the person to whom you will speak before you start talking.
- A woman's voice is often harder to hear than a man's, because of the pitch. Make a conscious effort to lower the pitch of your voice if you are a female. Speak in a lower pitched voice than normal. Raise the volume of your voice, if necessary, but avoid shouting. If a person wearing a hearing aid does not understand you, try raising the pitch of your voice slightly.

- Tell the patient what you are going to talk about.
- Avoid abrupt changes of subject or interjecting small talk into your conversation, as the patient will likely use context to a considerable degree in trying to comprehend what you are saying.
- In a group situation, seat the patient where he or she can see all parties.
- Write down key words, if necessary. Use communication boards or other adaptive equipment, if available.
- If the patient has difficulty with letters and numbers, try "M as in Mary," "2 as in twins," "B as in boy." Say each letter and number separately. Remember these sound-alikes: m and n, 2 and 3, 56 and 66, b, c, d, e, t, and v.
- Some patients benefit from placing a stethoscope in their ears, which amplifies the sound when you speak into the diaphragm.
- If the patient does not understand a word, use a different word instead of repeating what you said more loudly.
- Keep conversations brief and limited to a single topic.
- Do not convey impatience by your body language.
- If you do not understand what a person who is deaf or has a speech impairment says, asking him or her to repeat it is acceptable.
- If an interpreter is helping you, speak to the patient, not the interpreter.
- Inform the patient when you are finished speaking. Do not just walk away, leaving the patient to think that you don't care.
- Tell the patient when you are leaving the room. Make sure the patient is comfortable and safe, with the call signal and needed personal items within reach.

FIGURE I-I2 Techniques to use with patients who have problems that interfere with communication and care.

Caring for Hearing Aids

- The hearing aid is fragile. Avoid dropping it. Hold it over a soft surface or table when cleaning it.
- Keep the hearing aid clean. Remove it daily and wipe off any dust, earwax, or body oil with a tissue. Avoid using alcohol, acetone, or ether-based products to clean it.
- If the hearing aid is the cannula type, remove earwax from the speaker opening with a pipe cleaner or special appliance cleaner. Ask the patient if he has a tool called a wax loop, and use this, if available. Never use a toothpick, paper clip, or other sharp object.
- When caring for a female patient, avoid spraying hair spray when the hearing aid is in place.
- Avoid getting the hearing aid wet. If it has an outer ear mold, the earpiece may be washed with mild soap and warm water. The part of the hearing aid containing the batteries should never get wet. Allow the mold to dry thoroughly before reattaching it to the unit.
- Remove the aid when bathing the patient or washing the hair.
- Turn the hearing aid off when it is not in the patient's ear. Opening the battery case when the aid is stored prevents unnecessary drain on the battery.
- Remove the battery at night and check it for leaks. Store the aid and battery in the case. Replace worn or leaking batteries. Wipe the battery gently with a clean cloth before reinserting it.
- Avoid temperature extremes. Do not store the aid in a cold area or on a heater, and do not place it in direct sunlight.
- If the hearing aid has a cord, check it for cracks or breaks.
- Insert the hearing aid properly. Sometimes the shape of the ear changes with aging and the hearing aid may have to be refitted. If the patient complains of pain or the aid is difficult to insert, this may be the problem. Advise the RN if this occurs.
- When communicating with the patient, follow the same guidelines that you use when communicating with a patient who has a hearing impairment.
- Check the bed linen carefully before placing it in the soiled linen hamper. A hearing aid is small, expensive, and easily lost. It will not survive a trip through the washer and dryer!
- After meals, check soiled meal trays for personal items, such as dentures, glasses, and hearing aids. Some patients wrap these sensory aids in napkins or paper towels and set them on trays. The costly items may become lost, accidentally thrown in the trash, or ruined in the dishwasher when the trays return to the dish room or kitchen.

Troubleshooting Hearing Aid Problems

- Never try to repair a hearing aid yourself. However, if the patient has problems with the aid, there are several things you can do that may resolve them.
- Check the aid to see if it is turned on. Some models have settings marked on them. These are "M" for microphone, "T" for telephone, and "O" for off. Set the switch to the "M" setting.
- Check the volume of the aid to be sure it is turned up loud enough for the patient to hear.
- Hold the hearing aid in the palm of your hand. Turn the volume up all the way. Cup the aid between your hands. You should hear a loud whistle. A weak or absent sound indicates that the battery is low.
- Before changing the battery, check the position of the old battery so you can put the new one in the same way.
- When inserting a new battery, place it in the unit gently. If you meet resistance, do not force it. Consult the RN.
- Check the ear mold for wax. If present, remove it.
- Ask the RN to check the patient's ears with an otoscope for wax buildup.
- If the hearing aid is in the patient's ear and makes a loud, whistling sound, check the position. The aid should be securely in the ear. Make sure that hair, earwax, or clothing are not interfering with the position. Check the tubing for cracks. Whistling usually indicates an air leak.
- If the hearing aid works intermittently or makes a scratchy sound, check for dirt under and around the battery. Also check the volume control and connections. If the hearing aid has a connecting wire, make sure it is plugged in tightly and is not cracked or bent.

Caring for Patients Who Have Problems with Language and Understanding

- Knock on the door and identify yourself by name and title before entering the room. Call the patient by the preferred name.
- Approach the patient in a friendly, courteous manner.
- Assist the patient with the use of glasses and hearing aids, if used.
- Explain what will be done.
- Use short, simple words. Pronounce them clearly and slowly.
- Focus on one topic and use short sentences.
- Use gentle touch to show that you care.
- Keep the conversation short, but frequent.
- Use your facial expression and gestures to convey your message.
- Allow adequate time for the patient to respond. Do not be tempted to complete a sentence for the patient.

FIGURE 1-12 Techniques to use with patients who have problems that interfere with communication and care—Continued

- Listen carefully to the response. Pay close attention to what the patient is saying.
- If you think you understand what the patient is saying, use paraphrasing to give the patient feedback.
- Allow the patient time to finish speaking. Don't cut him or her off.
- Monitor your body language. Avoid communicating frustration due to your inability to understand.
- Assume that the patient understands you if you are not sure and cannot get a response.
- Encourage the patient to point to things and use gestures.
- Use adaptive devices, such as picture boards, if available. The speech-language pathologist will often provide these devices and teach the patient to use them
- Tell the patient when you are leaving the room. Make sure the patient is comfortable and safe, with the call signal and needed personal items within reach.

COMMUNICATION ALERT

Sickness, medication, anesthesia, pain, aging, culture, and disease can affect the patient's ability to communicate. Practice empathy with patients by putting yourself in the patient's shoes and understanding how it feels. Be patient when speaking with patients whose primary language is not English. Some patients who cannot speak understand what is said to them. Some have limited writing skills, dictionaries, or adaptive devices to assist them in making their needs known. Show caring through your body language and demeanor.

Caring for Patients Who Have Cognitive Impairments (Confusion)

- Monitor your body language; make sure you are sending a suitable message.
- Monitor the patient's body language and expression for clues to the meaning of communications.
- Approach the patient in a calm, patient, and respectful manner. Be slow, calm, and deliberate in both your mannerisms and speech. Avoid making the patient feel rushed.
- Greet the patient by the preferred name. Avoid pet names, such as "Granny" or "honey." Make eye contact when speaking.
- Identify yourself by name and title and explain what you are going to do. Give simple instructions, one step at a time. You may need to explain several times during a procedure. Use gestures, if appropriate.
- Simplify tasks whenever possible.
  - Establish a routine and stick with it as much as possible.
  - Provide structure, consistency and direction in activities.
  - Keep the environment stable, with few changes and stimuli.
  - Limit decision making to simple choices. Avoid overwhelming the patient.
- Test the patient's understanding.
- Provide verbal reassurance. Touch the patient gently, if appropriate.
- Ask short, simple questions. Give the patient time to respond. Repeat if necessary.
- Use positive terms. Avoid words such as "can't," "don't," and "no."

- Use cues or signals such as gestures, pointing, touching, smiling, or placing an item in the patient's hand as you discuss using the item.
- Recognize when the patient is becoming frustrated, and try to help, if possible.
- Avoid quizzing the patient by asking questions, such as "Do you remember me?" Avoid trying to teach the patient to think or remember. Assist the patient to relate to people and memories that are familiar or pleasant.
- Provide care to meet the patient's basic human needs. For example, avoid assuming that the patient knows how to bathe, will remember to bathe, or can bathe. Provide reminders and assistance as necessary.
- Keep the patient's immediate environment quiet, simple, stable, and as free from change as possible.

DIFFICULT PATIENT ALERT

Patients who have coping and behavior problems usually have a behavior management care plan that lists steps to follow when the patient displays certain problems. Become familiar with the care plan. Carry out the approaches in the order listed. Modify your behavior in response to the patients behavior. Monitor how the patient responds to you, and then adjust your approach to achieve results. Vary routines and equipment, if necessary. Put yourself in the patient's shoes and try to understand what is happening.

Caring for Patients Who Resist Care

- Simplify care and routines as much as possible. Do tasks at the normal time of day for the activity. Try to do things the same way each day. Be calm and patient. Avoid rushing. Do not show impatience through your body language.

- Match the demands of care to the patient's abilities. Patients may resist care when the activity requires skills that the patient has lost.
- Be aware of how your care is affecting the patient.

FIGURE 1-12 Techniques to use with patients who have problems that interfere with communication and care—Continued

- All behavior has meaning. If you think you have identified the meaning of a patient's behavior, inform the RN. For example, yelling or grimacing upon movement suggests pain. Screaming when the light is off suggests fear of the dark. Fighting during incontinent care suggests that the patient perceives the activity as a sexual assault. Also, consider these common causes of behavior problems:
  - The patient may have unmet physical or psychosocial needs.
  - The complexity of the care may exceed the patient's ability to cope.
  - You may be expecting too much of the patient, rushing the patient, expressing your own anxiety or impatience to the patient, or sending mixed messages.
- Monitor the patient for signs of anxiety that suggest early resistance to care, such as restlessness, shifting position, clenching fists, wringing hands, or moaning.
- Stop the procedure at the first sign of distress, if you can safely do so.

- Meet unmet needs, if possible, to stop the problem behavior. Other approaches are:
  - Delaying the care until later
  - Simplifying the task
  - Providing additional assistance, instructions, or equipment
  - Slowing down
  - Adjusting your approach.

DIFFICULT PATIENT ALERT

Reward patients for positive behavior. Behavior that is rewarded is usually repeated. The goal is to show the patient a healthy way of directing energy. Verbal praise, positive feedback, and other signs of approval are rewards. Nonverbal rewards such as a hug, smile, or pat on the back may also be used, when appropriate. Snacks and privileges are sometimes used as rewards.

Caring for Patients Who Are Yelling or Screaming

- Distract the patient with a snack (hard candy or gum work well, if allowed). Try discussing a favorite topic or person. The patient cannot yell when eating or talking.
- Try to identify the cause(s) of the behavior. Common causes are over- or understimulation, boredom, fear, pain, unmet needs (hunger, thirst, and need to toilet).
- If you identify the cause, eliminate it.
- If the patient is alert, ask what the problem is. Use active listening skills and provide comfort.
- Realize that patients from some cultures scream with pain and grief. This is socially acceptable in the patient's culture.
- Ask the alert patient to verbalize his or her frustrations. Listen, but do not provide advice. Make comments such as, "I see you are upset." Show that you are interested in what the patient is saying.

- Monitor body language to see if the patient grimaces or shows other signs of pain.
- Try to distract the patient. Redirecting the behavior with a positive activity, such as a walk, or looking at a picture album, may be helpful.
- Eliminate or reduce environmental stimulation. Try moving the patient to a quiet area.
- Provide physical comfort measures, such as turning, positioning, or a backrub.
- Take the patient to the bathroom. Some confused patients scream from the discomfort of a full bladder.
- Ask the patient if you should leave and return later, as appropriate.

Caring for Patients Who Are Verbally or Physically Aggressive

- Remain calm and reassuring, and use nonthreatening body language. Speak in a soft, low, calm voice.
- Avoid yelling, becoming defensive, arguing, or reasoning with the patient.
- If aggressive behavior occurs in a public area, move the patient if it is safe to do so. If not, move others out of the way.
- Attempt to identify the cause of the behavior and eliminate it, if possible.
- Respect the patient's need for personal space.
- Take physical threats seriously and keep your distance.
- Watch the patient's eyes. They will usually focus on the part of the body to be attacked.
- Do not make the patient feel trapped or cornered.
- Do not turn your back on the patient. Monitor your body language. You should appear open and supportive, not hostile or defensive.
- Avoid touching the patient, as this may cause further agitation.
- Keep your distance. Remain at least one leg length from the patient. Do not let the patient block your path to the door.
- Show that you are interested in what the patient is saying.
- Show empathy and acknowledge the patient's feelings.
- Reassure the patient.
- Praise efforts at self-control.
- Try distraction to calm the patient.

- Try to identify the cause(s), such as pain, fear, anger, stress, feelings of helplessness, lack of privacy, misunderstanding, personality conflicts, and unmet needs.
- Call for assistance from others, if necessary.

DIFFICULT PATIENT ALERT

For many years, backrubs were almost a sacred routine part of nursing care. Over time, we have become much more dependent on technology. When we are busy or staffing is short, it seems as if there is no time for backrubs. However, calming the agitated patient who cannot sleep is time-consuming; the pregnant mother with a backache may use the call signal frequently; the patient with spasticity cannot get into a comfortable position. You may find that taking a few minutes to give a backrub will save you a great deal of time in caring for your patient. A good backrub is comforting and relaxing. Agitated patients often calm down. Uncomfortable patients become more comfortable and demand less attention. Do not omit this important part of nursing care that pays dividends in patient comfort and satisfaction. Over time, it may even make your job easier.

FIGURE 1-12 Techniques to use with patients who have problems that interfere with communication and care—Continued

Fear. Patients may react in a certain way because they fear the outcome of their illness or injury. Some fear the unknown. Infants and children often fear separation from their parents. Everyone fears what they do not understand. Encourage patients to talk about their fears. Offer support, but avoid giving the patient false hope. Allow patients to make choices and decisions about their care and routines. Encourage them to be as independent as possible. Totally dependent patients can exercise control by verbally directing their care. Being in control promotes positive self-esteem.

RESTORATIVE NURSING CARE

Restorative nursing care is based on a belief in the dignity and worth of each person. The patient's physical condition affects self-esteem. Providing restorative nursing care is important in every health care setting. Restorative nursing is given to assist each patient to attain and maintain the highest level of function possible considering his or her unique, individual situation.

Learning the principles of restorative nursing will help you understand the care you give, and why certain procedures have been ordered. The principles of restorative nursing are:

- *Begin treatment early.* Starting restorative care early in the disease or admission will improve the outcome (**Figure 1-13**).
- *Activity strengthens and inactivity weakens.* Keep the patient as active as possible, considering his or her medical condition. Encourage patients to be as independent as possible. Being partially independent is better than being completely dependent on others.
- *Prevent further disability.* Follow the care plan to prevent injury and deformity. Practice safety precautions appropriate to the patient's age, physical problems, and mental condition.
- *Stress the patient's ability and not the disability.* Emphasizing what the patient can do provides hope. Instead of saying, "You cannot use your right arm," say, "You can use your left arm."
- *Treat the whole person.* You cannot isolate the medical problem from the rest of the person. Consider the patient's entire situation. Use and build on strengths to

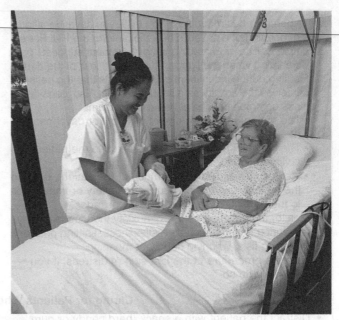

FIGURE 1-13 Beginning treatment early after an amputation will speed the patient's recovery.

overcome needs. Communicate strengths, so other team members can use them to help the patient as well.

Some patients have low self-esteem because they cannot care for themselves. Provide only the assistance necessary to complete the task. Set up the needed supplies. Give instructions, if necessary. Encourage the patient. Allow adequate time to complete the task. If the patient cannot complete the activity, offer to finish it. Provide positive feedback about the part of the task that the patient completed. Avoid making patients feel they have failed. Stressing the ability and not the disability is very important. This type of care takes patience and determination. However, it pays off in positive patient response. The approaches you use in providing restorative nursing are adjusted to the age of the patient, but restorative care is important to all age groups. Restorative nursing care improves self-esteem and satisfaction with care.

The patient's care plan or critical pathway will incorporate the principles of restorative nursing, and will guide you in the approaches to use. If you discover something that works for the patient, share the information with the RN. He or she will add it to the care plan. Good communication is an important part of restorative care!

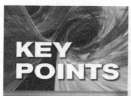

KEY POINTS

▶ Many changes have occurred in health care delivery and reimbursement since the mid-1980s.

▶ To improve efficiency, health care agencies combined departments and employee responsibilities. Workers learned to carry out procedures for which other departments were previously responsible.

▶ Health care facilities continuously evaluate and adjust care to meet patient needs. The process improvement committee conducts internal reviews to identify problems and find solutions to enhance services and care.

▶ Customer satisfaction is important in health care facilities.

▶ Patient-focused care brings services to patients, instead of bringing patients to services.

▶ Teaching health care workers new skills and procedures that were previously provided by other departments is called multiskilling or cross-training.

▶ UAPs are individuals who are trained to assist the licensed nurse in providing direct nursing care to health care consumers, as delegated by and under the supervision of the licensed nurse.

▶ The PCT is supervised by an RN or other licensed health care worker.

▶ The PCT's ability to perform procedures is determined by the state nurse practice act, state laws, facility policies, and job description.

▶ Standards of care are based on laws, facility policies and procedures, information learned in class, your job description, and published information. Standards may be defined by community, state, and national practices.

▶ Applying the standard of care involves doing what the reasonable, prudent worker would do based on his or her education and experience.

▶ Negligence is failure to meet the standard of care, or failure to exercise the degree of care that a reasonable person with equal qualifications would exercise in the same circumstances.

▶ Malpractice is negligence by a worker that results in harm or injury to a patient.

▶ The PCT must be competent in his or her responsibilities, to protect patient safety.

▶ Delegation is the transfer of responsibility for the performance of a nursing activity from a licensed nurse who is authorized to perform the activity to someone who does not already possess the authority.

▶ After an activity has been delegated, only the person given the authority may perform the procedure. He or she cannot delegate the activity to someone else.

▶ Nurses use the five rights of delegation as a guideline to decide whether it is appropriate to delegate a procedure.

▶ Delegation is inappropriate in some situations.

▶ Intradisciplinary teams are composed of workers from the same discipline.

▶ Interdisciplinary teams are made up of workers from different disciplines.

▶ Intradepartmental teams consist of workers from the same department.

▶ Interdepartmental teams are composed of workers from two or more different departments.

(continues)

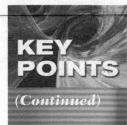

KEY POINTS
(Continued)

▶ The successful PCT is a team player who uses tact and diplomacy with others.

▶ Ethics are principles of conduct and moral values.

▶ Organizing your work involves setting priorities. Good organization improves the quality of care and makes the job easier.

▶ Responsible behavior is essential for health care workers. Responsible workers are dependable and trustworthy.

▶ Professional boundaries are unseen limits that define how health care workers act with patients. Being aware of boundaries and using good behavior, ethical practices, good judgment, and common sense will help workers to avoid crossing these boundaries.

▶ Boundary violations lead to inappropriate relationships with patients or families, and may cloud clinical judgment or lead to other serious consequences.

▶ Your attitude is reflected in your work. You display your attitude by your behavior, speech, and body language.

▶ Sympathy is a negative trait that involves feeling sorry for patients and taking on their feelings as your own. Empathy is a positive quality that involves understanding how patients feel, and connecting with and supporting patients when they work through difficult times.

▶ Family members are an extension of the patient, who must make adjustments when their loved one is admitted to the facility. This is a very emotional time for some family members.

▶ Communication is very important to the successful operation of the health care facility.

▶ Most communication is verbal, but people also communicate by listening, and through gestures, posture, body language, touch, and making eye contact.

▶ Sickness, medication, anesthesia, pain, aging, culture, disease, and physical distance affect the patient's ability to communicate.

▶ Developmental tasks are intellectual, social, and emotional skills that a person must accomplish at a certain age. Some patients will complete developmental tasks during their stay in the facility.

▶ Communication, safety, and personal care and comfort must be adjusted to the patient's age.

▶ Restorative nursing care is given to assist the patient to attain and maintain the highest level of function possible in light of his or her unique, individual situation.

CLINICAL APPLICATIONS

1. Stephen and Maria are nursing assistants at St. Mary's hospital. Several departments have been combined, and nursing assistants will be taking classes to learn how to draw blood, perform ECGs, and start intravenous feedings. Stephen believes it is against the law for nursing assis-tants to perform these procedures. Maria heard that another hospital in the community has im-plemented a multiskilling program. Where can they turn for more information?

2. As a PCT, Jenny is qualified to insert intravenous catheters (IVs). She is caring for Mrs. Long, a 51-year-old patient with heavy vaginal bleeding. The physician visits and orders an IV. The RN assigns

Jenny to care for another patient and states that he will start the IV on Mrs. Long. Jenny tells Amy that the RN does not trust her to start the IV. Do you think that the RN does not trust Jenny? List some reasons why the RN might want to start the IV on this patient.

3. As a PCT, you have been taught to catheterize patients. Mr. Hall is experiencing urinary retention. The nurse instructs you to insert a catheter. What information do you need before accepting this delegation?

4. The RN assigns you to admit the new patient in Room 531. What information do you need before accepting this delegation? After completing the admission procedure, what will you do first?

5. The nurse tells you that she is very busy and asks you to take Miss Roth her pain medication. She hands you a small cup with a pill in it. You have not been taught to give medications. How will you handle this situation?

6. You have set your priorities for your shift and are busy giving care. At 10:00 a.m., Mrs. Huynh's condition deteriorates, and the RN asks you to monitor her every 15 minutes. At 11:00 a.m., Mr. Mancini is discharged. At 1:15 p.m., a new patient is admitted to your section. You are frustrated and running behind with your work. What will you do?

7. A patient tells you that he dislikes all the other staff and you are the only one he trusts. He tells you he thinks his wife is cheating on him and he is feeling very anxious, stressed, and lonely. The patient gives you a $20 bill and asks if you can bring him a bottle of liquor tomorrow to help calm his nerves. How will you handle this situation to avoid a potential boundary and ethical violation?

CHAPTER REVIEW

Multiple-Choice Questions

Select the one best answer.

1. The purpose of workplace redesign is to:
   a. increase the PCT's responsibilities.
   b. operate the agency more efficiently.
   c. eliminate services and personnel.
   d. create more private rooms.

2. Teaching the nursing assistant to provide advanced technical skills is called:
   a. nurses training.
   b. specialization.
   c. multiskilling.
   d. competency evaluation.

3. The purpose of patient-focused care is to:
   a. bring services to patients.
   b. bring patients to services.
   c. provide more technical procedures.
   d. study facility practices.

4. In the hospital, the PCT is supervised by the:
   a. physician.
   b. nursing assistant.
   c. registered nurse.
   d. unit manager.

5. Nursing practice in each state is regulated by the:
   a. physician.
   b. nurse practice act.
   c. medical board.
   d. employer.

6. Standards of PCT care are based on:
   a. what the nurse thinks.
   b. information in books, journals, and laws.
   c. what the doctor would order in a similar situation.
   d. information provided by other workers.

7. The standard of care involves what the:
   a. average, reasonable worker in your position would do.
   b. best worker would do in a similar situation.
   c. nurse or doctor would do.
   d. worker with advanced education would do.

8. A negligent act:
   a. is always deliberate.
   b. involves a boundary violation.
   c. always causes injury or harm.
   d. may be accidental or deliberate.

9. Malpractice:
   a. involves negligence that harms a patient.
   b. does not apply to unlicensed workers.
   c. is a mistake that is easily corrected.
   d. involves adhering to the standard of care.

10. When determining whether to delegate a procedure to the PCT, the nurse must do all of the following *except*:
    a. know that the PCT is competent in the procedure.
    b. believe that the PCT will get the same or similar results as the nurse.

   c. believe that the patient's response to the
procedure is reasonably predictable.

   d. review each step of the task in the procedure
manual.

11. You are assigned to perform an unfamiliar
procedure. You should:
   a. say nothing and perform the procedure.
   b. ignore the assignment.
   c. tell the nurse that you have not been taught to
do the procedure.
   d. ask another PCT to perform the procedure.

12. A team composed of workers from different
departments, each with different training and
responsibilities, is an:
   a. interdisciplinary team.
   b. intradepartmental team.
   c. intradisciplinary team.
   d. interdepartmental team.

13. When providing age-appropriate care, the PCT
must consider all of the following *except:*
   a. tact, sympathy, and empathy.
   b. safety and security.
   c. personal care and comfort.
   d. communication.

14. The principles of restorative nursing care include:
   a. allowing the patient to rest as much as
possible.
   b. stressing the patient's disability.
   c. treating the whole person.
   d. exercising every two hours.

15. Professional boundaries:
   a. apply only to licensed nursing personnel.
   b. involve assisting patients with activities of daily
living.
   c. are part of the job description.
   d. are unspoken limits on relationships with
patients.

16. Health care workers who are at risk of having
inappropriate relationships with patients:
   a. are usually friendly and happy.
   b. may have financial or marital problems.
   c. exercise regularly to relieve stress.
   d. occasionally drink alcoholic beverages.

17. Sympathy involves:
   a. saying and doing things at the right time.
   b. being courteous, considerate, and polite.
   c. feeling truly sorry for the patient.
   d. understanding how the patient feels.

18. Empathy involves:
   a. connecting with and supporting a patient.
   b. being respectful to patients in thought and
deed.
   c. taking on a patient's feelings as your own.
   d. helping patients with their personal problems.

19. Developmental tasks are:
   a. barriers to personal growth and development.
   b. intellectual, social, and emotional skills.
   c. very private and personal thoughts and feelings.
   d. needed for healing and physical growth.

20. Process improvement involves:
   a. researching standards of care and negligence.
   b. ensuring that employees do not violate
boundaries.
   c. making sure employees treat patients with
respect and courtesy.
   d. evaluating care and practices to identify and
correct problems.

E X P L O R I N G   T H E   W E B

About.com	http://nursing.about.com
Age Specific Competency	http://www.dhmh.state.md.us/
American Health Quality Association	http://www.ahqa.org/
American Hospital Association Resources	http://www.hospitalconnect.com
American Nurses' Association	http://www.nursingworld.org
Best Practices Colorado	http://www.colorado.gov/bestpractices/
Biology Online	http://www.biology-online.org
Career Nurse Assistants Programs	http://www.cna-network.org
Center for Human Growth and Development	http://www.umich.edu
Center to Advance Palliative Care (CAPC)	http://64.85.16.230/educate/content/elements/membersofidt.html

Center to Advance Palliative Care (CAPC) U.S. Hospital Information	http://64.85.16.230/educate/content/elements/ushealthcare.html
Centers for Medicare and Medicaid Services (CMS)	http://www.cms.gov
Child Growth and Development	http://kidshealth.org
Consumer Coalition	http://www.consumers.org/
Department of Health and Human Services	http://www.hhs.gov
Developmental Psychology: Research on Human Development across the Life Span	http://www2.uni-jena.de/
Direct Care Alliance	http://www.directcarealliance.org
Fast Fact Hospital Statistics	http://www.hospitalconnect.com
General issues regarding ageing and technology	http://www.stakes.fi/
Health Care Disciplines and Education	http://www-hsl.mcmaster.ca
Healthy People, Healthy Communities	http://www.nnh.org
Human Growth and Development	http://www.webster.edu
Institute for Healthcare Improvement	http://www.ihi.org
Institute for Human Development Life Course and Aging	http://www.utoronto.ca
Interdisciplinary Team Issues	http://eduserv.hscer.washington.edu
Iowa Caregivers Association	http://www.iowacaregivers.org
Joint Commission on Accreditation of Healthcare Organizations (JCAHO)	http://www.jcaho.org
Kaiser Network	http://www.kaisernetwork.org
Meeting Religious and Spiritual Needs of Elder Residents	http://www.nursinghome.org
NA Resources on the Web	http://www.nursingassistant.org
National Clearinghouse on the Direct Care Workforce	http://www.directcareclearinghouse.org
National Council of State Boards of Nursing	http://www.ncsbn.org
Outline developmental issues	http://oz.plymouth.edu/~lsandy/
Paraprofessional Healthcare Institute	http://www.paraprofessional.org
The Platinum Rule	http://www.platinumrule.com
Registered Nurses of Ontario Best Practice Guidelines Program	http://www.rnao.org/bestpractices/
Seton Hall Gateway to Health Science Resources	http://library.shu.edu
Sharing Innovations in Quality	http://siq.air.org/
Teamwork	http://www.vta.spcomm.uiuc.edu
Ten Steps to Better Time Management	http://www.advancefornurses.com
You First Health Risk Assessment	http://www.youfirst.com

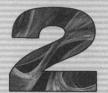

Observation, Documentation, and Reporting to the RN

OBJECTIVES:

After reading this chapter, you should be able to:

● Spell and define key terms.
● Differentiate between signs and symptoms.
● Differentiate between subjective and objective observations.
● Describe how to report and record patient information.
● Describe how to identify pain by making observations of facial expressions, gestures, movement, and body language.
● State the purpose of the medical record.
● List 10 guidelines for documenting in the medical record.

COMMUNICATING WITH OTHER MEMBERS OF THE HEALTH CARE TEAM

You will communicate with other members of the health care team frequently throughout your shift. Good communication is one of the keys to team success. Some communication is written. Some is verbal. Reporting and recording your observations and care are an important part of your job (Figure 2-1). Take this responsibility very seriously. You will report your care and observations to the RN who is your immediate supervisor.

Confidentiality and Privacy

As you know, the patient has a right to privacy with regard to his or her medical information. The medical record is a private and confidential document. All staff are responsible for protecting patient information and data from access by unauthorized persons. Likewise, you should not read patient charts out of curiosity. Medical records and other patient data should be accessed only by those with a need to know the information.

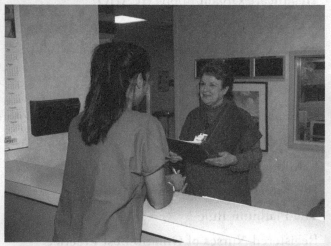

FIGURE 2-1 Report your observations to the RN in a timely manner. He or she will assess the patient and determine further action.

In 1996, Congress passed the **Health Insurance Portability and Accountability Act (HIPAA).** This law has many provisions. One portion concerns privacy, confidentiality, and medical records. The HIPAA rules:

● increase patients' control over their medical records

- restrict the use and disclosure of patient information
- make facilities accountable for protecting patient data
- require the facility to implement and monitor information release policies and procedures

The HIPAA regulations protect all individually identifiable health information in any form. The rules apply to paper, verbal, and electronic documentation, billing records, and clinical records. Because of this, patient information is provided to staff on a "need to know" basis. Information is disclosed only if staff members need it to carry out their duties. For example, the dietary department would need to know if a patient was on a diabetic diet. They would not need to know that the patient has an infectious disease. The PCT would need to know about both the diabetes and the infection. Facilities must monitor how and where they use patient information. Policies must protect patient charts, conversations and reports about patient information, faxing of patient documents, and disclosure of other personal information.

The HIPAA rules ask providers to analyze how and where patient information is used, and to develop procedures for protecting confidential data. This includes the areas where patient charts are stored, the places where patient information is discussed, and the ways in which patients' personal health information is distributed. The HIPAA policies and procedures for each facility are individualized to the facility.

OBSERVING THE PATIENT

You are responsible for making observations about the patient and reporting them to the RN. This is an important responsibility.

The PCT spends most of his or her time providing direct patient care. Because of the nature of your responsibilities, you are in a position to notice changes in the patient immediately. You will use your senses to make observations. Many changes are things that you can see. You may notice changes in movement (**Figure 2-2**), position, facial expression, or color. These changes may suggest pain or another problem. You will hear some changes, such as noisy breathing and things the patient tells you. Your sense of smell is useful to detect unusual odors that indicate a problem. You will note temperature changes or moisture on the skin with your sense of touch.

Observing the patient is a continuous process. If you see, feel, hear, or smell anything that seems ab-

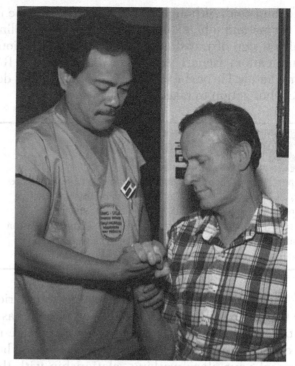

FIGURE 2-2 The patient has limited joint movement, and he complains of pain during range-of-motion.

normal, report your observations to the RN. Even changes that seem insignificant may indicate a problem. The nurse will select the course of action. You begin making observations the minute you enter the room. In addition to looking for changes in the patient's condition, you observe for safety, comfort, and other environmental factors. Bath time gives you the perfect opportunity to make observations of the patient's entire body and to note changes (**Figure 2-3**). For example, a red area on the skin may seem minor, but the area can quickly turn into a serious pressure ulcer. A patient who is receiving blood may complain

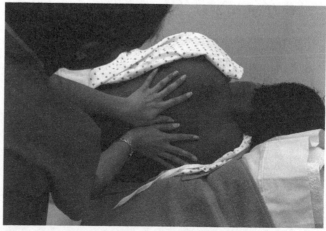

FIGURE 2-3 Bath time is an excellent time for making observations of the patient's overall condition.

of feeling cold. Although your first action may be to get the patient a blanket, you will learn that chilling is also a sign of transfusion reaction, a very serious complication. Report your observations to the RN immediately. He or she will assess the patient and decide what action to take.

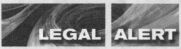
LEGAL ALERT

Reporting and recording your observations of patients are key PCT responsibilities. Pay attention to details. Practice good communication skills. You will learn which observations must be reported immediately, and which can wait until the end of the shift. An alert, observant PCT is invaluable in protecting patients' safety and well-being.

General observation and reporting summaries are listed throughout your book. Each patient has a certain normal condition and behavior. You are in an excellent position to notice these changes, because of your close working relationship with the patients and the nature of the care you give. Changes that occur suddenly may indicate an emergency. Report any changes from the patient's normal condition to the RN. The observations listed in Observe and Report provide an overview of changes to report for each body system.

In general, you should report:

- Changes in the patient's mood, behavior, or mental status (**Figure 2-4**)
- Changes in the patient's vital signs
- Comments or complaints the patient makes about his or her condition, such as pain, dizziness, numbness, and so forth
- Patient complaints
- Changes in the patient's body that you can see (**Figure 2-5**)

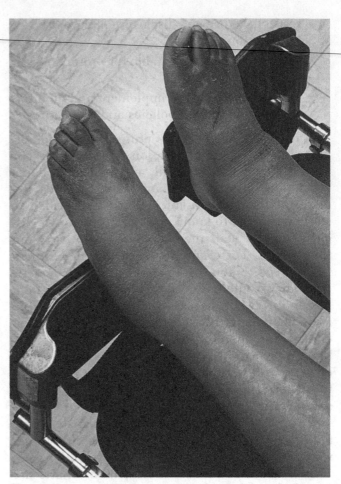
FIGURE 2-5 Always report changes in the patient's condition that you can see.

- What you observe using your senses of hearing, touch, smell, and sight
- Care that works well for the patient
- Approaches that are not working for the patient

If you report observations to the RN and the patient's condition seems to worsen, inform the RN again.

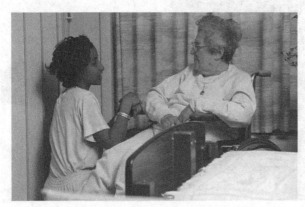
FIGURE 2-4 The patient's body language may be a key to her mood.

COMMUNICATION ALERT

You will develop proficiency in judging the priority of reporting your observations about patients as you gain experience. In general, high-priority items for reporting include abnormal vital signs, chest pain, difficulty breathing, change in color, change in mental status, bleeding, and pain. If you are in doubt about the urgency of reporting to the RN, report your observation immediately. If the patient's condition changes after you have reported your observations, inform the RN again. Do not assume that he or she knows of the change. Follow up and monitor the patient's safety until you receive further instructions from the RN. He or she may be busy and forget to assess the patient. If so, tactfully remind the RN of the observation.

Subjective and Objective Observations

Signs are things seen or observed by using your senses. Signs are usually indications of disease or abnormalities. The red area you noticed on the patient's skin during the bath is a sign. **Symptoms** are things patients notice about their conditions and tell you. They cannot be seen by others or detected by using your senses. Nausea is an example of a symptom. **Objective** observations are factual, and can be made by others. They are made by seeing, hearing, feeling, touching, and smelling. Subjective observations may or may not be factual. **Subjective** observations are based on what you think or information the patient gives you that may or may not be true. Reporting that the patient did not eat lunch is an objective observation. Reporting that the patient ate a large breakfast and probably was not hungry at lunchtime is subjective. It reflects what you think. In fact, the patient may have felt nauseated, had pain, been upset, or had another reason for not eating. Avoid making assumptions. Information reported to the RN should be objective.

Observe & Report

General Signs and Symptoms of Illness That Should Be Reported to the RN

Chest pain	Pain	Change in mental status
Shortness of breath	Nausea or vomiting	Excessive thirst
Difficulty breathing	Diarrhea	Lethargy
Weakness or dizziness	Cough	Unusual drainage from a wound or body cavity
Headache	Cyanosis or change in color	Changes in vital signs

SYSTEM OR PROBLEM	OBSERVATION TO REPORT
Signs/Symptoms of Infection	Elevated temperature
	Rapid pulse, rapid or noisy respirations
	Sweating
	Chills
	Skin hot or cold to touch
	Skin flushed, red, gray, or blue
	Inflammation of skin as evidenced by redness, edema, heat, or pain
	Drainage from wounds or body cavities
	Any unusual body discharge, such as mucus or pus

SYSTEM OR PROBLEM	OBSERVATION TO REPORT
Evidence of Pain	Chest pain
	Pain that radiates
	Pain upon movement
	Pain during urination
	Pain when having a bowel movement
	Splinting an area upon movement
	Grimacing, or facial expressions suggesting pain
	Body language suggesting pain
	Moaning or sighing
	Acute headache
	Complaints of binding pain or sensation around forehead
	"Splitting" headache
	Unrelieved pain after pain medication has been given
	Pain is not normal; all complaints of pain should be reported to the RN
Cardiovascular System	Abnormal pulse below 60 or above 100
	Pulse irregular, weak, or bounding
	Blood pressure below 100/60 or above 140/90
	Unable to palpate pulse or hear blood pressure
	Chest pain
	Chest pain that radiates to neck, jaw, or arm

(continues)

Observe & Report (Continued)

SYSTEM OR PROBLEM	OBSERVATION TO REPORT
Cardiovascular System, *continued*	Shortness of breath
	Headache, dizziness, weakness, vomiting
	Cold, blue, or gray appearance
	Cold, blue, painful feet or hands
	Shortness of breath, dyspnea, or abnormal respirations
	Blue color of lips, nail beds, or mucous membranes
Respiratory System	Respiratory rate below 12 or above 20
	Irregular respirations
	Noisy, labored respirations
	Dyspnea or Cheyne-Stokes respirations
	Shortness of breath
	Gasping for breath
	Wheezing
	Coughing
	Retractions
	Blue color of lips, nail beds, or mucous membranes
Integumentary System	Skin very dry or very oily
	Rash
	Redness
	Redness in the skin that does not go away within 30 minutes after pressure is relieved
	In dark- or yellow-skinned patients, spots or areas that are darker in appearance than normal skin color
	Pressure ulcers
	Irritation
	Bruises
	Skin discoloration
	Swelling
	Lumps
	Abnormal sweating
	Excessive heat or coolness to touch
	Open areas/skin breakdown
	Drainage
	Foul odor
	Complaints such as numbness, burning, tingling, itching
	Signs of infection
	Unusual skin color, such as blue or gray color of the skin, lips, nail beds, roof of mouth, or mucous membranes
	Skin growths
	Poor skin turgor/Tenting of skin
	Sunken, dark appearance around eyes
	Cuts, abrasions, skin tears, or other injuries
	Dry, chapped lips
	Dry mucous membranes inside mouth
Gastrointestinal System	Sores or ulcers inside the mouth
	Difficulty chewing or swallowing food
	Unusual or abnormal color or appearance of bowel movement
	Blood, mucus, or other unusual substances in stool
	Hard stool, difficulty passing stool
	Complaints of pain, constipation, diarrhea, bleeding
	Frequent belching
	Changes in appetite
	Excessive thirst
	Fruity smell to breath
	Complaints of indigestion or excessive gas
	Nausea, vomiting

Observe & Report (Continued)

SYSTEM OR PROBLEM	OBSERVATION TO REPORT
Gastrointestinal System, *continued*	Choking
	Abdominal pain
	Abdominal distention
	Coffee-ground appearance of emesis or stool
	Oral or rectal bleeding
	Abnormal condition of mouth or teeth, such as ulcerations; dental caries; pain; drainage; lesions on lips or inside mouth; abscesses; cracked, broken, or loose teeth; abnormalities such as bad breath or worn teeth
	Loose dentures or other denture problem
	Dry, chapped lips
	Dry mucous membranes inside mouth
Genitourinary System	Urinary output too low
	Oral intake too low
	Fluid intake and output not balanced
	Abnormal appearance of urine: dark, concentrated, red, cloudy
	Unusual material in urine: blood, pus, particles
	Complaints of difficulty urinating or inability to urinate
	Complaints of pain, burning, urgency, frequency, pain in lower back
	Urinating frequently in small amounts
	Sudden-onset incontinence
	Edema
	Sudden weight loss or gain
	Respiratory distress
	Change in mental status
Nervous System	Change in level of consciousness, orientation, awareness, or alertness
	Increasing mental confusion
	Progressive lethargy
	Loss of sensation
	Numbness, tingling
	Change in pupil size; unequal pupils
	Abnormal or involuntary motor function
	Loss of ability to move a body part
	Poor coordination
	Weakness
Musculoskeletal System	Pain
	Obvious deformity
	Edema
	Immobility
	Inability to move arms and legs
	Inability to move one or more joints
	Limited/abnormal range of motion
	Jerking or shaky movements
	Weakness
	Sensory changes
	Changes in ability to sit, stand, move, or walk
	Pain upon movement
	Decreased, unequal, or absent distal extremity pulses
Mental Status	Change in level of consciousness, awareness, or alertness
	Changes in mood or behavior
	Change in ability to express self or communicate
	Mental confusion
	Changes in orientation to person, place, time, season
	Excessive drowsiness
	Sleepiness for no apparent reason
	Sudden onset of mental confusion
	Threats of harm to self or others

(continues)

Observe & Report (Continued)

ACTIVITY	OBSERVATIONS TO REPORT
Activities of Daily Living	Loss of ability to perform an ADL independently
	Increasing need for assistance (note how much assistance, type of assistance)
	Inability to tolerate activity (does patient become fatigued, short of breath, etc.)
	Reduced tolerance to activity
	Weakness
	Pain during certain activities
	Lack of motivation, refusals of care
Dressing and Grooming	Increasing need for assistance
	Need for special services, such as shampoo, cutting of fingernails or toenails, dental services, podiatry services
Walking	Difficulty standing or sitting
	Need for an assistive device, such as a cane or walker
	Unsafe use of an assistive device
	Poor safety awareness
	Gait unsteady, shuffling, rigid, and so on
	Abnormal posture (leaning, pain)
	Sudden onset of falls, weakness, difficulty balancing
Position, Movement	Loss of ability to sit, stand, move, or walk
	Inability to position or reposition self
	Need for special positioning aids
	Presence of contractures, stiffness, or rigidity
	Deformity, edema
	Abnormal range of motion
	Loss of ability to move part or all of body
	Movements shaky, jerking, tremors, muscle spasms, other
	Spasticity (sudden, frequent, involuntary muscle contractions that impair function)
	Presence of pain upon movement
	Splinting, grimacing, or other body language suggesting pain on movement
Eating	Food likes and dislikes, refusals
	Lack of adherence to therapeutic diet
	Need for feeding assistance (note how much assistance, type of assistance needed)
	Consumed less than 75 percent of meal
	Difficulty chewing or swallowing, coughing, choking
Drinking	Inability to take a drink at will without assistance
	Inability to drink from straw, cup; need for special device
	Refuses water, if offered (note beverage preferences)
	Inadequate fluid intake
	Difficulty swallowing liquids, coughing, choking
Sleeping	Inability to sleep
	Sleeps constantly
	Sleeps during day, awake at night
	Difficult to awaken
	Needs to be repositioned by staff
	Need to be awakened for toileting
	Safety awareness upon awakening; does patient call for assistance before rising?
	Need for one or more side rails for positioning
	Need for other positioning aids

PAIN

Pain is not normal. If a patient complains of pain, inform the RN. Determining whether pediatric or cognitively impaired patients are in pain may be difficult because they cannot describe the nature of the problem. Cultural reactions to pain are listed in the Culture Alert.

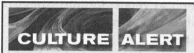

CULTURE ALERT

Patients from other cultures often have varying cultural beliefs about pain. Displaying outward signs of pain is considered to be a weakness and is unacceptable by people from some cultures. Monitor the patient's body language for signs and symptoms of pain. Although the patient may not display an outward appearance of pain, asking if he or she is having pain is the best way to find out.

Signs and Symptoms

Body language may be the first clue that a patient is having pain (**Figure 2-6**). This is particularly true with pediatric and cognitively impaired patients,

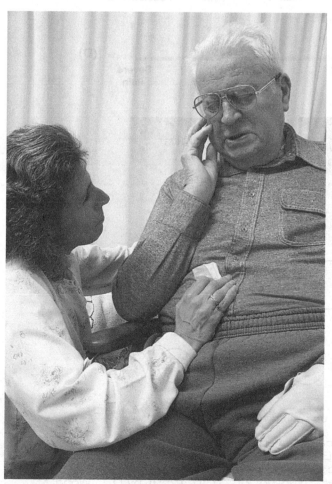

FIGURE 2-6 Pay close attention to the cognitively impaired patient's expression and body language.

those from other cultures, and patients who are comatose. Look for pain on movement, facial expressions, crying, moaning, and guarded positioning. The patient may withdraw when he or she is touched or repositioned. Watch for restlessness, irregular or erratic respirations, intermittent breath holding, dilated pupils, and sweating. The patient may favor one extremity. He or she may become irritable, fatigued, or withdrawn. The patient may refuse to eat, for no apparent reason. Often, the patient acts the opposite of normal. For example,

- A cognitively impaired patient who is normally very quiet becomes noisy
- A pediatric patient cries for no apparent reason
- A patient with garbled speech accurately describes his or her pain
- An agitated or combative patient becomes quiet and nonverbal
- A friendly and outgoing patient cries easily and withdraws
- A patient who is normally active becomes still and quiet

Always suspect pain if the patient's behavior changes. Report your observations to the RN compared with the normal behavior for the patient. If the behavior changes back to normal after the nurse administers an analgesic medication, this confirms that the change in body language or behavior was caused by pain.

AGE-APPROPRIATE CARE ALERT

The golden rule for pain relief is that whatever is painful to adults is painful to children unless proven otherwise. Pain control should be based on scientific facts, not personal beliefs or opinions. Never lie to a child when asked if a procedure will hurt. Admit that it will, but also tell the child that you will be there and that the child will be made as comfortable as possible.

Observation and Evaluation

Although many patients with pain display outward signs through their body language and behavior, avoid making assumptions about the presence or absence of pain if the patient is laughing, talking, or sleeping. For example, some health care workers assume that patients who are smiling or laughing cannot be in pain. These workers often believe that patients who are having pain should be grimacing, frowning, or crying. This is untrue. Some patients may appear comfortable while having severe pain. Once again, avoid judging the patient. His or her self-report of pain is the most accurate and reliable indicator of pain, and should be believed. Notify the RN of the patient's complaint of pain without passing judgment.

Pain management is an important part of patient care. Take complaints of pain seriously. Health care workers should not judge or disbelieve patient complaints about pain. The patients' right to pain assessment and management should be respected and supported. You are responsible for reporting the information to the RN, who will assess the patient and take the appropriate action.

The RN may use a pain scale to help assess and manage the patient's pain. The patient and the RN will establish a pain management goal, using the scale. The patient may refer to the goal in conversation with you, so you should become familiar with the scales used at your facility. More than one scale will be used. Different scales may be used for children and adults. The patient selects the scale that best helps him or her describe the pain. If a patient is having pain, the RN may also instruct you to use nursing measures, such as repositioning, supporting a body part on pillows, or providing a backrub, to help relieve the patient's pain.

Many different pain scales are used in health care (**Figure 2-7A, B, C, D, E, F, G**) as tools for assessing and managing patients' pain. These scales

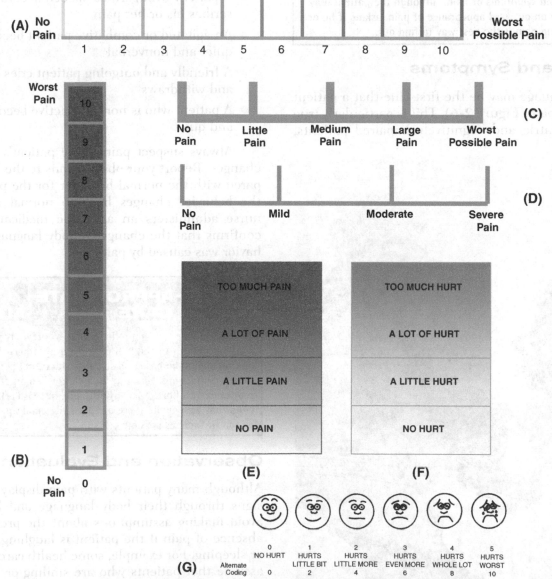

FIGURE 2-7 (A) Numeric pain scale (B) Numeric pain scale (C) Verbal pain scale (D) Verbal pain scale (E) Verbal pain scale (F) Verbal pain scale (G) The Wong-Baker FACES pain scale has become the standard of care for assessing pediatric pain. It is also useful for cognitively impaired adults and those whose primary language is not English. From *Wong's Essentials of Pediatric Nursing*, 7th ed. (p. 1259), by D. L. Wong, M. Hockenberry-Eaton, D. Wilson, M. L. Winkelstein, and P. Schwartz, 2005, St. Louis: Mosby, Inc. Copyright 2005 by Mosby, Inc. Used with permission.

are only examples. Your facility may use similar or different tools for evaluating pain. Pain scales use pictures, words, or numbers to help the patient describe pain intensity. Most scales range from no pain to very severe pain. Pictures use smiling faces, neutral faces, to frowns and tears. Some patients may not complain of pain and may appear to be comfortable. Asking them if they are having pain is not offensive. Always ask instead of making assumptions. Likewise, if a patient has been medicated for pain, but continues to complain, report this information to the RN. Do not assume that the pain has been relieved after a medication has been given, even if the patient is laughing or talking. Ask the patient. If he or she admits to continued pain, the RN must assess the patient further.

REPORTING OBSERVATIONS

Report observations and changes in condition promptly. You are responsible for reporting the information. The RN is responsible for interpreting it based on his or her further assessment of the patient. If the patient changes further after you have reported to the RN, report again. Don't assume that he or she knows there is a problem. Information reported to the RN must be objective. Specific changes for each body system are listed throughout this book.

You will also report to the RN when you leave the unit for any reason, and when you return. You will report off at the end of your shift. Likewise, you can expect to receive a report on your patients at the beginning of your shift, and periodically throughout the day if their conditions change.

RECORDING OBSERVATIONS ON THE MEDICAL RECORD

Documentation on the medical record is also a means of communication (Figure 2-8). Many individuals from many departments care for the patient. The physician and others read the medical record. The information advises others of the patient's problems, needs, solutions, and progress. This helps them plan their care.

The patient's **chart** is a notebook or binder containing the **medical record** (Figure 2-9). The medical record is a legal document. It can be subpoenaed and used in court. It is a record of the patient's true condition, progress, and care. Policies vary regarding who is responsible for recording information on the chart. You may be responsible for documenting information on various medical records. A common rule in health care is: "If it is not documented, it was not done." Documentation

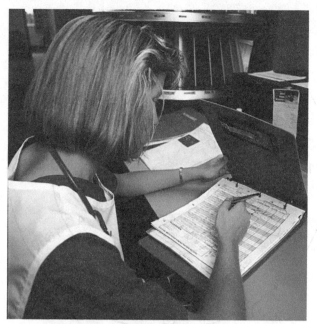

FIGURE 2-8 Documentation in the medical record is an important responsibility.

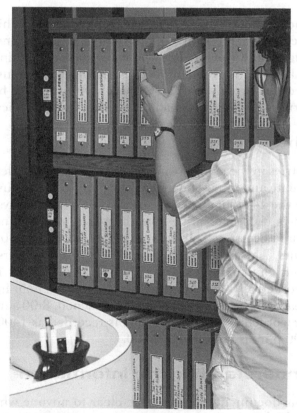

FIGURE 2-9 The medical record is an important legal document.

of care given is very important and should be taken seriously. Never document in advance. You can only document care that has already been given and observations you have already made.

Documentation on the medical record should be objective. It should be clear, concise, and easy to

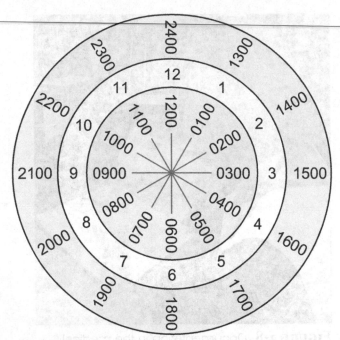

FIGURE 2-10 Most health care facilities document time using the 24-hour clock.

read. Many facilities use flow-sheet charting. This is common for vital statistics such as vital signs, height, and weight. Routine care, such as bathing and bowel movement records, is also commonly recorded on flow sheets. Other charting is done by narrative note. Know and follow your facility policy.

Charting Time

Entries in the chart are made in chronological order, by date and time. The time of the entry is written using the 24-hour clock (**Figure 2-10**). When this system is used, indicating times by noting a.m. or p.m. is not necessary. The day starts at midnight, or 2400 hours. This is the same as 12:00 a.m. For the first hour, only minutes are recorded. 12:25 a.m. is recorded as 0025. After the first hour, each hour increases by one until 24 hours are reached. 8:00 a.m. is recorded as 0800. 2:00 p.m. is recorded as 1400. 6:00 p.m. is recorded as 1800.

Understanding the Information

Your documentation must be clear to anyone who reads the chart. Use your words to paint a picture of the patients' conditions. Your entries must be legible. Illegible information is easily misinterpreted. If your handwriting is not legible, print. Your punctuation, grammar, and spelling must be correct. An accurate and concise record shows that you are conscientious. It implies that you have given quality care. Errors suggest that you are careless. If you

are careless with your documentation, the reader may assume that you are careless in performing other tasks and providing care.

Reimbursement

In some situations and facilities, reimbursement is based on documentation. This is common in skilled units, subacute care centers, and long-term care facilities that accept Medicare payment for services. The main purpose of documentation is to provide a record of the patients' care. However, the medical record may also be used to evaluate the level and value of the services the facility provides. The information on the record is used to set payment to the facility. Payment is denied if the documentation does not support the care given, or show that the patient required the care. The facility and its staff depend on reimbursement for survival. Reimbursement is what pays the bills and meets the payroll. Therefore, documentation is important for many reasons. Documentation requirements change as reimbursement changes.

Surveys

Health department and accreditation surveyors review documentation when they visit the facility. Complete, accurate documentation proves that workers have complied with the law. It shows that the patients have received good care. The record should show that the patients' risks and needs were identified and that care was given to meet them. Missing or absent documentation may cause problems during surveys. Surveyors may question staff about information in the chart, and about documentation policies and procedures (**Figure 2-11**).

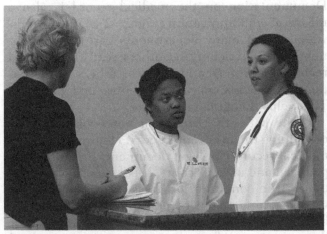

FIGURE 2-11 Surveyors may question you about your documentation.

LEGAL CONSIDERATIONS

Documentation is a legal record of the patient's care. As a legal document, the chart or medical record can be used in a court of law. The medical record may be read by lawyers, judges, juries, experts, and others. The notes are admitted as legal evidence. If a medical record is used in a trial, the documentation shows that care was or was not given. This has a major effect on the outcome of the trial. When a note from the chart is used in a lawsuit, the worker who wrote the note may also have to testify at the trial. Testifying is a frightening, stressful experience. Lawsuits move slowly through the courts. They often go to trial several years after care was given. You may not remember exactly what you did. Your notes must be complete to prove what you did. Thorough, concise notes help you defend your actions.

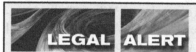

Documentation is a means of communication. Abbreviations must be clear and the meanings known by others for the communication to be effective and meaningful.

Accountability

Each person who cares for patients is responsible for documenting the services he or she provides. If you are unsure of how to describe the patient's condition, check with the RN. Each worker is responsible for what he or she has written. Every entry in the chart is evidence that care was given. Health care workers cannot document for each other. As you can see, the medical record is reviewed by many individuals.

Timeliness

Document your care as soon as possible after caring for the patient. Never chart before providing care. Sometimes you cannot document immediately after caring for the patient, so carry a small notebook. Record important information that you can transfer to the medical record notes later. If you forget to document something, and then remember later, follow facility policy for late-entry documentation. Usually, you will write the date and time the entry is made. You will begin the entry by writing, "Late entry for (date, time)."

Accuracy of the Medical Record

Avoid providing the opportunity for the record to be altered. For example, notes written in pencil or erasable ink can be changed. Avoid leaving blank lines. These provide space for someone to change the record. If there are blank spaces, draw a line through them. This prevents others from filling them in.

If you make an error, follow your facility policy for correcting it. In most facilities, you will draw a single line through the entry. Write the word "error" next to or above the entry. Do not erase, obliterate the original entry, or use correction fluid. It should be legible. Making and correcting an error is a minor problem, as long as the original entry is not altered. Sign the changes you make.

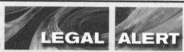

In health care, there is a maxim, "If it wasn't charted, it wasn't done." Although some facilities use a system called charting by exception, most adhere to the age-old maxim and chart all care given. The purpose of documentation is to communicate the care given and the patient's response. Documentation is a true record of the patient's care, and is the first line of defense in proving accountability for excellent care. Never chart care that you did not provide. For example, some assistants will chart that a patient was "turned every two hours" because they recognize that this is the care that is supposed to be given. Document only the facts. If you are unable to turn the patient every two hours, inform the RN early in the shift. Always chart after giving care. Never document on the medical record in advance. If you forget to document, follow your facility policy for making a late entry. Specify the exact date and time the entry was recorded, as well as the exact date and time the event occurred. Clearly mark your documentation as a late entry.

Incidents

If an incident occurs, document the details exactly. Be objective. Chart only the facts. Avoid emotion. Be as thorough as possible. State the patient's condition immediately after the incident. Describe your actions. Include whom you notified of the incident. Describe your follow-up monitoring. An incident report is completed for each unusual event. An incident report is a separate record, not part of the chart. Avoid mentioning the incident report in your notes.

Signing the Entry

Follow your facility policy for signing each entry. Some facilities require you to sign your complete legal signature. Others use the first initial and last name. Your name is followed by your title and/or certification. Flow sheets will have a key for the initials. Electronic medical records may also have a separate key for your signature. Make sure you sign the key so your entries can be identified.

COMPUTERS IN HEALTH CARE FACILITIES

Computers have become common in health care facilities (Figure 2-12). A large amount of information can be stored, processed, and retrieved easily by computer. Departments can communicate with each other by computer. The information is legible and easy to read. Patient information is readily available and easy to find. Using a computer saves a great deal of time. Statistics and data can be retrieved from the computer to identify problems and trends. Access to the computer requires the user to enter a password. Never give your password to anyone else. Some information in the medical records may not be available to all users.

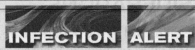

INFECTION ALERT

The computer is used by many individuals. It is a great potential source for cross-contamination. Always wash your hands immediately after using the computer. Some facilities cover the keyboard with a plastic cover, and users type through the plastic. If this is the case, the cover should be routinely disinfected. Wash your hands after typing on the plastic cover. When cleaning the computer and accessories, avoid products containing alcohol. Use only products that are recommended for the surface being cleaned.

Handheld Computers

Communication is essential to the interdisciplinary team. Handheld computers were first introduced in 1995. Since then, they have become essential tools for many health care workers. When first introduced, they sold faster than the VCR, color TV, cell phone, and personal (desktop) computer.

Guidelines for Charting

- Select the correct patient's chart.
- Document on the correct form.
- Charting must be accurate and legible. Follow your facility policy for using the computer, printing, or charting in script. Make sure that the entry is clear and easy to read.
- Know the meaning and correct spelling of words before you write them on the chart.
- Chart the facts. Be specific and objective. Avoid making judgments or charting your personal opinion.
- If you are charting on noncomputerized records, use the correct color pen with permanent ink. Never chart in pencil, erasable ink, or ink that runs when wet.
- Use short, concise phrases.
- Chart after an event occurs or care is given. Never chart in advance.
- Chart the exact time of the event.
- Leave no blank lines or spaces.
- If you make a mistake, do not erase or use correction fluid. Do not mark through the entry so it cannot be read. Draw a single line through the entry and write "error" and your initials.
- Sign your first initial, last name, and title immediately after your entry.

- Fill in all the boxes on flow-sheet charting. Blank spaces indicate that care was not given. Flow sheets are very important if the chart is used in a lawsuit.
- Read what you are documenting on flow sheets. It is easy to skip up or down a line. Be sure you are documenting on the correct line.
- Make sure the intake and output totals are accurate and recorded. If the fluid intake appears inadequate, notify the RN.
- Notify the RN if something is missing from a computerized flow sheet. The RN will add missing information that is listed on the patient's care plan or critical pathway. For example, your facility routinely charts that patients are turned and repositioned every two hours. You routinely turn and reposition Mrs. Li, according to her critical pathway. However, there is no place to document this important care on the flow sheet.
- Use only accepted abbreviations in your facility.
- Never chart for another person.
- Never chart care that you have not given.
- If you forget to chart something, follow your facility policy for making a late entry note on the chart.

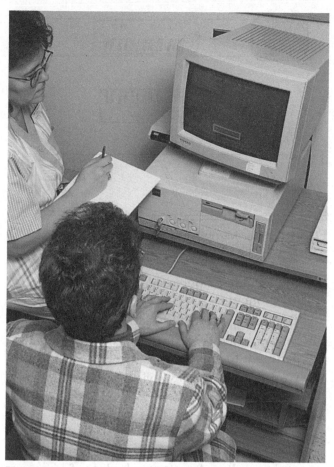

FIGURE 2-12 Your health care facility will teach you the computer program used for documentation on your nursing unit.

Two major classes of portable computing devices are being used with increasing frequency by health care workers. **Personal digital assistants (PDAs)** and **tablet PCs (TPCs)** are small handheld computers that have increased in popularity over the past few years. Many hospitals are using them as an integral part of their services, and professional and paraprofessional staff members have purchased them for personal, individual use. In addition to using the computer as an information resource at work, most individuals use them to hold personal information, such as appointments and a list of phone numbers. Most also have a calculator function. Using a computer has many benefits, and the portability of handheld models has made them a popular alternative.

Handheld computers use wireless Internet technology to transmit data. In many hospitals, handheld computers are used to transmit nursing notes and vital signs to the hospital's mainframe computer. Before handheld computer technology was available, nursing personnel often scribbled notes on the backs of their hands, on paper towels, and scraps of paper.

If the data were not subsequently lost, they were transferred to patient charts later in the shift. By using the handheld computer, personnel can record important data, then transmit it to the main computer. The keypad on the handheld computer is tiny and accessed with a stylus. Light pens and touch-screen data entry are also useful tools with some models. Data such as vital signs, intake and output values, and pain scale ratings can be readily entered by using the keypad. However, for longer narrative notes, the keypad may not be practical. The handheld computer may be plugged into a larger keyboard, which is easier and faster to use.

Because the handheld computer is portable, it is battery operated. If not regularly charged and maintained, it will lose data. *Hot-syncing* refers to linking the handheld computer to a full-size computer to update the information on both. Data are commonly transferred by placing the PDA into a cradle, which uploads data to the mainframe. This is essential for data preservation, especially if the handheld computer battery is running low. Many PDAs use rechargeable batteries, and placing the unit into the cradle also charges the battery.

Radio Frequency Emitting Devices

Your facility will have strict policies and procedures regarding the types of devices that may be used, and when and where they may be used. Become familiar with these policies and follow them. Radio frequency emitting devices have the potential to interfere with patient care and diagnostic, life support, and laboratory equipment. Most hospitals have banned cell phones or restricted their use to certain areas (Figure 2-13). The same is true regarding handheld computing devices. Some hospitals prohibit their use in highly instrumented clinical areas, such as the

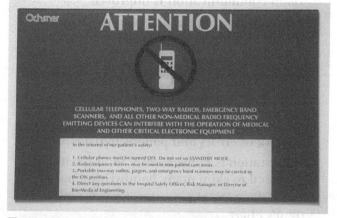

FIGURE 2-13 Cell phones and other electronic devices may interfere with medical equipment.

intensive care unit. Others prohibit their use within five feet of patient care and diagnostic equipment.

Computers and HIPAA Compliance

HIPAA affects all health care communication, especially information technology (IT). Because of this, hospital systems establish layers of access to patient medical records. For example, you will be able to access the records for only those patients listed in your assignment. Information will be limited to that which is essential to patient care. The IT department can track who is accessing any patient's record, and can readily identify misuse of the system. Most PDAs have the ability to access the Internet, so the hospital will construct a firewall to ensure that sensitive patient data are not being broadcast into cyberspace.

Advantages of Using Computers

There are many advantages to using computers in health care:

- Information access is rapid
- They are a ready source of decision trees, reference material and information
- They can provide warning messages, such as drug, allergy, and food interactions, alerting staff to potential negative side effects
- Documentation is faster and less time-consuming
- They enable users to manage patient and procedure information
- Bedside data entry can be done, before information is forgotten
- Data are available for research and teaching
- Team communication is improved
- Charges for supplies and services can be recorded immediately, so that charges are not lost
- Bar codes and other patient identification labels (Figure 2-14) can be created to track laboratory specimens, medications, and other items; using bar codes and scanners reduces the risk of errors and patient injuries
- Information is conveniently found, without the need to skim many handwritten pages
- They eliminate the need to hunt for a patient's chart
- There is no need to wait for others to finish using the chart you need

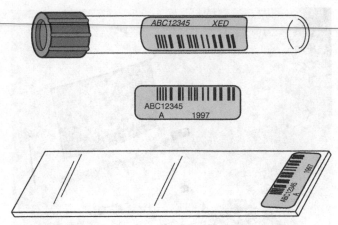

FIGURE 2-14 Many hospitals use bar codes to reduce the risk of errors.

- You can check personal work schedule and assignments
- Terminology and abbreviations are consistent
- Information is transferred easily from one department to another
- Worksheet or Kardex-style programs and forms are available
- You can check critical pathway and care plan information
- You can create checklists and worksheets, such as a list of patient schedules for the day
- Individual field data can be generated and database searches done (such as a list of baths, labs, surgery, and therapy)
- Computers are not as easily lost as written patient records
- Data and information are legible and easy to read
- They are portable and easy to use
- It is easy and helpful to check information at the bedside without going to the desk
- Computer use reduces errors and improves patient safety

Nursing personnel diagnose and treat the human response to illness. The physician's education is focused on the disease, illness, or injury, whereas nurses focus on how disease, illness, or injury affects the person. Having ready access to key nursing information is critical. Because of this, nursing diagnoses and classifications such as the Nursing Interventions Classification (NIC) and Nursing Outcomes Classification (NOC) are fully computerized, and data are readily available to nursing staff.

Nursing units do not use the normal word processing programs for recording patient information.

Special health care programs are available. These programs are usually simple to use, even for those with no computer experience. If you will be working with the computer, your facility will provide training for the programs you will be using. Don't be afraid of the computer. Becoming computer literate may be frustrating at first, but it can make your job much easier! Look at it as an opportunity to learn something new that will benefit you and allow you to spend more time with the patients.

Guidelines for Documentation on the Computerized Medical Record

- Remember that audit trails track the computer, user, date, time, and exactly which medical records are accessed, based on your user identification data.

- The electronic record must note whether manual records are also being used. If this is the case (such as during a storm or electronic system failure), the records must cross-reference each other. Most hospitals have policies, such as reverting to paper documentation if the computer is down for a designated period of time.

- Make sure you enter the patient's correct identification code.

- Turn or position the monitor so it is not visible to others.

- Select a password that is not easily deciphered.

- Do not give your identification code or password to others.

- Do not allow others to find your password. Do not write it down or leave it where it is easily found, such as under the mouse pad, keyboard, or in an electronic file. Regularly change your password. Change it immediately if you suspect it has been compromised.

- Never let someone look over your shoulder when you are signing in or accessing patient data.

- Access only information that you are authorized to obtain.

- Document only in areas you are authorized to use.

- Do not print information unnecessarily. Destroy printed copies that are not part of the permanent record. Placing them in the wastebasket is prohibited in many facilities because of privacy laws.

- Never delete information from the electronic medical record.

- Many computer programs place expert reminders, messages, and/or error codes on the screen. These may be annoying, but they are important. Read them and follow the directions.

- The procedure for late-entry and addendum documentation will be different from a narrative system. Know and follow your facility policies for this type of charting.

- Electronic documentation must be signed by the person giving care. Your facility will have a procedure for doing electronic signatures. These are valid as long as they are accessible only to the person identified by that signature.

- Protect patient data transmitted electronically, such as by using an e-mail encryption service. Never transmit nonsecure, identifiable patient information.

- Always log off when you have finished using the computer.

- Wash your hands after using the computer. Many people use it, so the keyboard is a huge potential source of cross-contamination. If your facility uses plastic keyboard covers, routinely disinfect the cover with the recommended product. Avoid products containing alcohol when cleaning the computer and accessories. Use only products that are recommended for the surface being cleaned.

- Stay current. Attend continuing education programs to learn how to maximize your use of computerized charting and information systems.

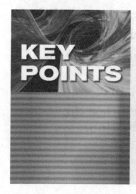
KEY POINTS

▶ Communication can be verbal or written; it is an important part of the PCT's job.

▶ The PCT reports his or her observations to the RN who is supervising the PCT.

▶ Patient observation is a continuous process; use your senses to make observations.

▶ Changes that occur suddenly may indicate an emergency; these should be reported to the RN immediately.

(continues)

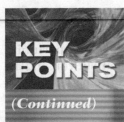

KEY POINTS

(Continued)

▶ Report to the RN:
  ▶ Changes in the patient's mood, behavior, or mental status
  ▶ Changes in the patient's vital signs
  ▶ Comments the patient makes, such as about pain, dizziness, numbness, and so forth
  ▶ Patient complaints
  ▶ What you observe using your senses of hearing, touch, smell, and sight
  ▶ Care that works well for the patient
  ▶ Approaches that are not working for the patient

▶ If you report observations to the RN and the patient's condition seems to worsen, inform the RN again.

▶ Signs are seen or observed by using your senses; they usually indicate disease or abnormalities.

▶ Symptoms are things patients notice about their conditions and tell you; they cannot be seen by others or detected by using your senses.

▶ Objective observations are facts that can be observed by others; they are made by seeing, hearing, feeling, touching, and smelling.

▶ Subjective observations may or may not be factual; they are based on what you think or information the patient gives you, which may or may not be true.

▶ Pain is not normal, and should always be reported to the RN.

▶ A patient's response to pain may be affected by age, cognitive status, and culture.

▶ Always suspect pain if the patient's behavior changes.

▶ Documentation on the medical record is a means of communication.

▶ The medical record is a legal document that can be subpoenaed and used in court.

▶ A maxim in health care is: "If it was not documented, it was not done."

▶ In some situations and facilities, reimbursement is based on documentation.

▶ Surveyors review documentation when they visit the facility.

▶ Each person who cares for patients is responsible for documenting the services he or she provides.

▶ Documentation must be clear to anyone who reads the chart.

▶ Errors in documentation suggest that you are careless, and the reader may assume that your carelessness in this area indicates carelessness in other areas too.

▶ Entries in the chart are made in chronological order, by date and time; the 24-hour clock is used.

▶ Care must be documented in a timely manner, after services are provided.

▶ Avoid providing any opportunity for the record to be altered.

▶ If an incident occurs, document the details exactly; avoid mentioning an incident report in the medical record.

▶ Sign each entry in the medical record with your name and title.

▶ Computerized documentation is common in health care facilities; the computer can easily store and retrieve a great deal of information.

CLINICAL APPLICATIONS

1. Miss Taber is cognitively impaired and nonverbal after a brain attack. She requires total nursing care. When you turn the patient on her side, she moans and grimaces. What does this suggest? What action will you take?

2. You answer the phone on your unit. A PCT from the previous shift is calling. She tells you that she forgot to document several things on Mr. Lanza's medical record, and asks you to add them. She says she was busy and her supervisor was angry with her today. She is afraid she will get in trouble if the RN discovers the missing documentation. What will you do in this situation? What will you tell the PCT?

3. Mrs. Frisch complains of chest pain. She tells you she thinks it is indigestion. Her color is pink and she does not appear to be in distress. What action will you take? Will you report this information to the RN? If so, when?

4. You are going off duty from the 3:00 p.m. to 11:00 p.m. shift when you remember that you did not document something on Mrs. Lopez's chart. You have already told the RN that you completed your charting for the shift. What action will you take?

5. The JCAHO surveyor is reviewing charts on your unit. She questions you about an abbreviation you used in your charting. She wants to know what the abbreviation means, and asks why you used it. The abbreviation is in your facility procedure manual and is accepted for use in charting. The surveyor makes you nervous. What will you tell her?

CHAPTER REVIEW

Multiple-Choice Questions

Select the one best answer.

1. A sign is an observation that you:
   a. detect with your senses.
   b. think.
   c. believe.
   d. should not report.

2. A symptom is:
   a. something you know to be true.
   b. what the patient tells you.
   c. what you think.
   d. never reported to the RN.

3. Objective means:
   a. something you think and feel.
   b. a complaint of pain.
   c. something you observe.
   d. a clinical judgment.

4. The medical record:
   a. is an ethical document.
   b. may not be used in court.
   c. should include only factual information.
   d. is a temporary record of care.

5. When using the 24-hour clock, 5:15 p.m. is:
   a. 0515 hours.
   b. 1515 hours.
   c. 1715 hours.
   d. 2015 hours.

6. The following is true about documenting in the patient's chart:
   a. Correction fluid should be used if you make a mistake.
   b. Factual information should be written on the chart.
   c. Charting is always done before care is given.
   d. Sign your first name, middle name, last name, and title.

7. Upon questioning, a patient from another culture admits that he is in pain. However, he is smiling and visiting with his family. You assume that the patient:
   a. is reacting according to his cultural norms.
   b. is having mild pain.
   c. is not in pain.
   d. has a language barrier.

8. A cognitively impaired patient is normally quiet. She is crying when you enter the room with her lunch tray. She refuses to eat. She shakes her head, "No." When you begin to lower the head of her bed, she grabs her abdomen and grimaces. You assume that the patient is:
   a. having pain.
   b. depressed.
   c. confused.
   d. constipated.

9. When documenting on the medical record, you should:
   a. always state what you think.
   b. be objective and avoid making judgments.
   c. always state your opinion.
   d. document only subjective findings and symptoms.

10. You accidentally documented information about Mr. Lincoln on Mrs. White's chart. You should:
    a. use correction fluid to remove the entry.
    b. scribble through the entry with your pen.
    c. mark over the entry with a heavy black marker.
    d. draw a single line through the entry and write "error."

EXPLORING THE WEB

American Academy of Pain Medicine	http://www.painmed.org
Care Plan Problem Statements	http://www.careplans.com
Change of Shift in the Computer Age	http://www.advancefornurses.com (see past articles 8/28/00)
City of Hope Mayday Resource Center	http://www.cityofhope.org
Comfort Theory	http://www3.uakron.edu
The Fifth Vital Sign	http://www.advancefornurses.com (see past articles 2/4/02)
General Comfort Questionnaire	http://www.uakron.edu
Hospice Comfort Questionnaire	http://www.uakron.edu
Hospital Soup	http://www.hospitalsoup.com
Intelihealth Pain Scales	http://www.intelihealth.com
Management of Chronic Pain in Older Persons (American Geriatrics Society)	http://www.americangeriatrics.org
Nurse Scribe	http://www.enursescribe.com
Nurses in Training	http://nursesintraining.8m.com
Nursing Documentation in the Medical Record	http://www.utmb.edu
Nursing Process and the CNA	http://www.nursingassistant.org
Nursing Process PowerPoint Slides	http://www.rsu.edu
Pain in Children and Adults	http://www.nursing.uiowa.edu
Pain.com	http://www.pain.com
Physical Exam Study Guides	http://www.medinfo.ufl.edu
Problem Oriented Care Plans	http://www.cnsonline.org
RN Central	http://www.rncentral.com
Student Nurse	http://studentnurse.hypermart.net

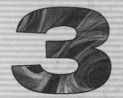

CHAPTER 3

Infection Control

OBJECTIVES:

After reading this chapter, you should be able to:

- Spell and define key terms.
- List seven ways in which infection is spread, and give an example of each.
- List the six factors in the chain of infection, and give an example of how to interrupt transmission in each link of the chain.
- List the times when the handwashing procedure should be performed, and demonstrate the handwashing procedure.
- Describe measures to take to prevent the spread of bloodborne pathogens and other infectious organisms to yourself and others.
- Describe the three types of transmission-based precautions and explain when each type is used.
- Demonstrate how to apply and remove personal protective equipment.

SPREAD OF INFECTION

The development of infection is dangerous for patients and very costly to the insurance carrier and the hospital. Prevention of infection is a major PCT function.

Infection is spread by many methods. The most common are by contact and in the air. The spread of infection by contact occurs in two different ways. Infections spread by **direct contact** are caused by touching an infected person. A handshake is an example of direct contact. You pick up the pathogen when you shake hands. Pathogens can enter your body through broken skin or the mucous membranes of your eyes, nose, mouth, or genital area. If a pathogen enters, you may develop an infection. Pathogens may also be spread by **indirect contact.** This involves touching environmental surfaces and **fomites** such as linen, supplies, or equipment that have pathogens on them (Figure 3-1). You pick up the pathogen on your hands and spread it to the inside of your body through nonintact skin or by touching your mucous membranes.

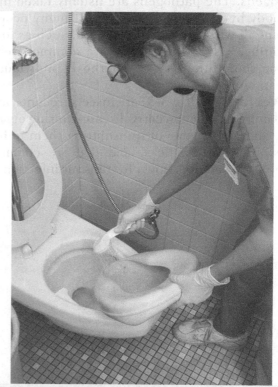

FIGURE 3-1 Your hands contact many unseen pathogens each day.

Infection is also spread by the **airborne** route. Pathogens spread by this method are very tiny and lightweight. They enter the air in respiratory secretions or drainage from the body. In this case, mucus from the nose and mouth contains the pathogens. A cough or sneeze expels them into the air. Because they are so light, they can travel long distances in the ventilation system, in dust, or on moisture in the air. Because of their weight, the pathogens stay suspended in the air for a long time. They are easily inhaled.

Pathogens may also enter the air and spread infection by the **droplet** method. Droplets are also respiratory secretions, such as those produced by sneezing or coughing. Pathogens spread by droplets are larger and heavier than those spread by the airborne method. Because of their size and weight, they remain within three feet of the host (Figure 3-2). They fall to the ground quickly. Understanding the difference between the airborne and droplet methods of transmission is important so you can follow proper procedures to prevent infection from spreading.

Infections can also be spread by a common **vehicle.** Examples of common vehicles are contaminated food, water, syringes used for some nursing procedures, and medication containing pathogens. The pathogens are usually taken into the body by eating and drinking. If many people become ill with the same condition, such as food poisoning, researchers look for a common vehicle, or something that all of the ill individuals have in common.

Vectors (Figure 3-3) are insects, rodents, and small animals that can carry disease-causing organisms, and are capable of transmitting them to humans. Mosquitoes, ticks, and lice are common examples of vectors known to transmit infection.

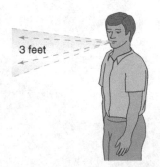

FIGURE 3-2 The droplets from a sneeze usually stay within three feet of the host.

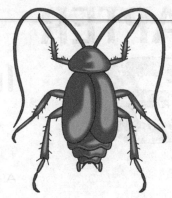

FIGURE 3-3 Vectors are often unseen. They carry pathogens from one place to another.

Chain of Infection

The **chain of infection** describes six factors necessary for an infection to develop. The **causative agent** represents the pathogen that causes disease. The **source** or **reservoir** is the place where the pathogen can grow. A **carrier** is a person who is infected with a disease that can be spread to others. The carrier may not know of the infection. The **mode of transmission** is the method by which the disease is spread. Some diseases can be spread by more than one of the methods listed earlier. The **susceptible host** is the person who can become infected. The **portal of entry** is where the microbe enters the body. Pathogens can enter the body through any opening, such as a tiny cut or crack in the skin. They can also enter through the mucous membranes of the eyes, nose, mouth, or genital area. The **portal of exit** is secretions, excretions, or droplets in which the pathogens travel when they leave the body. If any part of the chain of infection is broken, the disease will not spread. **Figure 3-4** shows breaks in each link of the chain of infection. Using one of the methods listed next to any link will break the chain and prevent the infection. The Observe and Report box lists general signs and symptoms of infection that you must report to the nurse.

HANDWASHING

In the health care facility, many infections are spread on the hands (Figure 3-5A and 3-5B). Because of this, you must pay special attention to hand hygiene. Keep the skin on your hands in good condition. When you are off duty, wear gloves for tasks that increase the risk of injury, such as gardening or washing dishes. Use hand lotion to keep the skin supple

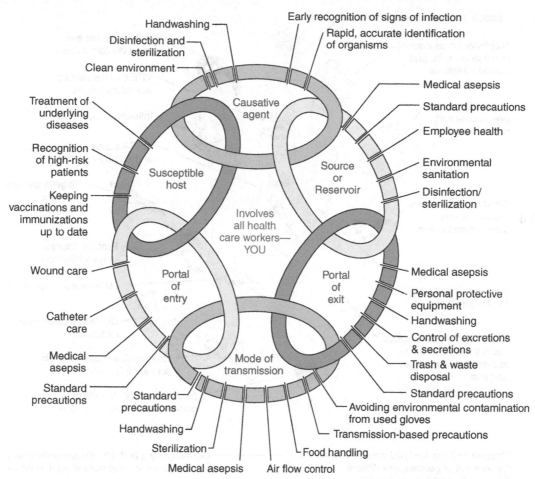

FIGURE 3-4 The circles represent the links in the chain of infection. Breaking a link by any of the methods listed will stop the infection from spreading.

and prevent drying and irritation. Most facilities do not permit caregivers to wear artificial fingernails of any type, including nail tips, overlays, silk wraps, gels, sculptured, or acrylic nails. Long nails (beyond the fingertips) are also not usually permitted. Keep natural nails tips less than one-quarter-inch long. Long and artificial nails have been proven to hold microbes and increase the risk of infection. They are difficult to clean and may cause gloves to tear. Avoid chipped nail polish as well. Chips and cracks in nail polish also hide germs. Wear only simple rings, such as a plain wedding band. Harmful pathogens can hide in rings with many stones and elaborate settings, and these rings are difficult to clean. Microbes may also hide under the rings. The stones and settings on rings may tear your gloves.

Handwashing is the most important method used to prevent the spread of infection. You can pick up microbes on your hands and introduce them to your own body. You can also transfer the microbes on your hands to patients. If your hands touch a clean object, you will transfer the microbes there. This is a potential source of indirect contact transmission. The purpose of handwashing is to clean the hands and prevent pathogens from spreading. Handwashing should take a minimum of 15 seconds. You must take longer if your hands are visibly soiled. The longer the handwashing, the more microbes are eliminated. The most important part of the handwashing procedure is the friction caused by rubbing your hands together. The friction removes the microbes from your hands. Quickly rinsing the hands with water, then drying them on a towel does not remove germs. Oils on your skin must be washed away, along with attached germs. This can be done only by using warm water, soap, and friction. You must spend enough time to wash the germs away.

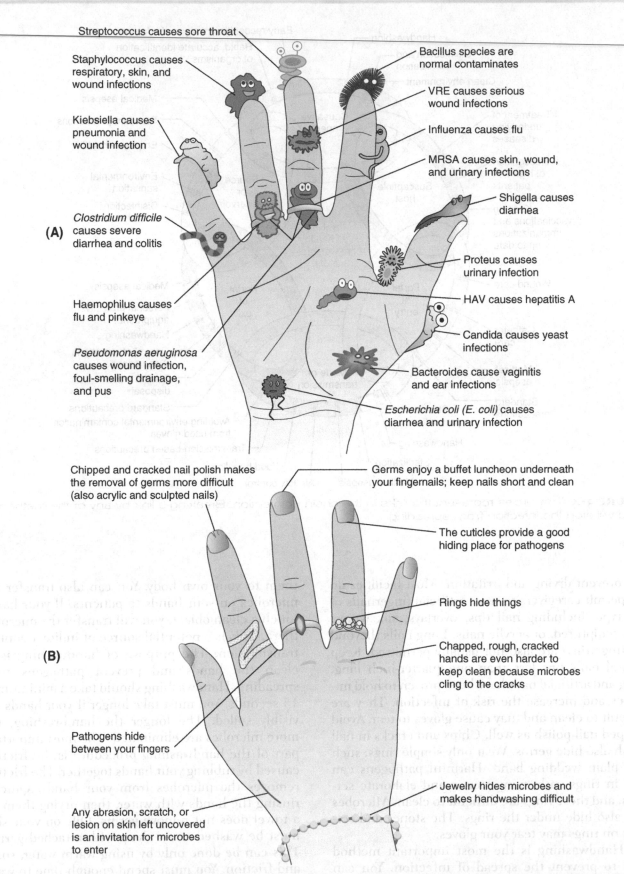

Streptococcus causes sore throat

Staphylococcus causes respiratory, skin, and wound infections

Kiebsiella causes pneumonia and wound infection

Clostridium difficile causes severe diarrhea and colitis

Haemophilus causes flu and pinkeye

Pseudomonas aeruginosa causes wound infection, foul-smelling drainage, and pus

Bacillus species are normal contaminates

VRE causes serious wound infections

Influenza causes flu

MRSA causes skin, wound, and urinary infections

Shigella causes diarrhea

Proteus causes urinary infection

HAV causes hepatitis A

Candida causes yeast infections

Bacteroides cause vaginitis and ear infections

Escherichia coli (E. coli) causes diarrhea and urinary infection

(A)

Chipped and cracked nail polish makes the removal of germs more difficult (also acrylic and sculpted nails)

Germs enjoy a buffet luncheon underneath your fingernails; keep nails short and clean

The cuticles provide a good hiding place for pathogens

Rings hide things

Chapped, rough, cracked hands are even harder to keep clean because microbes cling to the cracks

Jewelry hides microbes and makes handwashing difficult

Pathogens hide between your fingers

Any abrasion, scratch, or lesion on skin left uncovered is an invitation for microbes to enter

(B)

FIGURE 3-5 (A) Many infections are spread on the hands, so health care workers must pay close attention to good hand hygiene and eliminating areas where pathogens can hide. (B) Jewelry with many stones or complicated settings provides a hiding place for pathogens. Long fingernails, chipped nail polish, and acrylic nails also provide hiding places for microbes. Chapped, cut, cracked hands increase the risk of contracting an infection.

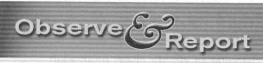

General Signs and Symptoms of Infection

SYSTEM OR PROBLEM	OBSERVATION TO REPORT
General Signs/ Symptoms of Infection	Elevated temperature (elderly persons can be very ill, but have a normal or below-normal temperature; they do not always have a fever because of aging changes to the immune system)
	Rapid pulse
	Rapid respirations
	Hypotension
	Fatigue
	New-onset mental confusion
	Sweating
	Chills
	Skin hot or cold to touch
	Skin flushed, red, gray, or blue
	Inflammation of skin as evidenced by redness, edema, heat, or pain
	Abnormal drainage from any part of the body
Respiratory System Infection	Rapid respirations
	Irregular respirations
	Noisy, labored respirations
	Dyspnea
	Coughing
	Blue color of lips, nail beds, or mucous membranes
Integumentary System Infection	Rash
	Redness
	Swelling
	Open areas/skin breakdown
	Drainage
	Foul odor
Gastrointestinal System Infection	Unusual or abnormal appearance or color of bowel movement
	Blood, mucus, or other unusual substances in stool
	Diarrhea
	Complaints of indigestion or excessive gas
	Nausea, vomiting
	Abdominal pain
Genitourinary System Infection	Urinary output too low or inability to urinate
	Oral intake too low
	Abnormal appearance of urine: dark, concentrated, red, cloudy
	Unusual material in urine: blood, pus, particles
	Complaints of pain, burning, urgency, frequency, pain in lower back
	Edema
	Sudden weight loss or gain
	Respiratory distress
	Change in mental status
Mental Status Problems	Change in level of consciousness, awareness, or alertness
	Changes in mood or behavior
	Change in ability to express self or communicate
	Mental confusion

Guidelines for Times When Handwashing Should Be Done

- When coming on duty
- After picking up anything from the floor
- Before and after caring for each patient
- Before applying and after removing gloves
- After personal use of the toilet or using a tissue to blow your nose
- After coughing or sneezing
- Before and after applying lip balm
- Before and after manipulating contact lenses
- Before and after eating, drinking, or smoking
- Before handling a patient's food and drink, passing trays, or feeding
- After contact with any equipment or environmental surface that might be soiled or contaminated
- Before handling any clean supplies
- Before treating a cut or break in your own skin
- After handling uncooked foods, raw meat, poultry, or fish

- After changing an infant's diaper or an adult incontinence brief
- After touching an animal (especially a reptile)
- After handling trash or garbage
- After touching anything that many people have handled
- Immediately before donning gloves to touch nonintact skin; if you are already wearing gloves, change them
- Immediately before donning gloves to touch mucous membranes; if you are already wearing gloves, change them
- After touching nonintact skin, mucous membranes, blood, or any moist body fluid, secretions, or excretions, even if gloves were worn during the contact
- Whenever your hands are visibly soiled
- Any time your gloves become torn
- Before going on break and at the end of your shift before you leave the facility

Rules for Handwashing

Never wash your gloved hands. Handwashing damages the gloves so they will not protect you. Remove gloves, wash your hands, then reapply a clean pair of gloves.

- Avoid leaning against the sink during the handwashing procedure. The inside of the sink and the faucet handles are contaminated. The outside of the sink may contaminate your uniform.
- Avoid splashing water on your uniform.
- Keep your fingertips pointed down.
- Bar soap can hold pathogens on its surface. Use liquid soap whenever possible.
- Turn the faucets on and off with a clean, dry paper towel.

Procedure 1

Handwashing

1. Turn on warm water using a paper towel.
2. Wet your hands. Keep your fingertips pointed down.
3. Apply soap from the dispenser.
4. Rub your hands together vigorously to create a lather. Rub the hands together in a circular motion for at least 15 seconds. Rub all surfaces of the hands. Pay particular attention to the area between your fingers. Keep your thumbs and fingertips pointed down (**Figure 3-6A**).

5. Rub the fingernails against the palm of the opposite hand. Clean the nails with a brush or an orange stick if they are soiled.
6. Rinse your hands from the wrist to the fingertips. Keep the fingers pointed down.
7. Dry your hands with a paper towel.
8. Use a clean, dry paper towel to turn off the faucet (**Figure 3-6B**). Do not touch the faucet handle with your hand.
9. Discard the paper towel.

(continues)

Procedure **1**, *continued*

Handwashing

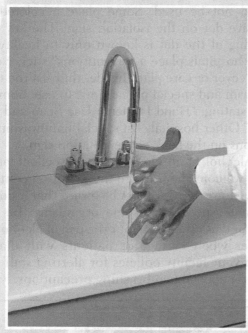

FIGURE 3-6(A) Rub your hands together to create a lather. Don't forget to wash the webs of your fingers and your thumbs.

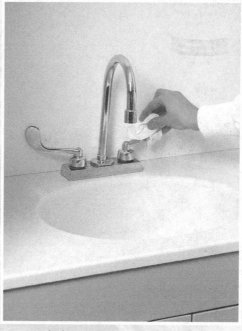

FIGURE 3-6(B) Turn the faucet on and off using a paper towel.

WATERLESS HAND CLEANERS

Many facilities provide dispensers containing waterless hand cleaners (**Figure 3-7**) in various locations in the facility. The hand cleaners contain an alcohol-based gel, lotion, or foam that is dispensed in dime- to quarter-sized portions (approximately 2 ml to 3 ml). Alcohol-based products are often less irritating to the hands than washing repeatedly with soap. Most alcohol solutions contain moisturizers that prevent drying of the skin. In addition, paper towels are not necessary when alcohol products are used. Paper towels contain wood fibers that can be very irritating to sensitive skin.

Each facility has directions for using the hand-cleaner product and policies and procedures for when waterless hand cleaners may be used. Waterless hand cleaner may be safely used instead of handwashing during most routine patient care. In fact, personnel are encouraged to use alcohol products before and after caring for each patient, except in certain circumstances. Washing at the sink should be done any time the hands are visibly soiled, and after personal use of the bathroom. To use the waterless cleaning product,

dispense the proper amount into the palm of your hand. Rub the product into the hands until it dries, making sure to rub all areas and surfaces, including the nail beds and between the fingers. This should take at least 15 seconds. Become familiar with the products used by your facility and their applications. They are very effective in reducing infection and eliminating pathogens from the hands.

Conditions Spread by Spores and Alcohol-Resistant Organisms

Some diseases, such as infectious diarrhea caused by *Clostridium difficile* (*C. difficile*, or *C. diff.*), are spread by spores. **Spores** are microscopic reproductive bodies that are very difficult to eliminate. They can survive in a dormant form until conditions are ideal for reproduction. The spores will multiply and continue to spread infection. Alcohol-based products will not eliminate spores. Handwashing at the sink is needed to eliminate them.

Rotavirus and *Norovirus* are other pathogens that cause infectious diarrhea. These conditions

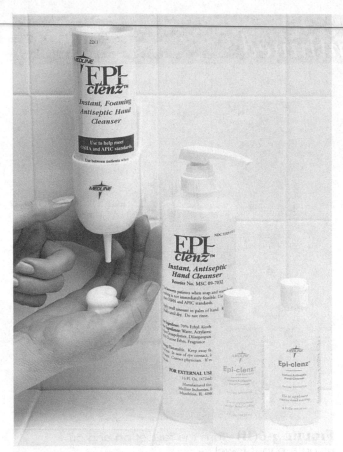

FIGURE 3-7 Alcohol-based hand cleaners may be safely used instead of washing at the sink unless your hands are contaminated with a protein substance, or you have cared for a patient with an infection that is spread by spores. (Courtesy of Medline Industries, Inc., Mundelein, IL. (800) MEDLINE.)

are also highly contagious. You may have heard of these viruses on the news. Diarrhea outbreaks caused by *Rotavirus* and *Norovirus* occurred on many cruise ships. Very few virus particles are needed to transmit infection. The pathogen originates in the stool. *Rotavirus* is plentiful throughout environments in which many young children spend time (such as day care centers), especially during the winter months. Both viruses are highly resistant to the disinfectants used for cleaning environmental surfaces. They are also highly resistant to alcohol-based handwashing agents. *Rotavirus* and *Norovirus* remain active on the hands for at least four hours, on hard dry surfaces for ten days, and on wet surfaces for weeks.

When caring for patients who are infected with *C. difficile, Rotavirus,* or *Norovirus,* you must do good handwashing. The friction and running water will remove spores and viruses from your hands. Because of HIPAA compliance, hospitals have become quite creative in alerting their personnel to the need for special precautions, such as not using alcohol

hand cleaner. Some hospitals post alerts to warn personnel that special handwashing measures are needed. In these facilities, a picture of alcohol hand cleaner may be posted, with a red circle and slash through it, indicating that alcohol hand cleaner should not be used. Some place a colored, self-adhesive dot on the isolation sign. The key to the meaning of the dot is known only to facility staff. Some hospitals place a "precautions" sticker on the chart cover or care plan. Inside, they list the type of organism and special precautions to use. Some post signs stating, "Hand Hygiene: Use Soap and Water Only." Other hospitals list special handwashing precautions on the back of the isolation sign.

Alcohol hand cleaner is an excellent product and a welcome addition to the infection control arsenal. However, you must be aware that it does not eliminate spores and some organisms. Be suspicious and ask the RN about the use of alcohol hand cleaner when caring for patients with diarrhea. Learn your facility policies for alerting staff to the need for special handwashing precautions.

INFECTION ALERT

You may use alcohol-based hand cleaner whenever handwashing is called for in this book unless:

- Your hands are visibly soiled with a proteinaceous substance
- The patient has a condition that is known to be spread by spores, such as Clostridium difficile or Bacillus anthracis
- The patient is known to be infected with Rotavirus or Norovirus

Use enough product, according to the manufacturer's directions. Make sure you take enough time and cover all surfaces of the hands and nail beds with the alcohol product. The procedure should take no less than 15 seconds. Your hands should be dry when done.
You should also wash your hands with soap and water before eating and after personal use of the restroom.

STANDARD PRECAUTIONS

Health care workers can take measures to prevent the spread of infection to themselves and others. These measures are called **standard precautions** (**Figure 3-8**). The purpose of using standard precautions is to prevent the spread of infection. You cannot tell whether someone has a disease or infection by appearance, so standard precautions are used in the care of all patients, regardless of their disease or diagnosis. Standard precautions protect workers against many diseases, including AIDS and hepatitis B and C.

STANDARD PRECAUTIONS FOR INFECTION CONTROL

Wash Hands (Plain soap)
Wash after touching blood, body fluids, secretions, excretions, and contaminated items. Wash immediately after gloves are removed and between patient contacts. Avoid transfer of microorganisms to other patients or environments.

Wear Gloves
Wear when touching blood, body fluids, secretions, excretions, and contaminated items. Put on clean gloves just before touching mucous membranes and nonintact skin. Change gloves between tasks and procedures on the same patient after contact with material that may contain high concentrations of microorganisms. Remove gloves promptly after use, before touching noncontaminated items and environmental surfaces, and before going to another patient, and wash hands immediately to avoid transfer of microorganisms to other patients or environments.

Wear Mask and Eye Protection or Face Shield
Protect mucous membranes of the eyes, nose, and mouth during procedures and patient-care activities that are likely to generate splashes or sprays of blood, body fluids, secretions, or excretions.

Wear Gown
Protect skin and prevent soiling of clothing during procedures that are likely to generate splashes or sprays of blood, body fluids, secretions, or excretions. Remove a soiled gown as promptly as possible and wash hands to avoid transfer of microorganisms to other patients or environments.

Patient-Care Equipment
Handle used patient-care equipment soiled with blood, body fluids, secretions, or excretions in a manner that prevents skin and mucous membrane exposures, contamination of clothing, and transfer of microorganisms to other patients and environments. Ensure that reusable equipment is not used for the care of another patient until it has been appropriately cleaned and reprocessed and single use items are properly discarded.

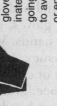

Environmental Control
Follow hospital procedures for routine care, cleaning, and disinfection of environmental surfaces, beds, bedrails, bedside equipment, and other frequently touched surfaces.

Linen
Handle, transport, and process used linen soiled with blood, body fluids, secretions, or excretions in a manner that prevents exposure and contamination of clothing, and avoids transfer of microorganisms to other patients and environments.

Occupational Health and Bloodborne Pathogens
Prevent injuries when using needles, scalpels, and other sharp instruments or devices; when handling sharp instruments after procedures; when cleaning used instruments; and when disposing of used needles.

Never recap used needles using both hands or any other technique that involves directing the point of a needle toward any part of the body; rather, use either a one-handed "scoop" technique or a mechanical device designed for holding the needle sheath.

Do not remove used needles from disposable syringes by hand, and do not bend, break, or otherwise manipulate used needles by hand. Place used disposable syringes and needles, scalpels, blades, and other sharp items in puncture-resistant sharps containers located as close as practical to the area in which the items were used, and place reusable syringes and needles in a puncture-resistant container for transport to the reprocessing area.

Use resuscitation devices as an alternative to mouth-to-mouth resuscitation.

Patient Placement
Use a private room for a patient who contaminates the environment or who does not (or cannot be expected to) assist in maintaining appropriate hygiene or environmental control. Consult Infection Control if a private room is not available.

FIGURE 3-8 Standard precautions. (Courtesy of BREVIS Corporation, Salt Lake City, UT)

Standard precautions involve using personal protective equipment (PPE) when performing certain tasks. *Personal protective equipment* is garments and apparel that protect you from contracting a disease from a patient. PPE also protects the patient from contracting a disease from a microbe passed from your hands.

Guidelines for Selection and Use of Personal Protective Equipment

Standard precautions are used anytime you anticipate contact with blood or any moist body fluid (except sweat), secretions, or excretions. They are also used anytime you anticipate contact with mucous membranes or nonintact or broken skin. Because there are many variables in patient care, no absolute guidelines exist. Think about the situation and use good judgment. You are responsible for applying the principles of standard precautions and selecting personal protective equipment according to the task. Equipment is worn during some direct patient care activities. However, use good judgment in your selection. Avoid overdressing. This is upsetting to the patient and is not necessary to protect you. If you are in doubt about your selection of PPE, check with the RN. You must also wear PPE during cleaning chores when contact with blood, body fluids, secretions, or excretions is likely.

Personal protective equipment will protect you only if it fits properly, if it is free from defects, and if you use it regularly. Never use equipment that is torn or has defects. You are responsible for using standard precautions to protect yourself and patients. Always follow the infection control policies and procedures of your facility.

Handwashing. Handwashing is done before all patient care and procedures. It is also done before applying and after removing gloves. Even when you are wearing gloves, it is possible to pick up microbes on your hands. Sometimes this occurs because of microscopic defects in the gloves. You can unknowingly contact microbes when your gloves are removed. Immediately wash your hands (or use alcohol-based hand cleaner) if you contact blood or any moist body fluid, secretions, or excretions. Wash your hands at the end of each procedure, after removing gloves.

Applying the Principles of Standard Precautions

Personal protective equipment is also called *barrier equipment*. Your facility will have PPE available in a variety of sizes in locations where use can be reasonably anticipated. Check the equipment before you use it. If it is cut or torn, it will not protect you, and should be replaced. Personal protective equipment is discarded, laundered, or decontaminated according to facility policy after use. Be sure to replace what you have used so it is available the next time it is needed.

Gloves

Applying precautions involves wearing gloves for handling or touching blood, any moist body fluid (except sweat), secretions, excretions, mucous membranes, or nonintact skin. If your gloves become visibly soiled, remove them, cleanse your hands, and apply a clean pair. Change your gloves *immediately* before contacting mucous membranes and nonintact skin. You may have to change your gloves and cleanse your hands several times during the care of one patient. Change gloves:

- before each patient contact
- after each patient contact
- *immediately before* touching mucous membranes
- *immediately before* touching nonintact skin
- after you touch a patient's secretions or excretions, before moving to care for another part of the body
- after touching blood or body fluids, before moving to care for another part of the body
- after touching contaminated environmental surfaces or equipment
- anytime your gloves become visibly soiled
- if your gloves become torn

Do not carry glove use to the extreme. Use gloves when necessary, but do not use them for all patient contact. Wearing gloves at all times sends a negative message. Touching is very important to all human beings. Gloves can be frightening to elderly and pediatric patients. Even when you are wearing gloves, it is possible to pick up microbes on your hands. Wear gloves when touching dressings, tissues, infective items, and contaminated surfaces or equipment. If you tear your gloves during a procedure, remove them as soon as possible. Wash your hands and put on a new pair of gloves before continuing. Avoid contaminating clean equipment, supplies, linen, or environmental surfaces with your gloves. This is easily done after a procedure. Think about what you are doing. If you have handled blood, body fluids, mucous membranes, secretions, or excretions with your gloves, do not touch anything with them! Remove one glove and use the ungloved hand to open doors and touch the environment. If absolutely necessary, you may also hold a paper towel or other clean item under a gloved hand to touch these surfaces. Avoid wearing two gloves in the hallways after performing a procedure. If wearing gloves is necessary, use the one-glove technique described here. Use your ungloved hand for touching environmental surfaces.

Cleaning Broken Glass. Always wear gloves for cleaning broken glass. Avoid picking up glass with your hands. Use a broom and dustpan, forceps, or other mechanical method. Protect your hands from being cut. Dispose of the broken glass in a puncture-resistant container.

Cleaning Blood and Body Fluid Spills. Follow your facility policy for cleaning up spills of blood or body fluid. Many facilities use an absorbent powder to soak up the fluid. After the fluid has been absorbed, sweep it up (**Figure 3-9**). Wipe the area with a facility-approved disinfectant. If your facility uses bleach as a disinfectant, mix it in a container using 1 part bleach to 10 parts water (1:10) or one part bleach to 100 parts water (1:100), according to facility policy. Label the container with the contents and the date it was mixed.

Discarding Trash. Items that have contacted blood or body fluids are biohazardous waste. Dispose of used PPE, linen, and trash contaminated with blood or body fluids according to your facility policy. These items must al-

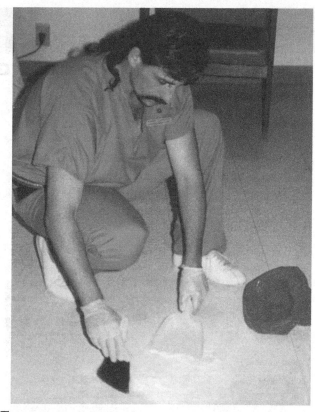

FIGURE 3-9 The absorbent powder has turned the body fluid spill into solid material that can be swept up. Wipe the floor with disinfectant after removing the powder.

ways be disposed of in leakproof, tightly closed containers. Biohazardous waste is stored in special areas until it is removed, and requires special handling during removal. This type of handling is very expensive, and storage space is often limited, so do not place non-biohazardous materials (such as disposable plastic catheter trays or other bulky, uncontaminated items) into the biohazard disposal containers.

Procedure 2

Applying Disposable Gloves

1. Wash your hands and dry them thoroughly.
2. Remove clean gloves from the box.
3. Put hands into the gloves, adjusting the fingers for comfort and fit.
4. Pull the cuff of gloves over the wrist, or sleeve of the gown, if worn.

Procedure 3

Removing Disposable Gloves

1. Grasp the outside of the glove on the nondominant hand at the cuff, just below the wrist. Pull the glove off so that the inside of the glove faces outward. Avoid touching the skin of your wrist with the fingers of the glove (Figure 3-10A).
2. Place this glove into the palm of the gloved hand.
3. Put the fingers of the ungloved hand inside the cuff of the gloved hand. Pull the glove off inside-out. The first glove removed should be inside the second glove.
4. Discard gloves into a covered container or trash, according to facility policy (Figure 3-10B).
5. Wash your hands.

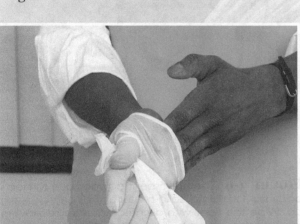

FIGURE 3-10(A) The left hand is clean, so avoid touching the outside of the glove. Insert your fingers inside the cuff, slipping the glove off.

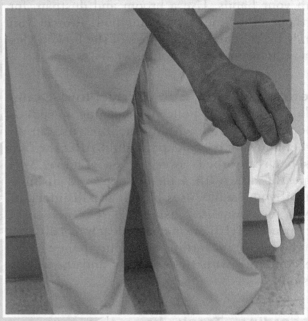

FIGURE 3-10(B) One glove is inside the other. Avoid touching the fingers or palm of the glove. Avoid touching environmental surfaces. Drop the gloves into the covered trash can.

Procedure 4

Applying a Gown

1. Wash your hands.
2. Hold the clean gown by the neck in front of you, letting it unfold (Figure 3-11A). Do not let the gown touch the floor.
3. Place your arms in the sleeves and slide the gown up to your shoulders (Figure 3-11B).
4. Slip your hands inside the neck band and grasp the ties. Tie them at the neck (Figure 3-11C).
5. Cover your uniform at the back with the gown and tie the waist ties (Figure 3-11D). The gown must completely cover your clothing.

(continues)

Procedure **4**, *continued*

Applying a Gown

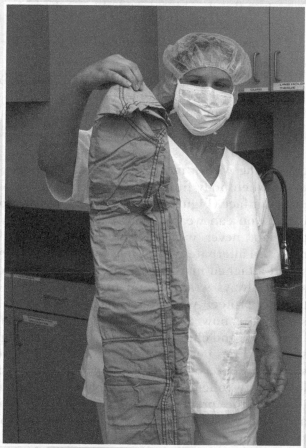

FIGURE 3-11(A) Hold the gown by the neck, away from your body, and let it unfold.

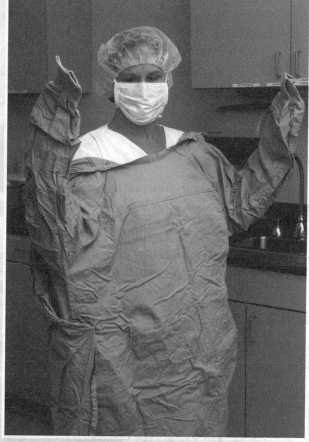

FIGURE 3-11(B) Slip your hands inside the gown, sliding it up to your shoulders.

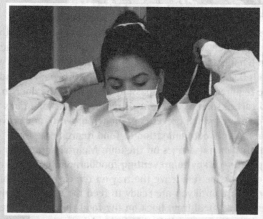

FIGURE 3-11(C) With your fingers inside the neck band, pull the gown up, adjusting the neck. Tie the neck ties.

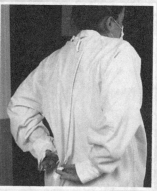

FIGURE 3-11(D) Cover your uniform completely with the gown, then tie the waist tie.

Procedure 5

Removing a Gown

1. Remove gloves, if worn.
2. Wash your hands.
3. If a mask is worn, untie the bottom ties of the mask, then the top ties.
4. Discard the mask, holding it only by the ties.
5. Untie the waist ties of the gown.
6. Untie the neck ties of the gown and loosen it at the shoulders by touching only the inside of the gown.
7. Grasp the neck ties and pull the gown off inside-out.
8. Roll the gown inward, away from your body. Discard according to facility policy.
9. Wash your hands.

Gowns

Wear a gown anytime your clothing may contact blood or any of the body fluids listed. The gown may be cloth or paper, but must be fluid-resistant. Many gowns are specially treated so they will resist fluid. Patient gowns are not appropriate in this situation, and will not protect you from contact with pathogens.

Face and Eye Protection

Facial barriers protect the mucous membranes in your eyes, nose, and mouth. A face shield or goggles, along with a mask, are worn during procedures when body fluids or secretions may splash into your face (**Figure 3-12**). A good rule to follow is that you can wear a mask without eye protection, but never wear eye protection without a mask. An alternate type of mask with a plastic eye shield attached may also be used. Eye protection should always wrap around to the sides of your face to protect you from splashes. Large face shields are now available that cover the entire face, neck, and chin. Because of the shield design, some facilities permit employees to wear this face shield without a mask, depending on the task. Follow facility policies for the equipment you are using and the procedure being done. You must anticipate what PPE you will need and apply it before beginning a procedure.

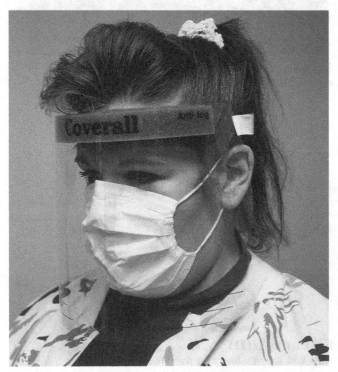

FIGURE 3-12 A mask is always worn with a face shield to protect your mucous membranes.

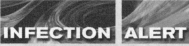

INFECTION ALERT

Keep the soiled linen hamper and housekeeping cart separated from the food cart by at least one room's width (approximately 12 to 16 feet). Some facilities remove the linen hampers and housekeeping carts from the hallway when food is being served. Know and follow facility policies and state requirements. When passing trays, close the door to the food cart as soon as each tray is removed. This maintains food temperature (which prevents pathogen growth), and prevents environmental contamination of food items. Serve food promptly when it arrives on the unit. Maintaining proper food temperature is key to preventing foodborne infection. If a patient must be fed, leave the tray on the cart to maintain temperature until you are ready to feed the patient. Avoid placing used meal trays back on the food cart until all fresh trays have been served. Avoid placing lab specimens in the refrigerator with food and beverages. Store these biohazardous items separately in a refrigerator or cooler marked with a biohazard label.

Procedure 6

Applying a Surgical Mask

1. Wash your hands. Remove a mask from the box by holding the ties (Figure 3-13A).
2. Cover your nose and mouth with the mask.
3. Pinch the metal nosepiece over the bridge of your nose until it fits comfortably (Figure 3-13B).
4. Tie the top tie (or stretch the elastic over the top of your head or ears, depending on the type of mask used).
5. Tie the bottom tie.
6. Wash your hands.

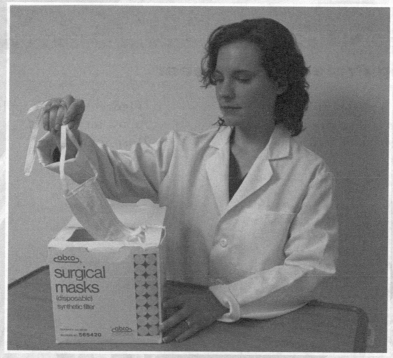

FIGURE 3-13(A) Carefully remove the mask, holding it only by the ties.

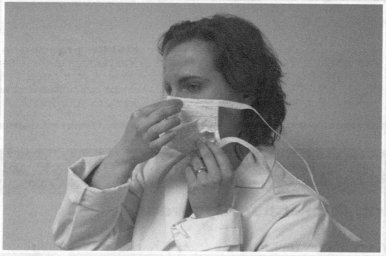

FIGURE 3-13(B) Pinch the metal band with your fingertips until the mask fits comfortably and securely.

Procedure 7

Removing a Surgical Mask

1. Remove gloves, if worn.
2. Wash your hands.
3. Untie the neck tie of the mask (or slip the elastic over your ears, depending on the type of mask worn).
4. Untie the upper tie.
5. Remove the mask by touching only the ties or elastic straps.
6. Discard according to facility policy.
7. Wash your hands.

Procedure 8

Applying Protective Eyewear

1. Wash your hands and apply the mask.
2. Apply the goggles and secure the elastic strap around the back of your head

(Figure 3-14), or apply the face shield. Adjust for comfort.
3. Wash your hands.

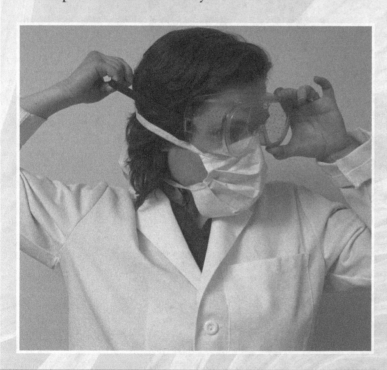

FIGURE 3-14 Holding the goggles with one hand, slip the elastic strap over the back of your head. Adjust the elastic straps on both sides so the goggles fit tightly to your face.

Procedure 9

Removing Protective Eyewear

1. Remove your gloves and wash your hands.
2. Lift the protective goggles or face shield away from your face.
3. Remove your mask.
4. Wash your hands.

Handling Needles and Sharps

Needle and sharp precautions are also used for all care. Handle needles, razors, and other sharp objects with care. Never cut, bend, break, or recap needles by hand. Always wear gloves when shaving patients with a disposable (nonelectric) razor, because of the high risk of contact with blood. The care plan will state special shaving measures to take for patients who are using blood-thinning medications, such as shaving with an electric razor only. Patients who are on blood thinners may bleed profusely from even a tiny cut.

Discard sharp objects in a puncture-resistant container. Avoid overfilling the sharps container. Close the cap when it is two-thirds to three-quarters full. The cap is designed so it cannot be snapped back off after it is closed. The sealed container is stored until it can be picked up with the biohazardous waste.

Accidental Exposure to Blood or Body Fluids

Accidental exposure to infectious blood or body fluids can be serious. If you accidentally contact blood or body fluids, secretions, or excretions with your skin, wash the area thoroughly as soon as possible. Your risk of contracting an infection increases if you have accidental mucous membrane or nonintact skin contact with blood, body fluids, secretions, or excretions. Wash the area thoroughly with soap and water. Flush mucous membranes well with water. Report the exposure incident to your supervisor. Your employer has policies and procedures for managing certain exposure incidents.

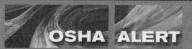

OSHA ALERT

Health care facilities are required to have an exposure control plan that describes what to do if you contact blood or body fluid. Immediately wash the area well. If something splashes into your eyes, flush them well with clear water. Report accidental contact with blood or body fluid to the RN immediately. You will be treated according to the established plan, have blood samples taken, and may begin drug therapy to prevent a bloodborne disease. Medical care and monitoring may continue over a long period of time.

ISOLATION MEASURES

Isolation measures are used when a pathogen is present in a patient. Isolation is used to prevent others from contracting the disease. Patients are also isolated to prevent them from contracting pathogens from others and from the environment.

When caring for a patient in isolation, remember that you are isolating the pathogen and not the person. Isolation can be very difficult for a patient emotionally. This is particularly true of the elderly. Pediatric patients will probably not understand the purpose of isolation. Many patients may feel unclean, unwanted, and untouchable. They may not like being confined to the room and separated from others. Some patients become depressed. Staff and visitors must wear personal protective equipment when they are in the room. Sometimes this is upsetting or frightening to the patient. Staff may not visit often because of the time needed for and difficulty of applying and removing the garments. This, too, can be difficult for the patient. A child may believe that he or she did something bad to cause the sickness. Children may also view isolation as punishment. Teach the patient about the purpose of the isolation. The least amount of isolation possible to contain the pathogen is used. Using extra precautions beyond those required to prevent the spread of disease is unnecessary. Check on patients in isolation frequently, and answer call signals promptly.

Transmission-Based Precautions

The **Centers for Disease Control and Prevention (CDC)** is a governmental agency that studies infectious diseases and makes recommendations to prevent their spread. The CDC recommends three types of **transmission-based precautions.** Standard precautions are used in addition to transmission-based precautions. The type of precautions is selected by the nurse manager, infection control nurse, and physician according to how the disease is spread. Transmission-based precautions are used because ordinary cleanliness and standard precautions may not prevent the spread of certain pathogens. A private room is used to confine the pathogen to the patient's unit. In certain situations, patients with the same disease may share a room.

Airborne Precautions. Airborne precautions (Figure 3-15) are used for patients whose disease is spread by the airborne method of transmission. The pathogen involved is very tiny and lightweight. It can be suspended on dust and moisture in the air and can travel for long distances in the ventilation system. Because of the mode of transmission, special precautions are used to contain the microbe. A private room is necessary. This room must have a special ventilation system. In a normal health care facility room, the air is forced downward from the ventilation system. In an airborne precautions room, the ventilation is reversed so that room air is

AIRBORNE PRECAUTIONS
(in addition to Standard Precautions)

VISITORS: Report to nurse before entering.

Patient Placement
Use **private room** that has:
Monitored negative air pressure,
6 to 12 air changes per hour,
Discharge of air outdoors or HEPA filtration if
recirculated.
Keep room door closed and patient in room.

Respiratory Protection
Wear an N95 respirator when entering the room of a
patient with known or suspected infectious pulmonary
tuberculosis.
Susceptible persons should not enter the room of
patients known or suspected to have **measles** (rubeola)
or **varicella** (chickenpox) if other immune caregivers are
available. If susceptible persons must enter, they should
wear an **N95 respirator.** (Respirator or surgical mask
not required if immune to measles and varicella.)

Patient Transport
Limit transport of patient from room to essential purposes
only. Use **surgical mask** on patient during transport.

FIGURE 3-15 Airborne precautions. (Courtesy of BREVIS Corporation, Salt Lake City, UT)

drawn upward into the vents. This creates a **negative pressure environment.** The ventilation is specially filtered or exhausted directly to the outside of the building. This room has 6 to 12 complete changes of air per hour. The door to the room is always kept closed. These precautions prevent the pathogen from escaping into the rest of the facility.

Some facilities do not have the special ventilation required for airborne precautions rooms. These facilities use portable units that are placed in the room to filter the air, creating a negative pressure environment. They are slightly noisier than the ventilation system, but are effective in eliminating the pathogen.

Staff entering the room must wear a special mask called a **high efficiency particulate air (HEPA) respirator** (Figure 3-16). This mask has very small pores that prevent the tiny pathogen from entering. The mask must be fit-tested by a qualified professional to be sure it fits the employee properly and does not leak. After fit-testing, you must also have a medical exam to be sure that wearing the HEPA mask is not dangerous to your health. Some individuals have underlying diseases that make working in the mask difficult or impossible. The medical examination is done to learn whether using the mask is safe for the worker. You must check for air leaks each time you apply the mask. Men with facial hair cannot wear

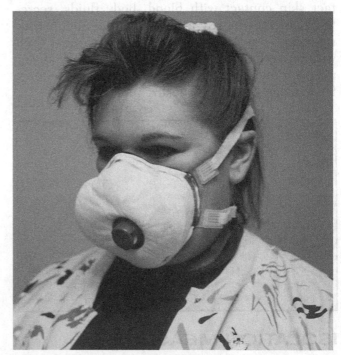

FIGURE 3-16 The HEPA respirator is reusable. Store it according to facility policy.

the HEPA mask because the facial hair causes air leaks. Special hoods can be worn instead of the mask. Facilities may select only certain employees to work

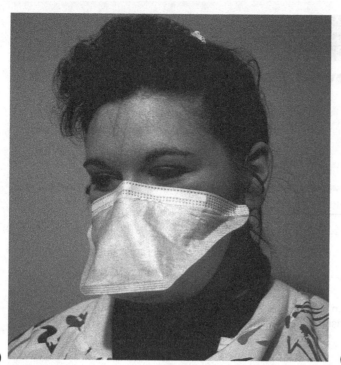

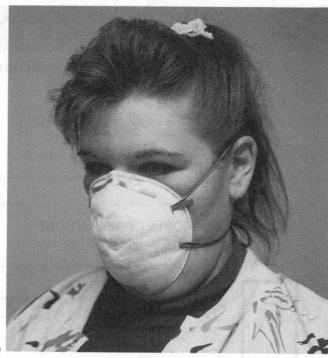

(A) **(B)**

FIGURE 3-17 (A) The PFR95 respirator is preferred by many health care workers because it is lightweight and comfortable. (B) The N95 respirator is disposable. In some facilities, personnel store it in a plastic bag and reuse it for one shift, then discard the mask at the end of the shift. Follow your facility policy.

in rooms where airborne precautions are used. Fit-testing and medical examinations are costly, and some facilities save money and limit worker exposure by designating only certain employees to work in airborne precautions. No other personal protective equipment is necessary unless it is needed to apply the principles of standard precautions.

The HEPA mask is not the only mask that can be used in an isolation room. Masks that are worn in airborne precautions rooms must be approved

by the **National Institute of Occupational Safety and Health (NIOSH)**. The **PFR95 respirator (Figure 3-17A)** or **N95 respirator (Figure 3-17B)** are approved alternatives. Some workers prefer these masks because they are lighter in weight and more comfortable to wear. Like the HEPA mask, there are fit-testing and health examination requirements. These masks are also tested for air leaks by the worker each time they are worn.

Procedure 10

Applying a NIOSH-Approved Respirator

1. Wash your hands.
2. Cup the mask upright in your hand, with the nosepiece in your fingertips. Allow the elastic straps to hang freely.
3. Position the mask under your chin. The nosepiece should be over the bridge of your nose.
4. Pull the upper elastic strap over the top of your head until it rests high on the back of your head.
5. Pull the bottom strap over your head. Position the strap low on the back of your head, below the ears.

6. Push the nosepiece inward with both hands, molding it to the shape of your nose. Next, push inward on the nosepiece with your fingertips so it fits securely.
7. Check the fit by placing both hands completely over the mask. Exhale. If you feel an air leak by the nose, repeat step 6. If air leaks around the edges of the mask, readjust the straps at the back of the head. Continue to check the fit and readjust until there are no air leaks.
8. Wash your hands.

Procedure 11

Removing a NIOSH-Approved Respirator

1. Wash your hands.
2. Cup the respirator in your nondominant hand.
3. Pull the lower strap up over your head.

4. Pull the upper strap up over your head.
5. Remove the respirator from your face and discard or store according to facility policy.
6. Wash your hands.

DROPLET PRECAUTIONS
(in addition to Standard Precautions)

VISITORS: Report to nurse before entering.

Patient Placement
Private room, if possible. Cohort or maintain spatial separation of **3 feet** from other patients or visitors if private room is not available.

Mask
Wear mask when working within **3 feet** of patient (or upon entering room).

Patient Transport
Limit transport of patient from room to essential purposes only. Use **surgical mask** on patient during transport.

FIGURE 3-18 Droplet precautions. (Courtesy of BREVIS Corporation, Salt Lake City, UT)

Droplet Precautions. Droplet precautions (**Figure 3-18**) are used for some patients whose infection is spread in the air. An example of a disease for which droplet precautions are used is influenza. The pathogen is spread by the droplets in mucus from oral, nasal, and respiratory secretions. The droplets usually remain within three feet of the patient. The secretions containing the pathogen are too large and heavy to be carried in air currents. A private room is necessary, but special ventilation is not used. Regular surgical masks are worn. The pathogen is too large to fit between the pores of the surgical mask. The door to the room can be left open, if this is the patient's preference. No other personal protective equipment is necessary unless it is needed to practice standard precautions.

Contact Precautions. Contact precautions (**Figure 3-19**) are used to contain pathogens that are spread by direct or indirect contact. The microbes that spread the disease or infection in patients in contact precautions are usually found in infections of the skin, urine, and fecal material. Apply gloves whenever you enter the room. No other personal protective equipment is necessary unless you anticipate having direct contact with the patient, linen, or environmental surfaces. Apply a gown when contact is expected. Standard precautions are used in addition to contact precautions.

Special Circumstances. Patients may have infections that are transmitted by more than one method. A patient may have an infection, such as a cold, that is spread by the droplet method. The patient may also have a separate infection of the skin. Some diseases are spread by more than one method. In this case, two types of isolation are used in addition to standard precautions.

CONTACT PRECAUTIONS
(in addition to Standard Precautions)
VISITORS: Report to nurse before entering.

Patient Placement
Private room, if possible. Cohort if private room is not available.

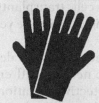

Gloves
Wear gloves when entering patient room.
Change gloves after having contact with infective material that may contain high concentrations of microorganisms (**fecal** material and **wound drainage**). Remove gloves before leaving patient room.

Wash
Wash hands with an **antimicrobial** agent immediately after glove removal. After glove removal and handwashing, ensure that hands do not touch potentially contaminated environmental surfaces or items in the patient's room to avoid transfer of microorganisms to other patients or environments.

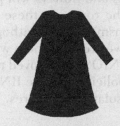

Gown
Wear gown when **entering** patient room if you anticipate that your clothing will have substantial contact with the patient, environmental surfaces, or items in the patient's room, or if the patient is **incontinent**, has **diarrhea**, an **ileostomy**, a **colostomy**, or **wound drainage** not contained by a dressing. **Remove** gown before leaving the patient's environment and ensure that clothing does not contact potentially contaminated environmental surfaces to avoid transfer of microorganisms to other patients or environments.

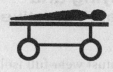

Patient Transport
Limit transport of patient to essential purposes only. During transport, ensure that precautions are maintained to minimize the risk of transmission of microorganisms to other patients and contamination of environmental surfaces and equipment.

Patient-Care Equipment
Dedicate the use of noncritical patient-care equipment to a single patient. If common equipment is used, clean and disinfect between patients.

FIGURE 3-19 Contact precautions. (Courtesy of BREVIS Corporation, Salt Lake City, UT)

Identifying Patients in Isolation. Most facilities post signs on the door to the room when a patient is in isolation. The sign provides directions on personal protective equipment to wear and describes precautions to take. Some facilities feel that posting signs on the door of the patient's room is an invasion of privacy. These facilities usually post a stop sign on the door that advises you to check with the RN before entering the room.

Expanded Precautions

At the time of this writing, the CDC is revising new isolation recommendations called *expanded precautions*.[1] Your facility will teach you how to use the ex-

[1]Draft CDC guideline for isolation precautions: Preventing transmission of infectious agents in healthcare settings 2004. (2004). Retrieved August 27, 2005, from http://www.cdc.gov/ncidod/hip/isoguide.htm

panded precautions when they are finalized and published. The new CDC precautions are needed because of the introduction of a new, serious disease called severe acute respiratory distress syndrome (SARS), and the spread of avian influenza (bird flu). The guidelines describe "Expanded Precautions," which place more emphasis on proper application and removal of PPE than previous guidelines. The CDC notes,

> There are two tiers of transmission precautions, Standard Precautions and Expanded Precautions. Standard Precautions are intended to be applied to the care of all patients in all health care settings, regardless of the suspected or confirmed presence of an infectious agent. *Standard Precautions* constitute the primary strategy for successful prevention of healthcare-associated transmission of infection among patients and personnel. Expanded Precautions are for patients who are known or suspected to be infected with important pathogens that require additional control measures to prevent transmission. More than one category may be used for diseases that have multiple routes of transmission (e.g., SARS). When used either singularly or in combination, they are always to be used in addition to Standard Precautions.

Protective Isolation

Normally, isolation measures and precautions are used when a pathogen is present in a patient. The purpose of isolation is to prevent the spread of disease to others. Years ago, the CDC had an additional isolation category called *protective isolation*. Some workers called this category *reverse isolation*. When standard precautions were first introduced, the CDC eliminated this isolation category, believing that standard precautions protected the patients who were formerly placed in protective isolation.

Patients with diseases of the immune system were frequently housed in reverse or protective isolation. These patients did not have any contagious diseases. Because of their immune system weakness, though, they could readily contract diseases. The isolation measures are used to prevent these patients from contracting pathogens from others and from the environment. Patients with other conditions, such as transplant patients, those with severe burns, and patients receiving cancer treatment, may also be placed in protective isolation. Many hospitals have retained the protective isolation category, so you must be familiar with it. The new expanded precautions list a "Protective Equipment" category for patients who have had stem cell transplants. The protective equipment precautions listed are very similar to reverse isolation.

The reverse isolation precautions are designed to meet the patient's specific needs. Staff entering the room of patients in protective isolation must put on protective garments. A gown and gloves are standard. A mask may also be required. Some patients in reverse isolation require special negative pressure rooms like those used for patients with tuberculosis. If this type of room is necessary, the door must be kept closed at all times, except when entering and leaving. Plants and flowers will probably not be permitted in the room, as these have been implicated in the transmission of pathogens. A patient leaving the negative pressure room will be required to wear a mask or NIOSH-approved respirator. Follow your facility policies and the RN's instructions in maintaining isolation measures.

Sequence for Applying and Removing Personal Protective Equipment

There are times when you must wear full isolation garments in a patient's room. If you will be using your watch in the room, you should remove it first and place it on a clean paper towel. You will carry the watch on the towel. The sequence in which you apply and remove your personal protective equipment is important. Follow the guidelines listed here.

Guidelines for Putting on Personal Protective Equipment

1. Wash your hands.
2. Put on the isolation gown (Figure 3–20).
3. Put on the isolation mask.

4. Apply goggles or face shield, if needed.
5. Put on the isolation gloves.

SEQUENCE FOR DONNING PERSONAL PROTECTIVE EQUIPMENT (PPE)

The type of PPE used will vary based on the level of precautions required; e.g., Standard and Contact, Droplet or Airborne Infection Isolation.

1. GOWN
- Fully cover torso from neck to knees, arms to end of wrists, and wrap around the back
- Fasten in back of neck and waist

2. MASK OR RESPIRATOR
- Secure ties or elastic bands at middle of head and neck
- Fit flexible band to nose bridge
- Fit snug to face and below chin
- Fit-check respirator

3. GOGGLES OR FACE SHIELD
- Place over face and eyes and adjust to fit

4. GLOVES
- Extend to cover wrist of isolation gown

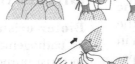
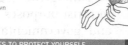

USE SAFE WORK PRACTICES TO PROTECT YOURSELF AND LIMIT THE SPREAD OF CONTAMINATION

- Keep hands away from face
- Limit surfaces touched
- Change gloves when torn or heavily contaminated
- Perform hand hygiene

SECUENCIA PARA PONERSE EL EQUIPO DE PROTECCIÓN PERSONAL (PPE)

El tipo de PPE que se debe utilizar depende del nivel de precaución que sea necesario; por ejemplo, equipo Estándar y de Contacto o de Aislamiento de infecciones transportadas por gotas o por aire.

1. BATA
- Cubra con la bata todo el torso desde el cuello hasta las rodillas, los brazos hasta la muñeca y dóblela alrededor de la espalda
- Átesela por detrás a la altura del cuello y la cintura

2. MÁSCARA O RESPIRADOR
- Asegúrese los cordones o la banda elástica en la mitad de la cabeza y en el cuello
- Ajústese la banda flexible en el puente de la nariz
- Acomódesela en la cara y por debajo del mentón
- Verifique el ajuste del respirador

3. GAFAS PROTECTORAS O CARETAS
- Colóquesela sobre la cara y los ojos y ajústela

4. GUANTES
- Extienda los guantes para que cubran la parte del puño en la bata de aislamiento

UTILICE PRÁCTICAS DE TRABAJO SEGURAS PARA PROTEGERSE USTED MISMO Y LIMITAR LA PROPAGACIÓN DE LA CONTAMINACIÓN

- Mantenga las manos alejadas de la cara
- Limite el contacto con superficies
- Cambie los guantes si se rompen o están demasiado contaminados
- Realice la higiene de las manos

SEQUENCE FOR REMOVING PERSONAL PROTECTIVE EQUIPMENT (PPE)

Except for respirator, remove PPE at doorway or in anteroom. Remove respirator after leaving patient room and closing door.

1. GLOVES
- Outside of gloves is contaminated!
- Grasp outside of glove with opposite gloved hand; peel off
- Hold removed glove in gloved hand
- Slide fingers of ungloved hand under remaining glove at wrist
- Peel glove off over first glove
- Discard gloves in waste container

2. GOGGLES OR FACE SHIELD
- Outside of goggles or face shield is contaminated!
- To remove, handle by head band or ear pieces
- Place in designated receptacle for reprocessing or in waste container

3. GOWN
- Gown front and sleeves are contaminated!
- Unfasten ties
- Pull away from neck and shoulders, touching inside of gown only
- Turn gown inside out
- Fold or roll into a bundle and discard

4. MASK OR RESPIRATOR
- Front of mask/respirator is contaminated — DO NOT TOUCH!
- Grasp bottom, then top ties or elastics and remove
- Discard in waste container

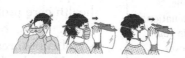
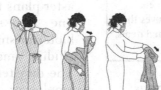
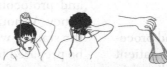

PERFORM HAND HYGIENE IMMEDIATELY AFTER REMOVING ALL PPE

SECUENCIA PARA QUITARSE EL EQUIPO DE PROTECCIÓN PERSONAL (PPE)

Con la excepción del respirador, quítese el PPE en la entrada de la puerta o en la antesala. Quítese el respirador después de salir de la habitación del paciente y de cerrar la puerta.

1. GUANTES
- ¡El exterior de los guantes está contaminado!
- Agarre la parte exterior del guante con la mano opuesta en la que todavía tiene puesto el guante y quíteselo
- Sostenga el guante que se quitó con la mano enguantada
- Deslice los dedos de la mano sin guante por debajo del otro guante que no se ha quitado todavía a la altura de la muñeca
- Quítese el guante de manera que acabe cubriendo el primer guante
- Arroje los guantes en el recipiente de deshechos

2. GAFAS PROTECTORAS O CARETA
- ¡El exterior de las gafas protectoras o de la careta está contaminado!
- Para quitárselas, tómelas por la parte de la banda de la cabeza o de las piezas de las orejas
- Colóquelas en el recipiente designado para reprocesar materiales o de materiales de deshecho

3. BATA
- ¡La parte delantera de la bata y las mangas están contaminadas!
- Desate los cordones
- Tocando solamente el interior de la bata, pásela por encima del cuello y de los hombros
- Voltee la bata al revés
- Dóblela o enróllela y deséchela

4. MÁSCARA O RESPIRADOR
- La parte delantera de la máscara o respirador está contaminada — ¡NO LA TOQUE!
- Primero agarre la parte de abajo, luego los cordones o banda elástica de arriba y por último quítese la máscara o respirador
- Arrójela en el recipiente de deshechos

EFECTÚE LA HIGIENE DE LAS MANOS INMEDIATAMENTE DESPUÉS DE QUITARSE CUALQUIER EQUIPO DE PROTECCIÓN PERSONAL

FIGURE 3-20 Sequence for applying and removing personal protective equipment. (Courtesy of Centers for Disease Control and Prevention. Atlanta, GA)

Guidelines for Removing Personal Protective Equipment

1. Untie the front waist tie of the isolation gown.
2. Remove your gloves.
3. Remove protective eyewear, if worn.

4. Untie the neck tie of the gown and remove the gown.
5. Remove your mask.
6. Wash your hands.

Exiting the Isolation Room. If you used your watch in the isolation room, pick it up after removing your protective equipment and put it on your wrist. Pick up the towel, holding the clean upper side, and discard it in the trash. Obtain a clean paper towel from the dispenser and use it to open the door of the room. After the door is open, discard the towel inside the room. The door may be left open in contact and droplet precautions if this is the patient's preference. It is a good idea to wash your hands again after leaving the room.

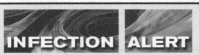

INFECTION ALERT

Make sure clean and soiled items are separated in patient rooms and storage areas. Keep the lids tightly closed on trash cans and linen hampers. Avoid throwing biohazard contaminated trash into open wastebaskets. When two or more patients share a room, make sure that all personal care items are labeled with each patient's name. Store personal items in the appropriate area. Store grooming supplies in a clean area. Avoid community areas such as bathrooms that increase the risk that personal care equipment and supplies will be used for the wrong patient(s). Wear gloves when removing bed linen that is wet or soiled. Place the soiled linen in a plastic bag or linen hamper. Follow facility policy for disinfecting the mattress. Allow it to dry. Cracks in the mattress are a potential source of odors and contamination. Report cracks in the mattress to the proper person in your facility. Discard your gloves and wash your hands. Never handle clean linen while wearing contaminated gloves. Wearing gloves is not necessary for handling clean linen. Avoid contaminating environmental surfaces with gloves that have handled soiled linen, trash, or other contaminated items. Remove one glove, if necessary.

BEGINNING AND ENDING PROCEDURE ACTIONS

Review the beginning procedure actions and procedure completion actions from your basic patient care or nursing assistant class. These are listed in the inside covers of this text for your convenience. Beginning actions are listed in **Table 3-1.** Comple-

tion actions are listed in **Table 3-2.** These steps are important, and are appropriate for all of the patient care procedures in this text.

BIOTERRORISM

Bioterrorism is the use of biological agents, such as pathogenic organisms or agricultural pests, for terrorist purposes. Since October 2001, state, local, and governmental public health authorities have been investigating cases of bioterrorism-related illness in the United States. Some individuals died of inhalation anthrax, a condition that was spread by a powdery substance sent through the mail. A number of other individuals developed the cutaneous (skin) version of this disease. Cutaneous anthrax is not fatal. Anthrax cannot be passed from person to person. It is transmitted only through contact with spores. In this case, the spores were spread in the powder. Fortunately, the number of workplaces and individuals contaminated was small, but it raised concerns regarding future terrorist attacks. Many individuals could be infected by a biological weapon before the exposure is detected and diagnosed. Some of the diseases that can potentially be used as biological weapons have been eradicated for years and today's health care professionals have never seen or treated them. Thus, bioterrorism potentially represents a significant threat.

Many health care facilities have developed disaster plans to address bioterrorism. The plans outline the steps necessary for responding to bioterrorism with the most common agents, including smallpox, botulism, anthrax, and plague. The disaster plan covers information for patients, employees, visitors, and public health precautions and protocols to follow in the event of an emergency. Although this need is a sad commentary on the state of world affairs, health care facilities must be prepared for potential terrorist actions in the future. Your facility will identify your role and responsibilities in such an emergency, and may conduct regular drills for emergency readiness.

Table 3-1 Beginning Procedure Actions

Beginning Procedure Action	Rationale
1. Wash your hands or use an alcohol-based hand cleaner.	Applies the principles of standard precautions. Prevents the spread of microbes and reduces the risk of cross-contamination.
2. Assemble equipment and take to the patient's room.	Improves efficiency of the procedure. Ensures that you do not have to leave the room.
3. Knock on the patient's door and identify yourself by name and title.	Respects the patient's right to privacy. Notifies the patient who is giving care.
4. Identify the patient by checking the identification bracelet.	Ensures that you are caring for the correct patient.
5. Ask visitors to leave the room and advise them where they may wait.	Respects the patient's right to privacy. Shows hospitality to visitors by advising them where to wait.
6. Explain what you are going to do and how the patient can assist. Answer questions about the procedure.	Informs the patient of what is going to be done and what is expected. Gives the patient an opportunity to get information about the procedure and the extent of patient participation.
7. Provide privacy by closing the door, privacy curtain, and window curtain.	Respects the patient's right to privacy. All three should be closed even if the patient is alone in the room.
8. Wash your hands or use an alcohol-based hand cleaner.	Applies the principles of standard precautions. Prevents the spread of microorganisms.
9. Set up the equipment for the procedure at the bedside. Open trays and packages. Position items in a location for convenient reach. Avoid positioning a container for soiled items in a manner that requires crossing over clean items to access it.	Prepares for the procedure. Ensures that equipment and supplies are conveniently positioned and readily available. Reduces the risk of cross-contamination.
10. Raise the bed to a comfortable working height.	Prevents back strain and injury caused by bending at the waist.
11. Position the patient for the procedure. Ask an assistant to help, if necessary, or support the patient with pillows and props. Make sure the patient is comfortable and can maintain the position throughout the procedure. Drape the patient with a bath blanket for modesty.	Ensures that the patient is in the correct position for the procedure. Ensures that the patient is supported and can maintain the position without discomfort. Respects the patient's modesty and dignity.
12. Apply a gown if your uniform will have substantial contact with linen or other articles contaminated with blood, moist body fluid (except sweat), secretions, or excretions.	Applies the principles of standard precautions. Protects your uniform from contamination with bloodborne pathogens.

(continues)

Table 3-1 Beginning Procedure Actions (Continued)

Beginning Procedure Action	Rationale
13. Apply a mask and eye protection if splashing of blood or moist body fluid is likely.	Applies the principles of standard precautions. Protects the nursing assistant's mucous membranes, uniform, and skin from accidental splashing of bloodborne pathogens.
14. Apply gloves if contact with blood, moist body fluids (except sweat), secretions, excretions, or nonintact skin is likely.	Applies the principles of standard precautions. Protects the nursing assistant and the patient from transmission of pathogens.
15. Lower the side rail on the side where you are working.	Provides an obstacle-free area in which to work.

Table 3-2 Procedure Completion Actions

Procedure Completion Action	Rationale
1. Check to make sure the patient is comfortable and in good alignment.	All body systems function better when the body is correctly aligned. The patient is more comfortable when the body is in good alignment.
2. Remove gloves.	Prevents contamination of environmental surfaces from the gloves.
3. Replace the bed covers, then remove and discard any drapes used.	Provides warmth and security.
4. Elevate the side rails, if used, before leaving the bedside.	Prevents contamination of the side rail from used gloves. Supports the patient's right to a safe environment. Prevents accidents and injuries.
5. Remove other personal protective equipment, if worn, and discard according to facility policy.	Prevents unnecessary environmental contamination from used gloves and protective equipment.
6. Wash your hands or use alcohol-based hand cleaner.	Applies the principles of standard precautions. Prevents the spread of microorganisms.
7. Return the bed to the lowest horizontal position.	Supports the patient's right to a safe environment. Prevents accidents and injuries.
8. Open the privacy and window curtains.	Privacy is no longer necessary unless preferred by the patient.
9. Leave the patient in a position of comfort and safety, with the call signal and needed personal items within reach.	Prevents accidents and injuries. Ensures that help is available. Eliminates the need to call or reach for needed personal items.

(continues)

Table 3-2 Procedure Completion Actions (Continued)

Procedure Completion Action	Rationale
10. Wash your hands or use an alcohol-based cleaner.	Although the hands were washed previously, they have contacted the patient and other items in the room. Wash them again before leaving to prevent potential transfer of microorganisms to areas outside the patient's unit.
11. Remove procedural trash and contaminated linen when you leave the room. Discard in appropriate container or location, according to facility policy.	Prevents the spread of microbes and reduces the risk of cross-contamination. (Although the hands were washed previously, they have contacted the patient and other items in the room. Wash them again before leaving to prevent potential transfer of microbes to other patients, equipment, and surfaces outside the patient's unit.)
12. Inform visitors that they may return to the room.	Shows courtesy to visitors and the patient.
13. Report completion of the procedure and any abnormalities or other observations.	Informs the supervisor that your assigned task has been completed so further care can be planned and you can be reassigned to other duties. Notifies the licensed nurse of abnormalities and changes in the patient's condition for further assessment.
14. Document the procedure and your observations.	Ongoing progress and care given are documented. Provides a legal record. Provides a record of what has been done for other members of the interdisciplinary team.

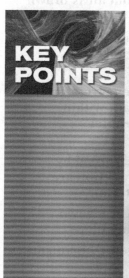

KEY POINTS

▶ Infections are spread by direct contact and indirect contact; in the air by the airborne and droplet methods; by common vehicles; and by vectors.

▶ The chain of infection describes six factors necessary for an infection to develop. Breaking any link in the chain will prevent an infection from developing.

▶ The causative agent is the germ that causes disease.

▶ The source or reservoir is the place where the pathogen can grow.

▶ The susceptible host is the person who can become infected by pathogen exposure.

▶ A carrier is a person who is infected with a disease that can be spread to others. He or she may not know of the infection.

▶ The mode of transmission is the method by which the disease is spread.

▶ The portal of entry is the place where the microbe enters the body.

(continues)

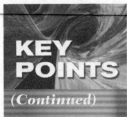

KEY POINTS

(Continued)

▶ The portal of exit is secretions, excretions, or droplets in which the pathogens travel when they leave the body.

▶ Handwashing is the most important method used to prevent the spread of infection. Because infection is readily spread on the hands, PCTs must wash their hands frequently when on duty.

▶ An alcohol-based waterless hand cleaner may be used instead of routine handwashing except when the hands are visibly soiled, or the patient has a condition that is known to be spread by spores, such as *Clostridium difficile* or *Bacillus anthracis*.

▶ Spores are microscopic reproductive bodies that remain dormant until conditions are ideal for reproduction. The spores will then multiply and continue to spread infection. Alcohol-based hand cleaners will not eliminate spores.

▶ Standard precautions are used in the care of all patients, regardless of disease or diagnosis, to prevent the spread of infection.

▶ Standard precautions are used anytime you anticipate contact with blood or any moist body fluid (except sweat), secretions, or excretions. They are also used during contact with mucous membranes and nonintact skin.

▶ Personal protective equipment will protect you only if it fits properly, if it is free from defects, and if you use it regularly and correctly.

▶ Isolation measures are used when a pathogen is present in a patient. Isolation is used to prevent others from contracting the disease.

▶ Transmission-based precautions are used for isolation because ordinary cleanliness and standard precautions may not prevent the spread of certain pathogens.

▶ Standard precautions are always used in addition to transmission-based precautions.

▶ Airborne precautions are used for patients whose disease is spread by the airborne method of transmission. The pathogen involved is very tiny and lightweight. It can be suspended on dust and moisture in the air and travel for long distances in the ventilation system.

▶ A negative pressure environment is used in an airborne precautions room. In this type of system, the ventilation is reversed so that room air is drawn upward into the vents.

▶ A NIOSH-approved respirator is used by staff working in an airborne precautions room. Special fit-testing and medical examination requirements apply to use of this type of respirator.

▶ The pathogen involved in droplet infection is spread in mucus from oral, nasal, and respiratory secretions. The droplets usually remain within three feet of the patient. Personnel caring for patients in droplet precautions wear a surgical mask.

▶ Contact precautions are used to contain pathogens that are spread by direct or indirect contact. The pathogens that spread the infection are usually found in infections of the skin, urine, and fecal material.

▶ Wear gloves when entering a contact precautions room. Wear a gown when directly contacting the patient, bed linen, or environment.

▶ Bioterrorism is the use of biological agents, such as pathogenic organisms or agricultural pests, for terrorist purposes.

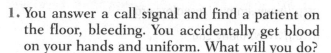

CLINICAL APPLICATIONS

1. You answer a call signal and find a patient on the floor, bleeding. You accidentally get blood on your hands and uniform. What will you do?

2. You are assigned to provide incontinent care for a patient who is in airborne precautions. What personal protective equipment will you wear?

3. An incontinent patient on your unit is moved into a contact precautions room for a urinary infection. You have cared for this patient and are worried that you have been exposed to the pathogen. Based on your knowledge of the chain of infection and standard precautions, list some routine practices that you should use to protect yourself when caring for an incontinent patient when you do not know that the patient has an infection.

4. You are bathing a dependent patient. She has old bruises and open skin tears on her arms. Will you wear personal protective equipment when washing her arms? If so, what? When will you put it on? When will you remove it?

5. You are caring for an incontinent patient. Your gloves become heavily soiled with excretions. The side rail on the bed is down, and the patient cannot be left alone. What will you do?

CHAPTER REVIEW

Multiple-Choice Questions

Select the one best answer.

1. Susan sneezes, covering her nose and mouth with her hands. A minute later, she shakes hands with Harold. An infection that is spread by shaking hands is spread by the:
   a. droplet method.
   b. indirect contact method.
   c. direct contact method.
   d. airborne method.

2. Many people become ill with a type of food poisoning called salmonella. Food poisoning is spread by the:
   a. indirect contact method.
   b. fomite method.
   c. direct contact method.
   d. common vehicle method.

3. Karen has hepatitis B, but doesn't know of the infection. She:
   a. can transmit the infection to others.
   b. cannot transmit the infection to others.
   c. is more susceptible to colds.
   d. probably shows signs of serious illness.

4. The germ that causes disease is the:
   a. host.   c. reservoir.
   b. causative agent. d. portal of exit.

5. Before caring for a patient, wash your hands for a minimum of:
   a. 2 to 3 seconds.   c. 15 seconds.
   b. 5 seconds.   d. 60 seconds.

6. When caring for a patient with AIDS, always use:
   a. contact precautions.
   b. droplet precautions.
   c. airborne precautions.
   d. standard precautions.

7. Change your gloves before:
   a. leaving each patient's room.
   b. touching mucous membranes.
   c. touching intact skin.
   d. washing your hands.

8. You are asked to assist with a procedure. The RN tells you that secretions may splash into the air during this procedure. You will wear:
   a. a face shield and mask.
   b. eye goggles.
   c. a HEPA respirator.
   d. a mask only.

9. You are entering a room in which contact and airborne precautions are being used. Which protective garment will you put on first?
   a. Gloves   c. Gown
   b. Mask   d. Eye shield

10. After caring for a patient in isolation, which will you do first?
   a. Remove the gloves
   b. Put your watch on your wrist
   c. Wash your hands
   d. Remove the mask

EXPLORING THE WEB

100% Immunization Campaign	http://www.immunizeseniors.org
All the Virology on the WWW	http://www.tulane.edu
American Academy of Pediatrics, Head Lice in Children	http://www.medem.com
Association of Professionals in Infection Control (APIC)	http://www.apic.org
Bad Bug Book	http://vm.cfsan.fda.gov
Care Tech Labs	http://www.caretechlabs.com
Categories of Acquired Immunity	http://www.wisc-online.com
Caught Dirty Handed	http://www.microbe.org
CDC Evolution of Isolation Practices	http://www.cdc.gov
CDC Guidelines and Recommendations	http://www.cdc.gov
CDC Guidelines for Handwashing	http://www.cdc.gov
CDC Guidelines for Long Term Care	http://www.cdc.gov
CDC Issues in Healthcare Settings	http://www.cdc.gov
CDC National Prevention Information Network	http://www.cdcnpin.org
Centers for Disease Control and Prevention (CDC)	http://www.cdc.gov
Clean Hands Campaign	http://www.washup.org
Doctor Fungus	http://www.doctorfungus.org
Gastrointestinal Viruses	http://www.ncsu.edu/student_health
GloGerm	http://www.glogerm.com
Guidelines for Control of MRSA	http://goapic.org/MRSA.htm
Guideline for Handwashing and Hospital Environmental Control	http://www.cdc.gov
Guideline for Isolation Precautions in Hospitals	http://www.cdc.gov
Guidelines for Prevention of Tuberculosis in Healthcare Settings	http://www.cdc.gov
Hand Hygiene Resource Center	http://handhygiene.org
Henry the Hand	http://www.henrythehand.com
Hepatitis Neighborhood	http://www.hepatitisneighborhood.com
Herpes Web	http://www.herpesweb.net
Hopisafe	http://www.hopisafe.ch/next.html
Hidden Killers: Deadly Viruses	http://library.advanced.org
HIV InSite	http://hivinsite.ucsf.edu
Infectious Diseases Syllabi	http://www.kcom.edu

National Foundation of Infectious Diseases	http://www.nfid.org
National Institutes of Health (NIH)	http://health.nih.gov
National Pediculosis Association	http://www.headlice.org
National Tuberculosis Center	http://www.umdnj.edu
OSHA Bloodborne Pathogen Fact Sheets	http://www.osha.gov
Overview of the Seven CDC Guidelines on Prevention of Healthcare Associated Infections	http://www.cdc.gov
A Primer on Bioterrorism	http://www.advancefornurses.com
Recommendations for Immunization of Health Care Workers	http://www.cdc.gov
Supercourse	http://www.pitt.edu
Walter Reed Hospital Infection Control Manual Policies and Procedures	http://www.wramc.amedd.army.mil

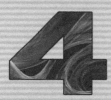

CHAPTER 4

Surgical Asepsis

OBJECTIVES:

After reading this chapter, you should be able to:

● Spell and define key terms.

● Define sterile technique and explain why it is used.

● List the guidelines for sterile procedures.

● Describe the purpose of a sterile field and demonstrate how to establish a sterile field.

● Explain when to use sterile gloves, and describe how to use them without contamination.

STERILE TECHNIQUE

Sterile technique is a microbe-free method used for performing procedures within body cavities and during certain dressing changes. Many procedures in this book require the use of sterile technique. Common nursing procedures in which sterile technique is used are:

● all invasive procedures

● procedures in which the skin is broken, such as injections, and inserting intravenous needles or catheters

● procedures in which body cavities are entered, such as catheterization and tracheal suctioning

● changing surgical dressings

● changing dressings on central intravenous catheters

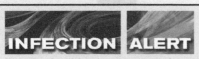

INFECTION ALERT

In some facilities, personnel are instructed to bring extra supplies to the room in case they are needed during a procedure. For example, personnel commonly contaminate sterile gloves, or need extra sterile urinary catheters. Once supplies have been taken into a patient's room, they cannot be returned to stock and used in the care of another patient. Thus, if the sterile supplies are not used, they must be discarded. This is costly, in terms of both replacement supplies and waste disposal. Know and follow your facility policies for bringing extra supplies into patients' rooms in anticipation of need during sterile procedures. Do so only if permitted by facility policy, and obtain directions for how to dispose of unused sterile items.

● procedures involving patients with severe destruction of the skin, such as burns (**Figure 4-1**) and trauma

An item or area is *sterile* if it is free from all microorganisms and spores. Sterile technique may also be called **surgical asepsis.** Only sterile supplies contact the patient's body during sterile procedures. Sterile gloves are worn.

Packaging Sterile Supplies

Many sterile supplies are disposable. These are purchased in sterile packages. Extra items in the package are thrown away at the end of the procedure. Reusable items, such as instruments, may be sterilized in your facility. After sterile items or trays are prepared, they are placed into an **autoclave,** or sterilizer, for a period of time. The heat and steam from the autoclave eliminate all microbes, sterilizing the item. Before sterilizing supplies in an autoclave, the outer wrapper is sealed with special tape. The tape changes color during autoclaving, indicating that the contents of the package are sterile (**Figure 4-2**). Do not use a sterile package unless the outside wrapper is intact. Avoid using it if the outside has become wet. Avoid using the contents if the autoclave tape has not changed color. Many sterile items have dates listed on the package. Avoid using them if it is after the date listed on the package.

Handwashing

Personnel in the operating room have traditionally done a 10-minute scrub, using an antimicrobial

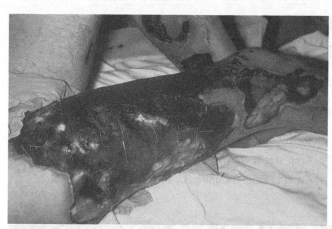

FIGURE 4-1 Sterile technique is always used when caring for patients with serious burns. (Courtesy of Emory University Hospital, Atlanta, GA)

soap and a brush, prior to assisting with a surgical procedure. The 2002 CDC guidelines have modified the recommendations for surgical hand antisepsis. The CDC recommends:

- Removing watches, rings, and jewelry before beginning a surgical hand scrub.
- Using a nail cleaner and running water to remove debris from fingernails.
- When using antimicrobial soap and water, scrub for the length of time recommended by the manufacturer, usually two to six minutes.
- When using an alcohol-based product:
  - Wash hands and forearms well with soap and water.
  - Dry thoroughly.
  - Apply the alcohol-based product to hands and forearms and rub well, according to the product manufacturer's directions. Allow to dry thoroughly before applying sterile gloves.

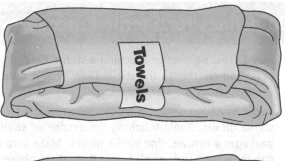

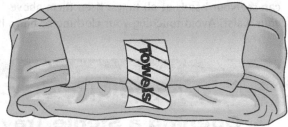

FIGURE 4-2 Package of towels before and after autoclaving. The stripes on the package indicate that it was exposed to a high temperature in the autoclave.

Environmental Conditions

Before using a sterile item or creating a sterile field, check the environment. The surface on which you open the package must be clean, dry, flat, and stable. The area must be free from airborne contamination. Masks are worn during some sterile procedures. Follow the guidelines in Procedure 6 for applying the mask. In some procedures, the patient also wears a mask. In others, a mask is not necessary. Check with the RN if you are not sure whether to wear a mask.

Patients can accidentally contaminate sterile supplies and trays. Explain the procedure to the patient before beginning. Instruct him or her to avoid touching sterile supplies, crossing over the sterile field, or talking, coughing, or sneezing over sterile articles. Reinforce and remind the patient during the procedure, as necessary.

Guidelines for Sterile Procedures

- Always wash your hands or use an alcohol-based cleanser before beginning a sterile procedure.
- If the sterility of an item is in doubt, consider it unsterile and avoid using it.
- If a sterile item contacts an unsterile item, the sterile item is contaminated.
- If a sterile package is cracked, cut, or torn, it is contaminated and should not be used.
- If a sterile item or package becomes wet, it is contaminated.
- Do not use a sterile package beyond the expiration date.

- Follow your facility policy. You may be asked to sanitize and dry the table or other surface that the sterile supplies will be placed on before establishing a sterile field.
- The outside of a sterile wrapper is not sterile. It may be handled with your hands. Avoid touching the inside of the wrapper or items inside the package with your hands.
- The inside of a sterile package can be used as a sterile field.
- Never turn your back on a sterile field.

(continued)

Guidelines for Sterile Procedures (Continued)

- Avoid crossing over or touching a sterile field. If you must add an item to the sterile field, drop it onto the field from the sterile package.

- Avoid touching unsterile articles when wearing sterile gloves. Avoid touching the outside of sterile packages when wearing sterile gloves. Make sure you can see your hands at all times. Keep them above your waist. Avoid touching your clothing or body. If the gloves become torn or contaminated, change them immediately.

- If sterile gloves touch an unsterile item, such as the outside of a package, they are contaminated. Change them before proceeding.

- Keep sterile items above waist level.

- Avoid talking, coughing, or sneezing over a sterile field.

Procedure 12

Opening a Sterile Tray

1. Wash your hands.
2. Check the seal and outside of the package to ensure that they are intact.
3. Remove the tape or package seal.
4. Touch only the outside of the package.
5. Open the package away from your body.
6. Open the **distal** flap of the package by touching only the corner. The distal flap is the farthest away from your body (**Figure 4-3A**).
7. Open the right-hand flap by touching only the corner (**Figure 4-3B**).

8. Open the left-hand flap by touching only the corner (**Figure 4-3C**).
9. Open the **proximal** flap by touching only the corner, then lifting the flap up and pulling it toward you, allowing it to drop over the edge of the counter or table. The proximal flap is the one closest to your body (**Figure 4-3D**). Avoid touching the inside of the wrapper or the contents of the package.
10. Wash your hands.

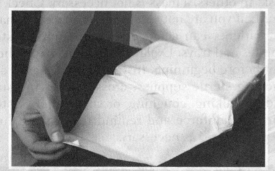

FIGURE 4-3(A) Touching only the corner, open the distal flap away from your body.

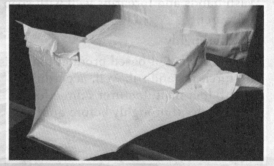

FIGURE 4-3(C) Carefully grasp the wrapper, opening the left side of the package.

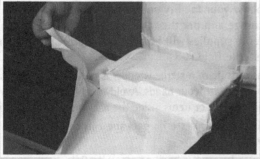

FIGURE 4-3(B) Open the right side. Avoid touching or crossing over the center of the package.

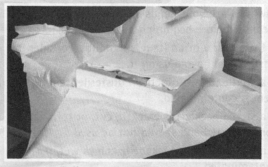

FIGURE 4-3(D) Open the proximal flap toward you. Avoid touching the flap with your clothing.

Procedure 13

Opening a Sterile Package

1. Wash your hands.
2. Grasp the upper edges of the package securely.
3. Using your thumbs, slowly peel the edges back and downward, exposing the contents.
4. When opened, the inside of the wrapper provides a sterile field, or the contents can

be placed on a commercially made drape (Figure 4-4).

5. If assisting with a procedure, hold the exposed sterile item toward the RN so he or she can grasp it with sterile gloves.

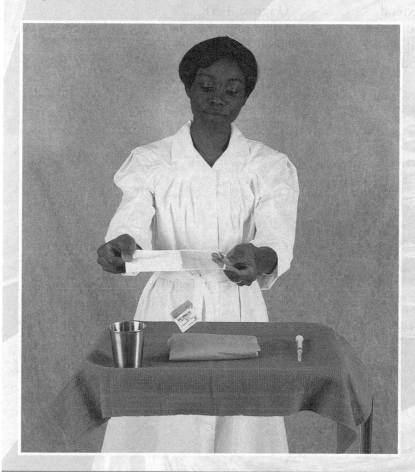

FIGURE 4-4 Peel the sides of the package back, dropping the item onto the sterile field.

SETTING UP A STERILE FIELD

A **sterile field** is a sterile surface that you create to use as a work area for sterile procedures. A one-inch border around the outside edge of the field is considered not sterile. Avoid placing sterile items in this border area. Only the top surface of the work area is considered sterile. A sterile drape often hangs over the edges of the table. The area below the table top is not sterile. Sterile supplies can touch only the sterile field. Avoid touching the field or items on it with your hands.

If a small surface is needed, the inside of a sterile package can be used as a sterile field. If a larger surface is needed, a sterile drape is used as the foundation for the sterile field.

Procedure **14**

Setting up a Sterile Field Using a Sterile Drape

1. Wash your hands.
2. Open the sterile package containing the sterile drape.
3. With the thumb and index finger of your dominant hand, grasp the folded top edge of the drape.
4. Lift the drape out of the package. Extend your arm, holding the drape away from your body. Allow it to unfold. Make sure it does not touch any other surface, your body, or your clothing as it unfolds.

5. Pick up the top corner on the other side of the drape after it is unfolded. Avoid touching the drape to your body, clothing, or other surfaces.
6. Beginning with the side opposite your body, slowly lay the drape across the table (**Figure 4-5**).
7. Open the other packages and add necessary items to the sterile field.

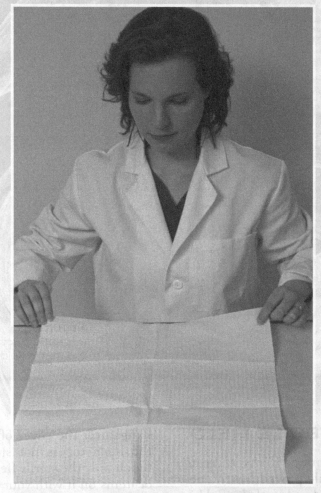

FIGURE 4-5 Cover the table from back to front. Make sure you can see the sterile drape at all times. Avoid touching your clothing or other objects.

Procedure 15

Adding an Item to a Sterile Field

1. Wash your hands.
2. Open the sterile package.
3. With one hand, grasp the package from the bottom. Using your free hand, pull the sides of the package away from the sterile item (**Figure 4-6**).
4. Drop the sterile item onto the sterile field. Avoid touching the sterile field with the package wrapper.
5. Discard the wrapper.
6. Perform your procedure completion actions.

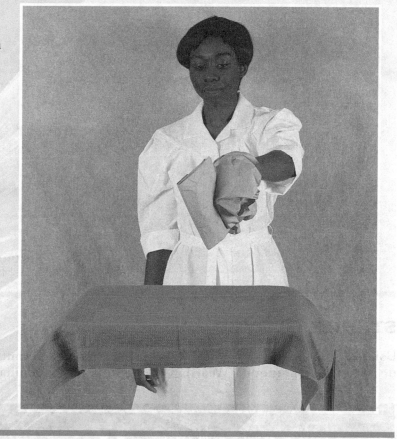

FIGURE 4-6 Fold the wrapper back, holding it away from the sterile item. Make sure that the bottom of the wrapper does not contact the sterile field.

Procedure 16

Adding Liquids to a Sterile Field

1. Wash your hands.
2. Inspect the container. The seal should be intact and the container should not be broken or cracked.
3. Open the container of liquid.
4. Place the cap upright on the table, with the outside of the cap resting on the table surface and the clean inner side facing up.
5. Pour a small amount of the solution into the sink or wastebasket to rinse the lip. When adding the solution to the sterile field, pour from the same side of the container. This is done to remove potential microbes.
6. Hold the bottle at an angle, 6 to 8 inches above the sterile bowl or other sterile container. Avoid crossing over the sterile field with your arm or hand.
7. From the clean side of the container, slowly pour the liquid to prevent splashing (**Figure 4-7**). If the liquid is spilled or splashed, the field is contaminated because moisture soaks through to the nonsterile surface beneath.
8. Replace the cap on the bottle.
9. Write the date and time the container was opened on the bottle. Write on the label, or use a separate piece of tape. Avoid writing directly on the plastic bottle. The ink from a pen or marker may bleed through the plastic, contaminating the solution.

(continues)

Procedure 16, *continued*

Adding Liquids to a Sterile Field

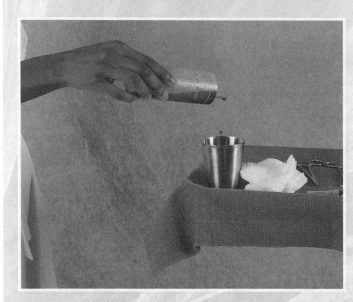

FIGURE 4-7 Pour the liquid slowly to prevent splashing.

STERILE GLOVES

Using sterile gloves is essential when using aseptic (sterile) technique. Wearing sterile gloves permits you to touch sterile items without contaminating them.

Procedure 17

Applying and Removing Sterile Gloves

1. Wash your hands.
2. Check the glove package for sterility.
3. Open the outer package by peeling the upper edges back with your thumbs.
4. Remove the inner package containing the gloves and place it on the inside of the outer package.
5. Open the inner package, handling it only by the corners on the outside (**Figure 4-8A**).
6. Pick up the cuff of the right-hand glove using your left hand (**Figure 4-8B**). Avoid touching the area below the cuff.
7. Insert your right hand into the glove. Spread your fingers slightly, sliding them into the fingers. If the glove is not on correctly, do not attempt to straighten it at this time.
8. Insert the gloved fingers of your right hand under the cuff of the left glove (**Figure 4-8C**).
9. Slide your fingers into the left glove, adjusting the fingers of the gloves for comfort and fit. Because both gloves are sterile, they may touch each other. Avoid touching the cuffs of the gloves.
10. Insert your right hand under the cuff of the left glove and push the cuff up over your wrist (**Figure 4-8D**). Avoid touching your wrist or the outside of the cuff with your glove.
11. Insert your left hand under the cuff of the right glove and push the cuff up over your wrist. Avoid touching your wrist or the outside of the cuff with your glove.
12. You may now touch sterile items with your sterile gloves. Avoid touching unsterile items.

(continues)

Procedure **17**, *continued*

Applying and Removing Sterile Gloves

To remove the gloves:

13. Grasp the outside of the glove on the nondominant hand, at the cuff. Pull the glove off so that the inside of the glove faces outward. Avoid touching the skin of your wrist with the fingers of the glove.

14. Place this glove into the palm of the gloved hand.

15. Put the fingers of the ungloved hand *inside* the cuff of the gloved hand. Pull the glove off inside-out. The first glove removed should be inside the second glove.

16. Discard the gloves into a covered container or trash, according to facility policy.

17. Wash your hands and perform your procedure completion actions.

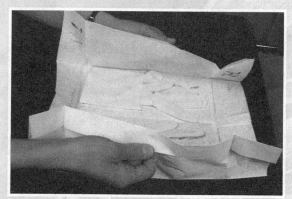

FIGURE 4-8(A) Fold the edges of the package back carefully without touching the inside of the package or gloves.

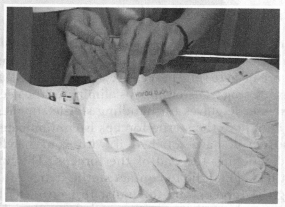

FIGURE 4-8(B) Lift the edges of the cuff with your fingertips, and slide your hand into the glove.

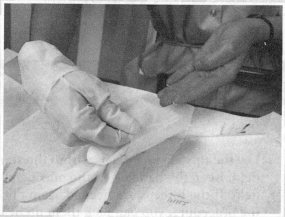

FIGURE 4-8(C) Protecting your right-hand glove with the cuff, slide your fingers into the glove. Adjust the fingers for comfort and fit.

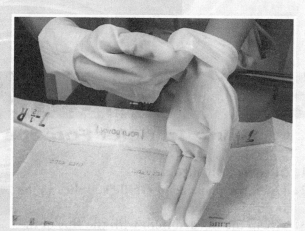

FIGURE 4-8(D) Adjust the cuffs carefully. Avoid touching your wrists.

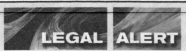
Transfer Forceps

Some facilities use sterile transfer forceps to add supplies to a sterile field (**Figure 4-9**). The forceps are used for one procedure, then sterilized after use. Using transfer forceps eliminates the need to use sterile gloves for handling sterile supplies. The handle to the sterile forceps is contaminated because you have touched it with your hands. Avoid touching the end of the forceps. The tips must be kept sterile to contact sterile items. After using the forceps, the tips must rest on a sterile surface to keep them sterile until the end of the procedure.

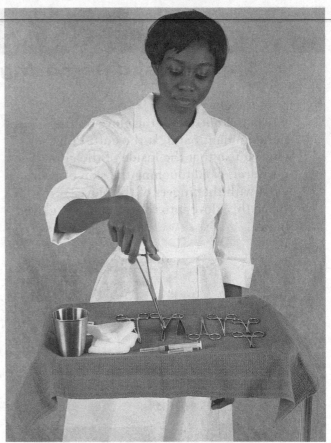

FIGURE 4-9 Sterile ring forceps or transfer forceps may be used to add items to or rearrange items on a sterile field. Leave the inner part of the forceps on the sterile field so they may be used again, if needed. Hang the handles over the edge to prevent contaminating the field. Do not allow the tips of the forceps to touch unsterile surfaces or objects.

Procedure 18

Using Transfer Forceps

1. Wash your hands.
2. Open the package of sterile supplies in the normal manner.
3. Grasp the needed item with the tips of the forceps.
4. Pick the item up, moving it to the sterile field.

5. Lay the tips of the forceps within the sterile field. Keep the handles on the outside of the field. If the forceps are needed again during the procedure, you can pick them up by the handles to use them again.

STERILIZATION

Steam sterilization is the most common method of sterilizing instruments and other items in the hospital. As a rule, most sterilization is done under controlled conditions in the central service depart-

ment. There are times, however, when a procedure called **flash sterilization** is necessary. *Flash sterilization* is a quick method of sterilizing essential items, such as a one-of-a-kind instrument that was dropped on the floor. This procedure is almost always performed when personnel are rushed and stressed, and the risk of error is great. Flash sterilization is safe only if proper procedures are followed. Without these processes in place, both patients and workers are at risk. If you are responsible for sterilizing items, make sure you are permitted to sterilize instruments and other items in your facility, and know the proper procedures for the equipment you are using.

Before instruments are sterilized, they must be scrubbed clean. Resist the temptation to rinse the instrument under water. Take it to the sink in the soiled utility area and scrub it with a brush, or according to the manufacturer's directions. An enzymatic cleaner may be necessary to remove protein substances. Holding the instrument and the brush under the water level will prevent splashing or spraying of pathogens. After washing, treat the instrument with a water-soluble lubricant. This product is often called "milk" because it is white in color. The lubricant protects the instrument's surface and prolongs its life. Allow the lubricant to air-dry.

Items with many parts must be disassembled for washing. Leave them disassembled during the sterilization procedure to allow the steam to contact all instrument surfaces. Leave hinged instruments open. Flush instruments that have lumens with sterile distilled water immediately before sterilization. Flash sterilization may be done with the device unwrapped, or by wrapping with a single wrapper. The unwrapped method is the most common. However, preventing recontamination after sterilization is a great concern. Some sterilizers have containers that totally contain the instrument during and after sterilization.

To sterilize the item, follow the instructions for the equipment you are using. In most cases, sterilization will take from 3 to 10 minutes. Document the procedure on the flash sterilization log. Logs are available with each sterilizer and are used to trace items in the event of a sterilizer malfunction.

Improper flash sterilization technique is a common cause of survey deficiencies. Make sure to wash instruments well and follow all facility policies for using the flash sterilizer. Pay close attention to your technique and use all quality controls required by your facility.

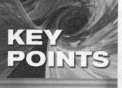

KEY POINTS

▶ Sterile technique is a microbe-free technique.

▶ A sterile item is free from all microorganisms and spores.

▶ Sterile technique is used during procedures within body cavities and for certain dressing changes.

▶ An autoclave is used to sterilize reusable supplies, such as instruments.

▶ The surface on which you open a sterile package must be clean, dry, flat, and stable. The area must be free from airborne contamination. Masks are worn during some sterile procedures.

▶ Always wash your hands or use an alcohol-based hand cleaner before beginning a sterile procedure.

▶ If the sterility of an item is in doubt, consider it unsterile and do not use it.

▶ If a sterile item contacts an unsterile item, it is contaminated.

▶ If a sterile package is cracked, cut, torn, or wet, it is contaminated.

▶ If a sterile package is dated, do not use it beyond the expiration date.

▶ The outside of a sterile wrapper is not sterile.

▶ The inside of a sterile package can be used as a sterile field.

▶ Never turn your back on a sterile field.

▶ Avoid crossing over or touching a sterile field.

▶ If sterile gloves touch an unsterile item, they are contaminated. Change them before proceeding.

▶ Keep sterile items above waist level.

▶ Avoid talking, coughing, or sneezing over a sterile field.

▶ A one-inch border around the outside edge of the sterile field is considered not sterile.

(continues)

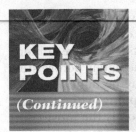

KEY POINTS
(Continued)

▶ Only the top surface of the work area is considered sterile.

▶ Sterile supplies may be handled with sterile forceps. Touch the forceps only by the handle, so that the tip remains sterile. The forceps are sterilized after each use.

▶ Flash sterilization must be done correctly to be effective.

CLINICAL APPLICATIONS

1. You are asked to set up a sterile field for the RN. She tells you she will need sterile gauze sponges, a #14 straight urethral catheter, sterile gloves, skin disinfectant solution, and a specimen collection cup. Describe how you will establish a sterile field, and how you will add the supplies to the field without contaminating them.

2. You will be assisting with a sterile dressing change to a central intravenous catheter that was inserted yesterday. The RN tells you that both you and the patient must wear masks. How will you explain the mask to the patient?

Why do you think it is necessary for the patient to wear a mask?

3. You are assigned to set up a sterile tray. The package has a stain on it. It is wrinkled and looks like it may have gotten wet. What will you do?

4. You are alone in the room, setting up a sterile tray. You accidentally brush against the tray with your uniform. You do not know if you have contaminated the tray. What will you do?

5. You are wearing sterile gloves, performing a sterile procedure. Without thinking, you accidentally drop your hands below your waist. What should you do?

CHAPTER REVIEW

Multiple-Choice Questions

Select the one best answer.

1. Sterile technique is free from:
   a. pathogens only.
   b. spores only.
   c. all microbes and spores.
   d. some harmful microbes.

2. The surface on which you set up a sterile field should be:
   a. covered with a drape.
   b. moist from disinfectant.
   c. at least three feet away from the patient.
   d. clean, dry, and flat.

3. Which of the following can be used to set up a sterile field?
   a. The inside of a sterile package
   b. A clean towel
   c. The outside of the wrapper for a sterile package
   d. A clean drawsheet or underpad

4. When wearing sterile gloves, keep your hands:
   a. at your sides.
   b. above your waist.
   c. below your waist, in front of your body.
   d. on the sterile field at all times.

5. Open the outer wrapper of a sterile package using:
   a. sterile gloves.
   b. your hands.
   c. sterile forceps.
   d. exam gloves.

6. To add an item to a sterile field:
   a. put on a mask.
   b. use transfer forceps.
   c. pick up the item with your hand.
   d. wear clean disposable gloves.

7. When wearing sterile gloves, you can:
   a. open the outer wrapper of the sterile package.
   b. touch surfaces below the table top that are covered with a sterile drape.
   c. touch items on the inside of the sterile package.
   d. hold your hands below your waist.

8. The border around a sterile field is considered not sterile for approximately:
   a. one-quarter inch from the edges.
   b. half an inch from the edges.
   c. three-quarters inch from the edges.
   d. one inch from the edges.

9. If a sterile item gets wet, it:
   a. is contaminated.
   b. is sterile.
   c. must be used right away.
   d. must be used within 24 hours.

10. The equipment used to sterilize supplies in the health care facility is a:
   a. fomite.
   b. common vehicle.
   c. vector.
   d. autoclave.

EXPLORING THE WEB

Aseptic Technique	http://www.bmb.psu.edu
Aseptic Technique & the Sterile Field	http://www.infectioncontroltoday.com
Aseptic Technique: The ABCs of Infection Control	http://www.iceinstitute.com
NCBON CNAII Sterile Technique	http://www.ncbon.com
Principles of Aseptic Technique	http://www.laras-lair.com
Principles of Sterile Technique for the OR	http://www.lhsc.on.ca
Sterile Technique	http://structbio.vanderbilt.edu
Sterile Technique & Personal Protective Equipment	http://www.texashste.com
Sterile Technique Flashcards	http://www.flashcardexchange.com
Sterile Technique Information Links	http://www.fp.ucalgary.ca

CHAPTER 5

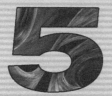

Wound Care

OBJECTIVES:

After reading this chapter, you should be able to:

- Spell and define key terms.
- Identify the structures of the skin affected by Stage I, Stage II, Stage III, and Stage IV pressure ulcers.
- List at least seven systemic factors and seven local factors affecting wound healing.
- Describe how to remove a dressing and observations to make of the underlying wound.
- Demonstrate how to cleanse a linear wound and a circular wound, and explain why you will clean a wound from the most clean to least clean areas.
- Define dressings and bandages, and describe when each is used.
- Demonstrate how to apply dressings to wounds with and without drains.
- State the indications for using transparent film dressings, hydrocolloid dressings, and wet-to-dry dressings.
- Demonstrate pin care.
- Demonstrate suture and staple removal.

THE SKIN

As a PCT, you will be exposed to many different types of wounds from many causes. These include trauma and accidental injury, burns and other thermal injuries, surgical incisions, and pressure ulcers. Pressure ulcers are common, and understanding the anatomy of the wound will help you understand the anatomy and care of all wounds.

The skin (**Figure 5-1**) is the largest organ of the body. It serves primarily as protection for the underlying organs and structures. It is also used for excretion of wastes and regulation of body temperature. The outer, protective layer of skin is the *epidermis*. Beneath this layer is the *dermis*, which contains nerves, hair follicles, sweat glands, and oil glands. Beneath these two layers is subcutaneous tissue or fat. This layer serves as a covering for muscles, tendons, and bone.

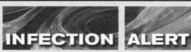

INFECTION ALERT

Become familiar with the appearance of scabies, head and body lice on the skin. Scabies and body lice are microscopic parasites that appear to be numerous, tiny scabs on the skin surface. They are often linear, with the lines following the blood vessels. The scabbed areas itch, and the patient may scratch them. If the patient has multiple, tiny, scab-like areas, wear gloves for skin contact. When performing hair care, check patients for nits. Nits are tiny, oval-shaped eggs that are yellow-white. They look like dandruff, but are firmly attached to the hair and are usually very difficult to remove. Head lice are tiny brown insects about the size of a sesame seed that are visible to the eye. They can run very fast, but head lice do not hop, jump, or fly. They move away from light quickly. Report abnormal skin lesions or head lice to the RN.

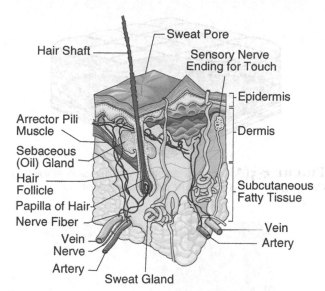

FIGURE 5-1 Cross-section of the skin

Pressure Ulcers

Pressure ulcers are classified by stage, as determined by the depth and degree of involvement of the underlying structures. The stages are:

- Stage I (**Figure 5-2 A & B**): Nonblanchable erythema of intact skin, the heralding lesion

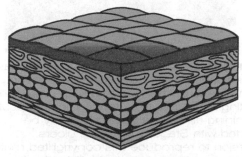

FIGURE 5-2(A) Cross-section of the skin showing damage from a Stage I pressure ulcer.

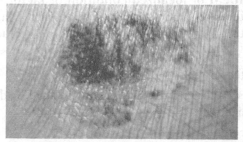

FIGURE 5-2(B) A Stage I pressure ulcer has nonblanchable erythema of intact skin, the heralding lesion of skin ulceration. In individuals with darker skin, discoloration of the skin, warmth, edema, induration, or hardness may also be indicators. (Permission to reproduce this copyrighted material has been given by the owner, Hollister, Inc.)

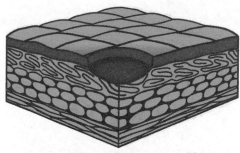

FIGURE 5-3(A) Cross-section of the skin showing damage from a Stage II pressure ulcer.

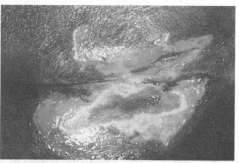

FIGURE 5-3(B) A Stage II pressure ulcer has partial-thickness skin loss involving epidermis, dermis, or both. The ulcer is superficial and presents clinically as an abrasion, blister, or shallow crater. (Permission to reproduce this copyrighted material has been given by the owner, Hollister, Inc.)

of skin ulceration. In individuals with darker skin, discoloration of the skin, warmth, edema, induration, or hardness may also be indicators.

- Stage II (**Figure 5-3 A & B**): Partial-thickness skin loss involving epidermis, dermis, or both. The ulcer is superficial and presents clinically as an abrasion, blister, or shallow crater.
- Stage III (**Figure 5-4 A & B**): Full-thickness skin loss involving damage to or necrosis of subcutaneous tissue that may extend down to, but not through, underlying fascia. The ulcer presents clinically as a deep crater with or without undermining of adjacent tissue.
- Stage IV (**Figure 5-5 A & B**): Full-thickness skin loss with extensive destruction, tissue necrosis, or damage to muscle, bone, or supporting structures (e.g., tendon, joint capsule). Undermining and sinus tracts also may be associated with Stage 4 pressure ulcers.

When skin integrity is disrupted, the patient is at high risk of infection, pain, and other complications. It is essential to try to heal wounds as quickly

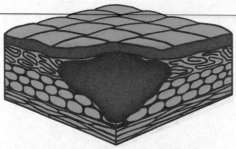

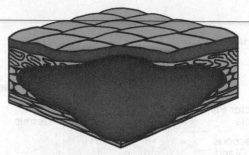

FIGURE 5-4(A) Cross-section of the skin showing damage from a Stage III pressure ulcer.

FIGURE 5-5(A) Cross-section of the skin showing damage from a Stage IV pressure ulcer.

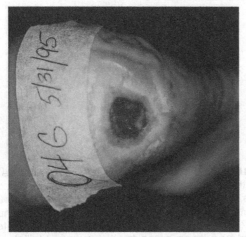

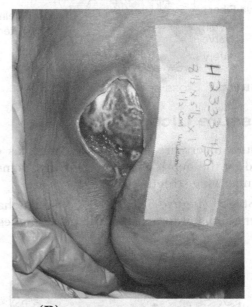

FIGURE 5-4(B) A Stage III pressure ulcer has full-thickness skin loss involving damage to or necrosis of subcutaneous tissue that may extend down to, but not through, underlying fascia. The ulcer presents clinically as a deep crater with or without undermining of adjacent tissue. (Permission to reproduce this copyrighted material has been given by the owner, Hollister, Inc.)

as possible. Local and systemic factors must be addressed to optimize the patient's ability to heal.

FACTORS AFFECTING WOUND HEALING

A **systemic** condition or factor is something that affects the entire body, rather than its single individual parts. Systemic factors that affect wound healing are:

- age
- nutritional status
- body build
- presence or absence of chronic disease
- circulatory problems
- weakened immune system
- radiation therapy

FIGURE 5-5(B) A Stage IV pressure ulcer has full-thickness skin loss with extensive destruction, tissue necrosis, or damage to muscle, bone, or supporting structures (e.g., tendon, joint capsule). Undermining and sinus tracts also may be associated with Stage IV pressure ulcers. (Permission to reproduce this copyrighted material has been given by the owner, Hollister, Inc.)

A **local** or localized condition or factor is one that affects only one system or body part. Many local factors affect wound healing. These include:

- moist wound environment
- infection
- **necrotic tissue** (tissue that is dead or devitalized)
- foreign objects in the wound
- trauma
- edema
- pressure on the wound
- incontinence and presence of excretions contaminating the wound

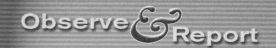

The elderly do not heal as rapidly as younger patients. Good nutrition and hydration are important for wound healing. Body build also affects healing. Obese patients and those who are emaciated do not heal as rapidly. Some chronic diseases and conditions impair wound healing. Patients with a weakened immune system, cigarette smokers, and those receiving radiation therapy do not heal as well.

Wounds heal best, and are less painful, in a moist environment. Avoid pressure on wounds, and keep them free from body excretions from incontinence. Also avoid trauma and pressure on the wound. If necrotic tissue is present, notify your supervisor. This is dead tissue that is usually brown or black in appearance. It must be removed for proper wound healing.

Infection Control

An infected wound will not heal. The infection must be eliminated to promote healing. Signs and symptoms of infection are listed in the Observe & Report box.

PPE. Infection control is an area in which you cannot afford to cut corners. When caring for patients who have breaks in the skin, you must be careful to avoid introducing pathogens into the wound(s). Likewise, you must avoid picking up a pathogen from a patient and carrying it. Care providers usually apply gloves and other PPE to protect themselves. Remember that the gloves and other apparel protect the patient and others as well.

Always plan your work carefully, and think about what you are doing. Before beginning, set your supplies up in a manner that makes it easy for you and prevents contamination. Make sure you use good clean or sterile technique and excellent, frequent handwashing. Avoid contaminating the patient or the environment with your used gloves. If necessary, remove one glove and use the ungloved hand to touch environmental surfaces. You should not touch the side rails, doorknobs, faucets, or other surfaces with gloves you have worn during a treatment procedure. Discard gloves correctly.

Treatment Cart. The surface and drawers of the treatment cart should always be kept clean and free from spills. The cart should be well stocked. Replace and charge all items that you use for patient care. Restock the cart regularly. Avoid bringing the unit's treatment cart into a patient's room. Leave the cart in the hallway. Make sure the cart is locked, and that no harmful liquids or sharp items are available on the top. If the cart is inadvertently contaminated with a soiled glove, dressing, or other item, disinfect it with a facility-approved cleanser.

Work Surface. The surface you set up to hold your clean supplies during procedures must be clean and dry. The overbed table is used only for clean items. It should not be used for bedpans, urinals, or soiled supplies. Wipe your work surface with facility-approved disinfectant and allow it to dry, if needed. You may also cover the work surface with a disposable underpad or other clean barrier or drape.

Multiple Dressings. Some patients have more than one wound that requires dressing. If this is the case, care for each wound separately. Use a new pair of gloves for each, and wash your hands in between wounds. Always work from the cleanest to the least clean wound.

Bandage Scissors. Bandage scissors are a potential source of serious cross-contamination. Many nursing personnel carry bandage scissors in their pockets when on duty, and use them one or more times each shift. Wash your scissors well with soap and water, then dry them after each use. If they are used during both the soiled and clean portions of a procedure such as a dressing change, wash and dry the scissors each time you wash your hands.

Trash Disposal. Make sure that you position your plastic bag or other trash receptacle in an area that will not contaminate clean supplies. The end of the bed works well for this purpose. Never cross over the trash with clean or sterile supplies. When you are finished with the procedure, discard trash in the proper area. Avoid leaving it in the open wastebasket in the patient's room. Tie plastic bags closed and take them with you. Gloves and items that have contacted blood, body fluids, nonintact skin, mucous membranes, secretions, or excretions are considered biohazardous waste. Discard these items in the designated area on your unit, as they require special handling. Avoid placing items such as empty plastic catheter and dressing trays, empty plastic bottles, and other bulky items in the biohazardous waste. These things do not require special trash handling. Biohazardous waste handling is quite expensive, and storage space is usually limited. Filling the biohazardous trash with nonessential items will increase the facility's costs.

Stock Supplies of Liquid Solutions. Another area of potential contamination is stock supplies of skin cleansers, such as povidone iodine and normal saline. These usually come in large bottles.

Never take floor-stock bottles into patients' rooms. If the stock supplies are needed, dispense only as much as you will need into a cup or smaller container, and take that into the room. Consult the nurse about ordering an individual supply for a patient who uses an item regularly. Never share a tube of ointment or cream between patients.

Become familiar with the liquid cleansers you are using. Some are no-rinse products; others must be rinsed and allowed to dry before the dressing is applied. Products such as peroxide and povidone iodine are not recommended for care of open wounds, such as pressure ulcers, because they destroy **granulation tissue.** This is a specialized tissue created by the body in response to injury. It contains many tiny blood vessels, and may appear like a small, red, beadlike mass. It has also been described as appearing deep pink or red with an irregular, "berry-like" surface.

Always place the lid to a bottle with the sterile, top, inner side facing up to prevent contamination. When opening a new, sealed bottle of liquid, such as normal saline, write the date and your initials on the bottle. Remember that ink will bleed through soft plastic bottles, so use a label or tape to affix the date, if necessary. Each facility has policies regarding how long open solution bottles may be used. Some items, such as normal saline, must be discarded within a period ranging from 24 hours to 7 days. Other products may be discarded after a longer period of time. You must learn and adhere to the time frame required by your facility for discarding bottles of solution to prevent contamination.

REMOVING A DRESSING

Before applying a clean or sterile dressing, the old dressing must be removed. Wash your hands and apply clean gloves before removing the soiled dressing. Carefully loosen the edges of the tape, pulling the tape ends toward the wound while holding traction on the skin with your other hand. Lift the dressing off. If the dressing sticks to the wound, pour a small amount of sterile saline on the dressing to loosen it. Let it sit for a minute, then gently pull the dressing off, holding gentle traction on the skin above the wound. Note the color, odor, and amount of drainage on the dressing. Discard the soiled dressing in a plastic bag, or according to facility policy. Keep the soiled dressing away from clean and sterile supplies. If traces of adhesive remain on the skin, remove them with tape remover or baby oil.

Observing the Wound

After the dressing is removed, observe the wound. If signs or symptoms of infection are present, or if you suspect there is another problem, call the nurse to the bedside to assess the patient before you cover the wound with a dressing. Leaving the wound uncovered to find the RN is not appropriate. Remain at the bedside and use the call signal.

CLEANSING THE WOUND

Always clean the wound before applying a dressing. Many products are available for wound cleansing. Normal saline is also safe and effective. Many antiseptic cleansing products are **cytotoxic.** These products harm healing tissue, and should not be used. Products that are pH neutral are preferred. Follow the physician's order, facility policies, and your supervisor's directions.

A wound is cleaned to remove debris and bacteria. Cleaning must be done gently to prevent pain and trauma to healing tissue. Always work from the clean area near the wound outward to less clean areas. This will prevent you from accidentally introducing skin microbes into the wound. Use each gauze or swab for one stroke, then discard it. Avoid contaminating the cleansing solution with used swabs or gauze.

> **HEALTH CARE ALERT**
>
> Gauze sponges are commonly used for cleansing and covering wounds. Select gauze sponges very carefully. Some are soft and absorbent. Others are rough and irritating. Check the fiber and ensure that it is kind to skin. Gauze can be very traumatic, irritating, and harmful to tender, healing tissue.

To clean a wound, use sterile gauze pads and the cleansing solution. Apply the cleansing solution to the gauze, then squeeze the pad so it is not dripping. Cotton swabs are used to clean some wounds. Use the swab on the wound and discard it. If more solution is necessary, use a clean swab. Never dip a used swab into a bottle of cleansing solution. Some wound cleansers must be rinsed off using sterile normal saline solution. Others do not have to be rinsed. Read the product directions and the physician's orders for guidance. If in doubt, rinse the cleanser from the wound with a moist gauze sponge and pat dry.

Cleanse a linear wound or surgical incision from top to bottom. Work from clean to less clean areas. Use a new gauze pad for each stroke. Work outward from the wound in parallel lines (**Figure 5-6**). Avoid rubbing back and forth. Rinse, if necessary, using the same technique.

To cleanse an open wound, such as an injury or pressure ulcer, work in half circles or full circles (**Figure 5-7**). Begin in the center of the wound and work outward. Clean at least one inch beyond the edge of the dressing. If no dressing will be applied, clean at least two inches beyond the wound margins. Use a new gauze pad for each circle. Rinse, if necessary, using the same technique.

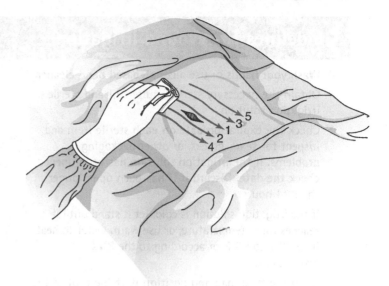

FIGURE 5-6 Begin next to the wound. Work from top to bottom. Use a new pad for each stroke.

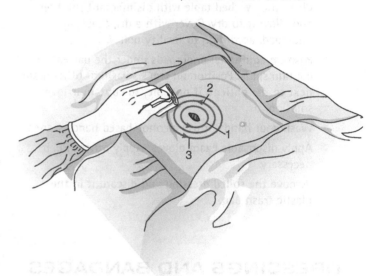

FIGURE 5-7 Begin close to the wound, working outward in full or half circles.

After removing the soiled dressing and cleaning the wound, remove and discard your gloves. Wash your hands or use alcohol-based hand cleaner before continuing. This prevents cross-contamination and infection.

Wound Irrigation

Irrigation removes bacteria and debris from the wound. In some facilities, antibiotic or antiseptic solutions are used to irrigate the wound. Many solutions are harmful to healing tissue. Irrigation with medicated solutions must be done by a nurse. Strict sterile technique must be used. Some wounds are packed after irrigation.

Guidelines for Wound Irrigation

- Wash your hands or use alcohol-based hand cleaner.
- Obtain the necessary sterile equipment and sterile irrigation solution.
- Check the expiration date on each sterile item and inspect for tears, cracks, or other packaging problems. If the irrigation solution has been opened, check the date. Discard if it has been open longer than 24 hours.
- If the irrigation solution is cold, let it stand until it reaches room temperature, or use warm water to heat it to 90°F to 95°F, or according to the RN's instructions.
- Open the trash bag and position it at the foot of the bed. Make sure you will not have to reach across the sterile field to discard trash.
- Clean the overbed table with disinfectant solution and allow it to dry. Cover with a disposable underpad, according to facility policy.
- Position additional underpads under the patient to contain spills. Position an emesis basin or other basin next to the patient, if possible, to contain irrigant solution.
- Wash your hands or use alcohol-based hand cleaner.
- Apply disposable exam gloves. Apply other PPE, if necessary.
- Remove the soiled dressing and discard it in the plastic trash bag.
- Remove your soiled gloves and discard them in the plastic trash bag.
- Wash your hands or use alcohol-based hand cleaner.
- Open sterile equipment and establish a sterile field.
- Pour the irrigation solution into a sterile basin.
- Apply sterile gloves and other PPE, if indicated.
- Withdraw the irrigation solution into a 35-mL piston syringe. Avoid using a bulb syringe, if possible. Connect an 18- or 19-gauge intravenous catheter to the syringe, if needed to irrigate small cavities.
- Slowly and gently instill the irrigating solution into the wound until the syringe is empty. Direct the flow of fluid from the cleanest area of the wound to the dirtiest area of the wound to prevent contamination. Make sure to irrigate all areas of the wound.
- Refill the syringe and repeat the irrigation until the prescribed amount of solution has been used.
- Rinse the wound with sterile normal saline. Pat dry gently, or allow to air-dry.
- Apply a sterile dressing to the wound.
- Remove and discard gloves and other protective equipment.
- Wash your hands or use alcohol-based hand cleaner.
- Discard the catheter, syringe, and other trash according to facility policy.

DRESSINGS AND BANDAGES

Caring for surgical wounds, injuries, and ulcers is very important. **Dressings** are gauze, film, or other synthetic substances that cover a wound, ulcer, or injury. Some dressings have an adhesive backing. Some are held on with tape. Many different types of tape are available in the health care facility. Some patients need special **hypoallergenic tape,** which reduces the incidence of skin reactions in patients who are allergic to the adhesive on the back of the tape. **Bandages** are sometimes used to hold dressings in place. These are fabric, gauze, net, or elasticized wrappings used to cover the dressing and keep it securely in place. Bandages are available in different sizes and shapes. Gauze bandages are commonly used to cover dressings. Elastic bandages are used to reduce edema and support injured body parts. When applying bandages, avoid wrapping them so tightly that they restrict circulation.

Occasionally, **Montgomery straps** (Figure 5-8) are used to hold dressings in place. These are long strips of adhesive attached to the skin on either side of the wound. After the dressing is in place, the straps are tied to hold the dressing securely. Binders (**Figure 5-9**) may also be used to hold dressings in place.

Elastic mesh and tubular gauze bandages are sometimes used to cover dressings on various parts of the body. These are available in small sizes, such as would be used for a finger, and range up to very large sizes that may be used to cover legs, arms, and the torso. Manufacturers' directions for the large bandages show how to fold and cut the bandage to fashion devices such as underwear to hold a dressing on the perineum or buttocks. The elastic mesh and tubular bandages make it easier to dress wounds and provide versatility for difficult-to-bandage parts of the body.

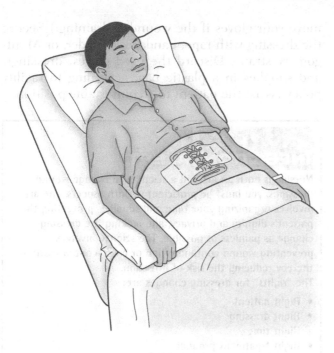

FIGURE 5-8 Montgomery straps may be used to hold dressings securely in place, reducing the irritation of tape on the skin.

STERILE TECHNIQUE AND CLEAN TECHNIQUE

Any break in the skin increases the risk of infection. Wounds are most susceptible to infection during the first four days, although infection can begin at any time. Dressings protect the wound, preventing contamination. They also increase comfort and prevent further injury. Some dressings are used to apply pressure to the wound to control bleeding. Always apply the principles of standard precautions when caring for wounds.

The RN will instruct you regarding which type of dressing to apply. Dressings covering burns, surgical sites, drains, and deep or extensive wounds are always sterile. Sterile dressings and supplies are used. You will use aseptic, or sterile, technique to apply the dressing that contacts the wound directly.

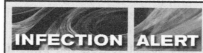

INFECTION ALERT

Make sure you have an order to open a tube or drain or remove a dressing. Document that sterile technique was used.

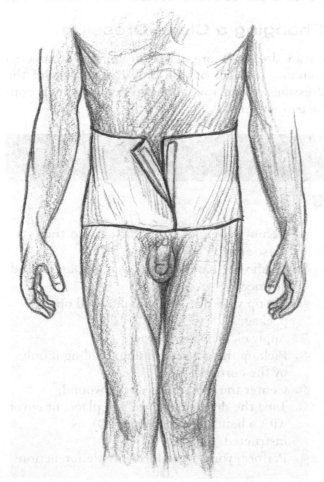

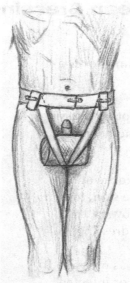

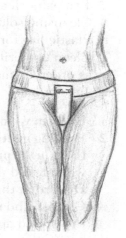

FIGURE 5-9 Various binders

In most cases, a clean outer bandage can be used to hold the dressing in place. Check with your supervisor for the type of outer bandage to use if you are unsure.

Clean technique may be used for superficial pressure ulcers and other minor wounds. Clean dressing supplies may be used in an emergency to stop bleeding in any wound.

APPLYING A DRESSING

Before applying the dressing, check the wound care order. Gather your supplies. Select a dressing that will extend at least one inch beyond the borders of the wound. If gauze dressings are used, several layers may be necessary to protect the wound and collect drainage. Wounds with heavy drainage may need additional composite dressings over the gauze. Extra dressings may be applied to some wounds for protective padding. This prevents discomfort and trauma to the wound.

It may be necessary to reposition the patient for the procedure. Assist the patient into a position that he or she can maintain for the entire procedure without discomfort. Dressing changes for some wounds and surgical incisions are uncomfortable. The nurse may administer pain medication 30 to 60 minutes before the dressing change.

After you have applied the dressing and the wound is covered, you can remove your gloves, if necessary, so tape does not stick to them. (Do not re-move your gloves if the wound is draining.) Secure the dressing with tape, bandage, a binder, or Montgomery straps. Discard the used gloves, dressings, and supplies in a plastic bag, according to facility policy. Assist the patient to a comfortable position.

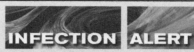

INFECTION ALERT

Nursing is both an art and a science. To change wound dressings, you must be proficient in both aspects. The art involves organizing your time and supplies, protecting the patient's dignity and privacy, and making the dressing change as painless as possible. The science involves preventing wound contamination or cross-contamination, thereby reducing the risk of infection.

The "rights" for dressing changes are:

- Right patient
- Right dressing
- Right time
- Right treatment product
- Right amount/quantity
- Right environment
- Right technique
- Right documentation

Changing a Clean Dressing

Clean dressings are used on minor, uninfected wounds. You will handle only the corners of the dressings. Avoid touching the center, which contacts the wound.

Procedure 19

Changing a Clean Dressing

Supplies needed:
- Two pairs clean, disposable exam gloves
- Cleansing solution
- Plastic bag for used supplies
- Clean or sterile gauze pads or other dressing, as ordered, and according to facility policy
- Tape or bandage material

1. Perform your beginning procedure actions.
2. Holding gentle traction on the skin, loosen the tape by pulling the ends toward the wound, and then remove the dressing. Discard in the plastic bag.
3. Cleanse and rinse the wound as ordered. If the wound appears abnormal or infected, notify your supervisor.
4. Remove the gloves and discard in the plastic bag.
5. Wash your hands or use alcohol-based hand cleaner.
6. Set up your dressing supplies and open packages.
7. Apply clean exam gloves.
8. Pick up the gauze dressing, holding it only by the corners.
9. Center the dressing over the wound.
10. Tape the dressing securely in place, or cover with a bandage (Procedure 20), as instructed.
11. Perform your procedure completion actions.

Procedure 20

Applying a Bandage

1. After applying the dressing, apply the bandage. Most bandaging materials are conforming, self-adhering gauze. Brand name products, such as Kling® and Kerlix®, or generic products, such as conforming gauze, are commonly used in health care facilities.

2. The bandage must cover the dressing completely. Begin by holding the bandage in your dominant hand. Hold the bandage against the skin with your nondominant thumb, approximately one inch below the dressing.

3. Wrap the bandage around the extremity two or three times to hold it securely in place.

4. Wrap the bandage from distal to proximal, in overlapping spiral turns (**Figure 5-10**). Each turn should overlap ½ to ¾ of the previous turn. The bandage should be snug so it does not fall off. However, it must not be so tight that it restricts blood flow.

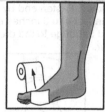

Foot and ankle Use 3-inch width. Hold foot at right angle to leg. Start bandage on ridge of foot just back of the toes.

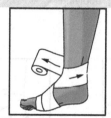

Pass bandage around foot from inside to outside. After two or three complete turns around foot, ascending toward the ankle on each turn, make a figure eight turn by bringing bandage up

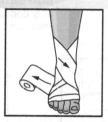

over the arch–to the inside of the ankle–around the ankle–down over the arch–and under the foot.

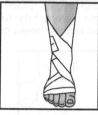

Repeat the figure eight wrapping two to three times. Fasten end by pressing the last 4 to 6 inches of unstretched bandage to the preceding layer.

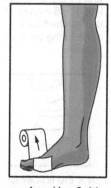

Lower leg: Use 3-4 inch width depending on the size of the leg. A leg wrap requires two rolls of bandage. Hold foot at right angle to leg. Start bandage on ridge of foot just back of the toes.

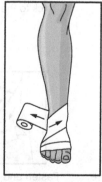

Pass bandage around foot from inside to outside. After two complete turns around foot, make a figure eight turn by bringing bandage up over the arch–to the inside of the ankle– around the ankle–

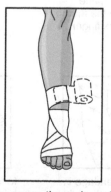

down over the arch–and under the foot. Start circular bandaging, making the first turn around the ankle. To begin the second roll of bandage, simply overlap the unstretched ends by 4 to 6 inches, press firmly, and continue wrapping.

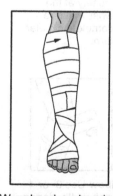

Wrap bandage in spiral turns to just below the kneecap. Fasten end by pressing the last 4 to 6 inches of unstretched bandage to the preceding layer.

FIGURE 5-10 Bandage-wrapping techniques. Always wrap from distal to proximal using spiral, circular, and figure-eight turns. (Courtesy Becton Dickinson, and Co., Rutherford, NJ)

(continues)

Procedure **20**, *continued*

Applying a Bandage

5. Wrap the bandage at least one inch above the top of the dressing. Wrap it completely around the extremity twice, then cut the end. Tape the end to the bandage, not the skin.

6. Assess the circulation distal to the bandage to ensure that the circulation is adequate.

7. Perform your procedure completion actions.

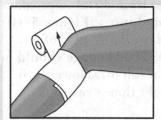

Knee: Use 4 inch width. Bend knee slightly. Start with one complete circular turn around the leg just below the knee.

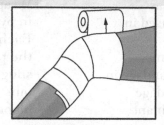

Start circular bandaging, applying only comfortable tension. Cover kneecap completely.

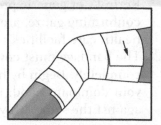

Continue wrapping to thigh just above the knee. Fasten end by pressing the last 4 to 6 inches of unstretched bandage to the preceding layer.

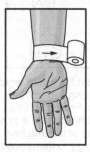

Wrist Use 2- or 3-inch width. Anchor bandage loosely at the wrist with one complete circular turn.

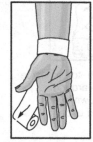

Carry the bandage across the back of the hand, through the web space between the thumb and index finger

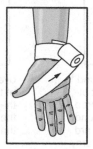

and across palm to the wrist, Make a circular turn around

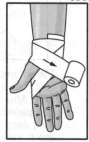

the wrist and once more carry the bandage through the web space and back to the wrist.

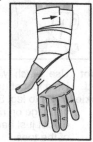

Start circular bandaging, ascending to the wrist. Fasten the end by pressing the last 4 to 6 inches of unstretched bandage to the preceding layer.

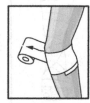

Elbow Use 3- or 4-inch width, depending on the size of the arm. Two rolls of bandage are required to complete the wrap. Start with a complete circular turn just below the elbow.

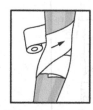

Wrap bandage in loose figure eights

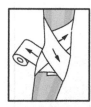

to form a protective bridge across the front of the elbow joint.

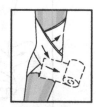

Fasten end by pressing 4 to 6 inches of unstretched bandage to preceding layer. Start second bandage with a circular turn below the elbow

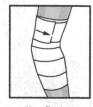

over the first wrap. Continue spiral bandaging over the elbow, ascending to the lower portion of the upper arm. Fasten end with circular turn.

FIGURE 5–10 Bandage-wrapping techniques. Always wrap from distal to proximal using spiral, circular, and figure-eight turns—Continued

Procedure **20**, *continued*

Applying a Bandage

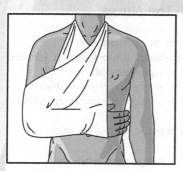

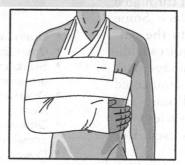

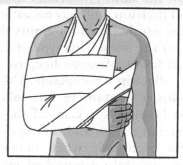

Shoulder A shoulder wrap is used to provide additional support for an arm in a sling. Use 4- or 6-inch width. One or two rolls of bandage may be used. Start under the free arm.

Carry the bandage across the back, over the arm in the sling, across the chest and back under the free arm in complete circular, overlapping turns. Fasten the end by pressing 4 to 6 inches of unstretched bandage to underlying bandage.

Additional support can be obtained with a second bandage. Start at the back just behind the flexed elbow in the sling. Carry the bandage under the elbow, up over the forearm, around the chest and back, and repeat. Fasten end.

FIGURE 5-10 Bandage-wrapping techniques. Always wrap from distal to proximal using spiral, circular, and figure-eight turns—Continued

Procedure **21**

Applying a Sterile Dressing

Supplies needed:
- One pair disposable exam gloves
- One pair sterile gloves
- Cleansing solution
- Plastic bag for used supplies
- Sterile gauze pads or other dressing
- Tape or bandage material

1. Perform your beginning procedure actions.
2. Holding gentle traction on the skin, loosen the tape by pulling the ends toward the wound, and then remove the dressing. Discard it in the plastic bag.
3. Cleanse and rinse the wound as ordered. If the wound appears abnormal or infected, notify your supervisor.
4. Remove the gloves and discard in the plastic bag.

5. Wash your hands or use alcohol-based hand cleaner.
6. Set up your sterile field and prepare sterile dressing supplies. Arrange the field so that you do not have to cross over it when reaching for supplies.
7. Cut the tape, if used. Place on the edge of the overbed table, if permitted by your facility policy.
8. Apply sterile gloves.
9. Pick up sterile dressings, holding them only by the corners. Center them over the wound.
10. Tape the dressing securely in place, or cover with a bandage (Procedure 20). You may remove your gloves to apply the tape, if desired.
11. Perform your procedure completion actions.

MANAGING WOUNDS WITH DRAINS

Drains may be placed in wounds during surgical procedures. These will drain fluids that collect below the skin. The drain exits the skin through a small incision and may be sutured in place. Some drains are hollow and empty directly to the outside of the body. This type of drain requires additional layers of gauze because the drainage does not collect in a receptacle. Others are connected to closed containers for collecting fluids, and must be emptied. Care of the device varies with physician orders and the type of drain used. Use sterile technique when managing drains. Consider the drain a portal of entry through which the patient can contract an infection. Always apply the principles of standard precautions. Observations of drains to make and report are listed in the Observe & Report box.

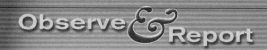

Observe & Report

Drain Observations to Report to the Nurse

- Drain is not intact or not patent
- Drain appears blocked, dislodged, or kinked
- Surrounding skin appears abnormal (erosion, red, hot, swollen, macerated)
- Drainage is eroding surrounding, healthy skin
- Drainage is purulent, cloudy, or foul-smelling
- Drainage color changes or appears abnormal
- Amount of drainage decreases markedly or stops entirely
- Amount of drainage increases markedly
- Patient has fever, tachycardia, hypotension
- Urinary output decreases

Procedure 22

Applying a Dressing Around a Drain

Supplies needed:
- One pair disposable exam gloves
- Two to Three pairs sterile gloves
- Gown, mask, and eye protection if copious drainage or splashing of blood or body fluids is anticipated
- Plastic bag for used supplies
- Cleansing solution
- Small sterile bowl (optional)
- Sterile forceps (optional)
- Sterile towel or drape
- Sterile cotton applicators (optional)
- Sterile gauze pads or other dressings
- Sterile precut drain gauze
- Tape or bandage material

1. Perform your beginning procedure actions.
2. Holding gentle traction on the skin, loosen the tape by pulling the ends toward the wound, and then gently remove the dressing.
3. Cleanse and rinse the skin surrounding the incision, as ordered. If the wound appears abnormal or infected, notify your supervisor. Visually check the drain to ensure that it is attached to the skin securely. Avoid disturbing the drain at this time. Cleanse only the wound.
4. Remove your gloves and discard them in the plastic bag.
5. Wash your hands or use an alcohol-based hand cleaner.
6. Set up your sterile field and prepare sterile dressing supplies. Pour liquid solution into the sterile basin, if necessary. Arrange the field so that you do not have to cross over it when reaching for supplies.
7. Cut the tape, if used. Place on the edge of the overbed table, if permitted by your facility policy.
8. Apply sterile gloves.
9. Cleanse the incision itself, as ordered. Use a sterile applicator or gauze sponge. Wipe from cleanest to less clean, in a single downward stroke. Discard the applicator or gauze sponge. If another is needed, use a

(continues)

Procedure 22, *continued*

Applying a Dressing Around a Drain

second applicator. Avoid contaminating the solution with a used applicator.

10. Rinse the skin.

11. Pat dry with a gauze sponge, if necessary.

12. Cleanse the area surrounding the drain. Use a circular motion, beginning at the center and working outward (**Figure 5-11**). Handle the drain as little as possible. Lift it using a sterile applicator or your finger.

13. Apply at least two layers of precut drain gauze, or as ordered. Cover with two layers of uncut gauze.

14. If your gloves are visibly contaminated with drainage, remove them, wash your hands, and reapply new sterile gloves before proceeding.

15. Pick up the sterile cover dressings by holding them only by the corners. Center them over the wound and drain, or dress each area separately, according to location and physician's orders.

16. Tape the dressing securely in place.

17. Perform your procedure completion actions.

(Also see Appendix D, "Caring for a Patient with a T-Tube.")

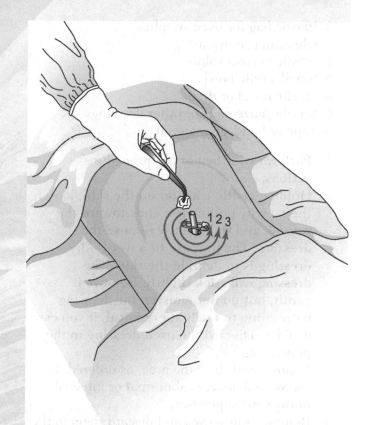

FIGURE 5-11 Begin close to the drain, working outward in full or half circles.

WET-TO-DRY DRESSINGS

Wet-to-dry dressings are used for healing surgical incisions. They are occasionally used for removing necrotic tissue from pressure ulcers. This is a dated method of treatment, and other, less traumatic methods are now more commonly used. "Damp to dry" might be a more accurate name for this type of dressing. The dressing is damp, but is not dripping wet when it is applied to the wound. This is a sterile procedure. Remember that a sterile field is contaminated if it gets wet. Avoid contaminating sterile items with solution or wet items.

Procedure 23

Changing Wet-to-Dry Dressings

Supplies needed:

▸ One pair disposable exam gloves
▸ One pair sterile gloves

▸ Gown, mask, and eye protection if copious drainage or splashing of blood or body fluids is anticipated

(continues)

Procedure 23, *continued*

Changing Wet-to-Dry Dressings

- Plastic bag for used supplies
- Cleansing solution
- Sterile normal saline
- Small sterile bowl
- Sterile towel or drape
- Sterile gauze pads or other dressings
- Tape or bandage material

1. Perform your beginning procedure actions.
2. Holding gentle traction on the skin, loosen the tape by pulling the ends toward the wound, and then gently remove the dressing. The purpose of a wet-to-dry dressing is to debride the skin. The dressing will stick slightly. Remove it gently, but do not moisten the dressing with saline to facilitate removal, if you can avoid it. Discard the used dressing in the plastic bag.
3. Cleanse and rinse the area, as ordered. If the wound appears abnormal or infected, notify your supervisor.
4. Remove your gloves and discard them in the plastic bag.
5. Wash your hands or use an alcohol-based hand cleaner.
6. Set up your sterile field and prepare sterile dressing supplies. Pour liquid solution into the sterile basin, if necessary. Arrange the field so that you do not have to cross over it when reaching for supplies.
7. Place sterile gauze sponges in the basin and pour sterile normal saline over them. The gauze may be packaged in a plastic tray. The inside of the tray is sterile, and saline may be poured into this container, if desired.

8. Cut the tape, if used. Place on the edge of the overbed table, if permitted by your facility policy.
9. Apply sterile gloves.
10. Cleanse the incision itself, as ordered. Use a sterile applicator or gauze sponge. Wipe from cleanest to less clean, in a single downward stroke. Discard the applicator or gauze sponge. If another is needed, use a second applicator. Avoid contaminating the solution with a used applicator.
11. Pick up the moist gauze sponges, one at a time. Squeeze them so they are damp and not dripping. Open and unfold the dressings. Avoid touching other surfaces or the patient's skin when opening the gauze sponges. Place the dressings over the wound. Cover the wound completely.
12. Pick up the sterile cover dressings, holding them only by the corners. Cover the damp dressings and wound completely.
13. Tape the dressing or bandage securely in place (**Figure 5-12**).
14. Perform your procedure completion actions.

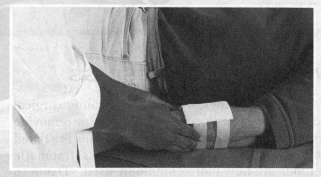

FIGURE 5-12 Tape the dry, outer dressing in place.

TRANSPARENT FILM AND HYDROCOLLOID DRESSINGS

Transparent film dressings are adhesive membranes of various sizes and thicknesses. Select a dressing size that allows at least 1¼ inch of dressing surrounding the entire wound. The dressing is eas-ily molded over various parts of the body. These dressings are waterproof and protect the wound from bacteria. They maintain a moist environment that promotes healing.

One benefit is that the dressings are changed infrequently: every three to seven days or according to physician's orders. Transparent dressings are used for minor pressure ulcers and superficial injuries such as abrasions, blisters, and wounds on elbows, heels, and flat surfaces. They work well as a secondary dressing (cover dressing) instead of tape over a gauze dressing, and promote a moist wound environment, which enhances and promotes healing and debrides superficial necrotic tissue. They should never be used if infection is present or suspected. Some of the newer transparent films are marked specifically for IV use. These were designed to promote visualization, while keeping intravenous insertion sites dry. *Never cover a wound with a dressing designed strictly for intravenous use.*

Because these dressings are transparent, the nurse can evaluate progress in wound healing. No cover dressing is used. They are not recommended for infected or draining wounds. Transparent dressings are not used for patients with very fragile skin, as they increase the risk of skin tears. Patients can bathe or shower with a transparent dressing in place. Some types are difficult to handle and stick together after the paper backing is removed.

Hydrocolloid dressings are made of materials such as gelatin and pectin. They are self-adhesive and come in various sizes and thicknesses. They conform to areas that are difficult to dress with other types of dressings and bandages. Select a dressing size that allows at least 1¼ inch of dressing surrounding the entire wound. Hydrocolloids provide a moist environment for wound healing. The dressings are used for pressure ulcers and some other wounds. They can be used for wounds with light to moderate drainage. Hydrocolloid powders and pastes may be used with the dressing to increase absorbency. The dressing will debride necrotic tissue. Hydrocolloids should not be used on patients with fragile skin. They are not used on deep or infected wounds, or on wounds in which tendon or bone is exposed. The dressing is left in place for up to seven days. The frequency of dressing change is determined by physician's order and type of dressing. Some hydrocolloids curl at the edges and must be taped. They protect the wound from contamination and require no cover dressing. You cannot see through this type of dressing, so the nurse cannot assess the wound with a hydrocolloid dressing in place.

Check with your supervisor if the patient is allergic to adhesive tape before applying a transparent film or hydrocolloid dressing. Some patients with tape allergies can use these dressings successfully. Others have allergic reactions. A rash, hives, redness, and heat in the area are signs of an allergic reaction to the dressing. Report these signs to the RN. Overall, the incidence of allergies to these dressings is low.

Procedure 24

Applying a Transparent Film Dressing

Supplies needed:
- Two pairs disposable exam gloves
- Normal saline or cleansing solution
- Sterile gauze sponges
- Transparent dressing
- Plastic bag for used supplies

1. Perform your beginning procedure actions.
2. If placing the dressing for the first time, clipping or shaving the hair may be necessary. Check with your supervisor. Remove oil from skin surrounding the wound, if present, with alcohol. Avoid contacting an open wound with alcohol. Allow to dry.
3. Apply disposable exam gloves.
4. Holding gentle traction on the skin, press down on the skin, then loosen the adhesive in one corner, and remove the dressing by peeling it back. Stretch the dressing horizontally, gently lifting it over the open area. The stretching helps to break the adhesive bond. Always remove the dressing by pulling in the direction of hair growth. If the skin is not hairy, the corners on opposite sides of the dressing can be lifted. Stretch the dressing from the edges toward the center and lift off. Discard in the plastic bag.
5. Cleanse the wound with normal saline or skin cleansing solution, as ordered. Rinse.
6. Pat the skin dry with sterile gauze sponges.

(continues)

Procedure **24**, *continued*

Applying a Transparent Film Dressing

7. Remove gloves and discard in plastic bag.
8. Wash your hands or use alcohol-based hand cleaner.
9. Open the package by peeling the tabs back. Remove the dressing.
10. Grasp the tabs on the underside of the dressing and peel them back approximately one inch.

11. Center the dressing over the wound, then gently lower it, smoothing the center portion in place.
12. Peel away the backing paper slowly from one side at a time, while gently smoothing the film in place. Gently smooth out wrinkles as you go.
13. Perform your procedure completion actions.

Procedure **25**

Applying a Hydrocolloid Dressing

Supplies needed:
- Two pairs disposable exam gloves
- Normal saline or cleansing solution
- Sterile gauze sponges
- Hydrocolloid dressing
- Adhesive or other bandage tape, if needed
- Plastic bag for used supplies

1. Perform your beginning procedure actions.
2. If placing the dressing for the first time, clipping or shaving the hair may be necessary. Check with your supervisor. Remove oil from skin surrounding the wound, if present, with alcohol. Avoid contacting an open wound with alcohol. Allow to dry.
3. Apply disposable exam gloves.
4. Holding gentle traction on the skin, press down on the skin, loosening the adhesive in one corner. Continue pressing and lifting around the edges of the dressing until all are loose. Carefully peel back the remainder of the dressing, in the direction of hair growth. Discard in the plastic bag.

5. Cleanse the wound with normal saline or skin cleansing solution, as ordered. Rinse.
6. Pat the skin dry with sterile gauze sponges.
7. Remove your gloves and discard them in the plastic bag.
8. Wash your hands or use alcohol-based hand cleaner.
9. Open the package by peeling the tabs back. Remove the dressing.
10. Separate the backing paper on the back side of the dressing. Peel back approximately one inch.
11. Center the dressing over the wound, then gently lower it, smoothing the center portion in place.
12. Peel away the backing paper slowly from one side at a time, while gently smoothing the dressing in place. Gently smooth out wrinkles as you go.
13. Place the palm of your hand over the dressing and hold for 30 to 45 seconds. This warms the dressing, promoting adherence.
14. Tape the edges, if necessary.
15. Perform your procedure completion actions.

PIN CARE

Metal pins may be used to hold the bone in place in some surgical procedures. These pins may protrude from the skin, and are often attached to traction. The pins must be kept clean to prevent infection. An infection on the skin near the pin insertion site can move down from the skin into the underlying tissues and bone. This will cause serious problems. Some physicians order dressings over the pin insertion site.

After the site is healed, the physician allows it to remain open to the air. Pin care is done to prevent infection. Although it has been performed for years, no standard guidelines describe the procedure. The guidelines presented here were published in a nursing journal in 1999,[1] but your agency or facility may use a different procedure. The author recommends use of sterile technique while the patient is hospitalized. Notify the nurse if signs and symptoms of infection, such as redness, heat, edema, tenderness, and purulent drainage, are present. Report loosened pins. Also, report to the RN if crusts are present at the pin insertion site. Some facilities remove these to promote free drainage. Others leave the crusts in place, believing they prevent infection from entering the insertion site.

[1]McKenzie, L. L. (1999). In search of a standard for pin site care. *Orthopaedic Nursing, 18*(2), 73–77.

Procedure 26

Pin Care

Supplies needed:
- Sterile gloves
- Sterile normal saline or prescribed cleansing solution
- Sterile applicators
- Sterile gauze dressings, if ordered
- Plastic bag for used supplies

1. Perform your beginning procedure actions.
2. Moisten an applicator with normal saline or prescribed cleansing solution.
3. Beginning with the skin closest to the insertion site, wipe the skin in a circle around the pin. Discard the applicator.
4. With a second moistened applicator, wipe the skin around the pin in a second circle, working outward from the pin insertion site. Discard the applicator.
5. Continue wiping outward, using one applicator for each circle, until you have cleansed a 1½-inch area surrounding the insertion site. Use each applicator for one circle only. Avoid contaminating the cleansing solution with used applicators.
6. Apply sterile dressings as ordered. A healed pin insertion site may be left open to the air.
7. Perform your procedure completion actions.

REMOVING SUTURES AND STAPLES

Sutures and staples are used to close surgical wounds and large lacerations. The sutures used to hold muscle and tissue below the skin surface are made of absorbable material, and are not removed. Sutures and staples holding the skin surface together are removed in 7 to 10 days, depending on the location of the wound and the progress of healing. Leaving them in longer increases the risk of infection. **Interrupted sutures** (Figure 5-13A) are most commonly used. In this type of suture, each thread is tied off and knotted separately. In **continuous sutures** (Figure 5-13B), a single thread is used to close an open area of skin. Staples may be used to close abdominal and chest wounds. Patients may be apprehensive about suture and staple removal because of pain. Explain that there may be slight discomfort when each is removed, but it is not painful.

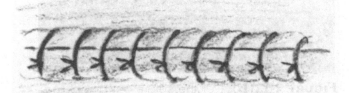

(A)   **(B)**

FIGURE 5-13 (A) Interrupted sutures (B) Continuous sutures

Procedure 27

Removing Sutures

Supplies needed:

- ▶ Suture removal kit or sterile suture removal scissors and sterile forceps
- ▶ Sterile normal saline solution or other cleansing agent
- ▶ Sterile gauze for wound cleansing and removing sutures from forceps
- ▶ Sterile dressings as necessary for covering the wound after suture removal
- ▶ Disposable exam gloves
- ▶ Sterile gloves
- ▶ Butterfly® bandage, steri-strips®, or other skin adhesive, as needed
- ▶ Plastic bag for used supplies

1. Perform your beginning procedure actions.
2. Open the suture removal kit and set up dressing supplies.
3. Apply exam gloves.
4. Remove the dressing and discard in the plastic bag.
5. Remove your gloves and discard them in the plastic bag.
6. Wash your hands or use alcohol-based hand cleaner.
7. Apply sterile gloves.

8. Cleanse the incision line with normal saline or prescribed cleansing solution.
9. Remove every other suture by lifting the suture up, away from the skin, with the tweezers. Cut the suture close to the skin (Figure 5-14A).
10. With the tweezers, lift the suture up by the knot, and pull it through the skin in one piece (Figure 5-14B).
11. Discard used sutures on a gauze pad. Then discard all the sutures and the pad in a plastic bag after all sutures are removed.
12. Remove every other suture. Evaluate the skin to determine if the edges are separating. If so, stop and notify the nurse before proceeding. If the skin separates at any time during the procedure, notify the nurse.
13. Cleanse the skin with the skin cleanser, allowing it to dry.
14. Apply a butterfly® or steri-strip® to the skin where each suture was removed.
15. Remove the remaining sutures.
16. Apply a butterfly® or steri-strip® to the skin where each suture was removed.
17. Dress the wound as ordered.
18. Perform your procedure completion actions.

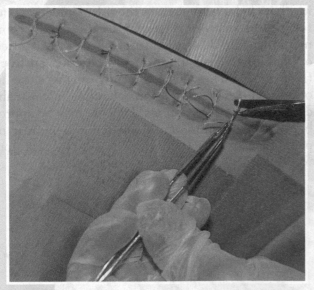

FIGURE 5-14(A) Cut the suture close to the skin.

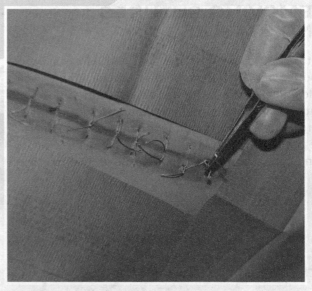

FIGURE 5-14(B) Pull the suture out by holding the knot with the tweezers.

Procedure 28

Removing Staples

Supplies needed:

- Staple removal kit or sterile staple extractor
- Sterile normal saline solution or other cleansing agent
- Sterile gauze for wound cleansing and removing staples from forceps
- Sterile dressings as necessary for covering the wound after staple removal
- Disposable exam gloves
- Sterile gloves
- Butterfly® bandage, steri-strips® or other skin adhesive, as needed
- Plastic bag for used supplies

1. Perform your beginning procedure actions.
2. Open the staple removal kit and set up dressing supplies.
3. Apply exam gloves.
4. Remove the dressing and discard in the plastic bag.
5. Remove your gloves and discard them in the plastic bag.
6. Wash your hands or use alcohol-based hand cleaner.
7. Apply sterile gloves.
8. Cleanse the incision line with normal saline or prescribed cleansing solution.
9. Slide the staple remover under the staple (Figure 5-15A). Squeeze the handles (Figure 5-15B). Gently lift the staple out.
10. Discard used staples on a gauze pad, then discard all the staples and the pad in the plastic bag after all staples are removed.
11. Remove every other staple. Evaluate the skin to determine if the edges are separating. If so, stop and notify the nurse before proceeding. If the skin separates at any time during the procedure, notify the nurse.
12. Cleanse the skin with the skin cleanser, allowing it to dry.
13. Apply a butterfly® or steri-strip® to the skin where each staple was removed.
14. Remove the remaining staples.
15. Apply a butterfly® or steri-strip® to the skin where the remaining staples were removed.
16. Dress the wound as ordered.
17. Perform your procedure completion actions.

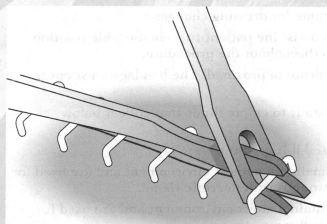

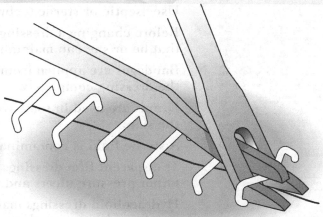

FIGURE 5-15(A) Insert the staple extractor gently.

FIGURE 5-15(B) Squeeze the handles, then lift the staple up.

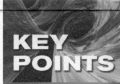

KEY POINTS

▶ The skin is the largest organ of the body. It protects underlying structures, excretes wastes, and helps regulate body temperature.

▶ The outer, protective skin layer is the epidermis. Beneath this layer is the dermis, which contains nerves, hair follicles, sweat glands, and oil glands. Beneath these two layers is subcutaneous tissue or fat. This layer serves as a covering for muscles, tendons, and bone.

▶ Systemic factors affecting wound healing are age, nutritional status, body build, presence or absence of chronic disease, circulatory problems, weakened immune system, and radiation therapy.

▶ Good nutrition and hydration affect wound healing.

▶ Local factors affecting wound healing are moist wound environment, infection, necrotic tissue, foreign objects in the wound, trauma, edema, pressure on the wound, and incontinence and presence of excretions contaminating the wound.

▶ Necrotic tissue must be removed before wound healing will take place.

▶ When removing a dressing, note the color, odor, and amount of drainage.

▶ Normal saline is a safe and effective wound cleanser. Some wound cleansers are cytotoxic.

▶ Read the product directions carefully for the cleanser you are using.

▶ Cleanse wounds from most clean to less clean areas, using a single stroke. Use a clean gauze pad for each stroke.

▶ Change gloves and wash hands after removing the soiled dressing, before applying a new dressing.

▶ Some patients have tape allergies and need a special hypoallergenic tape.

▶ Dressings are placed on the skin and wound for protection. Bandages are used to hold dressings in place, reduce edema, and support body parts.

▶ A break in the skin increases the risk of infection.

▶ Use aseptic or sterile technique for dressing changes.

▶ Before changing a dressing, assist the patient to a comfortable position that he or she can maintain throughout the procedure.

▶ Bandages are applied from distal to proximal. The bandage must cover the dressing completely.

▶ Drains are used in some wounds to empty fluids that collect below the skin.

▶ A sterile field is contaminated if it gets wet.

▶ Transparent film dressings maintain a moist environment and are used for minor pressure ulcers and wounds with necrotic tissue.

▶ Hydrocolloid dressings maintain a moist environment and are used for uninfected pressure ulcers and some other wounds.

▶ Pin care is done at the insertion site of metal pins, to prevent infection.

▶ Sutures and staples usually remain in place for 7 to 10 days before removal.

CLINICAL APPLICATIONS

1. Mr. Hoover, a 72-year-old patient, picked at his breakfast and lunch. He ate 25 percent of breakfast and 35 percent of lunch. He tells you he just "didn't feel like eating." Mr. Hoover has a large pressure ulcer on his right hip and an incision from recent abdominal surgery. Explain to Mr. Hoover why eating his meals is important. Will you report Mr. Hoover's appetite to the RN? Why or why not?

2. You are doing daily dressing changes to Miss Hayes's pressure ulcer. Today you notice some black tissue around the edges of the wound. What could this be? Should you report this change in wound appearance to the RN?

3. When you perform pin care on the insertion site of Mr. Tsai's skeletal traction, you observe a large amount of purulent drainage that appears to be coming from the underside of the pin. What action will you take?

4. You are changing the dressing on Mrs. Strong's abdominal incision. When you cleanse the incision with normal saline, Mrs. Strong asks you to use hydrogen peroxide instead. She says she always uses this to clean wounds to prevent infection. How will you respond to this patient? What action will you take?

5. You will be removing Mrs. Hernandez's sutures. She confides in you that she fears it will hurt. How will you respond to her concerns?

C H A P T E R   R E V I E W

Multiple-Choice Questions

Select the one best answer.

1. Which of the following affect wound healing?
   a. hunger
   b. thirst
   c. nausea and vomiting
   d. presence of infection

2. Wounds heal best in a:
   a. dry environment.
   b. moist environment.
   c. wet environment.
   d. wet-to-dry environment.

3. Necrotic tissue is:
   a. dead, devitalized tissue.
   b. an indication that the wound is healing.
   c. a sign of infection.
   d. swollen tissue.

4. When removing a soiled dressing:
   a. pull the ends of the tape away from the wound.
   b. pull the tape in the direction away from hair growth.
   c. pull the edges of the tape toward the wound.
   d. loosen the tape with adhesive remover first.

5. You are removing a dressing that is sticking to the center of the incision line. You should:
   a. quickly pull the dressing away from the incision.
   b. loosen the dressing with adhesive remover.
   c. notify the RN immediately.
   d. pour a small amount of normal saline on the area.

6. A product that is cytotoxic:
   a. is safe and effective for wound care.
   b. is harmful to healing tissue.
   c. should be used when caring for infected wounds.
   d. should be used when caring for wounds with eschar.

7. When cleansing a wound, always:
   a. work from the wound outward.
   b. work from the area surrounding the wound inward.
   c. scrub back and forth gently to remove pathogens.
   d. apply an alcohol-based cleanser.

8. Signs and symptoms of infection include:
   a. red tissue.
   b. black tissue.
   c. drainage with an odor.
   d. clear wound drainage.

9. A dressing:
   a. holds the bandage in place.
   b. is used only if pressure is needed on the wound.
   c. contacts the wound directly.
   d. is never used if infection or necrosis is present.

10. A hydrocolloid or transparent film should not be used:
    a. for minor pressure ulcers.
    b. on the heel or ankle.
    c. on the buttocks.
    d. in the presence of infection.

E X P L O R I N G   T H E   W E B

AHCPR Clinical Practice Guidelines: Pressure Ulcers in Adults: Prediction and Prevention	http://www.ncbi.nlm.nih.gov
AHCPR Clinical Practice Guidelines: Treatment of Pressure Ulcers	http://www.ncbi.nlm.nih.gov
Applying a Dressing to a Minor Skin Tear	http://www.in.gov
Australian Wound Management Association (AWMA)	http://www.awma.com.au
Convatec Skin and Wound Care	http://www.convatec.com
Decubitus Foundation	http://www.decubitus.org
Dermatology Image Atlas	http://dermatlas.med.jhmi.edu
External Fixators and Care of Your Pin Sites	http://www.newcastle-hospitals.org.uk
How to Remove Surgical Sutures and Staples	http://www.findarticles.com
How to Use Transparent Films	http://www.findarticles.com
Importance of Nutrition in Wound Care	http://www.woundnutrition.com
Information About Decubitus Ulcers	http://www.ldhpmed.com
National Pressure Ulcer Advisory Panel	http://www.npuap.org
Nursing Issues in Therapy of Chronic Osteomyelitis—Pin Care	http://www.uchc.edu
Nursing the Patient with an External Fixator	http://www.nursing-standard.co.uk
Pin Care	http://patienteducation.upmc.com
Practicing Smart Wound Care	http://www.infectioncontroltoday.com
Procedure for Pin Care	http://www-nmcp.med.navy.mil
Removing Stitches	http://www.emedicinehealth.com
Removing Sutures and Staples	http://www.findarticles.com
Suture and Staple Removal	http://www.spaceref.com
3M Skin Health—Skin Health Products and Practices at 3m.com	http://www.3m.com
Transparent Film Dressing Procedure	http://devweb3.vip.ohio-state.edu
Transparent Film Dressings	http://wound.smith-nephew.com/uk
When to Use Transparent Films	http://www.findarticles.com
WOCN Position Statement Clean Versus Sterile	http://www.wocn.org
World Wide Wounds	http://www.worldwidewounds.com
Wound Care/Dressing Protocol—Skin Tear	http://www.kendallhq.com
Wound Care Product Selection	http://www.uspharmacist.com
Wound Glossary	http://www.edu.rcsed.ac.uk
Wound Healing	http://www.lef.org
Wound, Ostomy and Continence Nurses Society (WOCN)	http://www.wocn.org
Wounds Research	http://www.woundsresearch.com
Wounds1.com	http://www.woundcare1.com

CHAPTER

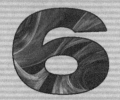

6

Phlebotomy

OBJECTIVES:

After reading this chapter, you should be able to:

- Spell and define key terms.
- List some factors that affect the condition of the veins.
- Describe how to select a vein for venipuncture.
- Describe how to cleanse and puncture the skin.
- Explain why standard precautions are used during phlebotomy procedures, and list the PPE to wear.
- Explain the similarities and differences between the vacuum-tube and syringe and needle methods of drawing blood.
- List eight precautions to take regarding venipuncture site selection.
- List two common complications of venipuncture.
- Describe the purpose of a centrifuge and list precautions to take when using a centrifuge.
- Demonstrate how to:
  - apply a tourniquet, dilate a vein, and perform a venipuncture.
  - collect a specimen using the vacuum-tube system, needle and syringe, and butterfly and syringe methods.
  - collect a blood culture.
  - collect a specimen from a capillary.
  - measure bleeding time.

PHLEBOTOMY

Phlebotomy means collecting blood. **Venipuncture** is the act of puncturing a vein with a needle. Venipuncture is done for drawing blood, starting intravenous infusions (IVs), and administering some medications. You will perform venipuncture for the purpose of collecting blood. Before performing this procedure, check the requisition slip and make sure you understand the procedure you will be using. Gather all necessary equipment or supplies in advance.

To perform venipuncture, you must first select a vein. Age, illness, dehydration, and previous needlesticks all affect the condition of the veins. Young adults often have many veins to choose from. Veins in the elderly are often limited. They may roll or break upon puncture. Avoid drawing blood from the legs and feet in the elderly. This increases the risk of **thrombophlebitis,** or inflammation of a vein with blood clot formation. Finding a vein in children may also be difficult. Children often move during this procedure. Ask another PCT to assist you in immobilizing the child.

> ### HEALTH CARE ALERT
>
> Prioritize your work if you must draw specimens from multiple patients. "Stat" specimens have the highest priority, and should be obtained immediately. The next priority is patients who are fasting and cannot eat breakfast until blood has been drawn. Routine requests are your third priority.

Cleansing the Skin

Before puncturing the skin, you must prepare it by cleansing it with alcohol or povidone-iodine. Alcohol is most commonly used to disinfect the skin. However, if you are drawing a blood culture or test for blood alcohol, povidone-iodine must be used. Many facilities use a product called chlorhexidine, which is an excellent product for eliminating germs, for all skin punctures.

The povidone-iodine discolors the skin, making it more difficult to visualize the veins. Avoid wiping it off with alcohol before drawing the specimen. However, you may cleanse the skin with alcohol to remove the iodine after the specimen is collected. If you are removing the skin prep after the procedure, avoid wiping the needle insertion site directly, as this will cause discomfort.

To prepare the skin, begin wiping in the area of the proposed needle insertion site. Wipe in a circular motion, moving outward with each circle. Prepare an area 2 to 3 inches in diameter surrounding the needle insertion site. Allow the skin to dry thoroughly before beginning the procedure.

Opening Packages

Needles, lancets, and other items used for drawing blood are packaged in sterile packages or plastic tubes. Do not use a package that is torn, damaged, has become wet, or is past the expiration date. To open the package, hold the top edge with the thumb and forefinger of each hand, and peel it back. To open a tube, twist the top until the paper seal is broken. Avoid touching the needle, as that will cause contamination. Also, avoid touching the open hub end where the needle connects to a syringe. This will also cause contamination. The needle must be kept sterile for a blood draw. If it is accidentally contaminated, discard and replace it. If your first attempt at entering the vein is not successful, use a new needle or setup before continuing. Remember, you should not change the needle with your hands, so you may have to obtain a new tube holder, depending on the type of system and needle being used.

Needles

A hollow needle (**Figure 6-1**) is used any time a vein is entered. With some intravenous devices, the needle is withdrawn after a plastic catheter is threaded into the vein. However, a needle is always necessary to puncture the skin. Needles come in a variety of sizes, from very small to very large. The length of the needle

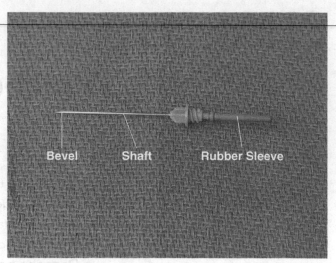

FIGURE 6-1 The needle for a vacuum-tube system is sharp at both ends. One end pierces the patient's vein. The other pierces the vacuum tube, causing it to fill with blood.

also varies. The gauge of the needle determines the inside diameter of the needle, or the **lumen.** The size of the lumen of the needle decreases as the gauge number increases. Thus, a 12-gauge needle is very large, and a 27-gauge needle is tiny. The **bevel** is the slant or inclination at the end of the needle.

Blood is a thick solution, so larger needles are necessary to withdraw a sample from the body. Drawing blood through a needle with a small lumen will cause **hemolysis,** breaking of the fragile blood cells. In most situations, a 20- to 23-gauge needle is used. The needle is 1 or 1½ inches long. The length of the needle is selected by the user. To penetrate the vein, the needle is inserted just below the skin. The length affects your ability to position the needle. Try both lengths and select the one that is most comfortable to use. Select a safety needle (**Figure 6-2**) whenever possible.

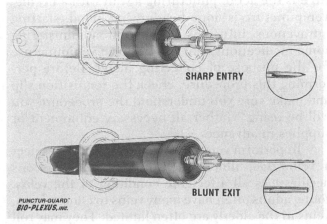

FIGURE 6-2 A safety blood collection needle (Courtesy of BioPlexus, Inc., Tolland, CT)

The same technique is used whether entering a vein for venipuncture or starting an intravenous infusion. Always insert the needle in the direction of the heart. Never insert the needle facing the distal extremity. Sometimes you will pierce the skin, but be unsuccessful in piercing the vein. If you cannot enter the vein readily, withdraw the needle and try again at another site. Avoid digging for the vein, as this may cause damage to nerves and blood vessels. On your next attempt, use a new, sterile needle. Never puncture the skin twice with the same needle. Never recap a used needle. Needles are always discarded uncapped in the puncture-resistant sharps container.

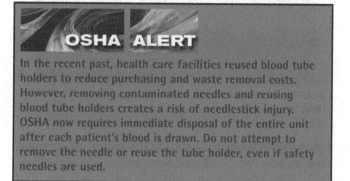

OSHA ALERT

In the recent past, health care facilities reused blood tube holders to reduce purchasing and waste removal costs. However, removing contaminated needles and reusing blood tube holders creates a risk of needlestick injury. OSHA now requires immediate disposal of the entire unit after each patient's blood is drawn. Do not attempt to remove the needle or reuse the tube holder, even if safety needles are used.

STANDARD PRECAUTIONS

Always apply the principles of standard precautions when performing the procedures discussed in this chapter. Most health care facilities require workers

to wear long-sleeved lab coats or gowns when drawing blood. These must be fluid-resistant. Always wear gloves. Pull the cuffs of the gloves over the cuffs of your sleeves. Follow your facility policy and the RN's directions. Wear a gown, mask, and eye protection if this is your preference, facility policy, or if you have reason to believe that splashing or spraying of blood will occur. The risk of contamination is increased if you must transfer blood from one container to another, such as from a syringe to a test tube. When performing this procedure, wearing full personal protective equipment (PPE) is recommended.

METHODS OF DRAWING BLOOD

Several different methods are used for drawing blood. One method involves using a vacuum tube, often called a **vacutainer,** with a needle attached (**Figure 6-3**). This is the safest and easiest method. Select a special safety needle and tube holder (**Figure 6-4**) whenever possible to reduce your risk of injury. Blood can also be withdrawn using a needle and syringe. Check with the RN if you have questions about which method to use.

Vacuum-Tube Method

In this method of drawing blood, a dual-headed needle is attached to a plastic holder. A tourniquet is applied to the arm and the needle is inserted into

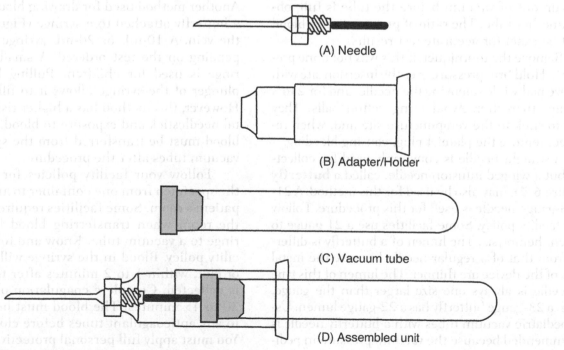

(A) Needle

(B) Adapter/Holder

(C) Vacuum tube

(D) Assembled unit

FIGURE 6-3 Parts of the vacuum tube for drawing blood

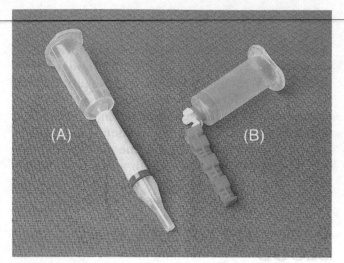

FIGURE 6-4 (A) Safety needle and holder (B) Locking cover

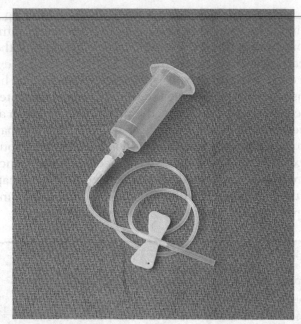

FIGURE 6-5 A butterfly needle can be used for drawing blood.

the vein. Upon entering a vein, stabilize the needle holder so it does not move, and push the inner end of the needle through a test tube.

The rubber stopper on the end of a vacuum test tube is color-coded. You must draw each test using the proper color tube, in the proper sequence. Set out tubes within reach, in the proper order, before beginning. The vacuum inside the test tube allows blood to flow freely, filling the tube. When the tube is full, stabilize the needle holder and gently remove the test tube, inserting the next tube. Continue until all tubes have been filled. The tubes will fill three-quarters full. They will not fill completely. If you run out of vacuum before the tube is full, obtain another tube. The ratio of preservative to blood must be exact for accurate test results.

Remove the tourniquet, if this was not done previously. Hold firm pressure over the insertion site with a gauze pad while removing the needle, and for 2 to 3 minutes thereafter. Avoid using cotton balls. They tend to stick to the venipuncture site and, when removed, remove the platelet plug, causing bleeding.

A straight needle is commonly used for collecting, but a winged infusion needle, called a **butterfly** (**Figure 6-5**), may also be used for this method. A 21- or 23-gauge needle is used for this procedure. Follow your facility policy. Some facilities use a 21-gauge to prevent hemolysis. The lumen of a butterfly is different from that of a regular needle because the metal walls of the device are thinner. The lumen of this type of needle is always one size larger than the gauge. Thus, a 23-gauge butterfly has a 22-gauge lumen. Using pediatric vacuum tubes with a butterfly needle is recommended because the vacuum pressure in pedi-

atric tubes is lower than that in the larger, adult tubes. This makes vein collapse or specimen damage less likely. The plastic tube holders are disposable and should be discarded in the sharps container upon procedure completion. Some newer brands have needles that retract into the barrel to reduce the risk of accidental needlestick.

Syringe Method

Another method used for drawing blood is to insert a butterfly attached to a syringe (**Figure 6-6**) into the vein. A 10-mL or 20-mL syringe is used, depending on the test ordered. A smaller, 5-mL syringe is used for children. Pulling back on the plunger of the syringe allows it to fill with blood. However, this method has a higher risk of accidental needlestick and exposure to blood, because the blood must be transferred from the syringe to the vacuum tubes after the procedure.

Follow your facility policies for transferring the specimen from one container to another in the patient's room. Some facilities require you to leave the room when transferring blood from the syringe to a vacuum tube. Know and follow your facility policy. Blood in the syringe will **coagulate,** or clot, within 1 to 2 minutes after the specimen is collected. Complete coagulation occurs within 30 to 45 minutes. The blood must be transferred to any anticoagulant tubes before clotting begins. You must apply full personal protective equipment

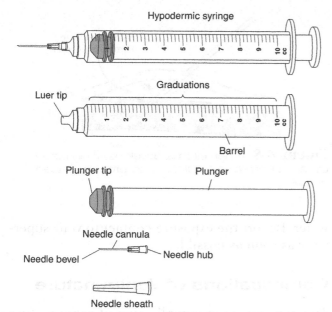

FIGURE 6-6 Parts of an assembled syringe

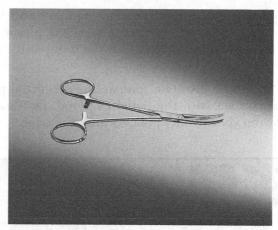

FIGURE 6-7 The Kelly clamp and other similar instruments can be used to remove needles. (Courtesy of Medline Industries, Inc., Mundelein, IL. (800) MEDLINE)

before transferring the blood. If you will be leaving the room, you must remove the needle first, to prevent accidental needlestick. To change the needle, always use an instrument. The **Kelly clamp** (Figure 6-7) is commonly used for this purpose. This is a curved clamp with teeth that grip the hub of the needle. Never change a used needle with your fingers. Replace the needle with a blood transfer device.

Precautions to Take

When drawing blood, you must take certain precautions to prevent complications or injury to the patient. You should avoid drawing blood from:

- An arm in which an intravenous solution or blood is being administered
- An infected or edematous area
- An area with a rash
- An extremity with a dialysis access device, shunt, or graft
- An existing intravenous line or heparin lock
- The affected arm of a stroke or mastectomy patient
- The site of previous injury or hematoma
- Any burned or scarred area
- The leg and foot veins, whenever possible (check with the RN before considering these veins)

Other precautions to take:

- Always use aseptic technique.
- Avoid injecting air into a vein. The venous system is a closed system, filled with blood. Accidentally injecting air can create serious problems.
- Immobilize the vein with the thumb of your opposite hand before inserting the needle.
- Position the needle with the bevel facing up.
- Always insert the needle in the direction of blood flow, facing the heart.
- Avoid sticking the patient more than twice. If you cannot puncture the vein in two needle-sticks, inform the RN.
- Keep the tourniquet on the arm for less than 2 minutes. Leaving it on longer than this increases the risk of complications. Prepare the skin, then release the tourniquet, allowing the alcohol or skin prep to dry before reapplying the tourniquet.
- Ensure that the vessel you are entering does not have a pulse. A pulse indicates that you are entering an artery.
- Remove the tourniquet as soon as blood flows freely. If blood flow is sluggish, leave the tourniquet in place, but always remove it before withdrawing the needle.
- Label all tubes after blood has been collected.
- Discard needles in a puncture-resistant container. Carry this container to the bedside with you. Never recap a used needle.

● Transport tubes of blood to the laboratory in a special test tube holder, or a sealed, plastic transport bag labeled with the biohazard emblem.

You must also take precautions to avoid personal contact with the patient's blood. Do this by following your facility policies and procedures.

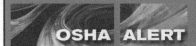

Select the equipment that best protects you. For example, if a needleless system is available, use it instead of a needle. If plastic test tubes are available instead of glass, use them. The risk of blood exposure is greater with venipuncture than with many other procedures. Always think safety and protect yourself.

Do not take shortcuts. Select the personal protective equipment appropriate to the procedure. Never recap a needle used to puncture the skin or draw blood. Drop the uncapped needle into the puncture-resistant sharps container. If you accidentally puncture your skin with a used needle, or have mucous membrane contact with a patient's blood, wash the area immediately. Use soap and water on a puncture wound, and scrub thoroughly. Flush mucous membranes well with cool, clear

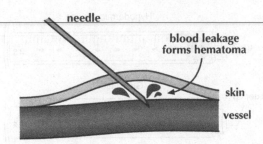

FIGURE 6-8 A hematoma develops when blood escapes from a vein due to an improperly placed needle.

water. Report the exposure contact to your supervisor as soon as possible.

Complications of Venipuncture

The most common complication of venipuncture is **hematoma** (Figure 6-8). This is a blood-filled bruise, caused when a blood vessel breaks. It may also develop if inadequate pressure is placed on the insertion site after a needle is withdrawn. To prevent hematoma, hold pressure on the needle insertion site with your gloved hand for 2 to 3 minutes with a gauze pad after the needle has been removed. You can ask the patient to hold pressure on the area, if he or she is able. Elevate the extremity and apply firm pressure to the area. Stop the procedure immediately if a hematoma develops. In-

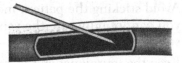

Correct — blood flows freely into the needle

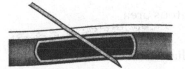

Incorrect — bevel against the upper wall impedes flow

Incorrect — bevel against the lower wall impedes flow

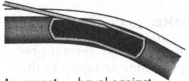

Incorrect — needle is inserted too far

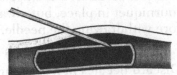

Incorrect — needle partially inserted, causing hematoma

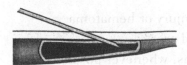

Incorrect — a collapsed vein

FIGURE 6-9 Improperly placed needles

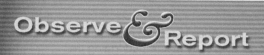

Observe & Report

Complications of Venipuncture to Report to the RN

- Bleeding from the venipuncture site
- **Ecchymosis** (bruise)
- Hematoma, a collection of blood under the skin
- Signs and symptoms of phlebitis and localized infection, including redness, swelling, or a red streak at the needle insertion site, or drainage from the venipuncture site
- Signs and symptoms of generalized infection, including malaise, fever, and chills
- Signs and symptoms of air embolus, including respiratory distress; cyanosis; weak, rapid pulse; decreased blood pressure; loss of consciousness; cardiac arrest

struct the patient not to bend the arm. Doing so will keep the vein open, causing blood to leak into the surrounding tissue and form a hematoma. Improper needle placement can also cause other problems, including collapsed veins and inability to draw blood despite having the needle in the vein (**Figure 6-9**). If the patient is taking blood-thinning medications called **anticoagulants,** maintain pressure for at least 5 minutes. Patients who take aspirin and ibuprofen regularly may also bleed for a prolonged period of time. These medications prevent blood from clotting, so it takes longer to control bleeding after a needlestick.

Infection is another complication of venipuncture. This can be serious, and is often caused by improper technique. You are entering the patient's bloodstream. Take your infection control responsibilities very seriously.

Observations that should be reported to the nurse are listed in the Observe & Report box.

SELECTING A VEIN AND PERFORMING THE VENIPUNCTURE

In most cases, the veins in the forearm are used for drawing blood (**Figure 6-10**). These veins are usually larger and straighter than those in other areas of the body. For drawing blood from adults, the veins in the **antecubital space,** or area in front of the elbow, are commonly used. If you cannot find a vein in the forearm, you may be able to use the hand. To draw blood, you must be able to see or feel a vein. Avoid probing randomly with a needle. Visualizing a vein may be easier in indirect lighting than

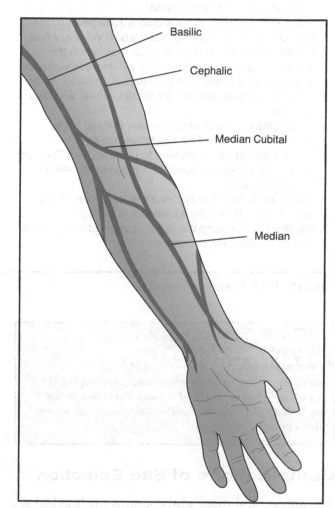

FIGURE 6-10 Veins of the forearm

in bright, direct lighting. However, some veins can be palpated but not visualized. Additional useful information for performing a venipuncture is listed in **Figure 6-11.**

- Always check the patient's allergies before beginning.
  - Make sure the patient is not allergic to latex, if a latex tourniquet is used. You must also avoid latex gloves.
  - Make sure the patient is not allergic to the iodine in a skin-prep solution.
- Monitor tourniquet position. It should be at least 2 to 3 inches away from the planned venipuncture site.
- Avoid pinching the patient's skin with the tourniquet. This is easily done in elderly patients and people with excess loose skin, such as patients who have lost weight.
- A "good" vein stands out when the tourniquet is tightened and goes down when the tourniquet is released.
  - When palpated, the vein should feel springy. If the tissue over the vein is scarred, or the vein feels hard or tough, avoid it if possible. A vein may stand out very well but be damaged. This problem commonly occurs in drug addicts and patients who have had repeated venous cannulation.
- If you are having difficulty finding a suitable vein, ask the patient. He or she may know which veins are best.
- Disinfect the proposed needle insertion site in the direction of the venous flow. This will improve vein filling by pushing the blood past the internal one-way valves.
- Use the nondominant arm for starting an IV, whenever possible.
- If **petechiae** develop under or near the site of the tourniquet, notify the RN. *Petechiae* are tiny hemorrhagic spots of pinpoint to pinhead size. They are caused by escape of blood from the vessels into the surrounding skin.
- Check the pulse after applying the tourniquet. If you cannot feel a pulse, the tourniquet is too tight. In addition to increasing the risk of complications, you will also have poor vein distention.

- Allow the antiseptic to remain on the insertion site and to air-dry completely before performing the venipuncture. Never wipe a povidone-iodine prep off with alcohol.
- Leave the tourniquet on for no more than 2 minutes; 1 minute is best. In addition to increasing the risk of complications, leaving the tourniquet on for a prolonged period increases the risk of causing hemoconcentration, which will alter the patient's lab values. Release the tourniquet after this length of time to allow veins to refill. Leave the tourniquet off for at least 2 minutes before reapplying it.
- If the patient's skin is sticky from previous use of adhesive and dressings, rub the tape with alcohol to soften the adhesive. Pick up an edge of the tape, then peel the tape back slowly in the direction in which the hair lies down.
- Avoid overfilling or underfilling the collection tube. The exact quantity of blood drawn into each tube will vary slightly with altitude, ambient temperature, and venous pressure. Fill tubes with additives completely to ensure a proper ratio of blood to additive, and then mix well to distribute the additive.
- If you are certain you are in the vein, but no blood flows into the tube, consider trying another tube before removing the needle. Occasionally tubes lose their vacuum.
- After two unsuccessful sticks, ask another worker to draw the blood. Make sure the tourniquet is removed when you are finished. Serious injury will occur if a tourniquet is left in place for a prolonged period of time.
- Use vacutainer tubes at room temperature. Protect tubes from extreme temperatures and store them in a cool place.
- Do not use expired tubes.

FIGURE 6-11 Venipuncture tips

HEALTH CARE ALERT

Gently rotate the patient's wrist while palpating the skin. The rotation will move the vein away from tendons and bones, reducing the risk of accidentally puncturing them with a needle.

Complications of Site Selection

The antecubital space also contains the brachial artery (**Figure 6-12**). You palpate the brachial pulse in this location when taking blood pressure. The patient may be injured if the artery is accidentally punctured. Arteries are usually larger and more elastic than veins. Avoid this blood vessel by checking for the presence of a pulse.

The median nerve, as well as other nerves and tendons, is also located in the antecubital space. Permanent damage can result if these structures are injured. Inserting the needle at the proper angle and not digging to locate a vein will help prevent damage to these structures. Make sure that you locate the vein before performing the needlestick. Before piercing the skin, you should be able to feel the vein, even if you cannot see it. Veins are near the skin surface, feel rubbery, and will rebound slightly when touched. They are not hard to the touch and do not pulsate.

Applying a Tourniquet

To select a vein, you must first apply a tourniquet (**Figure 6-13**). The tourniquet causes the veins to fill with blood. Apply the tourniquet tightly

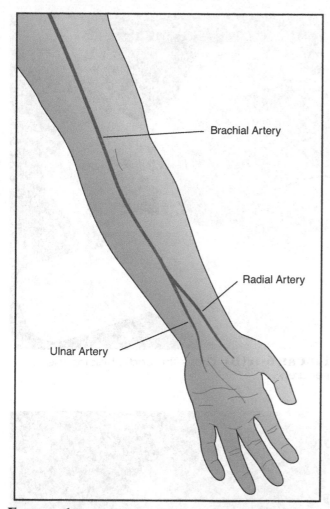

FIGURE 6-12 Arteries of the forearm

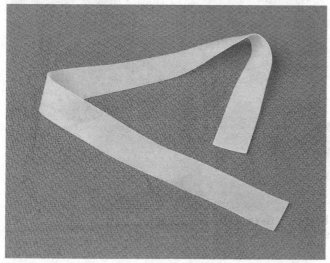

FIGURE 6-13 A latex tourniquet. Some hospitals are latex-free, so comparable nonlatex tourniquets are used.

enough to make the veins stand out. It should not be so tight that it stops the arterial blood flow. Make sure the pulse distal to the tourniquet is

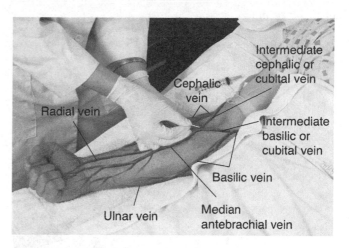

FIGURE 6-14 Carefully select the vein for venipuncture.

palpable. After you have selected a vein, release the tourniquet until you are ready to begin the procedure.

The veins in the arm are pictured in **Figure 6-14.** Extend the patient's arm and support it on the bed or other surface. Make sure the patient is comfortable and can maintain the position for the duration of the procedure. The median and cephalic veins are the safest choice. Use the basilic vein only if the median and cephalic veins cannot be located. Avoid veins on the underside of the wrist. The anatomy of this area presents a high risk of nerve damage.

Begin looking for a vein by applying the tourniquet approximately 2 to 3 inches above the elbow. Stretch the tourniquet and encircle the arm (Figure 6-15A). Cross the straps over tightly (Figure 6-15B), holding them in place with your nondominant thumb. Tuck the lower strap (Figure 6-15C) under the top strap and forward, forming a loop, with the ends facing the shoulder (Figure 6-15D). Check the radial pulse. If you cannot palpate the pulse, the tourniquet is too tight. Release it and reapply.

PROCEDURE ALERT

A "good" vein stands out when the tourniquet is applied, and immediately goes down when the tourniquet is removed. Touch is more important than sight when selecting a vein. If possible, use a vein that feels "springy" to touch. Some veins stand out well but are not suitable. This is particularly true in patients who have experienced repeated needlesticks.

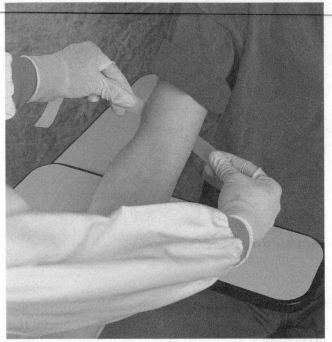

FIGURE 6-15(A) Wrap the tourniquet around the arm.

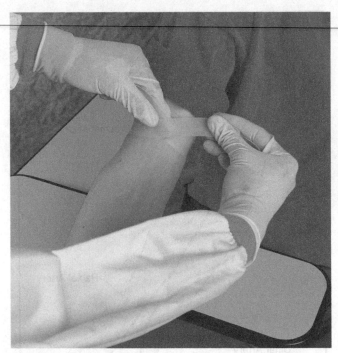

FIGURE 6-15(B) Cross the ends, holding them securely.

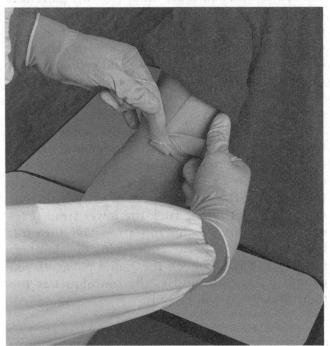

FIGURE 6-15(C) Tuck one end under the other, forming a loop.

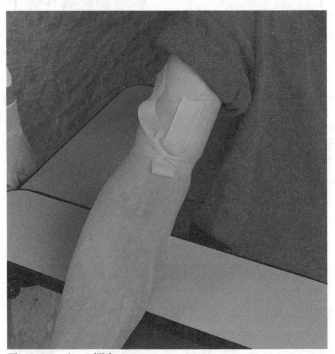

FIGURE 6-15(D) The ends of the tourniquet should point toward the shoulder.

The pressure from the tourniquet should cause the veins to stand up so they can be seen or palpated. Gently palpate the area with your index finger (Figure 6-16). If you cannot see or feel the vein, ask the patient to open and close his or her fist a few times. Instruct him or her to open and then release the fist slowly. Avoid a rapid, pumping motion, which may damage the specimen. Dangling the extremity over the edge of the bed may also dilate the vein. Rubbing or patting the area of the vein gently toward the tourniquet with your finger may also distend it. Massaging the forearm may also help dilate

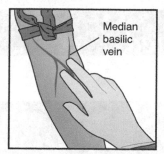

FIGURE 6-16 Palpate the vein.

a vein. If these techniques are ineffective, applying a warm compress to the area for 5 to 10 minutes may distend the vein. Release the tourniquet while the compress is in place. A warm, wet towel covered with plastic can be used. Follow your facility procedure for warm, moist compresses.

After the vein is selected, release the tourniquet by pulling the upper loop *downward*. Prepare your equipment and prep the skin. Allow the skin to dry. Then reapply the tourniquet and perform the venipuncture.

Tourniquets and Infection Control. Tourniquets are a great potential source of infection transmission. They easily become soiled with blood and other body fluids. A study in Great Britain resulted in a recommendation for discarding the tourniquet after each use. However, in the United States, the CDC has made no formal recommendation beyond noting that the device must be clean. Hospitals are handling this in different ways. Most discard a tourniquet after a single use. Some provide a new tourniquet for each patient that is kept in the patient's room and discarded upon discharge. Some have procedures for wiping used tourniquets with alcohol or otherwise disinfecting them. Your instructor will inform you of your facility policies for tourniquet use. Do not ignore this potential source of serious cross-contamination and infection. For procedures in which tourniquets are used, discarding or disin-

fecting the tourniquet should be part of your routine procedure completion actions.

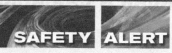

SAFETY ALERT

Tourniquets that remain on limbs for extended periods of time can cause serious nerve and circulatory damage, leading to amputation. The literature describes a patient nerve injury that occurred when a phlebotomist who was interrupted by a phone call left a tourniquet in place for 10 minutes (see Exploring the Web). A root cause analysis of tourniquet-related events resulted in many recommendations, such as using bright, fluorescent-colored tourniquets. Of all their suggestions, the bottom line is that workers must always check to make sure the tourniquet is removed after venipuncture.

AGE-APPROPRIATE CARE ALERT

For a pediatric or apprehensive patient, tell that patient that you will count to three. When you reach three, the patient should take a deep breath. When the patient begins to inhale the deep breath, quickly insert the needle. Do not hesitate. The patient will be thinking of the deep breath, not the needlestick. When you are ready to withdraw the needle, instruct the patient to take another deep breath.

HEALTH CARE ALERT

Avoid bandaging the puncture site until bleeding has stopped. Check to see if a hematoma is forming. If so, document it and inform the RN. Direct pressure is best for preventing a hematoma. Keep your finger on the gauze and apply gentle pressure (you can ask the patient to do this). Avoid bending the arm up, as this increases the risk of hematoma development.

Procedure 29

Performing a Venipuncture

Supplies needed:
- Disposable exam gloves
- 2 × 2 gauze pads
- Alcohol or povidone-iodine sponges
- Tourniquet
- Puncture-resistant needle disposal container

(continues)

Procedure **29**, *continued*

Performing a Venipuncture

▶ Syringe method:
  —10-mL syringe
  —Sterile needles: 20- to 21-gauge for adults, or 23-gauge butterfly
▶ Vacuum-tube method:
  —Vacuum tube with needle holder
  —Sterile double-needles: 20- to 21-gauge for adults, 23- to 25-gauge for children
▶ Plastic bag for used supplies
▶ Adhesive bandage

1. Perform your beginning procedure actions.
2. Apply a tourniquet and locate a vein. Select the largest, most stable vein in the area. When palpated, the site will feel firm and rebound slightly.
3. Release the tourniquet.
4. Cleanse the site with alcohol. Wipe in a circular motion. Begin in the center of the venipuncture site and extend the circle out 2 inches in diameter.
5. Allow the alcohol or other skin prep to dry thoroughly.
6. Reapply the tourniquet, taking care not to bump or touch the prepped skin area.
7. Remove the needle cover, holding the needle bevel facing up in your dominant hand.
8. Stabilize the vein by holding the skin taut with your nondominant thumb, approximately 1 inch below the puncture site (**Figure 6-17A**). Warn the patient that he or she will feel a stick.
9. With the needle at a 15° angle, slowly enter the patient's vein (**Figure 6-17B**). You will feel a change of pressure when it enters the vein. Slowly advance the needle 1/4 inch.
10. Release the tourniquet (**Figure 6-17C**) by pulling the upper end downward, before removing the needle. If you are releasing the tourniquet while filling tubes, hold the collection device securely. Avoid pulling upward, as this may cause the needle to come out of the patient's arm. If you are drawing one tube of blood, you may release the tourniquet as soon as the tube begins filling. If you are drawing multiple tubes,

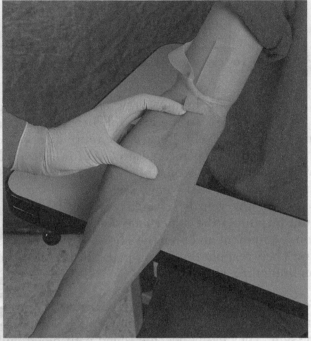

FIGURE 6-17(A) Hold the vein taut with your nondominant hand before making the venipuncture.

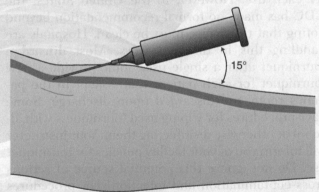

FIGURE 6-17(B) Insert the needle at a 15° angle.

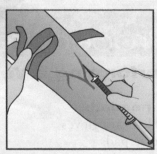

FIGURE 6-17(C) Release the tourniquet.

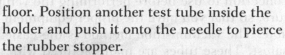

Procedure **29**, *continued*

Performing a Venipuncture

wait until the last tube is filling before releasing the tourniquet. For an elderly person, it may be best to wait until immediately before the needle is removed to release the tourniquet. Releasing it sooner may change the pressure, causing the vein to collapse.

11. Hold the needle steady. Continue the procedure by obtaining the blood specimen with the syringe or vacuum method or starting the intravenous infusion. Gently push the evacuated tube onto the needle inside the plastic holder. Keep the patient's arm and the tube pointed down while the tube is filling. If it is necessary to change tubes, gently remove the first tube from the holder. Set it where it will not roll onto the

floor. Position another test tube inside the holder and push it onto the needle to pierce the rubber stopper.

12. Place a 2 × 2 gauze pad over the insertion site (**Figure 6-17D**). Avoid using cotton balls. Cotton balls tend to stick to the venipuncture site and, when removed, remove the platelet plug, causing bleeding.

13. Quickly withdraw the needle. Immediately apply pressure on the insertion site. Maintain the pressure for 2 to 3 minutes, or longer, until bleeding stops (**Figure 6-17E**).

14. Cover the puncture site with an adhesive bandage.

15. Discard the needle and syringe or tube holder in the puncture-resistant container.

16. Perform your procedure completion actions.

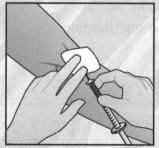

FIGURE 6-17(D) Hold gentle pressure on the sterile pad while removing the needle.

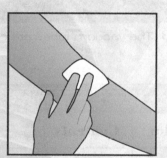

FIGURE 6-17(E) Apply pressure until bleeding stops. The patient may be able to do this.

HEALTH CARE ALERT

In addition to causing potential harm to the patient, prolonged tourniquet application (more than 1 to 2 minutes) will alter the results of many blood tests. For example, the total protein, aspartate aminotransferase (AST), total lipids, cholesterol, and iron values will be increased. Prolonged tourniquet application also affects packed cell volume and other cellular elements. Remove the tourniquet as quickly as possible. Avoid leaving it in place for more than 1 minute, if possible. If you must reapply the tourniquet, allow the vein to rest and refill for at least 2 full minutes.

HEALTH CARE ALERT

If the patient feels dizzy or faint in the middle of the venipuncture procedure, stop what you are doing immediately. If the patient is seated in a chair, have the patient place his or her head between the knees. After a brief rest, have the patient lie down. Check the blood pressure before continuing. If the patient is hypotensive (below 100/60), check with the RN. Document the situation and your findings.

COLLECTING A BLOOD SPECIMEN USING THE VACUUM-TUBE SYSTEM

You must determine which method of specimen collection to use before performing the venipuncture, so that you have the proper equipment available. The vacuum-tube method is the easiest and safest. These tubes are manufactured with a vacuum inside. Some contain preservatives, separators, and other additives necessary for certain laboratory tests (Figure 6-18). You must know which tests you are drawing specimens for so that you can select the proper tubes. The types of preservatives in the various tubes are listed in **Table 6-1.** Your facility will have a chart listing tube colors to use for specific tests. If a tube contains preservatives, you must mix the blood in the tube. Do this by inverting the tube 5 to 10 times (**Figure 6-19**). Avoid shaking, which can break the blood cells. Do not invert tubes without additives.

Another important consideration is the order in which multiple tubes of blood are drawn. Additives can be carried over from one tube to another, altering test results. Tubes should be filled in this order, regardless of whether the vacuum tube or syringe method is used:

- Blood culture bottles or tubes
- Citrate/light blue top tube (PT, PTT)
- Serum/nonadditive tube (red, gold, or tiger top tubes)
- Heparin/green top tube
- EDTA/lavender top tube
- Oxalate/gray top (fluoride)

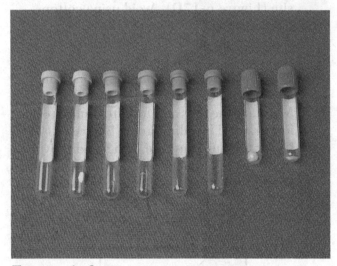

FIGURE 6-18 The vacuum tubes are color-coded.

Table 6-1 Overview of Vacuum Tubes		
Tube Color	**Contents**	**Tests**
Red	No additives or preservatives.	Used for serum samples.
Black	Contain sodium oxalate.	Used for coagulation studies.
Lavender	Contain EDTA.	Used for testing whole blood samples.
Yellow	Contain acid-citrate-dextrose (ACD) solution.	Used for testing whole blood samples.
Green	Contain heparin, an anticoagulant or blood thinner.	Used for testing plasma samples.
Gray	Contain a glycolytic inhibitor (could be sodium fluoride, powdered oxalate, or glycolytic/microbial inhibitor).	Used for blood sugar or glucose determinations.
Marble top	Contain silicone gel.	Used for serum separation.
Blue	Contain sodium citrate and citric acid.	Used for coagulation studies.

Each tube has an expiration date. The vacuum and contents are guaranteed through this date. This closed system prevents contamination. Always check the date, and avoid using tubes that are past the expiration date.

Another consideration is that several different types of vacuum systems are available. The components are not interchangeable. Make sure that the

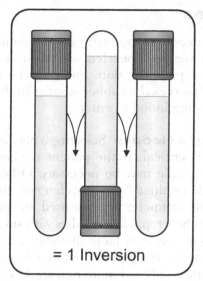

FIGURE 6-19 Inverting the tube down, then up, is one inversion. Avoid shaking, as shaking will damage the specimen.

equipment you select is all made by the same manufacturer. Always select a safety system, if available (**Figure 6-20**).

Saf-T-Clik® Shielded Blood Needle Adapter

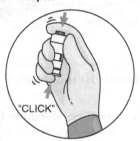

Instructions For Use
PREPARATION

1. Before attaching needle, push ends of Saf-T-Clik® together to ensure outer sleeve is seated.

2. Open needle cartridge. Twist to break the tamperproof seal. Remove cartridge cap to expose rear needle with threaded hub. Do not remove front needle cover. Use up to 1½" blood collection needle.

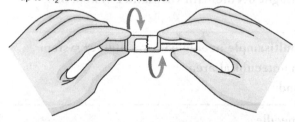

3. Attach needle to Safety Adapter. Screw needle into Safety Adapter until firmly seated.

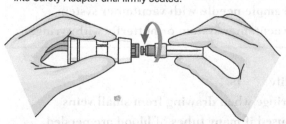

AFTER VENIPUNCTURE

4. When sampling is complete, grasp the Safety Adapter's outer sheath sliding it forward over the exposed contaminated needle until a distinctive "CLICK" is heard. "LOCKED, LOCKED" is visible when Adapter is locked. The contaminated needle is now safely covered.

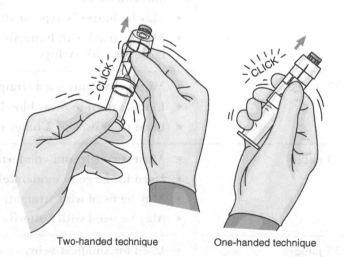

Two-handed technique   One-handed technique

5. Discard the Safety Adapter/Contaminated Needle Assembly according to hospital procedures. Do not reuse needle/Safety Adapter.

FIGURE 6-20 Instructions for using the Saf-T-Clik® shielded needle adapter. (Courtesy of MPS Acacia)

Needles

A special needle is used with the vacuum-tube system. This needle is beveled at both ends. One end pierces the patient's skin, entering the vein. The other end pierces the rubber stopper in the vacuum tube, allowing blood to enter.

Selecting a Needle. Selecting a needle of proper diameter is critical. If the patient is obese, a long (1½-inch) needle may be necessary. Otherwise, the length is determined by user preference. Remember that needle diameter is measured by gauge. The higher numbers represent needles with smaller diameters. Needles with a large diameter are more uncomfortable for the patient, but enable you to draw large volumes of blood more quickly. Use **Table 6-2** to assist in selecting the proper needle size.

Tube Holders

To use the vacuum-tube system, the needle and test tube must be inserted into a carrier or holder (Figure 6-21). Newer holders are designed to offer protection against accidental needlestick injuries (Figure 6-22). Older holders offer no protection. If your health care facility has several types available, always select the one that offers you the most protection. The holders have a flange on each side to support your fingers when piercing tubes.

After the Specimen Is Collected

After collecting the specimen, position the tubes so they do not roll off a table. Standing them upright in a carrier is best. One documented case of HIV infection occurred as a result of a needlestick that happened when the nurse was trying to stop tubes of blood from rolling off a table. In trying to catch the tubes, the nurse accidentally pricked her finger with a needle.

Discard the needle and tube holder in the sharps container. Avoid manipulating, recapping, or attempting to remove the tube from the holder. In previous years, the holder was reused. The Occu-

Table 6-2 Needle Sizes and Uses	
Needle Type/Size	**Suggested Use**
19 gauge	• Need to draw a large volume of blood (10 to 20 tubes) using the vacutainer system • Consider using a butterfly, which is most comfortable for the patient
21 gauge	• Commonly used for moderate to large veins, particularly those in the antecubital area • May be butterfly-type or straight, multisample needle • May be used with butterfly or straight needle with vacutainer system or butterfly with syringe
22 gauge	• Most commonly used straight, multisample needle with vacutainer system • Usually used to draw blood from antecubital area • Used to draw 1 to 3 tubes of blood
23 gauge	• Most versatile and comfortable needle • Used for large to moderately small veins • May be used with straight, multisample needle with vacutainer system • May be used with butterfly with vacutainer system or butterfly with syringe
25 gauge	• Used for smallest veins • Used for veins that collapse readily • Best used with a butterfly and syringe when drawing from small veins • Butterfly and vacutainer may be used if many tubes of blood are needed, but this increases the risk of vein collapse

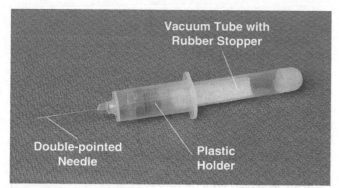

FIGURE 6-21 The evacuated blood collection system

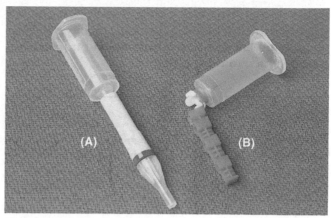

FIGURE 6-22 (A) Safety needle (B) Locking cover

pational Safety and Health Administration (OSHA) has made its position on reusing tube holders quite clear. This is summarized in **Figure 6-23.**

Label the tubes in the patient's room after collecting the specimen. Before leaving, check the patient's arm to ensure that bleeding has stopped and

there is no hematoma. Report procedure completion to the RN immediately after leaving the room. This is necessary because the patient may have restrictions on eating, drinking, and medications before the

Standard Interpretations
06/12/2002–Reuse of blood tube holders.
Standard Number: 1910.1030(d)(2)(vii)(A)
Question: What is OSHA's position regarding the use of blood tube holders, specifically removing a needle in order to reuse a tube holder? Must each blood tube collection device be disposed of with the needle attached each time they are used?

OSHA's Bloodborne Pathogens Standard (29 CFR 1910.1030, paragraph (d)(2)(vii)(A)) provides: "Contaminated needles and other contaminated sharps shall not be bent, recapped, or removed, unless the employer can demonstrate that no alternative is feasible or that such action is required by a specific medical or dental procedure." More specifically, our new compliance directive, CPL 2-2.69 at XIII.D.5, states, "removing the needle from a used blood-drawing/phlebotomy device is rarely, if ever, required by a medical procedure. Because such devices involve the use of a double-ended needle, such removal clearly exposes employees to additional risk, as does the increased manipulation of a contaminated device." *In order to prevent potential worker exposure to the contaminated hollow bore needle at both the front and back ends, blood tube holders, with needles attached, must be immediately discarded into an accessible sharps container after the safety feature has been activated.*

Using a syringe to collect blood would be an example of a situation where clinical or medical necessity would dictate the need for transferring the collected blood to a test tube before disposing of the contaminated blood collection device. If drawing blood with a syringe is necessary, engineering controls (engineered sharps injury protection) and safe work practices (including mechanical means of removal if available) must be used and needleless blood transfer devices must be implemented.

Removing contaminated needles and subsequently reusing blood tube holders poses multiple potential hazards. The increased manipulation required to remove a contaminated needle from a blood tube holder is unnecessary and may result in a needlestick from either the front or back end of the needle. According to information available from the International Health Care Worker Safety Center at the University of Virginia, injuries occurring in phlebotomy are among the highest-risk for transmitting bloodborne pathogens such as HIV, HCV and HBV, because they involve hollow-bore, blood-filled needles.

Further, improper disposal of used, unprotected needle devices potentially affects more than just the user. According to data presented by the California Department of Health Services (January 2002), close to half of all injuries from contaminated sharps occur to those who are not in immediate control of the device, but to those who come in contact with the unprotected needle downstream (e.g., nursing assistants, housekeepers, maintenance personnel). Therefore, disposing of single-use safety-activated blood collection devices decreases potential injuries downstream.

While patient safety is not within the scope of OSHA's mission, we recognize that tube holder reuse poses a potential health hazard to patients. Some clinical studies show that 50–80% of blood tube holders may be contaminated after just one use (Advance/Laboratory, p. 70, January 2000). While it may be difficult to document a patient-to-patient cross-contamination exposure, the risk does exist and should be weighed when making decisions regarding overall safety.
Source: http://www.osha.gov/OshDoc/Directive_pdf/CPL_2-2_69.pdf

FIGURE 6-23 OSHA position on reuse of blood tube holders

test is drawn. After the sample is collected, the RN will lift the restrictions. Follow your facility policy for completing laboratory requisitions and transporting the specimen to the laboratory.

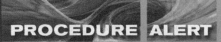

PROCEDURE ALERT

A full vacutainer will provide enough blood to test the specimen. Tubes that are less than half full may be inadequate, necessitating that the specimen be redrawn.

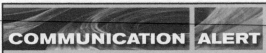

COMMUNICATION ALERT

Label the specimen at the bedside immediately after the procedure. Include the:
- Patient's last and first name
- Patient's ID or medical record number
- Requisition number
- Date of collection

Never prelabel a tube, because unused tubes may accidentally be used for another patient, resulting in a potentially serious error.

Procedure 30

Collecting a Blood Specimen Using the Vacuum-Tube System

Supplies needed:
- Disposable exam gloves
- 2 × 2 gauze pads
- Alcohol or povidone-iodine sponges
- Tourniquet
- Blood collection tubes
- Labels for collection tubes
- Permanent black pen for labeling tubes
- Laboratory requisition forms
- Puncture-resistant needle disposal container
- Vacuum tubes with needle holder
- Sterile double-needles: 20- to 21-gauge for adults, 23- to 25-gauge for children
- Plastic bag for used supplies
- Bandage

1. Perform your beginning procedure actions.
2. Assemble the needle and tube holder.
3. Check the requisition slip to determine what test to collect. Select the proper tubes. Position the specimen collection tubes in the order in which they will be drawn.
4. Apply a tourniquet and locate a vein. Select the largest, most stable vein in the area. When palpated, the site should feel firm and rebound slightly.
5. Release the tourniquet.
6. Cleanse the site with alcohol. Wipe in a circular motion. Begin in the center of the venipuncture site and extend the circle out 2 inches in diameter.

7. Allow the alcohol or other skin prep to dry thoroughly.
8. Reapply the tourniquet, taking care not to bump or touch the prepped skin area.
9. Remove the needle cover, holding the needle bevel facing up in your dominant hand.
10. Stabilize the vein by holding the skin taut with your nondominant thumb, approximately 1 inch below the puncture site. Warn the patient that he or she will feel a stick.
11. With the needle at a 15-degree angle, slowly enter the patient's vein. You will feel a change of pressure when the needle enters the vein. Slowly advance the needle 1/4 inch.
12. Rest your dominant hand on the patient's arm. Gently insert the first collection tube into the holder, and push forward gently to pierce the rubber stopper. Make sure that the needle does not move. Blood should begin to flow.
13. Release the tourniquet as soon as blood begins to flow. Hold the collection device securely, then pull the upper end of the tourniquet *downward*. Avoid pulling upward, as this may cause the needle to come out of the patient's arm.
14. When the tube has finished filling, grasp the end of the tube, pushing off the flange with your thumb.

(continues)

Procedure **30**, *continued*

Collecting a Blood Specimen Using the Vacuum-Tube System

15. Gently invert additive tubes 10 to 12 times, then insert the next tube. Repeat until all tubes are filled with blood.
16. Remove the last tube drawn from the holder.
17. Place a 2 × 2 gauze pad over the insertion site. Avoid using cotton balls. Cotton balls tend to stick to the venipuncture site and, when removed, remove the platelet plug, causing bleeding.
18. Quickly withdraw the needle. Immediately apply pressure on the insertion site. Maintain the pressure for 2 to 3 minutes, or longer, until bleeding stops.
19. Cover the puncture site with a bandage.
20. Discard the needle and blood tube holder in the puncture-resistant container.
21. Label the tubes according to facility policy.
22. Perform your procedure completion actions.

COLLECTING A BLOOD SPECIMEN WITH A WINGED INFUSION SET (BUTTERFLY) AND SYRINGE

A butterfly needle is useful for collecting specimens from children and adults with very small or fragile veins. The butterfly needle has a plastic tube attached, with a bulb at the end (**Figure 6-24**). This hub is attached to the syringe. A 23-gauge butterfly is commonly used for blood collection. Smaller needles may damage the blood cells in the sample. Check with the RN before using a smaller butterfly needle. The method of collecting the specimen is almost identical to using a vacuum tube, but the equipment is slightly different.

Formerly, a syringe and regular needle were used for drawing blood. This is no longer considered a safe practice, and this method should not be used. If a needle is necessary to draw blood from small or collapsing veins, a butterfly needle is the safest method to use. Transfer the blood to the vacutainer tube using a transfer device (**Figure 6-25**) that is specifically made for this purpose.

Coagulation Tubes. A special procedure is necessary when a coagulation tube is used with a winged-tip, butterfly needle. A **coagulation tube** has a blue stopper, and is used when drawing blood for coagulation (clotting) studies, such as prothrombin time (PT). The blue-topped coagulation tube should not be the first tube drawn. If a series of tubes is being drawn, the coagulation tube should be drawn as the second or third in the series. If the coagulation tube is the only tube to be drawn,

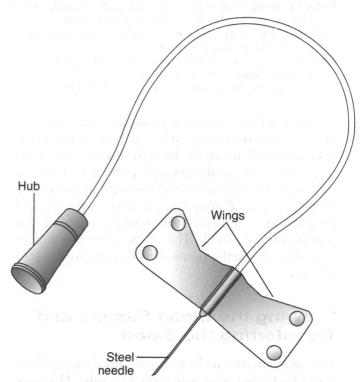

FIGURE 6-24 The winged infusion needle, or butterfly. The lumen of a butterfly needle is one size larger than the gauge.

draw a few milliliters of blood into another tube, such as a red-topped tube, before attaching the blue-topped coagulation tube. After you have finished, discard the red-topped tube.

Preparing the Needle and Syringe

To prepare the needle and syringe, select a 21- to 23-gauge sterile butterfly and a 10-mL syringe. To comply with OSHA regulations, only locking syringes

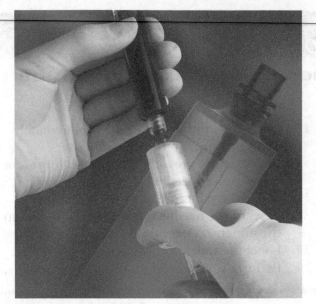

FIGURE 6-25 Transfer the blood to the vacutainer tube using a transfer device that is specifically made for this purpose. Never connect the syringe directly to the evacuated tube, which greatly increases the risk of splashing and aerosilization of blood. (Courtesy of Becton, Dickinson and Company, Franklin Lakes, NJ. (201) 847-6800)

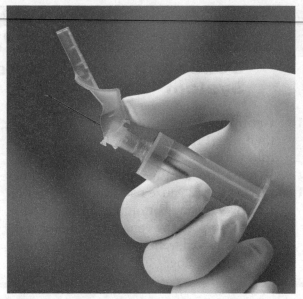

FIGURE 6-26 A luer lock twists the needle into place, reducing the risk that the needle and syringe will separate during use. (Courtesy of Becton, Dickinson and Company, Franklin Lakes, NJ. (201) 847-6800)

(those that fasten to the needle with a luer lock device) (**Figure 6-26**) should be used. Open the sterile packaging and attach the butterfly securely to the syringe. With the needle covered, pull back on the syringe plunger, then push it all the way forward so that no air remains. Pulling and pushing on the plunger breaks the seal inside the syringe, enabling the plunger to move freely. This reduces the risk of accidentally piercing the vein wall while manipulating the plunger.

Drawing the Blood Sample and Transferring the Blood

The venipuncture technique used for drawing blood is similar to that used with a vacuum tube. However, the blood sample must be transferred from the syringe to a test tube. The potential for accidental needlestick and exposure to blood is greatly increased. For this reason, drawing blood through a syringe is the least desirable method. This method should be used only if a blood transfer device is available. The blood transfer device is specially engineered to reduce the risk of exposure to blood and eliminates the risk of needlestick injury to the caregiver.

When transferring blood from the syringe to a vacuum tube, wear full personal protective equipment, including face mask or goggles, mask, long-sleeved gown or lab coat, and gloves.

Fill the tubes in the same order as you would use when drawing blood:

- Blood culture tubes
- Nonadditive tubes (red)
- Coagulation tubes (blue)
- Additive tubes
  - gel tubes (serum separator)
  - heparin (green)
  - EDTA tubes (lavender)
  - fluoride tubes (gray)

Using a safety shield is the safest method for transferring blood from one container to another. To transfer blood from a syringe to a test tube, use the shield. Place the tubes upright in a rack, or attach them to the syringe with the safety shield. Puncture the rubber top of the test tube with the transfer device. After the transfer device has pierced the rubber stopper, the tubes will fill readily because of the inner vacuum. Avoid forcing the plunger down, as this will cause blood cell breakage. Forcing blood into the tube causes hemolysis and increases the risk of overfilling, which also destroys the sample. After filling the tubes, discard the transfer device, with syringe attached, in the puncture-resistant sharps container. Gently invert the tubes to mix the sample. Avoid shaking the tubes, which causes hemolysis.

Procedure 31

Collecting a Blood Specimen Using a Butterfly Needle and Syringe

Supplies needed:

▶ Disposable exam gloves, 2 pairs
▶ Face shield or goggles
▶ Surgical mask
▶ Fluid-resistant gown or lab coat
▶ 2 × 2 gauze pads
▶ Alcohol or povidone-iodine sponges
▶ Tourniquet
▶ 10-mL syringe
▶ Sterile 23-gauge butterfly needle
▶ Sterile transfer device
▶ Bandage tape to secure the butterfly in place
▶ Blood collection tubes
▶ Labels for collection tubes
▶ Permanent black pen for labeling tubes
▶ Laboratory requisition forms
▶ Puncture-resistant needle disposal container
▶ Plastic bag for used supplies
▶ Bandage

1. Perform your beginning procedure actions.
2. Check the requisition slip to determine what specimen to collect. Select the proper tubes.
3. Assemble the needle and syringe. Uncoil the butterfly tubing. Move the plunger back and forth to break the seal.
4. Apply a tourniquet and locate a vein. Select the largest, most stable vein in the area. When palpated, the site should feel firm and rebound slightly.
5. Release the tourniquet.
6. Cleanse the site with alcohol. Wipe in a circular motion. Begin in the center of the venipuncture site and extend the circle out 2 inches in diameter.
7. Allow the alcohol or other skin prep to dry thoroughly.
8. Reapply the tourniquet, taking care not to bump or touch the prepped skin area.
9. Remove the needle cover, holding the needle by the wings, with the bevel facing up, in your dominant hand.
10. Stabilize the vein by holding the skin taut with your nondominant thumb, approximately 1 inch below the puncture

site. Warn the patient that he or she will feel a stick.

11. With the needle at a 15-degree angle, slowly enter the patient's vein. You will feel a change of pressure when the needle enters the vein. Slowly advance the needle ¼ inch.
12. Rest your dominant hand on the patient's arm. Make sure that the needle does not move. Blood should begin to flow into the attached tubing.
13. Gently tape the butterfly wings against the skin to hold the needle in place.
14. Release the tourniquet as soon as blood is obtained. Pull the upper end of the tourniquet *downward*. Avoid pulling upward, as this may cause the needle to come out of the patient's arm.
15. Holding the syringe with the dominant hand, slowly pull back on the plunger, filling the syringe with blood.
16. Place a 2 × 2 gauze pad over the insertion site. Avoid using cotton balls. Cotton balls tend to stick to the venipuncture site and, when removed, remove the platelet plug, causing bleeding.
17. Quickly withdraw the needle. Immediately apply pressure on the insertion site. Maintain the pressure for 2 to 3 minutes, or longer until bleeding stops.
18. Cover the puncture site with a bandage.
19. Remove the butterfly and tubing from the syringe. Carefully discard them in the puncture-resistant container.
20. Open the package for the transfer device and attach the device to the syringe.
21. Perform your procedure completion actions.
22. After leaving the room, apply full personal protective equipment.
23. Transfer the blood to the vacuum tubes in a rack by inserting the transfer device through the rubber stopper, allowing the tube to fill. Allow the rack to support the tube.
24. Fill the tubes in the order of the draw.

(continues)

Procedure **31**, *continued*

Collecting a Blood Specimen Using a Butterfly Needle and Syringe

25. Gently invert the tubes several times to mix the samples. Avoid shaking.
26. Discard the syringe and transfer device in the puncture-resistant container.
27. Label the tubes according to facility policy.
28. Transport the blood to the lab, following facility policy.

Procedure **32**

Using the Blood Transfer Device

Supplies needed:
▶ Disposable exam gloves and other protective equipment (mask, eye protection, gown) as required by facility policy
▶ Sterile transfer device
▶ Sharps container

1. Perform your beginning procedure actions.
2. Engage the safety shield on the butterfly needle.
3. Carefully remove the needle and place it in the sharps container.
4. Peel back the sterile package for the transfer device.
5. Insert the tip of the syringe into the blood transfer device. Turn clockwise to secure.
6. With the syringe held vertically and tip pointing down, center the tip of the vacutainer and press it up into the holder portion of the transfer device.
7. The tube will fill until the vacuum is used. Do not depress the plunger to the syringe. This will cause hemolysis of the blood sample and increases the risk of blood spattering.
8. Separate the vacutainer tube from the transfer device and syringe. Discard the syringe into the sharps container.
9. Label or sticker the tube of blood.
10. Perform your procedure completion actions.

BLOOD CULTURES

A **blood culture** is drawn to test the blood for the presence of a systemic infection. This infection may also be called **septicemia.** Several blood cultures are usually drawn over a period of time. Different collection sites are used to obtain the specimens. Never collect this specimen through a vascular access device or intravenous line. The specimen must be drawn directly from the vein to be accurate. The cultures are usually drawn when the patient has a fever and is chilling. The RN will inform you if the patient is re-ceiving antibiotics. If so, he or she may ask you to draw the blood immediately before the next dose is administered.

A 20-mL syringe is used for this procedure. One sample is drawn, then separated into bottles for two tests. The test for **aerobic** microbes is done to look for pathogens that can live only in the presence of oxygen. The test for **anaerobic** microbes monitors for pathogens that live without oxygen. Because this sample is used to test for the presence of microbes, sterile gloves are worn to prevent accidental contamination. Strive to use flawless sterile technique for this procedure.

Blood collected for this test must be transferred to another container. Regardless of the location of the transfer, the needle must be changed before the specimen is injected into the culture bottles. Remove the butterfly and attach a sterile transfer device. Always use a sterile needle for this portion of the procedure.

A blood culture bottle has a snap-off cap (Figure 6-27). The area under the cap is sterile. Avoid touching the rubber stopper with your hands, as this causes contamination. Cleanse this stopper with alcohol. Avoid using povidone-iodine, which causes deterioration of the bottle top. Allow the prep solution to dry completely before transferring the blood.

For this procedure, you will use a 20-mL syringe. Withdraw enough blood for both bottles. Transfer the appropriate amount to each culture bottle. The amount may vary, depending on the manufacturer of the bottles. This will provide a dilution ratio of 1:10 when mixed with the solution inside the bottles. After the blood is transferred to the culture bottles, the bottles should be transported to the laboratory immediately in plastic transport bags, or according to facility policy.

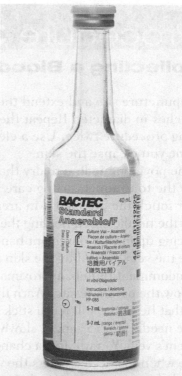

FIGURE 6-27 Blood culture bottle. (Courtesy of Becton, Dickinson and Company, Franklin Lakes, NJ. (201) 847-6800)

Procedure 33

Collecting a Blood Culture

Note: Documented incidences of contamination with inaccurate culture results have occurred as a result of improperly disinfected blood culture bottles. Each facility has a specific procedure with designated antiseptics to use for cleansing the bottle tops. All surfaces must be thoroughly disinfected before the specimen is drawn. Your instructor will inform you of the proper procedure and disinfectants to use in your facility.

Supplies needed:
- Sterile gloves
- Disposable exam gloves
- Face shield or goggles
- Surgical mask
- Fluid-resistant gown or lab coat
- 2 × 2 gauze pads
- Alcohol sponges, povidone-iodine, or blood culture prep kit
- Tourniquet
- 20-mL syringe
- Sterile needles: 20- to 22-gauge or 23- to 25-gauge butterfly
- Sterile blood transfer device
- Blood culture collection bottles
- Labels for collection bottles
- Permanent black pen for labeling bottles
- Laboratory requisition forms
- Puncture-resistant needle disposal container
- Plastic bag for used supplies
- Bandage

1. Perform your beginning procedure actions.
2. Check the requisition slip to determine what specimen to collect. Select the proper supplies.
3. Assemble the needle and syringe. Move the plunger back and forth to break the seal.
4. Apply a tourniquet and locate a vein. Select the largest, most stable vein in the area. When palpated, the site should feel firm and rebound slightly.
5. Release the tourniquet.
6. Cleanse the site with povidone-iodine. Wipe in a circular motion. Begin in the center of

(continues)

Procedure **33**, *continued*

Collecting a Blood Culture

the venipuncture site and extend the circle out 3 inches in diameter. Repeat the cleansing procedure twice. Use a clean swab each time you cleanse the skin.

7. Allow the povidone-iodine to dry thoroughly.

8. Reapply the tourniquet, taking care not to bump or touch the prepped skin area.

9. Remove the needle cover, holding the needle bevel facing up in your dominant hand.

10. Stabilize the vein by holding the skin taut with your nondominant thumb, approximately 1 inch below the puncture site. Warn the patient that he or she will feel a stick.

11. With the needle at a 15° angle, slowly enter the patient's vein. You will feel a change of pressure when the needle enters the vein. Slowly advance the needle ¼ inch.

12. Rest your dominant hand on the patient's arm. Make sure that the needle does not move. Blood should begin to flow into the hub of the needle.

13. Release the tourniquet as soon as blood is obtained. Hold the collection device securely, then pull the upper end of the tourniquet *downward*. Avoid pulling upward, as this may cause the needle to come out of the patient's arm.

14. Holding the syringe with the dominant hand, slowly pull back on the plunger with the nondominant hand, withdrawing the required amount of blood.

15. Place a 2 × 2 gauze pad over the insertion site. Avoid using cotton balls. Cotton balls tend to stick to the venipuncture site and, when removed, remove the platelet plug, causing bleeding.

16. Quickly withdraw the needle. Immediately apply pressure on the insertion site. Maintain the pressure for 2 to 3 minutes, or longer until bleeding stops.

17. Cover the puncture site with a bandage.

18. Engage the safety shield on the butterfly needle. Carefully remove the needle and discard it in the sharps container.

19. Peel back the sterile package for the transfer device.

20. Insert the tip of the syringe into the blood transfer device. Turn clockwise to secure.

21. Apply full protective equipment, including gown, face shield, mask, and gloves.

22. Snap the caps off the culture bottles.

23. Cleanse the rubber stoppers well, using alcohol. Wipe in a circular motion. Use a new sponge for each bottle. Allow to dry thoroughly.

24. With the syringe held vertically and the tip pointing down, center the tip of the anaerobic culture bottle and press it up into the holder portion of the transfer device. The bottle will fill until the vacuum is used.

25. Remove the anaerobic bottle and follow the same procedure to center the aerobic bottle and press it into the blood transfer device. The bottle will fill until the vacuum is used.

26. Carefully remove the syringe and transfer device from the bottle. Discard them in the sharps container.

27. Label the bottles according to facility policy.

28. Perform your procedure completion actions.

29. Transport the samples to the laboratory immediately in a plastic transport bag, or according to facility policy.

DRAWING BLOOD USING A LANCET FOR A MICRODRAW OR INFANT HEEL STICK

A **microdraw** is a small skin puncture used for collecting blood specimens. Many tests can be performed by this method, despite the fact that the sample is very small. Blood drawn through a micro-draw is a mixture of venous, capillary, and arterial blood. It most closely resembles arterial blood.

Lancets

A **lancet** (Figure 6-28) is a tiny, sharp, sterile device used to puncture the skin to collect small blood samples. One end is plastic. You will hold this end when

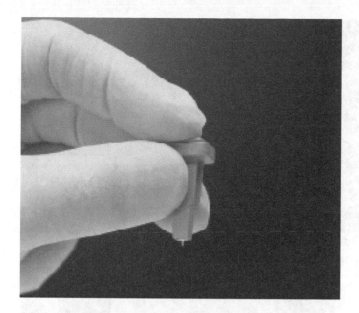

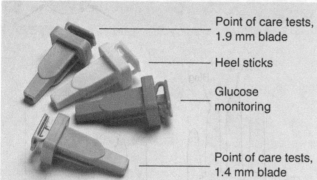

Point of care tests, 1.9 mm blade

Heel sticks

Glucose monitoring

Point of care tests, 1.4 mm blade

FIGURE 6-28 MICROTAINER safety lancets. Depress the plunger to puncture the skin, then release immediately. The needle is retractable, reducing the risk of needlestick injury. Discard in the puncture-resistant container. (Courtesy of Becton Dickinson VACUTAINER System, Franklin Lakes, NJ. (201) 847-6800)

performing the procedure. A tiny needle protrudes from the other end with which to puncture the skin. Some lancets have the needle exposed. Others require the user to activate a trigger to pierce the skin. This type reduces the risk of accidental needlestick. Lancets are available in several sizes. Depending on the manufacturer, both the blade width and puncture depth will vary. The smaller sizes are used for specimen collection from infants. Larger lancets are used for adults. Use the size of device recommended by your facility.

Capillary Tubes

When blood is collected from a lancet skin puncture, it is tested on a reagent strip or is drawn into a **capillary tube** (Figure 6-29) for further testing in the laboratory. The capillary tube is a slender, short, hollow tube.

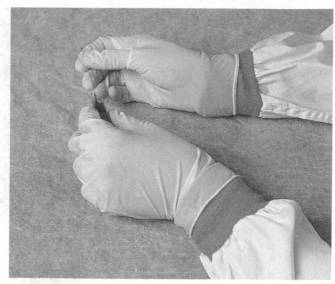

FIGURE 6-29 Filling a capillary tube with blood

For years, health care facilities used glass capillary tubes to collect blood for these tests. The hollow tubes are open at both ends, and are sealed with a clay or putty-like substance after being filled with blood. The tubes are very fragile, and the incidence of injury related to breakage is high. This often occurs in the process of sealing the tube, although breakage can occur at any step during the collection and testing process. In at least one instance, HIV was transmitted in this manner; the physician who was accidentally injured by the broken capillary tube died from AIDS. In 1999, as a result of the high risk of accidental tube breakage, the government agencies that regulate health care facility safety recommended the use of capillary tubes that:

- are not made of glass, or
- are wrapped in puncture-resistant film, or
- use a method of sealing that does not require manually pushing one end of the tube into putty to form a plug, or
- allow the blood to be tested without centrifugation.

Because of this government directive, the procedures in this book describe the use of the **microvette collection device.** This is a closed system capillary tube that complies with the federal recommendations.

The microvette collection device is similar to a capillary tube, and is used to collect the blood. Two types are available. The purple-capped collector is used for obtaining blood counts, and contains EDTA. The collector with a red cap contains no preservatives. It may have a serum separator inside. When collecting

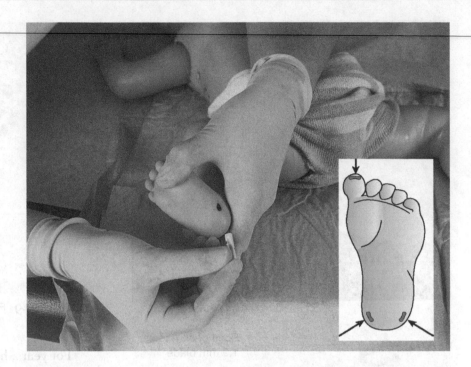

FIGURE 6-30 Proper method of holding the infant's foot for capillary puncture, and safe areas for infant specimen collection.

samples using both tubes, collect the purple-capped tube first. The tubes hold 1 mL of blood. Follow facility policy for filling the tubes. Laboratory policies usually require you to fill the tubes three-quarters or two-thirds full. The purple-topped tube is filled with slightly less, so that it can be mixed properly.

Skin Puncture Site

You will select the location for the specimen collection. In an infant or child under 1 year of age, use the medial or lateral heel (**Figure 6-30**). The heel is the preferred site, but the great toe may also be used. The sides of the fingers are used to collect the sample from adults. Use the middle and ring fingers (**Figure 6-31**). Puncturing the skin perpendicular to the fingerprint will cause a drop of blood to form. Puncturing the skin horizontal to the fingerprint will cause the blood to run down the finger instead of forming a drop.

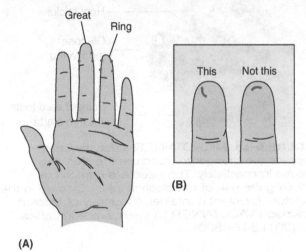

FIGURE 6-31 (A) In adults, collect capillary blood from the sides of the great and ring fingers. (B) Correct direction of puncture.

Avoid the other fingers. Avoid the pad in the center of the fingers. Earlobes may also be used. However, the earlobe is not as desirable as other areas, and should not be used if other sites are available. These sites are recommended because they have fewer nerve endings and are less painful. If multiple specimens are collected, rotate the sites. Avoid sites that are edematous, infected, swollen, scarred, or cyanotic. Do not puncture the same site repeatedly. In recent years, many new devices have been marketed for checking blood sugar in diabetic patients. Some of these advocate using the forearm and other areas for making the capillary puncture. Follow the instructions for the equipment you are using.

AGE-APPROPRIATE CARE ALERT

When doing a fingerstick capillary test on a child or adult, instruct the patient to wash his or her hands under warm, running water. This reduces the risk of infection and increases blood flow to the hand. After piercing the skin with the lancet, squeeze lightly to stimulate blood flow. Avoid prolonged pressure, as this may cause erroneous results by introducing tissue fluids. The fingerstick should be deep enough so that hard pressure is not required. If gentle pressure is not effective to start blood flow, repeat the puncture.

Do not try to collect a capillary sample if the skin is cool. The blood vessels are constricted, making it difficult to bring a drop of blood to the skin surface. You may wish to apply a warm washcloth to the area for 3 to 5 minutes before collecting the sample. The patient may also run the hand under warm water. This dilates the blood vessels, bringing blood to the surface and making the sample easier to collect.

Procedure 34

Drawing Blood Using a Lancet for a Microdraw or Infant Heel Stick

Supplies needed:
- Disposable exam gloves
- Alcohol or povidone-iodine sponges
- Lancets
- Microvette collection devices
- 2 × 2 gauze pads
- Labels for collection devices
- Permanent black pen for labels
- Laboratory requisition forms
- Puncture-resistant needle disposal container
- Plastic bag for used supplies
- Bandage or spot adhesive bandage

1. Perform your beginning procedure actions.
2. Check the requisition slip to determine what specimen to collect. Select the proper supplies.
3. Identify the specimen collection site.
4. Cleanse the site with alcohol. Wipe in a circular motion. Begin in the center of the puncture site and extend the circle out 2 inches in diameter.
5. Allow the alcohol or other skin prep to dry.
6. Hold the plastic end of the lancet in your dominant hand. With your nondominant hand, break the plastic cover off the end to expose the needle.
7. Hold the lancet at a 45° angle. With the sharp end of the lancet, pierce the skin. For an adult fingerstick, make the stick perpendicular to the lines in the fingerprints. Follow the directions for the type of lancet you are using. If the lancet has a plunger, depress it to pierce the skin while holding pressure on the site.
8. Remove the lancet. Discard it in the puncture-resistant sharps container.
9. Wipe the first drop of blood away with a sterile 2 × 2 sponge. You will need the rest to fill the containers.

10. Hold the collection tube near the puncture site. Position the tube almost horizontally, with the end slightly down. Squeeze the skin *slightly*, allowing blood to flow into the tube. Do not squeeze hard, as this forces tissue fluid into the sample, diluting it. If blood does not flow freely, create suction by placing your gloved finger over the end of the capillary tube, or by squeezing the small bulb. Fill the tube approximately ⅔ to ¾ full. Usually, two or three tubes are filled.
- If you are instructed to collect a sample on a filter paper test card, fill each circle by dropping a hanging drop of blood over it (Figure 6-32). Do not smear the blood into the circles.
11. Apply gentle pressure with the 2 × 2 gauze to the skin to prevent painful bleeding inside the tissues. The patient can hold the gauze sponge in place until the bleeding stops. Avoid using cotton balls. Cotton balls tend to stick to the puncture site and, when removed, remove the platelet plug, causing bleeding.

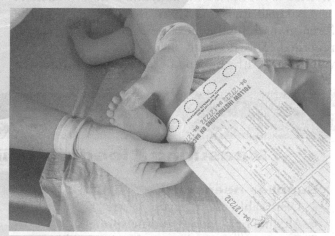

FIGURE 6-32 Transfer drops of blood from the capillary puncture to all circles on the filter paper card.

(continues)

Procedure **34**, *continued*

Drawing Blood Using a Lancet for a Microdraw or Infant Heel Stick

12. Wipe any remaining blood from the skin, and cover with an adhesive bandage.

13. Label the sample while in the patient's room.

14. Perform your procedure completion actions.

AGE-APPROPRIATE CARE ALERT

The bottom of the newborn infant's heel contains the best capillary bed. Avoid sites that were previously (recently) punctured. Puncture the skin on the flat bottom surface of the foot. Avoid the curve at the back of the heel. The heel bone (calcaneus) is very close to the skin in this area, and puncturing it could damage nerves or the bone, and increase the risk of infection. Warming the heel with a warm, moist washcloth will increase blood flow, but do not leave the washcloth in place for more than 2 to 3 minutes, or it will begin cooling the skin. Prep the skin and perform the capillary stick as soon as the washcloth is removed.

MEASURING BLEEDING TIME

The bleeding time test (**Figure 6-33**) measures how long it takes bleeding to stop. For this test, a small incision is made in the skin. The test is done for patients with a family history of bleeding disorders. It is also commonly used to screen patients for bleeding problems before surgery. Three methods of performing this test are used. The Mielke method is the most common, and is described here.

A small incision, 3 mm deep, is made in the forearm, and the time it takes for bleeding to stop is recorded. This normally takes 1 to 9 minutes. The values vary with the type of study used. Inform the patient that this procedure will result in a tiny scar on the forearm, which may be visible after healing.

Before performing this test, the RN must question the patient about medication intake over the past week. Aspirin, ibuprofen, and anticoagulant medications will alter the test results. Double-check with the RN to ensure that he or she has assessed the medication history. He or she has probably already done so, but double-checking does not hurt. If the patient is having surgery, you may be instructed to proceed with the test despite the medication regimen. Note the patient's medication use on the laboratory requisition form, or follow facility policy.

The forearm is the preferred site for the bleeding time test. Never perform the test above the site of an intravenous infusion. Select an area that is free from superficial veins. Some facilities apply a warm, moist compress to the forearm for 5 to 10 minutes before the procedure to bring blood to the skin surface. If you are unable to obtain blood from the forearm, inform the RN. An alternate method of testing may be performed on a different site.

Bleeding should stop during the procedure. If it has not stopped within 15 minutes, discontinue the procedure. Apply pressure to the incision to stop the bleeding with a 2 × 2 sponge in your gloved hand. Apply a dressing. Notify the RN that the procedure was stopped. He or she will notify the physician.

Procedure **35**

Measuring Bleeding Time

Supplies needed:

- Disposable exam gloves
- Alcohol or povidone-iodine sponges
- Surgicutt®, template, spring-loaded blade, or similar device
- Tourniquet
- Blood pressure cuff
- Watch with second hand
- Filter paper
- 2 × 2 gauze pads
- Puncture-resistant sharps container
- Plastic bag for used supplies
- Steri-strips, butterfly bandage, or other bandage

(continues)

Procedure 35, *continued*

Measuring Bleeding Time

1. Perform your beginning procedure actions. Double-check the requisition slip.
2. Support the patient's arm on the bed or other surface, palm up. Make sure the patient is comfortable and can maintain this position for the duration of the procedure.
3. Apply the blood pressure cuff to the upper arm. Do not inflate it.
4. Apply gloves.
5. You will perform the test approximately 4 inches below the antecubital space. Cleanse the site with alcohol or povidone-iodine. Wipe in a circular motion. Begin in the center of the puncture site and extend the circle out 3 inches in diameter.
6. Allow the alcohol or other skin prep to dry.
7. Remove the Surgicutt®, template, or other product from the package. Twist off the tab on the side, taking care not to touch the blade or activate the trigger.
8. Inflate the blood pressure cuff until the gauge reads 40 mm Hg. You must start the test within 60 seconds of inflating the cuff.
9. Apply the Surgicutt® or other device to the prepared skin, approximately 4 inches below the antecubital space. Position the device so the blade is parallel to the bend in the elbow.
10. Depress the trigger while monitoring the second hand on your watch. Remove the blade from the skin within 1 second of depressing the trigger. Record the time. Discard the device containing the blade in the puncture-resistant container.
11. Absorb the blood with the edge of the filter paper. Position the paper near the incision, without touching the wound directly. Placing the paper directly on the incision will interfere with the results of the test.
12. With the filter paper, blot the bleeding every 30 seconds. When the blood no longer stains the paper, stop timing. Discard the filter paper in the plastic bag. Record the time the test ended.
13. Deflate the blood pressure cuff.
14. Wipe remaining blood from the skin.
15. Apply a steri-strip, butterfly bandage, or dressing to the incision.
16. Remove the gloves and discard in the plastic bag.
17. Remove the blood pressure cuff.
18. Perform your procedure completion actions.

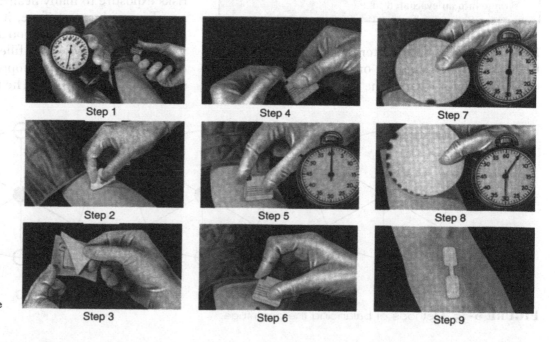

FIGURE 6-33
Surgicutt bleeding time procedure

Step 1   Step 4   Step 7

Step 2   Step 5   Step 8

Step 3   Step 6   Step 9

TRANSPORTING SPECIMENS TO THE LABORATORY

Blood specimens are considered biohazardous waste materials, and a biohazard label should be affixed to the test tubes. The samples should be transported to the laboratory in the test tube carrier. If this is not available, seal the tubes in a plastic bag for transport. Affix a biohazard label or color code, according to facility policy. Make sure the specimen is properly labeled. Ensure that the requisition slip does not become separated from the sample.

THE CENTRIFUGE

The **centrifuge** (Figure 6-34) is a device that holds and spins test tubes. This is done to separate liquids from solids within the tubes. Several different types of centrifuges are used. One type of centrifuge is used to spin test tubes, and another type is used for capillary tubes.

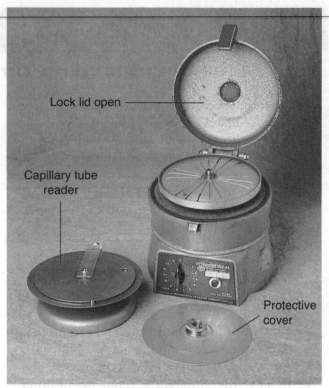

FIGURE 6-34 A tabletop centrifuge

Lock lid open

Capillary tube reader

Protective cover

PROCEDURE ALERT

Hemolysis results from breaking of red blood cells. Unfortunately, it may not be detected until the sample has been separated. Severe hemolysis interferes with many tests, and the sample must be redrawn. Hemolysis may occur when:
- Drawing blood from a vein with a hematoma
- Quickly pulling the plunger back on the syringe
- Using a needle with a small gauge
- Using a butterfly needle with a very large collection tube
- Frothing of blood because of air leak or improper fitting of needle on syringe
- Not using a blood transfer device; forcing blood from a syringe into an evacuated tube

Desktop and large, laboratory models are available. Keep the rubber stoppers on the tubes while centrifuging. Before using the centrifuge, check the

test tubes for cracks, scratches, or chips. The tubes must be intact, or they will break as they spin. If a tube breaks during the procedure, turn the centrifuge off immediately. Keep the lid to the unit closed until it stops spinning. The device spins at up to 3,000 revolutions per minute, so broken or open tubes will spray blood or body fluids. If a tube accidentally breaks, you must clean the unit following the manufacturer's directions. A soiled unit risks exposure to many health care workers.

To use the centrifuge, it must be counterbalanced. In other words, if you are testing a tube, you must place another tube, filled with approximately the same volume of water, opposite the tube you are spinning (Figure 6-35). The tube you are using as

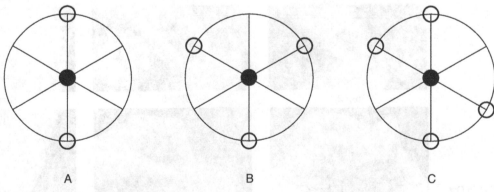

A   B   C

FIGURE 6-35 Methods of balancing the centrifuge

a counterbalance should be the same size as the blood-filled tube.

After the centrifuge stops spinning, remove the tubes and place them in a rack. Next, the rubber stopper must be removed so the specimen can be tested. If you will be responsible for this procedure, wear full protective apparel, including a long-sleeved lab coat or gown, gloves, a mask, and a face shield. Cover the rubber stopper with a gauze pad and twist it off, holding the end of the tube away from your face.

Methods of using the centrifuge vary with the type of test and type of tube in which the specimen is collected. The type of centrifuge and operating instructions vary from one facility to the next. Your employer will teach you to operate the unit if this will be one of your responsibilities.

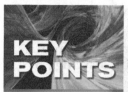

KEY POINTS

▶ Phlebotomy means collecting blood.

▶ Venipuncture is the act of collecting blood from a vein.

▶ Age, illness, dehydration, and previous needlesticks all affect the condition of the veins.

▶ The gauge of the needle determines the inside diameter of the needle, or the lumen.

▶ In most situations, a 20- to 23-gauge needle is used for drawing blood.

▶ The intravenous needle is always inserted in the direction of blood flow.

▶ A sterile needle is used each time the skin is penetrated.

▶ Always apply the principles of standard precautions when performing venipuncture.

▶ Blood can be withdrawn by using a vacuum-tube system, needle and syringe, butterfly and syringe, or butterfly and vacuum tube.

▶ Blood inside a syringe will begin to coagulate or clot within 1 to 2 minutes after the specimen is drawn.

▶ Always use an instrument to change needles.

▶ Never recap a used needle.

▶ Avoid drawing blood from: an arm in which an intravenous solution or blood is being administered; an infected or edematous area; an extremity with a dialysis access device, shunt, or graft; an existing intravenous line or heparin lock; the affected arm of a mastectomy patient; the site of previous injury or hematoma; any burned or scarred area; or leg or foot veins.

▶ Precautions to take when drawing blood include immobilizing the vein before performing venipuncture, positioning the needle with the bevel facing up, inserting the needle in the direction of blood flow, not sticking the patient more than twice, keeping the tourniquet on the arm for less than 2 minutes, ensuring that you are not entering an artery, labeling the tubes properly, discarding needles in a puncture-resistant container, and transporting tubes of blood in a tube holder or a sealed, plastic transport bag labeled with the biohazard emblem.

▶ Hematoma is the most common complication of venipuncture.

▶ Infection is a complication of venipuncture that is usually caused by improper technique.

▶ Select a large, straight vein for performing phlebotomy procedures. The antecubital space is commonly used.

▶ Never pierce the skin unless you can see or feel the vein.

▶ Veins are near the skin surface, feel rubbery, and will rebound slightly when touched. They are not hard to the touch and do not pulsate.

(continues)

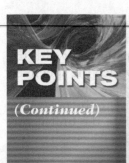

KEY POINTS

(Continued)

▶ Proper application of the tourniquet is important to the success of the procedure.

▶ Blood should be collected in this order: blood culture bottles, nonadditive tubes (red), coagulation (or citrate) tubes (blue), and additive tubes last.

▶ Always notify the RN after you have collected the patient's blood specimen so that restrictions on eating, drinking, and medication administration can be lifted.

▶ Wear a fluid-resistant gown, gloves, mask, and face shield when transferring blood from one container to another.

▶ A butterfly needle is useful for collecting blood from children, and from adults with small, fragile veins. This needle can be used with a syringe or vacuum-tube system.

▶ A blood culture is a sterile procedure performed to test for a systemic blood infection, or septicemia. The sample should be collected when the patient has a fever and is chilling.

▶ A microdraw is a small skin puncture used for collecting blood specimens.

▶ A microlance or lancet is used to pierce the skin for a microdraw.

▶ Blood from a microdraw is collected in a capillary tube. Glass tubes pose a very high risk of breakage, and should not be used.

▶ The microvette collection device is similar to a glass capillary tube, but does not carry the risk of breakage and contamination.

▶ A capillary specimen should be collected from the sides of the third or fourth finger in adults, or the sides of the heels in infants.

▶ If capillary specimens are collected frequently from a patient, use different puncture sites.

▶ The bleeding time test measures how long it takes bleeding to stop.

▶ Aspirin, ibuprofen, and anticoagulants prolong bleeding time.

▶ A tiny incision is made in the forearm to collect the bleeding time test. This may leave a small scar after it has healed.

▶ The centrifuge is a device that holds and spins test tubes.

▶ The centrifuge must be counterbalanced, and tubes must be intact to reduce the risk of breakage.

CLINICAL APPLICATIONS

1. An obese patient tells you she has blood drawn frequently in her doctor's office. You are having difficulty locating a vein. She points to her inner antecubital space and tells you she has a good vein there. What will you do?

2. You must draw blood from an infant. The child is very active. The parents are in the room. Do you need an assistant to perform this procedure? Why or why not? What is the best action to take?

3. You enter the room where Susan, another PCT, is attempting to remove a used needle from a sy-

ringe using her thumb and index finger. She explains that she contaminated the needle and is changing it before puncturing the skin again. The patient is listening and watching attentively. What action will you take?

4. After drawing blood with a butterfly needle and syringe, you must transfer the specimen to vac- uum tubes. What personal protective equipment will you wear?

5. You are assigned to draw blood from Mrs. Terensky. She tells you that her veins collapse easily. Her veins are visible and protrude above the skin surface without a tourniquet. State some techniques to use that will minimize the risk of vein collapse.

C H A P T E R   R E V I E W

Multiple-Choice Questions

Select the one best answer.

1. Which of the following affect the condition of the veins?
   a. Pulse rate   c. Fever
   b. Mental status   d. Dehydration

2. Avoid drawing blood from the feet and legs because this increases the risk of:
   a. hemorrhage.   c. infection.
   b. blood clots.   d. edema.

3. When collecting blood from an adult, select a:
   a. 12- to 14-gauge needle.
   b. 16- to 18-gauge needle.
   c. 20- to 23-gauge needle.
   d. 25- to 27-gauge needle.

4. The easiest and safest method of drawing blood involves using a:
   a. vacuum-tube collection system.
   b. needle and syringe.
   c. butterfly and syringe.
   d. plastic cannula and syringe.

5. When changing a used needle, always use:
   a. your fingertips.
   b. an instrument.
   c. the sharps container.
   d. a filter paper.

6. Mr. Huynh has an IV in his left forearm. His right hand is bandaged because of a hematoma from a previous IV. You must draw blood from this patient. It is safe to draw blood from the:
   a. left antecubital space.
   b. right antecubital space.
   c. left hand.
   d. right foot.

7. Apply the tourniquet so that the ends of the strap face the:
   a. shoulder.   c. chest.
   b. wrist.   d. wall to the
                            patient's right.

8. You have collected blood in a vacuum tube containing a preservative. You should:
   a. immediately transport the specimen to the lab.
   b. shake the tube vigorously.
   c. transfer the specimen to another tube.
   d. invert the tube 5 to 8 times.

9. When transferring blood from a syringe to a blood culture bottle, you should:
   a. shake the bottle vigorously.
   b. inject 1 mL of air into the bottle.
   c. use a sterile transfer device.
   d. use a butterfly needle.

10. Before inserting a test tube into the centrifuge, you should:
    a. check the tube for cracks and chips.
    b. remove the rubber stopper.
    c. fill a larger tube with water.
    d. wipe the unit with disinfectant.

EXPLORING THE WEB

Adult Venipuncture	http://www.pathology.unc.edu
CDC: Safety Devices for Phlebotomy Procedures	http://www.thebody.com
Dartmouth-Hitchcock Medical Center Laboratory Procedures Manual	http://labhandbook.hitchcock.org:591
Disposal of Contaminated Needles and Blood Tube Holders Used for Phlebotomy	http://www.osha.gov
Georgia Institute of Technology Biosafety Manual Policies and Procedures	http://www.safety.gatech.edu
Pediatric Venipuncture—Evacuated Tube Method	http://www.pathology.unc.edu
Phlebotomy CEU module for RNs, LPNs, Nurse Practitioners	http://www.nursingclasses.com
Phlebotomy Team Policies	http://www.medicine.uiowa.edu
Specimen Collection	http://www.crlcorp.com
Tidewater Naval Medical Center Laboratory Policies and Procedures Manual	http://www-nmcp.med.navy.mil
Tourniquet Left on Patient's Arm for Ten Minutes— Ulnar Nerve Damage—$154,000 Gross Kentucky Verdict.	http://www.hpso.com
WNCC Policies and Procedures Manual	http://www.wncc.edu

CHAPTER
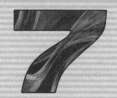

Intravenous Therapy

OBJECTIVES:

After reading this chapter, you should be able to:

● Spell and define key terms.
● Describe how to select the insertion site for IV therapy.
● List at least five factors influencing the type of device selected for venipuncture.
● List at least 10 precautions to take when starting an IV.
● Explain why immobilizing the insertion site is important.
● State the purpose of IV controllers and volumetric pumps and describe how each is used.
● Describe five common complications of IV therapy, and list signs and symptoms of each.
● State the purpose of a heparin lock.
● List considerations for pediatric IV therapy.
● State the purpose of a central intravenous catheter.
● Describe precautions to take when checking blood, and list signs and symptoms of a transfusion reaction.

INTRAVENOUS THERAPY

Intravenous (IV) therapy requires the venipuncture skills you learned in Chapter 6. The IV procedure involves inserting a needle into a vein for the purpose of administering fluids and medications. A physician's order is always necessary for this procedure. State laws vary regarding who can perform intravenous procedures. In some states, only RNs are allowed to perform these procedures. In others, LPN/LVNs can perform these procedures after completing a special training course. In some states, the nurse practice act and state laws do not address these procedures, so they can be performed by unlicensed personnel. Your instructor will guide you according to your state law and nurse practice act. You may not be allowed to perform some or all of the procedures in this chapter, depending on your facility policies and state regulations.

Intravenous solutions and supplies are always sterile. You must keep all parts of the system sterile to prevent infection, a serious complication. If a piece of intravenous equipment accidentally becomes contaminated, replace it.

Many different products are available for starting an IV. The most commonly used devices are catheters that are mounted over needles. The size of the device inserted in the vein is determined by the size of the vein and the type of the solution to be administered. The vein must be large enough to hold the catheter. A size 20- to 24-gauge catheter is used for most adults. Strict aseptic technique is used for this procedure. Your risk of needlestick injuries is high for the procedures in this chapter. Follow your facility policies and procedures for needle insertion and disposal, and exercise caution when handling these devices. Avoid recapping used needles. Avoid contact with catheters and other devices that have contacted the patient's blood.

Site Selection

You will select the site using the same principles you learned for phlebotomy. The age of the patient and how long the IV is to remain in place may influence your selection. Avoid the veins of the lower extremities. Avoid the scalp veins in infants unless you are specially trained in this procedure. Select a vein in the hand or forearm of the nondominant hand, if possible. If the patient is expected to have ongoing intravenous therapy, site selection is critical. Selecting a site low on the hand or arm allows for site rotation and subsequent venipuncture higher up on the arm. Avoid veins over joints whenever possible, particularly if the patient is restless or cannot be expected to cooperate. Choose the largest, straightest vein available.

Intravenous Needles and Catheters

The selection of an IV needle or catheter is determined by the patient's diagnosis, length of IV therapy, type of medication or other solution infused, and condition of the veins. Other considerations are the size of the patient's veins, the location of the IV insertion site, and the patient's activity level.

In general, the gauge of plastic intravenous catheters is denoted using an even number. The gauge of butterfly and steel needles for intravenous use is listed in odd numbers. Patient comfort is an important consideration. Catheters stay in the vein longer than needles, and permit more movement. In most cases, the health care worker selects the device to use. However, the physician may order a specific needle or catheter. Check with the RN for the correct device to use.

Most intravenous therapy is infused through flexible, plastic or Teflon catheters, or **over-the-needle catheters** (ONCs) (**Figure 7-1**). ONCs are used for short- or long-term IV therapy, and for restless patients. Many brand names are available, in an assortment of sizes. These are inserted into the vein with a needle or introducer. The catheter is threaded into the vein after the vein has been pierced by the needle. The needle is withdrawn, the catheter is connected to the fluid administration set, and the flow of intravenous solution is initiated.

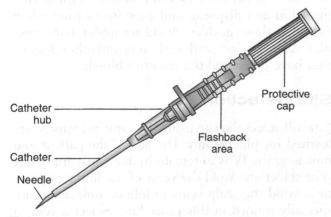

Catheter hub

Protective cap

Flashback area

Catheter

Needle

FIGURE 7-1 The over-the-needle catheter

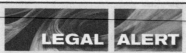

LEGAL ALERT

Nurses apply certain principles, practices, and safeguards to reduce the risk of medication errors. These are called the "six rights" of medication administration. You will apply these same six rights to intravenous initiation and administration. These are:
- Right solution
  - Compare the label to the MAR or order
  - Check the IV three times
  - Make sure you have the correct preparation
  - Always check the expiration date
  - Always check for allergies, especially for the prep solution, dressing, and tape. Make sure the patient is not allergic to alcohol, iodine, tape, or transparent dressings.
- Right strength
  - Always ask an RN to check your calculations of drip rates. Some IV solutions, such as dextrose and saline, are available in different concentrations. If you have any doubts about whether the solution you are using is correct, check with the RN.
- Right route
  - Make sure the preparation you are using is labeled for IV use.
  - Make sure all equipment is sterile and that flawless sterile technique is maintained.
- Right time
  - Check the order for correct time
- Right patient
  - Always check the patient ID band. Ask the patient to state his or her name.
  - If the patient does not have an ID band on, obtain one and apply it.
- Right documentation
  - Never chart IVs in advance.
  - Initial the IV record immediately after starting the IV.
  - Document other care (such as changing dressings or tubing) on the correct form.
  - If the patient is not on intake and output (I&O), place an I&O worksheet at the bedside and inform the RN so he or she can initiate I&O monitoring.
  - Document vital signs, such as pulse or blood pressure, and other monitoring as warranted by patient condition, physician orders, and facility policies.

The Intravenous Solution

Intravenous fluid is a prescription item, and must be ordered by a physician. The order must be followed exactly as written. The solution is packaged in a plastic bag or bottle. To infuse properly, the solution must hang at least 30 to 36 inches above the level of the heart. The solution is attached to an IV pole or IV standard at the patient's bedside. The standard is adjustable. The height of the IV standard affects the rate of flow of fluid. Fluid runs faster when the standard is elevated to the maximum height.

The Basic Infusion Set

Flexible, plastic tubing through which the solution flows is attached to the IV solution on one end, and the patient on the other. This is called the **administration set.** Several types of administration sets are used for special purposes. You will be starting IVs using the basic administration set (**Figure 7-2**). The design of the basic administration set varies slightly with the manufacturer. A manual or electronic device is used to control the flow of solution.

You must understand the purpose of the various parts of the basic administration set. The **piercing pin** pierces the plastic bag or bottle. The pin is sterile, and is covered with a plastic cap. The **drop orifice** is the entry to the **drip chamber** or drop chamber. The orifice controls the size of the drops of fluid. The drip chamber is a semi-rigid container that is filled halfway with fluid. It allows easy visualization of the flow rate.

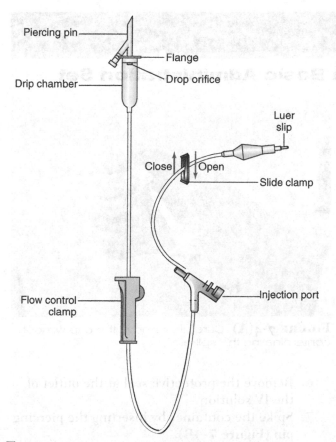

FIGURE 7-2 The basic IV administration set

Some administration sets have two **Y-sites,** and some have only one. This is a connection for administration of medications. The **flow control clamp** is a roller clamp used to regulate the speed or rate of fluid flow. The lower **slide clamp** is a plastic clamp used to stop or regulate the flow of fluid. It is used primarily during medication administration, but may be used to stop the fluid quickly, if necessary. Some administration sets do not have this clamp. The **Luer slips** at the bottom connect the tubing to the needle or IV catheter. The Luer mechanism provides a means of locking the tubing and needle or catheter together, making them more difficult to separate. The basic administration set should be made by the same manufacturer as the IV solution you are using.

Before initiating an IV, always prime the tubing with the IV solution so it is completely full of fluid and free from bubbles. This will reduce the risk of air entering the vein, which can kill the patient.

Special Considerations

Intravenous administration sets come in both **macrodrip** and **microdrip** versions. The macrodrip is most commonly used for adults. The microdrip is used for pediatric patients and for certain adults. The macrodrip sets deliver fluid in a larger volume, typically 10 to 20 drops per milliliter of fluid. The volume delivered in the macrodrip set varies with the manufacturer and the purpose of the tubing. The microdrip sets deliver fluid in smaller drops, usually 60 drops per milliliter. Always select the macrodrip unless directed otherwise by the RN.

The best way to prevent infection is to use standard precautions and strict aseptic technique, including good handwashing. However, some health care facilities attach in-line **filters** (Figure 7-3) to the administration set. Filters allow fluid to pass, but trap particles. Many agencies do not use them routinely, believing that they increase the infection rate and cause occlusion. If used, the filters are attached to the administration set. Know and follow your facility policy, which should address the use of filtering mechanisms.

The junctions of an intravenous infusion must be fastened together securely to prevent serious complications. They should not, however, be taped. Junctions in the administration set, filter, and between the insertion device and catheter or needle should be connected according to the manufacturer's directions. A heparin lock must also be fastened securely. (Use of heparin locks is described

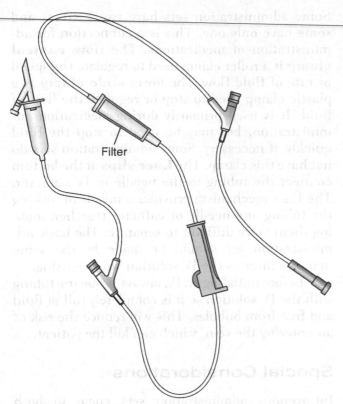

FIGURE 7-3 An in-line filter attached to the basic IV administration set

later in this chapter.) In most equipment, the two pieces of equipment are pushed together, then twisted tightly in a clockwise direction.

Marking the Container. Your facility will have policies regarding information to mark on the intravenous container, or the pharmacy may provide a label with some of this information. You may be asked to mark the container with the:

- Patient's name
- Room number
- Date and time
- Container number
- Flow rate ordered
- Duration of the infusion
- Your name or initials

Intravenous containers are made of various types of plastic. Never write directly on the container with a permanent marker or pen. The ink from a marker will bleed through the plastic container, contaminating the solution. Write on a label, then affix the label to the container. Avoid covering writing or markings on the container with the label.

Procedure 36

Assembling and Priming a Basic Administration Set

Supplies needed:
▶ Intravenous solution
▶ Basic administration set

1. Perform your beginning procedure actions.
2. Open the package and remove the administration set.
3. Close the roller clamp.
4. Hold the solution to the light and examine it for particles, cloudiness, or discoloration. Examine the container for cracks or chips. Do not use the solution if it contains particles, the fluid is cloudy, or the color is abnormal. Do not use a container that is chipped or cracked. Do not use a solution that is past the expiration date.
5. Remove the cover from the piercing pin (Figure 7-4A). Maintain sterility and avoid touching this device to other surfaces.

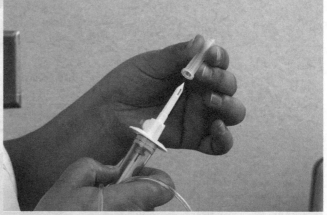

FIGURE 7-4(A) Carefully remove the cap without contaminating the spike.

6. Remove the protective seal at the outlet of the IV solution.
7. Spike the container by inserting the piercing pin (Figure 7-4B).

(continues)

Procedure **36**, *continued*

Assembling and Priming a Basic Administration Set

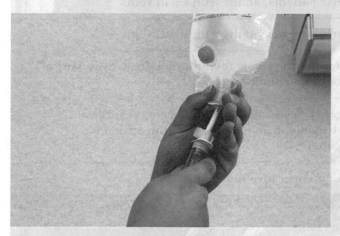

FIGURE 7-4(B) Pierce the bag or bottle with the spike.

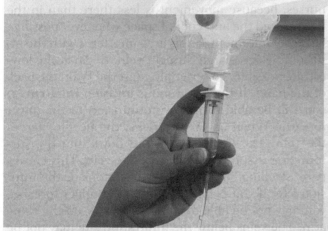

FIGURE 7-4(C) To fill the drip chamber, gently squeeze the sides, then release.

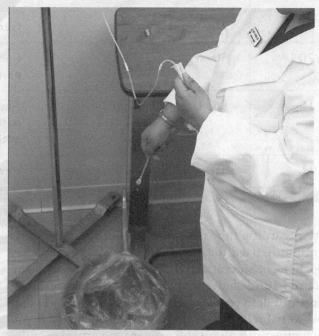

FIGURE 7-4(D) Open the roller clamp (or slide clamp), allowing fluid to flow through the tubing.

8. Hang the container of solution on an IV pole.
9. Squeeze the sides of the drip chamber gently until they meet (**Figure 7-4C**), then release them. This allows fluid to flow into the chamber to the halfway point.
10. Slowly open the roller clamp, allowing fluid to flow through the tubing (**Figure 7-4D**).

Leave the clamp open until all air is expelled from the tubing. The tube should be completely filled with fluid.
11. Close the roller clamp.
12. If the set has Y-connection sites, tap them gently to remove trapped air. Cover the distal end of the tubing with a cap, as appropriate, to maintain sterility.
13. Loop the tubing over the IV pole to keep it from touching the floor or other surfaces.
14. Prepare a label according to facility policy. Affix the label to the solution. Do not cover the markings on the container.
15. Perform your procedure completion actions or perform the venipuncture.

INSERTING A PERIPHERAL IV IN AN ADULT

The technique used for venipuncture in Procedure 29 is the same technique used for starting an IV. What is different, however, is the type of device used for fluid administration. Straight needles are seldom used, if ever. You will be using an over-the-needle catheter (ONC) or butterfly needle. For most adult fluid infusions, you will use a 20- to 24-gauge ONC. However, if the patient will be receiving blood, a larger gauge is used. Facility policies

Table 7-1 Catheter Selection Considerations

Gauge	Fluid Delivery Rate	Factors Influencing Selection
24	15–25 mL/minute	Geriatric patients, adults with small veins
22	26–36 mL/minute	Geriatric patients, adults with small veins
20	50–65 mL/minute	Long-term intravenous therapy, radiologic dyes, partial parenteral nutrition
18	85–105 mL/minute	Emergency department patients, general surgical patients, patients in which blood transfusion is anticipated
16	More than 105 mL/minute	Certain preoperative infusions

vary regarding the size, but an 18-gauge catheter is commonly used for blood. In addition to vein size, another consideration for catheter selection is the ordered fluid delivery rate. Suggested sizes, uses, and fluid delivery rates are listed in **Table 7-1**. Follow your facility policy. Check with the RN if you have questions about the proper type and size of device. Some facilities use prepackaged kits for starting IVs. Others use individual supplies.

Selecting the Vein

Follow the same precautions for site selection and needle insertion that you use for phlebotomy. Avoid:

- An infected or edematous area
- An area with a rash
- An extremity with a dialysis access device, shunt, fistula, or graft
- An existing intravenous line or heparin lock
- The affected arm of a mastectomy patient
- The affected arm of a paralyzed patient
- An arm with neurological or circulatory impairment
- The site of previous injury or hematoma
- Any burned or scarred area
- The leg and foot veins, whenever possible (check with the RN before considering these veins)

Ask the patient which is his or her dominant hand. If possible, start the IV in the opposite extremity. This allows maximum freedom of movement. Hand and forearm veins are most commonly used.

The veins of the hand and forearm are pictured in **Figure 7-5**. Forearm veins are preferred by some nurses, because movement is less there than in the hand. Avoid the antecubital space whenever possible, because movement in this area interferes with the infusion. Select a large, straight vein. Begin at the lowest site possible. For example, start the IV on the back of the hand. If the intravenous infusion **infiltrates,** you will be able to move the infusion to the lower forearm. When an IV infiltrates, the needle pierces the vein. The intravenous fluid flows into the surrounding tissue instead of into the vein. This causes pain, swelling, and other complications at the infusion site. If you begin therapy in the upper forearm, you may not be able to start another IV on the same arm. The veins below the infiltration site may not be usable. Follow your facility policy for site selection. If in doubt about vein availability, check with the RN.

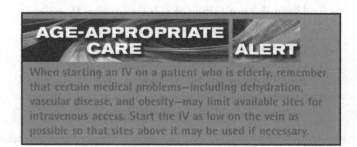

AGE-APPROPRIATE CARE — **ALERT**

When starting an IV on a patient who is elderly, remember that certain medical problems—including dehydration, vascular disease, and obesity—may limit available sites for intravenous access. Start the IV as low on the vein as possible so that sites above it may be used if necessary.

Patient Teaching

Patients may be anxious about IV insertion. The RN is responsible for patient teaching, but you must reinforce this teaching each time you perform a procedure. Make sure you explain the procedure well, and answer the patient's questions before be-

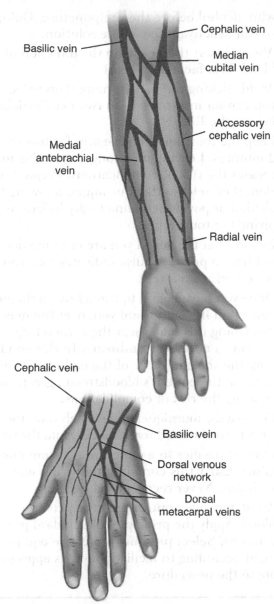

- Cephalic vein
- Basilic vein
- Median cubital vein
- Accessory cephalic vein
- Medial antebrachial vein
- Radial vein
- Cephalic vein
- Basilic vein
- Dorsal venous network
- Dorsal metacarpal veins

FIGURE 7-5 Hand and forearm veins

ginning. If the patient has questions that you cannot answer, notify the RN. When describing the intravenous procedure, explain that the solution may feel cold at first, but that this sensation will subside within a few minutes. Also explain signs of complications to the patient. Instruct him or her to report any discomfort, pain, or burning after the catheter is inserted and solution begins to flow. Also advise the patient to report swelling or leaking at the insertion site. Inform the patient to call if the solution stops dripping, suddenly slows down or speeds up, or if blood backs up in the tubing.

Advise the patient how to manage the intravenous infusion. Inform the patient of the purpose of the roller clamp, and instruct him or her to leave the clamp alone. Advise him or her not to remove the solution from the IV pole. Also explain that he or she should avoid pulling on the tubing, or lying on, kinking, or otherwise obstructing the tubing. If possible, instruct the patient to position the arm with the IV at heart level when in bed. When the patient is ambulating, instruct him or her to place the arm with the IV across the abdomen. Advise the patient not to comb hair or brush teeth with the arm with the IV. You should check the infusion and insertion site each time you are in the room, or according to facility policy.

Some facilities inject a small amount of anesthetic into the skin before IV insertion. Some facilities apply a patch of topical anesthetic cream, called EMLA cream (**Figure 7-6**), to the insertion site one hour prior to the venipuncture. These procedures will be done by the RN. If no anesthetic is used, explain that the patient will feel slight pain at the insertion site, but that the sensation will stop after the catheter is inserted.

Precautions to take when starting an IV include:

- Always use aseptic technique.

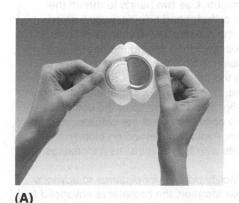
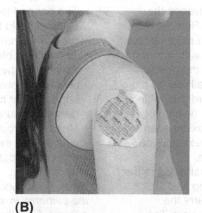
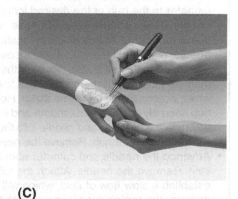

(A)   **(B)**   **(C)**

FIGURE 7-6 EMLA cream may be applied to the insertion site one hour prior to the venipuncture to numb the skin. (A) Remove the backing. (B) Apply the patch to the insertion site. (C) Label the dressing. (Courtesy of AstraZeneca LP, Wayne, PA)

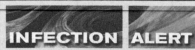

INFECTION ALERT

An IV infection can be very serious, because once inside the blood vessel, pathogens can move freely about the body. Most IV infections are caused by skin flora that are picked up during or after catheter insertion. Organisms on the skin at the insertion site may migrate on the inside or outside of the catheter. Contamination of the hub or connectors may also migrate into the catheter, causing infection.

- Avoid injecting air into a vein. Check the tubing to ensure that no air remains. If you will be using a syringe to start the IV, ensure that the plunger is pushed all the way in.
- Immobilize the vein with the thumb of your opposite hand before inserting the needle.
- Position the needle with the bevel facing up.

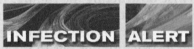

INFECTION ALERT

Never wipe the skin with alcohol after applying a povidone-iodine prep solution. The alcohol eliminates the beneficial effect of the povidone-iodine. Remember to check the patient's allergies. Iodine allergy is fairly common.

- Cleanse the skin with alcohol or povidone-iodine for one full minute. Avoid leaving iodine on an area that will come into contact with tape or a transparent dressing, as this may cause a chemical reaction, resulting in a burn. Wipe the area with an alcohol sponge to remove the iodine after the venipuncture has been completed. Never remove the iodine

with alcohol before the venipuncture. Doing so will deactivate the iodine solution.

- Always insert the needle in the direction of blood flow, facing the heart.
- Avoid sticking the patient more than twice. If you cannot insert the IV in two needlesticks, inform the RN.
- Keep the tourniquet on the arm for less than 2 minutes. Leaving it on longer than this increases the risk of complications. Prepare the skin, then release the tourniquet, allowing the alcohol or povidone-iodine to dry before reapplying the tourniquet.
- Ensure that the vessel you are entering does not have a pulse. A pulse indicates that you are entering an artery.
- Once you have begun to thread the catheter, never pull it back toward you, over the needle. Doing this may shear the catheter tip, creating a **catheter embolus.** In this condition, the sheared piece of the catheter floats freely in the patient's bloodstream, greatly increasing the risk of complications.
- Remove the tourniquet immediately after the catheter is threaded (or advanced) into the vein.
- Discard needles in a puncture-resistant container. Carry this container to the bedside with you. Never recap a used needle.
- Avoid personal contact with the patient's blood. Apply the principles of standard precautions. Select personal protective equipment according to facility policy, as appropriate to the procedure.

- Carefully advance the catheter and needle into the vein as a unit. When you reach the hub of the catheter, remove the needle.
- Hold the needle securely and carefully advance the catheter to the hub or the desired length. Remove the needle. If the catheter kinks or bends, you must remove it and restart the IV in a different location with a new needle. Never pull the catheter back over the needle.
- Hold the needle unit stable. Advance the catheter no more than 1/4 inch (or pull the needle back toward you 1/4 inch, which accomplishes the same thing). Hold the catheter hub securely between your thumb and index finger and advance the catheter and needle into the vein until you reach the catheter hub. Remove the needle.
- Advance the needle and catheter about halfway into the vein. Remove the needle. Attach the tubing and establish a slow flow of fluid, which will carry the catheter the remainder of the way into the vein. To be effective, the skin and vein must be securely anchored with one hand.

- One-handed technique: Use the index finger to advance the catheter, while simultaneously withdrawing the needle using the thumb and middle finger.
- Two-handed technique: Use two hands to thread the catheter. Hold the catheter and skin securely with one hand while removing the needle with the other hand.
- To minimize bleeding when removing the needle and connecting the tubing, hold the hub of the catheter securely between the thumb and index finger of your nondominant hand. Use the ring or small finger to apply gentle pressure slightly above the tip of the catheter. Make sure you are above the tip of the catheter, and not directly over the tip. Avoid this method on elderly persons, or patients with fragile veins, as it increases the pressure.

Note: Follow your facility policies for distance to advance the catheter. In some facilities, the catheter is advanced to 1/8 inch from the hub. This enables the RN to remove the catheter with forceps in the unlikely event it becomes separated from the hub.

FIGURE 7-7 Techniques for threading a catheter

Threading the Catheter

Once you have entered the vein, you must carefully thread the catheter and remove the needle without accidentally piercing the vein wall. When you have a flashback of blood, lower the needle slightly so it is almost even with the skin. Several different techniques may be used to advance the catheter. Use whichever method is easiest for you. These methods are listed in **Figure 7-7**. An alternate method used for removing a safety needle is shown in **Figure 7-8**.

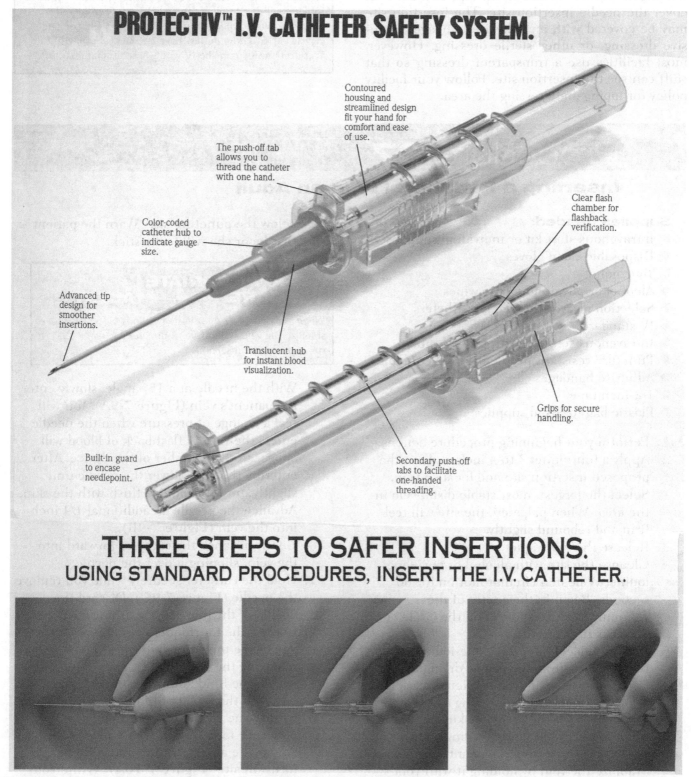

PROTECTIV™ I.V. CATHETER SAFETY SYSTEM.

Contoured housing and streamlined design fit your hand for comfort and ease of use.

The push-off tab allows you to thread the catheter with one hand.

Clear flash chamber for flashback verification.

Color-coded catheter hub to indicate gauge size.

Advanced tip design for smoother insertions.

Translucent hub for instant blood visualization.

Grips for secure handling.

Built-in guard to encase needlepoint.

Secondary push-off tabs to facilitate one-handed threading.

THREE STEPS TO SAFER INSERTIONS.
USING STANDARD PROCEDURES, INSERT THE I.V. CATHETER.

FIGURE 7-8 PROTECTIV™ IV Catheter Safety System. (Courtesy of Ethicon Endosurgery, a Johnson & Johnson Company)

Immobilizing and Dressing the Insertion Site

The needle insertion site must be immobilized with tape to prevent the catheter from moving. Movement is uncomfortable and increases the risk of dislodging the catheter. Position the tape so it does not cover the needle insertion site. The insertion site may be covered with an adhesive bandage, occlusive dressing, or other sterile dressing. However, most facilities use a transparent dressing so that staff can see the insertion site. Follow your facility policy for taping and dressing the area.

AGE-APPROPRIATE CARE ALERT

Immobilize the catheter well to prevent movement, which may cause skin tears and infiltration. However, you must follow your facility policies and documentation for use of restraints. In some situations, the device or method you use for immobilizing the insertion site may be considered a restraint. This is a particular problem with pediatric and elderly patients who do not have the mental capacity to keep from dislodging the IV without additional restraint.

Procedure 37

Inserting a Peripheral IV in an Adult

Supplies needed:
- Intravenous start kit or individual supplies
- Disposable exam gloves
- Tourniquet
- Alcohol or povidone-iodine wipes
- Selection of over-the-needle catheters
- IV standard
- Intravenous solution with primed tubing
- Puncture-resistant needle disposal container
- Adhesive bandages
- 1/2-inch tape
- Plastic bag for used supplies

1. Perform your beginning procedure actions.
2. Apply a tourniquet 3 to 4 inches above the proposed insertion site and locate a vein. Select the largest, most stable distal vein in the area. When palpated, the site will feel firm and rebound slightly.
3. Release the tourniquet.
4. Cleanse the site with alcohol or povidone-iodine. Wipe in a circular motion for 60 seconds. Begin in the center of the venipuncture site and extend the circle out 3 inches in diameter.
5. Allow the alcohol or povidone-iodine to dry thoroughly. While the skin is drying, cut the tape and place it in a convenient location.
6. Reapply the tourniquet, taking care not to bump or touch the prepped skin area.
7. Remove the needle cover, holding the needle bevel facing up in your dominant hand.
8. Stabilize the vein by holding it with your nondominant thumb, approximately 1 inch

below the puncture site. Warn the patient that he or she will feel a stick.

AGE-APPROPRIATE CARE ALERT

When starting an IV on a patient who is elderly, stabilize the vein well, as veins in elderly persons tend to roll upon needle insertion.

9. With the needle at a 15° angle, slowly enter the patient's vein (**Figure 7-9A**). You will feel a change of pressure when the needle enters the vein. A flashback of blood will appear in the chamber of the device. After entering the vein, lower the needle unit slightly until it is almost flush with the skin. Advance the needle an additional 1/4 inch into the vein (**Figure 7-9B**).
10. Gently advance the catheter forward into the vein, slipping it over the needle.
11. Hold the catheter securely while you remove the needle (**Figure 7-9C**). Discard the needle in the puncture-resistant container.
12. Release the tourniquet by pulling the upper end of the tourniquet *downward*, before removing the needle.
13. Attach the fluid administration set and establish the flow of fluid.
14. Secure the catheter according to facility policy, or tape by applying a piece of tape across the arm, 1/8 inch above the infusion site (**Figure 7-10A**). While you

(continues)

Procedure **37**, *continued*
Inserting a Peripheral IV in an Adult

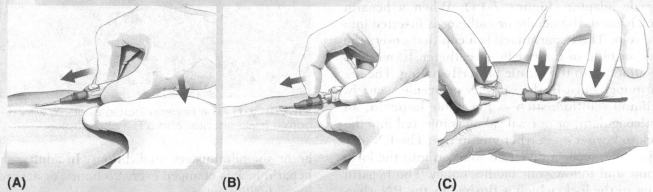

(A)   **(B)**   **(C)**

FIGURE 7-9 An over-the-needle catheter can be inserted using one or both hands. (A) The one-handed technique is shown in this picture. (B) The index finger is used to slide the catheter into the vein. (C) One hand stabilizes the vein while the other is used to remove the needle. (Courtesy of BD Medical Systems, Franklin Lakes, NJ)

continue to hold the catheter, insert a second piece of tape, sticky side up, under the needle. Cross it over the needle, securing it to the upper piece of tape on the opposite sides (**Figure 7-10B**). Attach one more piece of tape at the bottom (**Figure 7-10C**). Avoid taping the connections closed, and avoid covering the needle insertion site with the tape.

15. Regulate the drip rate or connect to a pump, according to facility policy.

16. Recheck the connections to the administration set, filter, and catheter to ensure that they are tight and secure.

17. Perform your procedure completion actions.

AGE-APPROPRIATE CARE   **ALERT**

In patients who are elderly, skin is often paper–thin and tears easily. Secure the catheter with hypoallergenic tape, or cover with an IV transparent dressing. Remove the tape or transparent dressing by pulling in the direction of hair growth. A transparent dressing is best removed by lifting opposite corners of the dressing and stretching.

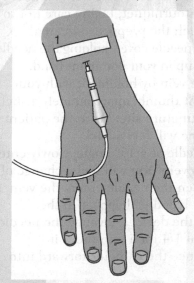

FIGURE 7-10(A) Apply a piece of tape across the arm, just above the insertion site.

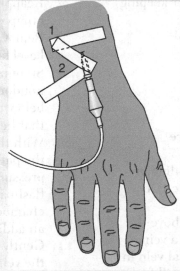

FIGURE 7-10(B) Cross the tape over, forming a "V," and secure the tape on opposite sides of the cannula or needle.

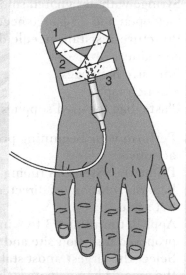

FIGURE 7-10(C) Attach a third piece of tape across the bottom. Avoid taping directly over the junction of the catheter and administration set.

HEPARIN LOCKS

A **heparin lock** may be used for patients who are receiving intravenous medications. Two types are available, one with a male adaptor and one with a female adaptor (**Figure 7-11**). When a heparin lock is used, the needle or catheter is inserted into the vein. The heparin lock is a cap that covers the end, or hub, of the needle or catheter. It may also be attached to the plastic butterfly tubing. The heparin lock must fit the catheter or needle securely. A liquid solution, such as injectable **heparin,** an anticoagulant, or normal saline is injected into the lock to keep it open when not in use. The RN may inject the heparin or saline solution into the lock. Know and follow your facility policy. The heparin stays in the lock, which is flushed by the RN when

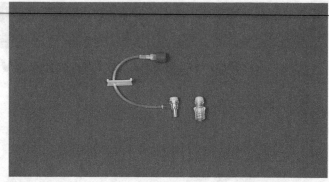

FIGURE 7-11 The heparin lock is available with both a male adaptor and a female adaptor.

he or she administers medications. In adults, the heparin lock is changed every 96 hours, or according to facility policy.

Procedure 38

Inserting a Heparin Lock

Supplies needed:
- Intravenous start kit or individual supplies
- Disposable exam gloves
- Tourniquet
- Alcohol or povidone-iodine wipes
- Selection of over-the-needle catheters
- Sterile 2 × 2 gauze pad
- Heparin lock to fit catheters
- Syringe with designated solution for keeping lock open and 25-gauge needle
- Puncture-resistant needle disposal container
- Adhesive bandages
- 1/2-inch tape
- Plastic bag for used supplies

1. Perform your beginning procedure actions.
2. Prime the extension tubing with saline or heparin solution, as directed by the RN. Set aside.
3. Apply a tourniquet 3 to 4 inches above the proposed insertion site and locate a vein. Select the largest, most stable distal vein in the area. When palpated, the site will feel firm and rebound slightly.
4. Release the tourniquet.
5. Cleanse the site with alcohol or povidone-iodine. Wipe in a circular motion for 60 seconds. Begin in the center of the venipuncture site and extend the circle out 3 inches in diameter.
6. Allow the alcohol or povidone-iodine to dry thoroughly. While the skin is drying, cut the tape and place it in a convenient location.
7. Reapply the tourniquet, taking care not to bump or touch the prepped skin area.
8. Remove the needle cover, holding the needle bevel facing up in your dominant hand.
9. Stabilize the vein by holding it with your nondominant thumb, approximately 1 inch below the puncture site. Warn the patient that he or she will feel a stick.
10. With the needle at a 15° angle, slowly enter the patient's vein. You will feel a change of pressure when the needle enters the vein. A flashback of blood will appear in the chamber of the device. Advance the needle an additional 1/4 inch into the vein.
11. Gently advance the catheter forward into the vein.
12. Place a sterile 2 × 2 gauze pad under the catheter.

(continues)

Procedure 38, *continued*

Inserting a Heparin Lock

13. Release the tourniquet by pulling the upper end of the tourniquet *downward,* before removing the needle.
14. Hold the catheter securely while you remove the needle. Discard the needle in the puncture-resistant container. Apply gentle pressure on the vein, approximately 1 inch above the insertion site.

15. Attach the heparin lock by removing the protective cover and twisting the lock gently into the IV catheter. After the lock is connected, release pressure on the vein. Recheck the connection to ensure that the lock is securely attached.
16. Secure the catheter according to facility policy.
17. Perform your procedure completion actions.

INSERTING AN IV USING A BUTTERFLY NEEDLE

In some situations, an intravenous infusion is initiated with a butterfly needle. These needles are shorter than many other IV needles. They are relatively easy to insert because of the short bevel and the wing design. Butterfly needles are commonly used in elderly patients and in children. The needle may be inserted for patients with small veins, or if the location of the vein is difficult to access with another type of device. They are useful for short-term therapy in adults, for administering medications, and for certain forms of cancer treatment.

The butterfly needle is not used for long-term therapy. The rate of infiltration is higher than with an ONC. However, studies have shown that the rate of infection with metal needles is lower than with plastic catheters. Avoid using the butterfly in veins that cross over joints.

Procedure 39

Inserting a Peripheral IV with a Butterfly Needle

Supplies needed:
- Intravenous start kit or individual supplies
- Disposable exam gloves
- Tourniquet
- Alcohol or povidone-iodine wipes
- Selection of butterfly needles
- IV standard
- Intravenous solution with primed tubing
- Puncture-resistant needle disposal container
- Adhesive bandages
- 1/2-inch tape
- Plastic bag for used supplies

1. Perform your beginning procedure actions.
2. Apply a tourniquet 3 to 4 inches above the proposed insertion site and locate a vein. Select the largest, most stable distal vein in the area. When palpated, the site will feel firm and rebound slightly.
3. Release the tourniquet.
4. Cleanse the site with alcohol or povidone-iodine. Wipe in a circular motion for 60 seconds. Begin in the center of the venipuncture site and extend the circle out 3 inches in diameter.
5. Allow the alcohol or povidone-iodine to dry thoroughly. While the skin is drying, cut the tape and place it in a convenient location.
6. Reapply the tourniquet, taking care not to bump or touch the prepped skin area.
7. Remove the needle cover, holding the needle bevel facing up in your dominant hand.

(continues)

Procedure 39, *continued*

Inserting a Peripheral IV with a Butterfly Needle

8. Stabilize the vein by holding it with your nondominant thumb, approximately 1 inch below the puncture site. Warn the patient that he or she will feel a stick.

9. Fold the wings of the butterfly up and grip them securely. With the needle at a 15° angle, slowly enter the patient's vein. You will feel a change of pressure when the needle enters the vein. A flashback of blood will appear in the tubing. Gently lift the device up and slowly advance the needle into the vein. Allow the tubing to fill with blood to purge the system of air.

10. Release the tourniquet by pulling the upper end of the tourniquet *downward,* before removing the needle.

11. Attach the fluid administration set to the butterfly and establish the flow of fluid.

12. Secure the needle according to facility policy, or apply a piece of tape vertically over each wing of the butterfly, forming an "H" shape (**Figure 7-12**). Avoid covering the needle insertion site.

13. Regulate the drip rate or connect to a pump, if permitted, according to facility policy.

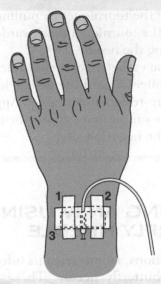

FIGURE 7-12 Apply tape vertically over each wing, then horizontally, forming an "H" shape. Avoid taping directly over the needle insertion site.

14. Recheck the connections to ensure that they are fastened tightly.

15. Perform your procedure completion actions.

INSERTING A PERIPHERAL IV IN A CHILD

When selecting a device for IV infusion in children, a 22- or 24-gauge over-the-needle catheter is preferable. Children are active, and a butterfly will easily come out of the vein. Children may be fearful of needlesticks. Before starting an IV, provide the child with an age-appropriate explanation of the procedure. Show him or her the equipment and describe what you will be doing. However, you must be honest. Avoid telling the child that the procedure will not hurt. Have an assistant available to help you, providing the child with distraction and emotional support. The assistant may

restrain the child if necessary. Depending on the size of the child, a papoose board may be used. The child is placed on the board and the Velcro straps are folded over his or her body. The extremity in which the IV is being started is not secured on the papoose board.

Try to select a site that will not interfere with the child's play activities. The Centers for Disease Control and Prevention (CDC) guidelines recommend using a hand in preference to a leg, arm, or the antecubital space. Depending on your facility policy and the location of the IV, the child's extremity may be secured on an arm board. For a child patient, attaching the arm board before beginning the procedure may be preferable.

Procedure **40**

Inserting a Peripheral IV in a Child

Supplies needed:
- Intravenous start kit or individual supplies
- Disposable exam gloves
- Tourniquet
- Alcohol or povidone-iodine wipes
- Selection of over-the-needle catheters and butterfly needles
- IV standard
- Intravenous solution with primed tubing
- Puncture-resistant needle disposal container
- Adhesive bandages
- 1/2-inch tape
- Plastic bag for used supplies

1. Perform your beginning procedure actions.
2. Apply a tourniquet 2 to 3 inches above the proposed insertion site and locate a vein. Select the largest, most stable distal vein in the area. When palpated, the site will feel firm and rebound slightly. Select a butterfly needle or over-the-needle catheter appropriate to the size and location of the vein.
3. Release the tourniquet.
4. Cleanse the site with alcohol or povidone-iodine. Wipe in a circular motion for 60 seconds. Begin in the center of the venipuncture site and extend the circle out 3 inches in diameter.
5. Allow the alcohol or povidone-iodine to dry thoroughly. While the skin is drying, cut the tape and place it in a convenient location.
6. Reapply the tourniquet, taking care not to bump or touch the prepped skin area.

7. Remove the needle cover, holding the needle bevel facing up in your dominant hand.
8. Stabilize the vein by holding it with your nondominant thumb, approximately 1 inch below the puncture site. Warn the child that he or she will feel a stick.
9. With the ONC or butterfly at a 15° angle, slowly enter the child's vein. You will feel a change of pressure when the needle enters the vein. A flashback of blood will appear. Slowly advance the catheter or needle into the vein. Discard the needle used to introduce the catheter, if used, in the puncture-resistant container. If a butterfly needle was used, allow the tubing to fill with blood to purge the system of air.
10. Release the tourniquet by pulling the upper end of the tourniquet *downward*, before removing the needle.
11. Attach the fluid administration set and establish the flow of fluid.
12. Secure the needle according to facility policy, or apply tape appropriate to the device used. Avoid covering the needle insertion site with tape. Avoid taping tubing connections.
13. Regulate the drip rate or connect to a pump, according to facility policy.
14. Immobilize the arm on an arm board, if not done previously.
15. Recheck the connections to ensure that they are fastened tightly.
16. Perform your procedure completion actions.

MONITORING INTRAVENOUS FLOW RATE

The IV flow rate is ordered by the physician, based on the length of time the solution will hang. The solution should infuse at a steady rate. The speed of the solution should not fluctuate from rapid to slow. Several factors affect the flow, or drip rate, including the type of administration set used; the type of solution; the size, placement, and patency of the needle; and the height of the IV solution. The IV flow rate will be calculated by the RN. Some facilities attach a piece of tape to the side of the intravenous container. The approximate fluid level for each hour is marked on the tape (**Figure 7-13**). Intravenous pumps and controllers are more commonly used to control the rate.

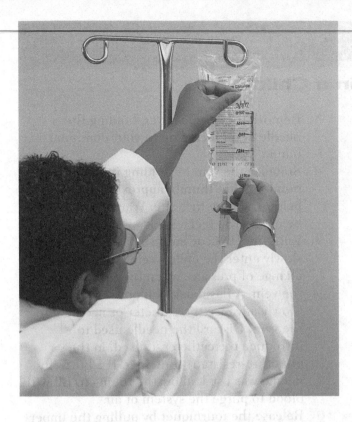

The pumps have a digital screen displaying the flow rate and volume delivered.

You may be responsible for periodically monitoring the IV flow rate and checking the infusion site. This may mean looking at the digital display or counting the drip rate, depending on the equipment being used. The RN will inform you of the designated drip rate. In some facilities, the PCT is permitted to adjust the flow. In others, changes to the flow rate must be done by the RN. Follow your facility policies and procedures for adjusting the flow rate.

Sometimes an IV will be administered at a very slow rate, which is just enough to keep the vein open. This may be called KO (keep open), TKO (to keep open), KVO (keep vein open), or some other facility abbreviation. When this rate is ordered, the patient does not need fluid. The infusion is used to keep the vein open for emergency use or administration of medications.

FIGURE 7-13 Apply the tape to the side of the container.

Procedure **41**

Monitoring the Intravenous Flow Rate

Supplies needed:
▶ Watch with second hand

1. Perform your beginning procedure actions.
2. Stand so that you can clearly see the flow of fluid into the drip chamber.
3. Hold your watch so that you can see it out of the corner of your eye. Look at the second hand and begin timing.
4. Begin counting each drop of fluid as it drops into the drip chamber (Figure 7-14).
5. Count the number of drops that fall into the drip chamber. Stop counting in exactly 30 seconds. Multiply this number by 2 to determine the total drip rate for 1 minute. Report deviations in the designated rate to the RN.
6. Perform your procedure completion actions.

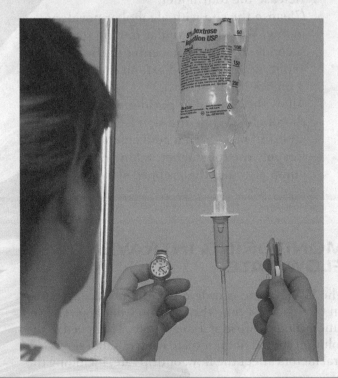

FIGURE 7-14 Count the drops entering the chamber for 30 seconds, then multiply by 2.

USING IV PUMPS AND CONTROLLERS

Most health care facilities administer intravenous solutions by using a controller or pump. These electronic devices fasten to the IV standard and operate by electricity. However, most automatically switch to battery mode in the event of a power failure. If you will be responsible for using pumps or controllers, your instructor will teach you about the devices being used by your facility. There are many manufacturers of these devices, and the operating instructions for each vary with the manufacturer. However, all controllers or pumps have alarms that sound for problems such as:

- Air in the line
- Line occlusion
- Problems that interfere with delivery of fluid at the designated rate
- Completion of the infusion
- Low battery

The alarm must always be in the "on" position when fluid is infusing. Never turn it off. Some pumps will change to a "keep vein open" rate if the alarm sounds. Some will shut off completely. Respond promptly to the alarm and take corrective action within the limits of your job description, or notify the RN promptly.

Volumetric intravenous pumps regulate the flow of IV fluids electronically. They are used to ensure accurate flow of IV solutions and drugs. Pumps measure flow of fluids in milliliters per hour of solution infused. **IV controllers** regulate gravity flow of IV fluids by counting drops of solution. Controllers count drops, which are not always of identical (equal) size. Because of this, they are not as accurate as using a pump.

To set up a pump or controller unit, assemble the IV solution as usual, and prime the tubing with the IV solution so it is completely full of fluid and free from air bubbles. The drip chamber should be approximately half full. At this point, you may need to attach a peristaltic tubing or controller to the IV tubing, depending on the unit being used. Follow the manufacturer's instructions for tubing placement or threading the tubing through the cassette. Position the IV standard on the same side of the bed as the IV. The tubing should never be draped across the patient or bed. To operate the unit, you should:

- Perform the venipuncture, if this has not already been done.
- Plug in the machine and attach the tubing to the IV catheter or needle.
- If you are using a controller, make sure the drip chamber is at least 30 inches above the insertion site.
- Turn the unit on and press the start button.
- Set the controls according to the manufacturer's direction. You may need to enter the drip rate and volume of the IV container. In some hospitals, 50 mL is subtracted from the container size. Thus, if you have a 1,000-mL IV bag, you would set the machine to read 950 mL. The alarm will sound when 50 mL of fluid remains in the bag. This will provide you with enough time to obtain and hang a new bag before the old one is empty.
- After setting the controls, verify the flow of fluid and drip rate, as appropriate. Monitor the insertion site for signs of infiltration.
- Turn the alarm on and explain its use and meaning to the patient.

Continue to check the insertion site each time you are in the room. Check the pump or controller to ensure it is operating correctly. Infiltration may develop quickly with these devices because of the increased pressure of the unit. Some facilities move the tubing every few hours to prevent tubing damage and compression. Change the tubing and cassette every 72 hours, or according to facility policy. Document the use of the controller or pump on the IV record and in your notes.

COMPLICATIONS OF IV THERAPY

Like all other medical procedures, IV therapy carries some risks. Some complications of IV therapy can be serious. You will check the IV each time you are in the room, or according to facility policy. Prompt identification of complications is best for the patient.

Table 7-2 lists tips for troubleshooting an IV. The RN should be asked to assess complaints of pain or burning at the insertion site. If you can quickly identify and correct one of the problems listed here, you should do so. However, if the patient is in distress, do not waste time troubleshooting. Inform the RN promptly.

Table 7-2 Troubleshooting an IV

Problem	Action
IV stops dripping	• Make sure there is fluid in the infusion container. • Check for kinks or obstructions of tubing. • Make sure all roller clamps and slide clamps are open. • Check for signs and symptoms of infiltration. • Lower the bag or bottle below heart level and check the tubing for blood return. • Make sure the IV pole and height of the bag are 30 to 40 inches above the insertion site. • Reposition the patient to see if this affects the flow of solution. • Continue to monitor the infusion frequently.
Flow rate too slow	• Check for signs and symptoms of infiltration. • Reposition the patient to see if this affects the flow of solution. • Check for kinks or obstructions of tubing. • Make sure all roller clamps and slide clamps are open. • Make sure the IV pole and height of the bag are 30 to 40 inches above the insertion site; try raising the pole to see if this affects the flow rate. • Reposition the catheter at the hub; elevate the hub slightly. Place one or more sterile 2 × 2 gauze pads under the hub and redress the site. • As a last resort, disconnect the tubing from the hub. If the fluid flows freely through the tubing, the problem is with the catheter. Discontinue it and restart the IV in another location. • Continue to monitor the infusion frequently.
Flow rate too fast	• Adjust the roller clamp to slow the rate. Time it to make sure it is accurate, as ordered by the physician.
Flow rate alternates between fast and slow	• Reposition the patient's arm; try elevating it on a pillow or lowering the arm. • Make sure the area under the IV is straight and still. • Monitor the flow rate for a few minutes. • Apply an arm board, if necessary. • Remove the dressing and reposition the catheter at the hub. Place one or more sterile 2 × 2 gauze pads under the hub and redress the site. • Continue to monitor the infusion frequently.

Hematoma

Hematoma is a complication that commonly occurs when the vein is injured during venipuncture. This can occur if you puncture the vein, or if inadequate pressure is placed on the insertion site after a needle is withdrawn. A hematoma looks like a bruise that fills rapidly with blood, causing swelling. Carefully observe the insertion site when entering a vein. With any venipuncture, stop the procedure immediately if a hematoma develops. Elevate the extremity and apply firm pressure.

Infiltration

Infiltration is also a common complication of IV therapy. This occurs when the catheter or needle comes out of the vein and fluid flows into the surrounding tissue. Signs and symptoms of infiltration are:

● Pain and/or burning at the insertion site
● Swelling at the insertion site
● Skin cool to touch; may be lighter in color at the insertion site

- Rigid, taut skin near the insertion site
- Infusion rate has slowed or stopped
- Dressing covering the insertion site is damp or wet
- No backflow of blood into IV tubing when the bag is lowered below the insertion site

Lowering the IV solution below the level of the heart should produce a blood return in the IV tubing. If there is no blood return, the IV has probably infiltrated. If you are unsure of the infiltration status of the IV, notify the RN.

Use an over-the-needle catheter whenever possible. The incidence of infiltration is higher with butterflies and other needle devices. Avoid inserting an IV over a joint, whenever possible, because movement increases the risk of infiltration. The incidence of infiltration is reduced by taping the device securely. Immobilizing the extremity on an arm board (**Figure 7-15**) to further limit movement is also beneficial.

Treatment for infiltration involves stopping the IV solution. The catheter or needle is removed and the IV is restarted in another location. The presence of fluid in the tissue may be painful for the patient. The RN may instruct you to apply warm, moist compresses to relieve discomfort and promote absorption of the fluid.

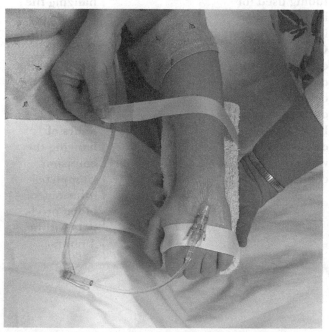

Figure 7-15 Immobilize the extremity using an arm board. Applying a piece of tape to the back of the middle third of each piece of tape will prevent discomfort caused by pulling hair when the tape is removed.

Phlebitis

Phlebitis is irritation of the vein. It may be caused by irritation from the IV device, or from the medication. Infection may also cause phlebitis, but this is less common than the mechanical reasons listed. An infection is usually the result of phlebitis, rather than the cause. Studies have shown that lower-extremity insertions have a greater risk of phlebitis than upper-extremity insertions. Hand veins have a lower risk of phlebitis than wrist and upper-arm insertions. Signs and symptoms of phlebitis are redness, warmth, swelling, and pain. The patient may have a red streak extending from the insertion site up the arm.

The risk of phlebitis can be reduced by using aseptic technique when priming the IV tubing, inserting the catheter or needle, and when manipulating the IV system. Taping the IV catheter or butterfly securely also reduces movement and irritation of the veins. Many facilities rotate the IV insertion site every 48 to 72 hours to reduce irritation to the wall of the vein. Treatment for phlebitis involves discontinuing the IV and restarting it in another location. Avoid insertion of subsequent IVs in the distal vein where the phlebitis developed. Elevate the extremity. Warm, moist compresses are used to relieve discomfort, as directed by the RN.

Air Embolus

Air embolus is a serious complication of IV therapy. Air can enter the system from any location, including the bag or bottle, administration set, a syringe, or from connections that become separated. Air embolus can be life-threatening. This condition occurs when air enters the vein, moving freely through the system. Signs and symptoms of air embolus are shortness of breath, cyanosis, weak, rapid pulse, decreased blood pressure, loss of consciousness, and cardiac arrest. If you discover a patient with signs of this condition, stay in the room and call for the RN by using the call signal. Turn the patient on the left side. This may trap the air, preventing it from moving into the pulmonary artery. The RN will administer oxygen and notify the physician. Follow his or her directions. This is a serious emergency that must be identified and treated quickly.

Catheter Breakage or Embolus

Loss of part or all of the catheter into the circulatory system causes a catheter embolus. This may be caused by shearing a piece from the catheter with

Table 7-3 CDC Recommendations for Peripheral Intravenous Fluids

Device	Replacement and Relocation of the Device (site rotation)	Replacement of Catheter Site Dressing	Replacement of Administration Set	Replacement of Heparin Lock	Hang Time for Fluids
Peripheral venous catheters	In adults, every 72 to 96 hours. Replace catheters inserted under emergency basis, and insert a new catheter at a different site, within 48 hours. In pediatric patients, do not replace catheter unless clinically indicated.	Replace dressing when the catheter is removed or replaced, or when the dressing becomes damp, loosened, or soiled. Replace dressings more frequently in diaphoretic patients. In patients who have large, bulky dressings that prevent palpation or direct visualization of the catheter insertion site, remove the dressing, visually inspect the catheter at least daily, and apply a new dressing.	Replace intravenous tubing, including piggyback tubing and stopcocks, no more frequently than at 72-hour intervals unless clinically indicated.	In adults, replace heparin locks every 96 hours.	No recommendation for the hang time of intravenous fluids, including nonlipid-containing parenteral nutrition fluids. Complete infusion of lipid-containing parenteral nutrition fluids (e.g., 3-in-1 solutions) within 24 hours of hanging the fluid. When lipid emulsions are given alone, complete the infusion within 12 hours of hanging the emulsion. Complete infusions of blood products within 4 hours.
			Replace tubing used to administer blood, blood products, or lipid emulsions within 24 hours of initiating the infusion. No recommendation for replacement of tubing used for intermittent infusions. Consider short extension tubing connected to the device as a portion of the device. Replace such extension tubing when the device is changed.		

the needle used for insertion. It can also occur if the catheter is not taped securely, causing the catheter to bend and break at the hub. Signs and symptoms of this condition are respiratory distress, chest pain, cyanosis, rapid pulse, and decreased blood pressure. The condition may cause unconsciousness. It may be difficult to differentiate this condition from an air embolus. Stay with the patient and use the call signal to notify the RN. He or she may instruct you to apply a tourniquet above the insertion site. The physician will be notified and an x-ray ordered. The circulating catheter must be removed surgically.

Infection

Infection is caused by contamination somewhere in the IV system, or by improper insertion technique. It may also occur if the connections between the catheter or needle and the administration set separate, allowing contaminants to enter. Signs and symptoms of localized infection are redness, swelling, heat, and pain at the insertion site. Foul-smelling drainage may be present. Signs of systemic infection are fever, chills, headache, and rapid respirations. Later, the blood pressure may decrease. If you observe these signs and symptoms, notify the RN immediately. If you are instructed to remove the IV catheter because of a suspected infection, do not discard it. Check with the RN to see if it should be sent to the laboratory for testing.

Infection is prevented by using good hand-washing technique, standard precautions, and aseptic technique when handling intravenous fluids, the infusion system, and materials for needle or catheter insertion. The CDC recommends routine changes of various components of the system to further reduce the risk of infection. These are listed in **Table 7-3.** Your facility may have additional policies and procedures, based on infection control committee recommendations, and intravenous and infection control nursing society guidelines.

Fluid Overload

Fluid overload occurs when fluids infuse too rapidly. This is a serious situation. Monitor the flow rate frequently and ensure that fluid is flowing at the proper rate. Signs and symptoms of this condition can be very serious, including respiratory distress and cardiac arrest. Early signs and symptoms are rapid respirations, shortness of breath, rapid pulse, increased blood pressure, and distended

AGE-APPROPRIATE CARE ALERT

Elderly and pediatric patients are at high risk for circulatory overload when IV fluids are given rapidly, making close monitoring necessary. Signs and symptoms to monitor and report to the RN are:
- Elevated blood pressure
- Rapid respirations
- Coughing, shortness of breath
- Signs and symptoms of pulmonary edema
  - Shortness of breath or difficulty breathing when lying flat
  - Awakening at night feeling breathless
  - A feeling of suffocating or drowning
  - Wheezing or grunting respirations
  - A productive cough with frothy, pink sputum
  - Excessive sweating
  - Pale or cyanotic skin color
  - Anxiety
  - Restlessness
  - Weight gain
  - Edema
  - Extremities that are cool to the touch
  - Rapid respirations
  - Tachycardia
  - Elevated blood pressure
  - Jugular vein distention
  - Retractions, use of accessory muscles of respiration

neck veins. Position the bed in Fowler's position. Stay with the patient and use the call signal to notify the RN immediately.

CHANGING A PERIPHERAL IV DRESSING

Most health care facilities have policies and procedures for dressing the intravenous insertion site. The techniques vary widely, but sterile technique and a sterile dressing are always used for this procedure. Some cover the insertion site with a sterile cover dressing. However, gauze dressings are not recommended, as the site cannot be visualized and there is risk of contamination from moisture. Likewise, roller gauze should not be used. If a gauze dressing is used, the insertion site should be evaluated daily. If the patient complains of pain at the insertion site, has a fever without an obvious cause, or shows signs of a localized or generalized infection, the dressing should be removed immediately and the site evaluated by the RN. Change the dressing immediately if it becomes wet, because of the high risk of infection.

Most facilities use a transparent film dressing to cover the insertion site. This type of dressing works well because you can easily visualize the insertion site. The patient can shower with the film in place, and it requires less frequent dressing changes than other types of dressings. This is an area of ongoing research.

The frequency of the dressing change also varies with facility policy. Dressings must always be changed when the device is removed or replaced, or if the dressing becomes soiled, damp, or loose. Frequent dressing changes may be necessary in diaphoretic (sweating) patients. Apply the principles of standard precautions, and avoid touch contamination of the catheter insertion site when the dressing is replaced.

Procedure 42

Applying a Transparent Film Dressing to an Intravenous Infusion Site

Supplies needed:
- Disposable exam gloves
- Alcohol or povidone-iodine wipes
- Sterile gauze sponges
- Transparent dressing
- Plastic bag for used supplies

1. Perform your beginning procedure actions.
2. If placing the dressing for the first time, clipping the hair may be necessary. Avoid shaving, which increases the risk of infection. Check with the RN if you are uncertain of the action to take. Remove oil from skin surrounding the insertion site, if present, with alcohol. Allow to dry.
3. Wash hands or use alcohol-based hand cleaner.
4. Apply disposable exam gloves.
5. Holding gentle traction on the skin, press down on the skin, then loosen the adhesive in one corner and remove the dressing by peeling it back, toward the insertion site. Hold the hub of the IV catheter in place when removing the dressing. Stretch the dressing horizontally, gently lifting it over the open area. The stretching helps to break the adhesive bond. You cannot use two hands to remove the dressing, so you may have to remove and stretch the edges by alternating movement in two opposite corners of the dressing. Always remove the dressing by pulling in the direction of hair growth. If the skin is not hairy, corners on opposite sides of the dressing can be lifted. Stretch the dressing from the edges toward the center, then lift off. Discard in plastic bag.
6. Evaluate the insertion site for redness, swelling, drainage, or other complications. If present, use the call signal to notify the RN.
7. Check the IV connections to ensure that they are fastened tightly.
8. Cleanse the skin with alcohol or povidone-iodine for 3 inches surrounding the insertion site. Begin at the insertion site, working outward.
9. Allow the skin cleanser to dry completely.
10. Remove gloves and discard in plastic bag.
11. Wash your hands or use alcohol-based hand cleaner.
12. Open the package by peeling the tabs back, and remove the dressing.
13. Grasp the tabs on the underside of the dressing, and peel them back approximately 1 inch. The dressing is sterile, and you must avoid touching the underside with your hands when opening the package or applying it to the insertion site.
14. Center the dressing over the catheter insertion site, then gently lower it, smoothing the center portion in place.
15. Peel away the backing paper slowly from one side at a time while gently smoothing the film in place. Gently smooth out wrinkles as you go.
16. Perform your procedure completion actions.

DISCONTINUING A PERIPHERAL IV

An IV is discontinued if complications such as infiltration occur. In this situation, it is restarted in another location, preferably the opposite extremity. An IV is also discontinued upon a physician's order.

Procedure 43

Discontinuing a Peripheral IV

Supplies needed:

- Disposable exam gloves
- Alcohol or povidone-iodine wipes
- Sterile 2 × 2 gauze pad
- Adhesive bandage
- Puncture-resistant container, if needle or butterfly removed
- Plastic bag for used supplies

1. Perform your beginning procedure actions.
2. Remove the dressing covering the insertion site. Loosen the tape on the needle and administration set tubing (**Figure 7-16**).
3. Apply gentle pressure over the insertion site with sterile gauze. Withdraw the needle or cannula at the same angle it was inserted. Observe the plastic cannula closely. If it appears to have broken off, do not discard it. Notify the RN immediately of this potentially serious complication.
4. Hold pressure on the insertion site until bleeding stops.
5. Cleanse the area with alcohol or povidone-iodine, if necessary. Avoid direct contact with the insertion site.
6. Cover the insertion site with an adhesive bandage or other dressing, according to facility policies.
7. Discard the needle, if used, in a puncture-resistant container. Discard other supplies contaminated by blood or body fluids in the plastic bag. Discard the IV solution and tubing according to facility policy, if the IV will not be restarted.
8. Perform your procedure completion actions.

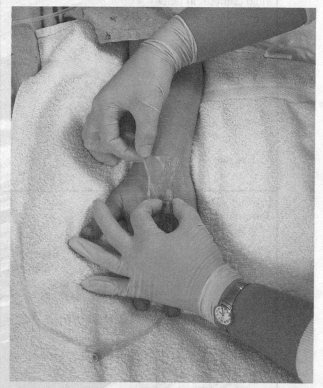

FIGURE 7-16 Gently loosen the transparent film (or tape).

ASSISTING THE RN WITH A CENTRAL INTRAVENOUS CATHETER DRESSING CHANGE

A **central intravenous catheter** (Figure 7-17) is a long catheter that is inserted into a vein in the shoulder or neck area. The tip of the catheter is in the superior vena cava or right atrium of the heart (Figure 7-18). This type of intravenous catheter is used for long-term IV therapy. Changing the dressing is a sterile procedure. Strict aseptic technique must be maintained. Like the peripheral catheter, the type of dressing and the

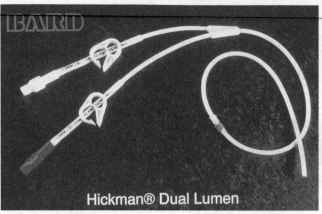
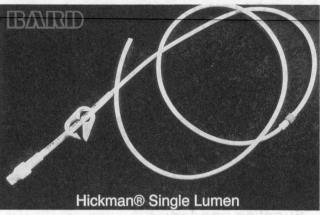

Hickman® Dual Lumen

Hickman® Single Lumen

FIGURE 7-17 The Hickman central intravenous catheter is commonly used. (Photo provided by Bard Access Systems. Hickman® is a registered trademark of Bard Access Systems)

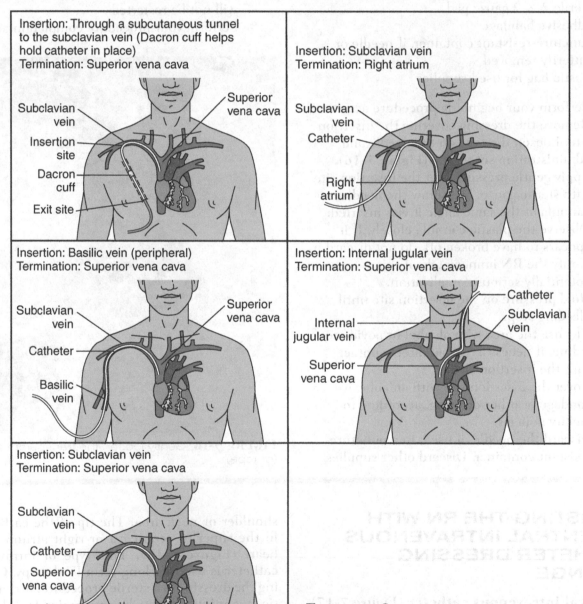

Insertion: Through a subcutaneous tunnel to the subclavian vein (Dacron cuff helps hold catheter in place)
Termination: Superior vena cava

Subclavian vein
Insertion site
Dacron cuff
Exit site
Superior vena cava

Insertion: Subclavian vein
Termination: Right atrium

Subclavian vein
Catheter
Right atrium

Insertion: Basilic vein (peripheral)
Termination: Superior vena cava

Subclavian vein
Catheter
Basilic vein
Superior vena cava

Insertion: Internal jugular vein
Termination: Superior vena cava

Catheter
Subclavian vein
Internal jugular vein
Superior vena cava

Insertion: Subclavian vein
Termination: Superior vena cava

Subclavian vein
Catheter
Superior vena cava

FIGURE 7-18 The central intravenous catheter is threaded through the vein until the tip reaches the superior vena cava or right atrium.

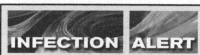

INFECTION ALERT

Central intravenous catheters have the greatest risk of infection of all IVs. Those that are completely implanted (such as ports) have the lowest risk. Catheters with multiple lumens have a higher risk than single-lumen catheters. The triple-lumen catheter has the greatest infection risk. The risk decreases for double and single lumens. The insertion site also affects the risk. These sites are listed respectively from highest to lowest risk for infection:
- Femoral
- Jugular
- Subclavian
- Peripheral sites

frequency of dressing change are determined by facility policy.

A mask is worn by the personnel performing this dressing change. Some facilities also require the patient to wear a mask. Know and follow your facility policy. Your responsibilities will be determined by the RN. In general, you will set up the sterile field, open sterile supplies and hand them to the RN, and discard used items following the procedure. Always follow the RN's directions.

Procedure 44

Assisting the RN with a Central IV Dressing Change

Supplies needed:
- Central IV dressing change kit or individual supplies
- Disposable exam gloves
- Sterile gloves, size to fit the RN
- Three masks
- Transparent film dressing or other sterile dressing
- Tape, if needed to secure dressing
- Sterile drape
- Three povidone-iodine applicator sticks
- Plastic bag for used supplies

1. Perform your beginning procedure actions.
2. Cleanse the table that will be used to establish the sterile field with alcohol or other disinfectant. Allow to dry.
3. Apply a mask. Instruct the patient to apply a mask, or turn the patient's head to the side opposite the insertion site, according to facility policy.
4. Wash your hands, or use alcohol-based hand cleaner.
5. Using the sterile drape, set up the sterile field. Open packages of sterile supplies, placing them on the sterile field. Avoid turning your back on the sterile field.
6. Apply disposable exam gloves and remove the soiled dressing. Discard in the plastic bag. Keep the soiled dressing and plastic bag well away from the sterile field. Avoid reaching over the field to discard the dressing.
7. Remove gloves and discard in the plastic bag.
8. Wash your hands, or use alcohol-based hand cleaner.
9. Open a package of povidone-iodine applicators, holding the end to the RN, who will use the applicator to cleanse the skin. If packaged in individual packages, repeat two more times. Three applicators are needed to cleanse the skin for this procedure. Hold the plastic bag open for the RN to discard each applicator.
10. After the skin dries, open the gauze dressing or transparent film dressing, holding it open for the RN. He or she will use it to cover the insertion site. Cut and hand tape to the RN, if a gauze dressing is used.
11. Hold the plastic bag open for the RN to discard his or her gloves.
12. Remove your mask. Assist the patient to remove his or her mask, if necessary. Discard the masks in the plastic bag.
13. Remove used supplies, and discard according to facility policy.
14. Perform your procedure completion actions.

BLOOD ADMINISTRATION

Blood or blood products may be administered to patients for many reasons. Commonly, patients with blood loss, and those with inadequate oxygen or nutrients in the blood, will receive a **transfusion.** This involves intravenous administration of blood. The procedure is the responsibility of the RN, but you may be asked to assist. You must also monitor the patient carefully for signs and symptoms of a transfusion reaction. Take your responsibilities seriously when a patient is receiving blood products. Complications of this procedure can be life-threatening.

Blood Groups and Types

Blood groups and types are designated using the ABO system and the Rh system. The purpose of these systems is to ensure that blood for transfusion matches or is compatible with the patient's own blood type. Incompatibilities can be life-threatening.

Four different types of blood are designated using the ABO system. These are:

- Type A
- Type B
- Type AB
- Type O

The Rh factor determines whether the blood is positive or negative for certain antigens, or foreign substances that cause an allergic reaction. Allergic reactions can be life-threatening. **Antigens** always stimulate an immune response. When an antigen is introduced into the body, the immune system develops substances called **antibodies.** Antibodies are a protective mechanism against foreign materials. The antibodies recognize the same substance the next time it is introduced into the body. An antigen-antibody reaction (AAR) occurs when the patient is allergic to the substance, in this case blood. Chemicals are produced within the body that cause signs of allergic reaction. To prevent a severe antigen-antibody reaction, or allergic reaction, the Rh factor of the donor blood must also be compatible with the patient's blood.

Type O blood is compatible with all other types of blood. Thus, this blood type is called the *universal donor.* Persons with any blood type may receive type O blood. Persons with type AB blood are considered *universal recipients* because they have no A

Table 7-4 Blood Type Compatibility

Patient Blood Type	Donor Blood Type
A	A, O
B	B, O
AB	AB, A, B, O
O	O

or B antibodies. However, universal donors and recipients are not considered except in emergency situations. Most donor blood is the same type and Rh as the patient's blood. Blood types and compatible donor types are listed in **Table 7-4.**

Obtaining Blood from the Blood Bank

The physician will order the blood or blood product for the patient. He or she will order a laboratory test called **type and cross-match.** This typing test identifies the patient's blood type and Rh. The cross-match test determines whether the patient's blood is compatible with the donor blood. The laboratory performs certain procedures to ensure that the blood cross-matched to the patient is identified properly.

Time is often critical, so this procedure must be performed immediately. The laboratory notifies the RN when the blood is available to be picked up from the blood bank, an area within the laboratory.

The RN will instruct you to pick up the blood from the laboratory. This is an important responsibility. Because of the urgency of the procedure, you must do this right away. However, you must check the blood carefully, and follow all facility policies and procedures for obtaining the correct blood for the patient. Two employees must check the blood before it leaves the blood bank, to reduce the potential chance for error. Do not be in such a hurry that you fail to check the blood correctly according to facility policy. One employee checks the blood requisition form and the other checks the blood product. The information on the form is read aloud and compared with the data on the blood bag.

Procedure 45

Obtaining and Checking Blood From the Blood Bank

Supplies needed:
- Blood requisition form

1. Wash your hands, or use alcohol-based hand cleaner.
2. Obtain the blood requisition form from the RN and take it to the blood bank.
3. Identify yourself to blood bank personnel and state that you have a requisition for blood.
4. Follow facility policy for checking the blood with a laboratory technician. One employee reads the following information aloud:
   - Patient's first name, middle initial, and last name
   - Patient's identification number
   - Patient's blood type
   - Patient's blood Rh

- The number of the blood donor
- The blood expiration date

While one employee reads the information on the requisition form, the other verifies the information on the bag of blood. After the information is confirmed, the laboratory employee will release the blood to you. He or she will also provide a blood identification band.

5. Obtain the blood and return immediately to your unit.
6. Upon return to the unit, inform the RN that you have obtained the blood. He or she will provide further instructions.
7. Wash your hands, or use alcohol-based hand cleaner.

Returning from the Blood Bank

After you return to the unit, give the blood and blood identification band to the RN, and follow his or her instructions. The blood must be checked one more time before it is administered to the patient. The RN may ask you to participate in this check. In some hospitals, two RNs must check the blood. Hanging the wrong blood is a serious error that can have grave consequences for the patient. Do not be offended if you are not allowed to perform this procedure.

Procedure 46

Checking Blood Products on the Nursing Unit

Supplies needed:
- Unit of blood
- Blood requisition
- Blood identification band from the laboratory

1. Go to the patient's room with the RN.
2. Wash your hands, or use alcohol-based hand cleaner.
3. Ask the patient to spell his or her name out loud. If the patient is unable, read the patient's name aloud from the identification band. The RN will compare this with the information on the blood slip. He or she will

also verify the information with the label on the bag of blood, or may ask you to do this.
4. Read the patient identification number aloud. The RN will compare this with the information on the blood slip. He or she will also verify the information with the label on the bag of blood, or may ask you to do this.
5. From the requisition, read aloud the blood bank identification number, blood expiration date, and patient's blood type. The RN will compare this with the information on the bag of blood.

(continues)

Procedure 46, *continued*

Checking Blood Products on the Nursing Unit

6. The RN will read aloud from the label on the bag of blood the blood bank identification number, blood expiration date, and patient's blood type. You will compare this with the information on the requisition form.

7. If a discrepancy is noted at any time during the procedure, inform the RN immediately. After the blood has been verified, you will both sign the blood requisition form.

8. Apply the blood identification band to the patient's wrist, according to facility policy. (In some facilities, this may be done at the time the blood is drawn for typing. If the bracelet comes off for any reason, another type and screen must be drawn and a new identification band applied.)

9. Wash your hands, or use alcohol-based hand cleaner.

Transfusion Reactions

A transfusion reaction is a serious complication that can occur at any time when blood is being administered. A patient can also have a reaction after the blood has infused completely. Close observation is indicated. The risk of reaction is greatest in the first 15 minutes of the infusion. However, vital signs are monitored carefully when blood is being administered, and periodically thereafter. In most facilities, vital signs are taken and recorded every 15 to 30 minutes while blood is infusing. Notify the RN immediately of changes in the patient's vital signs, or of signs and symptoms of a transfusion reaction listed in Observe & Report.

When you are checking the patient's vital signs, the RN may also ask you to check the flow rate of the blood. Follow the guidelines in Procedure 41. The RN will inform you of the designated rate. Notify the RN immediately if the blood is infusing at a different rate. Also inform the RN if the blood has stopped infusing, or if the bag is almost empty.

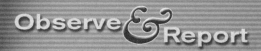

Signs and Symptoms of Transfusion Reaction

- Complaints of heat or a burning sensation in the vein through which blood is infusing
- Fever
- Chills
- Rapid pulse
- Decreased blood pressure
- Apprehension and anxiety
- Flushing of the face, or warm, flushed skin
- Chest pain
- Headache
- Lower back pain
- Shortness of breath

- Nausea and vomiting
- Diarrhea
- Abdominal cramping
- Coughing
- Rash or hives
- Itching
- Facial or throat edema
- Asthma reaction
- Muscular pain
- Blood in the urine
- Loss of consciousness
- Cardiac arrest

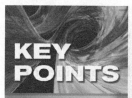

KEY POINTS

▶ Intravenous therapy requires a physician's order.

▶ Intravenous fluids are sterile solutions that must be administered using aseptic technique.

▶ The selection of an IV needle or catheter is determined by the patient's diagnosis, length of IV therapy, type of medication or other solution infused, size and condition of the veins, location of the IV insertion site, and the patient's activity level.

▶ Over-the-needle catheters are the product of choice for venipuncture in patients receiving long-term IV therapy.

▶ Intravenous fluids must be ordered by the physician, who will determine the length of time over which the fluids are administered.

▶ The height of an IV standard affects the rate of flow of the solution.

▶ IV fluid flows through the administration set, which is connected to the infusion device.

▶ A macrodrip administration set delivers fluid at 10 or 20 drops per mL.

▶ A microdrip administration set delivers fluid at 60 drops per mL.

▶ The best way to prevent infection in an IV is through using good handwashing, standard precautions, and strict aseptic technique.

▶ Filters in the administration set trap bacteria, air, and particles, preventing them from entering the patient.

▶ All connections in the infusion set, catheter or needle, heparin lock, and filter must be securely fastened to prevent air embolus, a serious complication.

▶ Avoid injecting air into a vein.

▶ Ink will bleed through plastic IV containers, so information is written on a label that is affixed to the container.

▶ Plastic over-the-needle catheters are most commonly available in even-numbered gauges and needles are usually available with odd-numbered gauges.

▶ When selecting a site for IV therapy, avoid an infected or edematous area; an area with a rash; an extremity with a dialysis access device, shunt, or graft; an existing intravenous line or heparin lock; the affected arm of a mastectomy or stroke patient; the site of previous injury or hematoma; or a burned or scarred area.

▶ Avoid starting an IV in the leg and foot veins.

▶ Start the IV in the patient's nondominant extremity, if possible.

▶ Start an IV in the largest, straightest vein possible. If the patient will receive long-term IV therapy, begin with the most distal site available.

▶ Teach the patient to position the arm with an IV at the level of the heart when in bed, and across the abdomen when ambulating.

▶ Teach the patient to avoid pulling on, kinking, or obstructing the IV tubing, and to avoid brushing teeth or combing hair with the arm that has the IV.

▶ Always insert an IV needle in the direction of blood flow.

▶ Remove an IV needle at the same angle at which the needle entered the vein.

▶ When inserting an IV, position the needle with the bevel facing up.

▶ Avoid sticking the patient more than twice.

▶ Keep the tourniquet on the arm for less than 2 minutes.

▶ Ensure that the blood vessel you are entering does not have a pulse.

(continues)

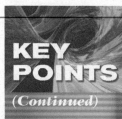

▶ Never pull an IV catheter back over the needle; doing so increases the risk of catheter embolus.

▶ Discard needles in a puncture-resistant container. Carry this container to the bedside with you. Never recap a used needle.

▶ The needle insertion site must be secured to prevent the catheter or needle from moving.

▶ Heparin locks are inserted into the IV catheter or needle for the purpose of medication administration.

▶ Butterfly needles may work best for IV therapy in children and elderly patients; they are not used for long-term IV therapy.

▶ Explain the IV procedure to children in an age-appropriate manner. Avoid telling them that the procedure will not hurt.

▶ Intravenous fluid should flow at a steady rate; the drip rate is determined by the length of time the container will hang.

▶ TKO, KO, and KVO are abbreviations used to designate a slow IV rate that keeps the vein open for emergencies and medication administration.

▶ Signs of infiltration are slowing or stopping of the flow of solution, swelling, cool skin temperature, and a white or pale skin color.

▶ Phlebitis is irritation of a vein caused by mechanical factors or infection.

▶ Air embolus is a life-threatening complication of IV therapy that occurs when air enters a vein.

▶ Signs and symptoms of localized infection are redness, swelling, heat, pain, and foul-smelling drainage at the insertion site.

▶ Signs of systemic infection are fever, chills, headache, rapid respirations, and decreased blood pressure.

▶ Fluid overload may occur when IV fluids infuse too rapidly.

▶ Apply the principles of standard precautions and use aseptic technique when changing an IV dressing.

▶ A central IV catheter is a long catheter threaded through the veins into the superior vena cava or right atrium. It is used for long-term therapy.

▶ Blood transfusion is used for patients with blood loss and those needing additional oxygen and nutrients in the blood.

▶ Complications of a transfusion can occur during and after a transfusion; some can be life-threatening.

▶ The type of blood may be group A, B, AB, or O.

▶ Type O blood is the universal donor; type AB is the universal recipient.

▶ The Rh factor designates whether the blood is positive or negative.

▶ Antigens cause allergic reactions.

▶ Two people must check blood before it is administered; the accuracy of this procedure is important.

▶ Signs and symptoms of transfusion reaction are complaints of heat or a burning sensation in the vein through which blood is infusing; fever; chills; rapid pulse; decreased blood pressure; apprehension and anxiety; flushing of the face or warm, flushed skin; chest pain; headache; lower back pain; shortness of breath; nausea and vomiting; diarrhea; abdominal cramping; coughing; rash or hives; itching; facial or throat edema; asthma reaction; muscular pain; blood in the urine; loss of consciousness; and cardiac arrest.

CLINICAL APPLICATIONS

1. You must start an IV on Mrs. Rosen. The nurse informs you that this patient will be receiving long-term IV therapy. The doctor has also ordered 2 units of blood. What type and size insertion device is the best choice for this patient?

2. You apply the tourniquet to Mrs. Rosen's forearm. She has a large, straight vein on the back of her hand. You notice another large, straight vein on the thumb side of the wrist. She has one more large, straight vein on the back of her forearm. All look large enough to hold the IV catheter you will be inserting. Of the veins listed, which is the best choice for beginning IV therapy?

3. Mrs. Rosen is active and moves freely in bed. She has bathroom privileges, and ambulates from the bed to the bathroom without assistance. What instructions will you give her regarding her activity to prevent complications with the IV?

4. You are instructed to change the transparent film dressing on Mrs. Rosen's infusion site. When you remove it, a small amount of clear fluid escapes from the dressing. The site does not appear red and the patient denies pain. What action will you take?

5. Mrs. Rosen is receiving her first unit of blood. She tells you she feels very cold. You feel warm, but have been very busy and are perspiring. What action will you take?

C H A P T E R   R E V I E W

Multiple-Choice Questions

Select the one best answer.

1. The IV solution should hang:
   a. at the level of the needle insertion site.
   b. at least 12 inches above the needle insertion site.
   c. below the level of the needle insertion site.
   d. at least 30 inches above the needle insertion site.

2. A macrodrip administration set delivers:
   a. 5 drops per mL.
   b. 6–8 drops per mL.
   c. 10–20 drops per mL.
   d. 60 drops per mL.

3. Avoid starting an IV in the:
   a. veins on the back of an arm with a rash.
   b. area above the site of a previous IV infusion.
   c. long veins in the forearm.
   d. veins on the back of the hand.

4. The selection of the insertion site is affected by the:
   a. length of time the device will remain in place.
   b. physician's preference.
   c. ability to use the IV for drawing blood.
   d. catheter size you want to use.

5. The IV catheter is immobilized:
   a. to prevent the patient from pulling it out.
   b. only for medication administration.
   c. to maintain a constant drip rate.
   d. to prevent catheter breakage.

6. A heparin lock is used for:
   a. routine administration of intravenous fluid.
   b. delivering medications only.
   c. emergencies only.
   d. keeping the vein patent in case it is needed.

7. When starting an intravenous infusion on a child:
   a. provide an age-appropriate explanation of the procedure.
   b. use the scalp veins whenever possible.
   c. always use a butterfly needle.
   d. reassure the child that it will not hurt.

8. A central IV catheter is commonly inserted for:
   a. medication therapy.
   b. pediatric patients.
   c. uncooperative patients.
   d. long-term IV therapy.

9. Signs and symptoms of transfusion reaction include:
   a. high blood pressure.
   b. back pain.
   c. mental confusion.
   d. runny nose.

10. Precautions to take when starting an IV include:
    a. using clean technique.
    b. applying the tourniquet for 5 minutes or less.
    c. inserting the needle in the direction of blood flow.
    d. immobilizing the skin lateral to the insertion site.

EXPLORING THE WEB

Helpful Hints on Preventing Transfusion Reactions	http://www.oahhs.org
Infection Control (skin prep)	http://www.aacn.org
Infusion Nurses Society	http://www.ins1.org
Intravenous Access Network	http://www.ivteam.plus.com
Intravenous Catheter Selection and Tip Termination: A Guide to Making the Best Choice	http://bbriefings.com
Rotherham Clinical Policies and Procedures	http://www.rotherhampct.nhs.uk
Royal College for Nursing Standards for Infusion Therapy Manual	http://www.rcn.org.uk
Standards of Safe Nursing Practice	http://www.clinnutr.org
Transfusion Procedures (University of Michigan Hospitals and Health Centers)	http://www.pathology.med.umich.edu
UTMB Nursing Practice Standards—Peripheral Intravenous Therapy	http://www.utmb.edu
Vancouver Hospital & Health Sciences Centre	http://www.vhpharmsci.com
Vanderbilt University Policies—Intravenous Therapy: Peripheral Vascular Access	http://vumcpolicies.mc.vanderbilt.edu
Where Did this Patient's I.V. Therapy Go Awry?	http://www.findarticles.com

CHAPTER

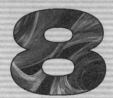

Urinary and Bowel Elimination

OBJECTIVES:

After reading this chapter, you should be able to:

- Spell and define key terms.
- State the purpose of reagents and describe how reagents are used.
- List some common urine tests that are performed using reagents.
- State the purpose of measuring the specific gravity of urine and describe how this test is performed.
- Differentiate an indwelling catheter from a straight catheter and list situations in which each is used.
- Explain why the prostate gland may interfere with catheterization, and identify the age group in which complications related to the prostate commonly occur.
- List the guidelines for disinfecting a urinary drainage bag and leg bag.
- State the purpose of the suprapubic catheter and describe PCT responsibilities in caring for patients with this device.
- State the purpose of the nephrostomy tube and describe PCT responsibilities in caring for patients with this device.
- List three types of dialysis and describe how each is used.
- Identify PCT responsibilities in caring for patients with peritoneal dialysis.
- State the purpose of bladder irrigation and describe three methods of performing this procedure.
- State the purpose of the rectal tube, cleansing enema, retention enema, and rectal suppository.
- List signs and symptoms of fecal impaction.
- Describe the purpose of an ostomy, and list general guidelines for ostomy care.

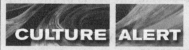

CULTURE ALERT

Cultural alerts are sometimes generalizations. Avoid stereotyping persons from other cultures because of their adherence to traditional practices. The cultural alerts in this chapter apply to elimination. Modesty and hygienic practices vary with age and how closely the individuals adhere to cultural beliefs and traditions.

ROLE OF THE PCT IN ASSISTING PATIENTS WITH ELIMINATION PROCEDURES

You have a very important responsibility in assisting patients with elimination procedures and tests. The circumstances of elimination are highly personal. Respect the patient's right to privacy. Always apply the principles of standard precautions when assisting patients with elimination. Wear personal protective equipment appropriate to the procedure. Wear a gown, eye protection, and face mask if splashing is likely. Use good judgment regarding when to apply and remove gloves. Avoid contaminating environmental surfaces with your gloves.

TESTING URINE

The physician can learn many things about body function and patient health from urine tests. Some of these tests are performed on the nursing unit. They must be performed correctly for the results to be accurate.

Reagent Strips

Special chemicals, called **reagents,** are used to perform certain tests on body fluids. These reagents come in tablets and strips. When the reagent contacts a body fluid, it reacts in a certain manner, providing information about the way the body is functioning. Reagents are commonly used for testing urine and blood on the nursing unit. All reagent products perform in the same manner, but the method of reading them varies. Strips impregnated with reagent are most commonly used. However, for certain tests, tablets are available (**Figure 8-1**). Reagent strips will not produce accurate results if the patient takes certain medications. In this situation, it may be possible to use a reagent tablet instead. Some reagent strips perform multiple tests (**Figure 8-2**); others perform single tests. Many hospitals test their employees for color-blindness before permitting them to interpret the results of reagent strip testing. Know and follow your facility

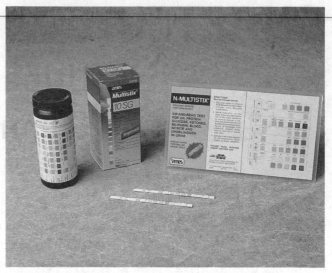

FIGURE 8-2 Multistix reagent strips are used to perform a wide variety of tests.

policies. If you know you are color-blind, inform your supervisor.

When performing reagent tests, you should:

- Store test strips at room temperature, between 15°C and 30°C.
- Store test strips in the original container. Do not remove the desiccant (drying agent) from the bottle.
- Do not expose the strips or bottle to direct sunlight.
- Remove only as many strips as required for testing. Immediately recap the container tightly.
- Avoid touching the test squares on the strip, as this may result in a false reading.
- Do not use strips beyond the expiration date.
- Read the directions for the product you are using.
- Apply the principles of standard precautions.
- Always collect and test a fresh urine specimen.
- Never let a specimen sit for a prolonged period before using it.
- Never collect urine from a catheter bag.
- Completely immerse reagent areas of the strip in fresh urine.
- Remove the strip immediately to avoid dissolving the reagent areas.
- While removing, tap the side of the strip against the rim of the urine container to remove excess urine.
- Compare each reagent area to its corresponding color block on the color chart and read

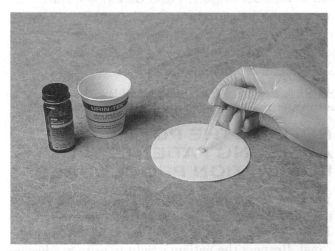

FIGURE 8-1 The acetest is a reagent tablet test used to check urine for the presence of ketones.

at the time specified. Proper read time is critical for optimal and accurate results.

- Obtain results by direct comparison with the color chart. Avoid guessing.
- Perform control testing, to ensure accuracy, at the frequency specified by facility policy. Document your findings.

Some reagent products are caustic and will damage mucous membranes. Avoid touching them with your fingers. These products cause serious injury if they are ingested, so they must be stored in a secure location or locked cupboard when not in use. Never leave reagent products where children or a cognitively impaired adult can reach them.

Reagents are used to measure levels of sugar and ketones in the urine. Normally, these substances are not present in the urine. In certain conditions, such as diabetes, their presence indicates an imbalance that must be corrected. The results of the urine tests help guide the physician in regulating the condition. Reagents are also commonly used to measure the **pH** of the urine. The pH is an indication of the acidity or alkalinity of a substance. When the pH of the urine is tested, it provides the physician with information about the function of the kidneys.

Urine Glucose and Ketone Testing with Reagent Strips

You will be testing the urine for the presence of glucose and ketones with reagent strips. Some reagent strips, such as Keto-Diastix, will perform both of these tests. Other strips measure these substances separately. If you are using a strip that performs multiple tests, hold the strip horizontally while it is processing. If the strip is vertical, the urine may cause the chemicals to run together, obscuring the results. Urine glucose testing may also be done with a paper tape that is impregnated with reagent. If desired, you may place the strips or tape on a paper towel while they are processing.

When testing a specimen for glucose, instruct the patient to void an hour before collecting the specimen. Ask him or her to drink several glasses of water. Return in an hour to collect a urine specimen. If the patient has orders to take nothing by mouth (is NPO), do not collect a double-voided specimen.

Apply gloves before handling the urine specimen. You will dip the reagent product into the urine (**Figure 8-3A**) and hold it for the length of time specified on the bottle. Remove the strip and tap off

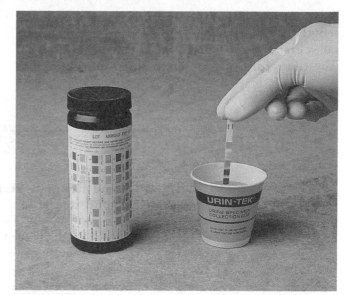

FIGURE 8-3(A) Dip the reagent strip into the urine specimen.

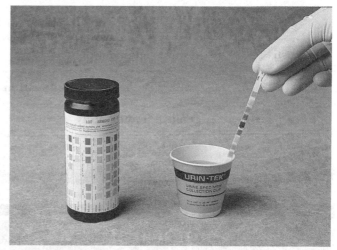

FIGURE 8-3(B) Remove the strip and tap it gently to remove excess urine.

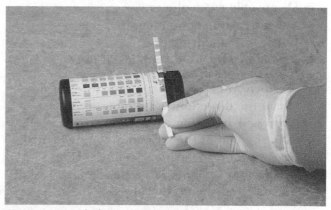

FIGURE 8-3(C) Compare the strip with the color chart on the container.

excess urine (**Figure 8-3B**). Wait the designated length of time, then compare the reagent to the color chart on the back of the bottle (**Figure 8-3C**). The times for some common glucose testing products are listed in **Table 8-1**. The color may continue to change after you take the reading. Ignore changes that occur after the designated time for reading the strip.

Product	Length of Time Reagent Strip Must Be Dipped in Urine	Length of Time to Wait After Removing Reagent Strip Before Comparing with Color Chart
Table 8-1 Testing Times for Urine Glucose and Ketone Reagent Strips		
Products for Glucose Testing		
Clinistix	2 seconds	10 seconds (ignore changes after 10 seconds)
Diastix	2 seconds	30 seconds (ignore changes after 30 seconds)
Tes-Tape	2 seconds	60 seconds (if the reading exceeds 0.5 percent, wait an additional 60 seconds and read again)
Products for Ketone Testing		
Ketostix	remove immediately	15 seconds (ignore changes after 15 seconds)
Products for Combination Glucose and Ketone Testing		
Keto-Diastix	remove immediately	ketone—read at exactly 15 seconds
		glucose—read at exactly 30 seconds

Procedure 47

Testing Urine with Reagent Strips

Supplies needed:
- Disposable exam gloves
- Specimen collection container
- Bottle of reagent strips
- Plastic bag for used supplies, if needed

1. Perform your beginning procedure actions.
2. Read the directions on the bottle for the strip you are using.
3. Dip the end of the strip impregnated with reagent into the urine specimen. Hold the strip in the sample for the designated length of time and then remove.
4. Wait for the length of time specified in the directions.
5. Hold the strip next to the color chart on the package. Compare the color. Record the reading, which is listed below each color on the chart.
6. Discard the strip and urine specimen according to facility policy.
7. Record the patient's intake and output, if applicable.
8. Perform your procedure completion actions.

Urine Specific Gravity

Urine specific gravity is a measure of how well the kidneys concentrate urine. This test provides useful diagnostic information for many different conditions. High quantities of glucose and protein in the urine can cause an elevated specific gravity. Specific gravity testing is done using a random urine specimen. You will not ask the patient to empty the bladder, then drink water, as you do with glucose testing. Specific gravity is most accurate if the specimen is collected after the patient has been NPO. As urine becomes more concentrated, the specific gravity increases.

For accurate results, the urine specimen should be room temperature when it is tested (approximately 71°F). Some facilities permit testing of specimens between 60°F and 100°F. Wait at least 20 minutes for the specimen to cool, particularly if the patient has a fever. Do not refrigerate it. Follow your facility policies for specimen collection and length of time to wait before performing the test.

The normal specific gravity in adults ranges from 1.010 to 1.035. Some facilities use a range from 1.002 to 1.025. Clinical norms for a 24-hour urine are 1.015 to 1.024. Values below 1.010 suggest very dilute urine, and are present in conditions such as serious renal infections and acute renal failure. Values above 1.025 suggest dehydration and congestive heart failure. Patients who have recently received contrast dyes can have falsely elevated values. The length of time for which the contrast dye affects the specimen will vary with the type and amount of dye used, and the patient's kidney function. Recent alcohol consumption may also affect the specific gravity reading. Monitoring the specific gravity may not be appropriate in these situations.

On the nursing unit, specific gravity may be determined using an instrument called a **urinometer** (Figure 8-4). A **refractometer** is a handheld unit that is used for checking specific gravity in many facilities. The refractometer is read by looking through the end (**Figure 8-5**), which is somewhat like a telescope. The reportable range for the TS meter, a commonly used refractometer, is 1.000 to 1.035. Other meters and devices may also be used for testing specific gravity in the laboratory. Some facilities use a reagent strip called Multistix for specific gravity testing. This strip is held in the urine

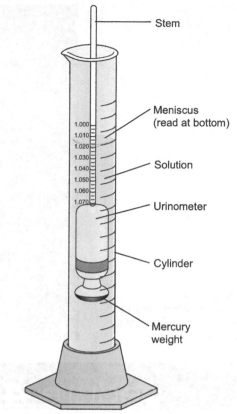

FIGURE 8-4 The urinometer is commonly used to measure urine specific gravity.

for 2 seconds. Tap the strip on the edge of the container to remove excess urine, then read the value immediately. Follow your facility policy for documenting your reading. Some facilities record the volume, color, odor, and appearance of urine in addition to the specific gravity.

For accuracy, the urinometer must be properly calibrated. The specific gravity test is done by comparing the weight of urine with the weight of distilled water. The weight of distilled water is 1.000, so urine is heavier. You may be asked to check the urinometer calibration and record your findings. Do this by performing the same procedure as you would for urine, using room-temperature distilled water. If the pH of the water is not 1.000, you will have to adjust the reading of the urine. This is done by adding 0.001 for every 5.4°F above the calibration temperature of 71.6°F, or subtracting 0.001 for every 5.4°F below the calibration temperature. Check with the RN or follow facility policy, if this is necessary. Your facility may have a chart available listing the conversions.

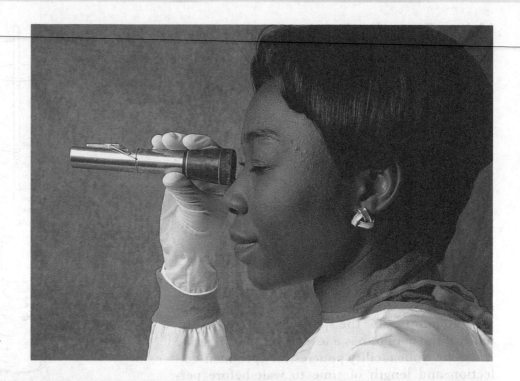

FIGURE 8-5 The refractometer is also used to determine the specific gravity of a urine specimen.

Procedure 48

Measuring Urine Specific Gravity with a Urinometer

Supplies needed:
- ▶ Disposable exam gloves
- ▶ Calibrated urinometer and cylinder
- ▶ Container for urine specimen

1. Perform your beginning procedure actions.
2. Carefully pour urine into the cylinder until it is 3/4 full.
3. Gently spin the urinometer, then drop it into the cylinder. If the device hits the side of the container and stops spinning, repeat this step.
4. Wait for the urinometer to stop bobbing, then read the value on the stem, or meniscus. Wait until the device stops moving, and make sure it does not touch the sides of the container, which will cause an inaccurate reading.
5. Position yourself so the meniscus is close to eye level (Figure 8-6). You should be able to clearly see the numbers and position of the meniscus. Take the reading on the lowest point of the scale.

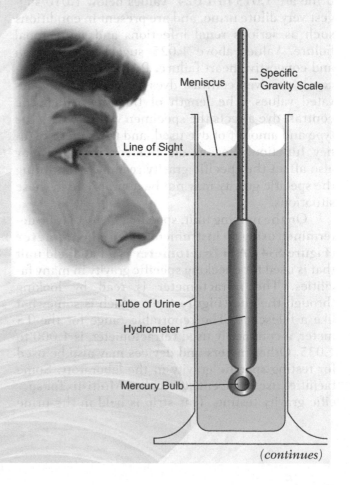

Meniscus

Specific Gravity Scale

Line of Sight

Tube of Urine

Hydrometer

Mercury Bulb

FIGURE 8-6 Read the urinometer stem at the meniscus, as close to eye level as possible.

(continues)

Procedure **48**, *continued*

Measuring Urine Specific Gravity with a Urinometer

6. Discard the urine.
7. Rinse the container with cool water. Avoid using warm water, which may

cause proteins in the urine to adhere to the container.
8. Perform your procedure completion actions.

Procedure **49**

Measuring Urine Specific Gravity with a Refractometer

Supplies needed:
- Disposable exam gloves
- Calibrated refractometer
- Container for urine specimen
- Eyedropper
- Lint-free tissue

1. Perform your beginning procedure actions.
2. Press the button on the back of the refractometer stand to turn on the light.
3. Place 1 to 2 drops of urine between the prism and the cover plate. Wait a few seconds to allow time for the urine to be drawn into the space between the two by capillary action.

4. Press the plastic cover gently but firmly to spread the urine in a thin, even layer over the prisms.
5. Read the specific gravity where the sharp boundary between the light and dark fields crosses the left-hand scale. If necessary, rotate the eyepiece to focus.
6. Lift the plastic cover plate up and wipe the sample from the prism and cover plate with a lint-free tissue.
7. Turn the light off.
8. Discard any remaining urine.
9. Perform your procedure completion actions.

Procedure **50**

Multistix Urine Testing

Supplies needed:
- Disposable exam gloves
- Test strips and bottle or color comparison chart
- Container for urine specimen

1. Perform your beginning procedure actions.
2. Collect the urine specimen. Pour the specimen into a container, such as a 30-mL plastic medicine cup.
3. Observe and note the urine color and appearance.

4. Briefly dip a Multistix test strip into the urine sample. Hold the strip in the urine for approximately 2 seconds.
5. Gently tap the strip on the side of the cup to remove excess urine. Never blot the test pads.
6. Read each color pad at the designated time printed on the color chart on the bottle or package insert. Reading the color at the indicated time is critical for optimal and accurate results. Color changes that occur after 2 minutes are of no diagnostic value.

(continues)

Procedure **50**, *continued*

Multistix Urine Testing

7. Urine color may cause the test strip to have a slightly different color compared with the color chart accompanying the test product.
   ▶ If the test strip color does not match a color square on the color chart, match the test strip to a color square of equal intensity.
   ▶ If the color development is slightly uneven, match the average color on the test pad.
   ▶ Save the strip so the RN can validate your findings.

8. Discard any remaining urine.
9. Perform your procedure completion actions.
10. Document your findings on a flow sheet, or according to facility policies. For example:
    ▶ Urine color: colorless, straw, yellow, amber, red, brown, blue, or green

▶ Urine appearance: clear, slightly cloudy, moderately cloudy, or turbid, sediment or mucus present
▶ Glucose: negative, 100, 250, 500, 1,000, or 2,000 mg/dL
▶ Bilirubin: negative, small, moderate, or large
▶ Ketone: negative, trace, small, moderate, or large
▶ Specific gravity: 1.000, 1.005, 1.010, 1.015, 1.020, 1.025, or 1.030
▶ Blood: negative, trace, small, moderate, or large
▶ pH: 5.0, 6.0, 6.5, 7.0, 7.5, 8.0, or 8.5
▶ Protein: negative, trace, 30, 100, 300, or 2,000 mg/dL
▶ Urobilinogen: negative or positive
▶ Nitrites: negative or positive
▶ Leukocytes: negative, trace, small, moderate, or large

CULTURE ALERT

Female patients from many cultures keep their bodies covered as much as possible. Special hospital gowns are available to cover women completely from shoulders to feet. If special gowns are not available in your facility, provide a long gown and robe when the patient is undressed, or assist the patient in fashioning a cover with a bath blanket. In some cultures, such as Islam, the female's body must be covered when members of the opposite sex are present. Some patients will refuse all care from members of the opposite sex. Some women prefer to wear a head covering. Patients of both genders from the Samoan culture may refuse to leave the room unless dressed in street clothes. Patients from the Gypsy culture are very modest and believe in separation of the sexes. They may resist or refuse a caregiver of the opposite sex. They have very high standards of personal hygiene. Cleanliness of the head is symbolic, and most believe that it helps keep them pure. These individuals usually shampoo the hair and request a clean pillowcase daily. Avoid touching their heads and pillowcases whenever possible. Gypsies believe in keeping the upper and lower body separate. Provide a separate towel, washcloth, and soap for each half of the body. Avoid contacting the upper body (or items that touch the upper body) with a bedpan.

CATHETERS

A *catheter* is a tube that is inserted into the bladder to drain urine. An indwelling catheter (**Figure 8-7**) remains in the bladder. This type of catheter may also

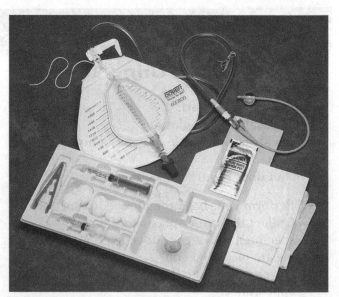

FIGURE 8-7 The indwelling catheter kit. (Courtesy of Sherwood-Davis & Geck)

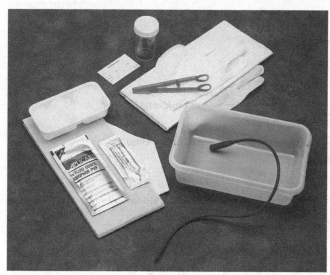

FIGURE 8-8 The straight catheter kit. (Courtesy of Sherwood-Davis & Geck)

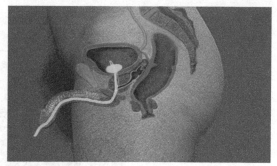

FIGURE 8-9 The inflated balloon holds the indwelling catheter in place in the bladder.

be called a *Foley,* or *retention, catheter.* Urine drains through a closed drainage system to a collection bag. To prevent infection, the system is not opened, except to empty the bag. An indwelling catheter is inserted during surgery, and for comfort in conditions in which the patient is unable to empty the bladder normally. A straight catheter (**Figure 8-8**) is used for obtaining a sterile urine specimen and in some medical conditions, such as multiple sclerosis, in which an indwelling catheter increases the risk of complications. The straight catheter is inserted and the bladder is emptied. The catheter is immediately removed. This type of catheterization may be called an *in-and-out catheterization.* Either type of catheter may be used to empty the bladder in conditions in which contact with urine would interfere with healing, such as burns or wounds.

Using an indwelling catheter is not a treatment for urinary incontinence. In this condition, it is a treatment of last resort. Because the indwelling catheter provides an open passageway to the bladder, the risk of infection is markedly increased. This risk is great in female patients because the urethra is short. The female urethra is 1 1/2 to 3 inches in length. The male urethra is approximately 6 to 7 inches in length. Although the risk of infection is lower in males, they may also contract an infection from catheterization.

Catheter Size

Catheters come in many different sizes, from very small to large. Like needles, the gauge of the catheter is determined by the size of the lumen. Unlike needles, however, low-number gauges indicate small catheters. A straight catheter has a single lumen. An indwelling catheter has a double lumen. One lumen is used to drain the urine. The second is connected to a balloon, which is inflated with sterile water or saline solution after the catheter is inserted. The balloon holds the catheter in the bladder (**Figure 8-9**). Some catheters have an additional lumen for medical treatments, such as continuous irrigation.

Depending on the make of the catheter, the abbreviation "Fr" may appear after the gauge number. This abbreviation stands for French, because catheters are sized using a French scale. The higher the gauge, the larger the catheter. For children, a 6-, 8-, or 10-gauge catheter is used. For adult females, a 14- or 16-gauge catheter is used. For adult males, a 14-, 16-, or 18-gauge catheter is used. The physician will order the catheter size. The RN will tell you which size to use.

Inserting a Catheter

Catheterization requires a physician's order. Because of the risk of infection, catheter insertion is a sterile procedure in the health care facility. Some patients self-catheterize themselves at home. In this situation, the patient may use clean technique. Sterile catheterization trays are available as complete units. You may have to add the proper size indwelling catheter. With some kits, you must also add the drainage bag. Contamination occurs easily during this procedure. Be very careful, and use good sterile technique. Good lighting is needed for this procedure. It may be necessary to ask an assistant to hold a flashlight so that you can see the urinary meatus in the female patient.

Catheterization is a very personal procedure. Provide complete privacy. Before beginning, provide an age-appropriate explanation, and then position the patient. Position the female patient as

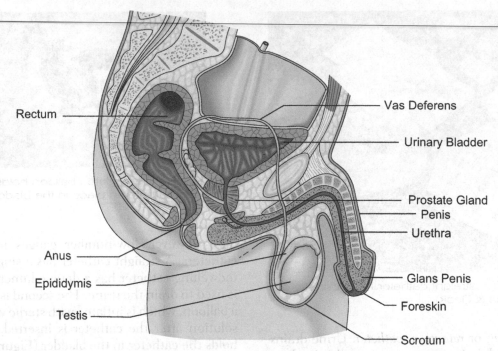

Rectum

Vas Deferens

Urinary Bladder

Prostate Gland

Penis

Urethra

Anus

Epididymis

Glans Penis

Testis

Foreskin

Scrotum

FIGURE 8-10 The prostate gland encircles the urethra. It commonly enlarges as the patient ages, causing partial or complete urinary obstruction.

you would for perineal care, with the knees up and feet flat on the bed. Children may not cooperate with this procedure, and an assistant may be necessary to keep the patient still and prevent contamination of the sterile field. You may also need an assistant for adults who cannot maintain the position necessary for catheterization. This is particularly true of patients with lower extremity disorders and elderly females.

Male patients may have an erection when the genitals are touched. Holding the penis firmly, rather than touching it gently, may eliminate the problem. If erection occurs, provide privacy. Tell the patient when you will return to complete the procedure, and leave the room. Avoid embarrassing the patient.

Elderly men often develop prostate problems. The prostate (**Figure 8-10**) is a gland that secretes fluid in semen. It surrounds the urethra just below the bladder in the male. As men age, the prostate gland enlarges and applies pressure to the urethra. This causes urinary retention, or inability to empty the bladder completely. Other problems related to the prostate are frequent dribbling of urine or inability to urinate at all. Problems with the prostate may make catheterization necessary. However, it may be difficult to insert a catheter because of the

enlarged prostate. If this is the case, a Coudé, a special catheter with a curved tip, will be used. This type of catheter must be inserted by the physician or an RN who is experienced in the procedure.

AGE-APPROPRIATE CARE **ALERT**

A straight catheter or Speci-cath is commonly used to obtain a urine specimen from an incontinent patient. Remember that incontinence is a medical problem. It is not a normal aging change. Loss of bladder control affects the patient's dignity and self-esteem. The problem is often one of communication, not a physical problem. The confused patient usually knows that he or she needs to use the toilet, but cannot communicate this need. Some patients will scream, yell, cry, or exhibit other behavior problems. These stop when the patient cannot contain the elimination and becomes incontinent. If seated on the toilet, such a patient almost always eliminates. Cognitively impaired patients may strike out because they interpret the genital manipulation as a sexual assault. Make every effort to assist elderly patients with toileting and maintaining normal bowel and bladder function. Avoid showing disgust. Be sensitive to the patient's feelings. Be tactful and empathetic. Use proper terms when referring to body parts or excretions.

Procedure 51

Inserting a Straight Catheter

NOTE: The guidelines and sequence for this procedure vary slightly from state to state and from one facility to the next. Your instructor will inform you if the sequence in your state or facility differs from the procedure listed here. Know and follow the required sequence for your state requirements and facility policies.

Supplies needed:
- Disposable exam gloves
- Bath blanket
- Washcloth
- Towel
- Incontinent pad
- Washbasin of warm water
- Soap
- Plastic bag for used supplies
- Catheterization tray
- Catheter size as directed by the RN

1. Perform your beginning procedure actions.
2. Place the incontinent pad under the patient's buttocks.
3. Position and drape the patient for perineal care.
4. Apply gloves.
5. Provide perineal care.
6. Discard used supplies.
7. Wash your hands, or use alcohol-based hand cleaner.
8. Adjust or position the lighting, if necessary.
9. Clean the overbed table. Disinfect the table, if soiled, or if required by facility policy.
10. Open the catheterization tray and establish a sterile field.
11. Open the catheter and place it on the sterile field.
12. Place the plastic bag for used supplies at the foot of the bed, or in a convenient location. Position the bag so that you do not have to cross over sterile supplies to discard soiled items.
13. Pick up the first drape. Stand away from the bed and hold the drape away from your body, allowing it to unfold.
14. Fold the drape back, over your gloves. Ask the patient to lift his or her buttocks.

Carefully slide the drape under the buttocks. Avoid touching the patient or the bed linen.
15. Pick up the next drape. Stand away from the bed and hold the drape away from your body, allowing it to unfold.
16. Position the hole in the center of the drape over the perineum. If it is necessary to lift the penis to position the drape, use your nondominant hand. This hand will be contaminated after touching the patient's skin and cannot be used to contact sterile supplies.
17. Apply sterile gloves.
18. Open the sterile packages on the sterile field, and arrange supplies as needed.
19. Inspect the catheter for cracks or rough spots. If found, replace the catheter.
20. Open the package of povidone-iodine or other antiseptic solution. Carefully pour the solution over the cotton balls or applicators.
21. Open the package of lubricant.
22. Lubricate the tip of the catheter. The lubricant should cover the catheter for approximately 2 inches for a female and 4 to 5 inches for a male.
23. With the forceps in the tray, pick up a cotton ball moistened with disinfectant solution. Cleanse the genitals:
Female patient: Separate the labia with the nondominant hand. This hand is now contaminated. You must keep the labia spread apart until the catheter has been inserted. If your hand accidentally slips, you must begin the cleansing procedure again if the sides of the labia contact each other. Wipe the labia from top to bottom, beginning with the center, with the cotton ball. Use one stroke, then discard the cotton ball. Next, pick up another cotton ball and repeat the procedure on the side opposite where you are standing (**Figure 8-11**). Discard the cotton ball. Pick up one more cotton ball, and cleanse the labia closest to you from top to bottom. Use the remaining cotton ball to pat the area dry. This

(continues)

Procedure **51**, *continued*

Inserting a Straight Catheter

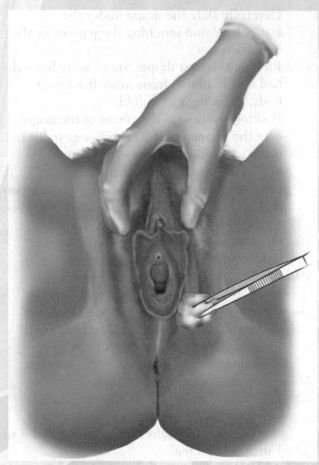

FIGURE 8-11 Cleanse the labia minora in a single stroke, from top to bottom.

reduces the stinging sensation caused by introducing the cleansing agent into the urethra with the catheter. Discard the cotton ball and forceps.

Male patient: Pick up the penis with the nondominant hand. This hand is now contaminated. Retract the foreskin of the penis. Beginning at the urinary meatus, wipe the penis in a circular motion. Discard the cotton ball. Next, pick up another cotton ball and repeat the procedure, cleansing outward from the meatus in a circle. Discard the cotton ball. Pick up one more cotton ball, and cleanse in a circle beyond the second circle. When done, you should have cleansed a large area. Use the remaining cotton ball to pat the area dry. This reduces the stinging sensation caused by introducing the cleansing agent into the urethra with the catheter. Discard the cotton ball and forceps.

24. Place the open end of the catheter into the specimen collection container or drainage basin positioned in front of the labia.
25. Pick up the catheter. Hold it approximately 1 1/2 to 2 inches from the tip.
26. Insert the catheter into the urethra.
Female patient: Visualize the urinary meatus **(Figure 8-12)**. Tell the patient you

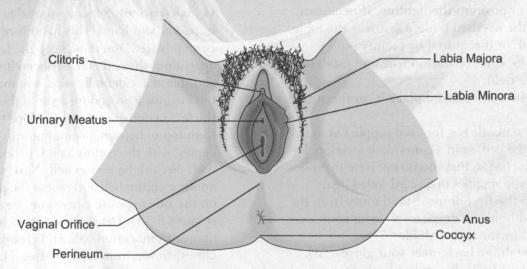

Clitoris

Urinary Meatus

Vaginal Orifice

Perineum

Labia Majora

Labia Minora

Anus

Coccyx

FIGURE 8-12 Insert the catheter into the urinary meatus. Visualize the structure carefully. It is difficult to see in some women.

(continues)

Procedure **51**, *continued*

Inserting a Straight Catheter

will be inserting the catheter now. Instruct the patient to cough, take a deep breath, or whistle. This will help relax the urinary sphincter. Insert the catheter into the urethra, threading it into the bladder (about 2 1/2 or 3 inches) until urine flows. If urine does not flow immediately, hold the catheter in place until urine drains. If no urine flows, the catheter may be in the vagina. Leave it in place. You must get fresh supplies and repeat the procedure. Leaving it in place will make it easier to find the urethra the next time. Remove it after the catheterization is successful. If an assistant is helping you, continue to hold the labia apart, and send him or her for another catheter. When he or she returns, have the assistant open the catheter. Grasp it with your sterile hand, and repeat the procedure.

Male patient: Hold the penis upright with your nondominant hand. Insert the catheter into the meatus (**Figure 8-13**). Tell the patient you will be inserting the catheter now. Instruct the patient to cough, take a deep breath, or whistle while you are inserting the catheter. The patient may also bear down, as if to urinate. Encourage him to continue throughout the procedure. Advance the catheter until urine flows. *Never force a catheter. If you meet resistance and are unable to advance the catheter, stop the procedure and notify the RN.*

27. Collect a specimen, if ordered. Collect approximately 30 to 50 mL of urine in the specimen cup, then pinch the catheter to stop the flow of urine. Move the cup to the side and position the drainage basin under the end of the catheter. Allow the bladder to empty into the basin. If 1,000 mL of urine drains

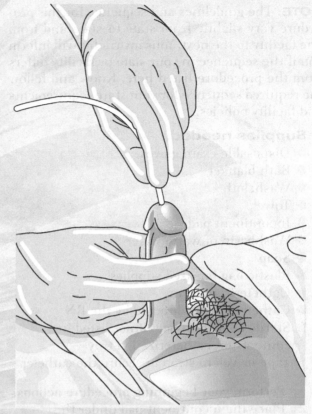

FIGURE 8-13 Hold the penis at a 90° angle. Insert the catheter gently 6 to 8 inches.

from the bladder and urine continues to flow, pinch the catheter and contact the RN. Some facilities require you to empty an overfull bladder over a period of time to prevent complications. Some facilities allow the bladder to empty completely. (This is a controversial area requiring further research.)

28. Slowly withdraw the catheter.
29. Replace the foreskin in the male patient.
30. Remove the drapes. Discard in the plastic bag.
31. Perform your procedure completion actions.

Procedure 52

Inserting an Indwelling Catheter

NOTE: The guidelines and sequence for this procedure vary slightly from state to state and from one facility to the next. Your instructor will inform you if the sequence in your state or facility differs from the procedure listed here. Know and follow the required sequence for your state requirements and facility policies.

Supplies needed:
- Disposable exam gloves
- Bath blanket
- Washcloth
- Towel
- Incontinent pad
- Washbasin of warm water
- Soap
- Plastic bag for used supplies
- Catheterization tray
- Catheter size as directed by the RN
- Sterile collection bag, if not listed in contents on catheterization tray
- Tape or Velcro strap to secure the catheter

1. Perform your beginning procedure actions.
2. Place the incontinent pad under the patient's buttocks.
3. Position and drape the patient for perineal care.
4. Apply gloves.
5. Provide perineal care.
6. Discard used supplies.
7. Wash your hands.
8. Adjust or position the lighting, if necessary.
9. Clean the overbed table. Disinfect the table, if soiled, or if required by facility policy.
10. Open the catheterization tray and establish a sterile field.
11. Open the catheter and place it on the sterile field.
12. Place the plastic bag for used supplies at the foot of the bed, or in a convenient location. Position the bag so that you do not have to cross over sterile supplies to discard soiled items.
13. Pick up the first drape. Stand away from the bed and hold the drape away from your body, allowing it to unfold.

14. Fold the drape back, over your gloves. Ask the patient to lift his or her buttocks. Carefully slide the drape under the buttocks. Avoid touching the patient or the bed linen.
15. Pick up the next drape. Stand away from the bed and hold the drape away from your body, allowing it to unfold.
16. Position the hole in the center of the drape over the perineum. If it is necessary to lift the penis to position the drape, use your nondominant hand. This hand will be contaminated after touching the patient's skin and cannot be used to contact sterile supplies.
17. Apply sterile gloves.
18. Open the sterile packages on the sterile field, and arrange supplies as needed. Attach the indwelling catheter to the drainage bag if no specimen will be collected. Check the clamp over the drainage spout to ensure that it is closed.
19. Inspect the catheter for cracks or rough spots. If found, replace the catheter.
20. Attach the saline-filled syringe to the inflation port on the catheter. Inject the fluid into the catheter to check the balloon for leaks (**Figure 8-14**). If the balloon will not inflate, or if leaks are present, replace the catheter. Pull back on the plunger of the syringe to deflate the balloon.
21. Open the package of povidone-iodine or other antiseptic solution. Carefully pour the solution over the cotton balls or applicators.
22. Open the package of lubricant.
23. Lubricate the tip of the catheter. The lubricant should cover the catheter for approximately 2 inches for a female and 4 to 5 inches for a male.
24. With the forceps in the tray, pick up a cotton ball moistened with disinfectant solution. Cleanse the patient:
    Female patient: Separate the labia with the nondominant hand. This hand is now contaminated. You must keep the labia spread

(continues)

Procedure 52, *continued*

Inserting an Indwelling Catheter

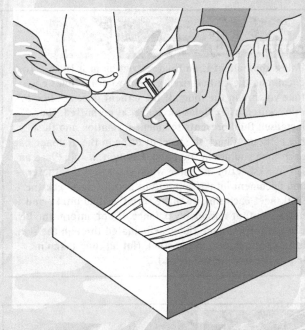

FIGURE 8-14 Insert the syringe into the catheter and inflate the balloon. Pull back on the plunger to deflate the balloon.

apart until the catheter has been inserted. If your hand accidentally slips, you must begin the cleansing procedure again if the sides of the labia contact each other. Wipe the labia from top to bottom, beginning with the center, with the cotton ball. Use one stroke, then discard the cotton ball. Next, pick up another cotton ball and repeat the procedure on the side opposite where you are standing. Discard the cotton ball. Pick up one more cotton ball, and cleanse the labia closest to you from top to bottom. Use the remaining cotton ball to pat the area dry. Discard the cotton ball and forceps.

Male patient: Pick up the penis with the nondominant hand. This hand is now contaminated. Retract the foreskin of the penis. Beginning at the urinary meatus, wipe the penis in a circular motion. Discard the cotton ball. Next, pick up another cotton ball and repeat the procedure, cleansing outward from the meatus in a circle. Discard the cotton ball. Pick up one more

cotton ball, and cleanse in a circle beyond the second circle. When done, you should have cleansed a large area. Use the remaining cotton ball to pat the area dry. Discard the cotton ball and forceps.

25. If a specimen will be collected, place the open end of the catheter into the specimen collection container or drainage basin positioned in front of the patient.

26. Pick up the catheter. Hold it approximately 1 1/2 to 2 inches from the tip.

27. Insert the catheter into the urethra.
Female patient: Visualize the urinary meatus. Tell the patient you will be inserting the catheter now. Instruct the patient to cough, bear down, or whistle. This will help relax the urinary sphincter. Insert the catheter into the urethra, threading it into the bladder (about 2 1/2 or 3 inches) until urine flows. If urine does not flow immediately, hold the catheter in place until urine drains. If no urine flows, the catheter may be in the vagina. Leave it in place. You must get fresh supplies and repeat the procedure. Leaving it in place will make it easier to find the urethra the next time. Remove it after the catheterization is successful. If an assistant is helping you, continue to hold the labia apart, and send him or her for another catheter. When he or she returns, have the assistant open the catheter. Grasp it with your sterile hand, and repeat the procedure.
Male patient: Hold the penis upright with your nondominant hand. Insert the catheter into the meatus. Tell the patient you will be inserting the catheter now. Instruct the patient to cough, bear down, or whistle while you are inserting the catheter. Encourage him to continue throughout the procedure. Advance the catheter until urine flows.
Never force a catheter. If you meet resistance and are unable to advance the catheter, stop the procedure and notify the RN.

(continues)

Procedure **52**, *continued*

Inserting an Indwelling Catheter

28. Collect a specimen, if ordered (Figure 8-15). Collect approximately 30 to 50 mL of urine in the specimen cup, then pinch the catheter to stop the flow of urine. Move the cup to the side and position the drainage basin under the end of the catheter. Allow the bladder to empty into the basin. If 1,000 mL of urine drains from the bladder and urine continues to flow, pinch the catheter and contact the RN. Some facilities require you to empty an overfull bladder over a period of time to prevent complications. Some facilities allow the bladder to empty completely. (This is a controversial area requiring further research.)

29. Pick up the syringe and attach it to the inflation port in the catheter. Slowly push the plunger to inflate the balloon.

30. Attach the collection bag to the catheter, if this was not done previously.

31. Hang the collection bag on the bed frame. Do not let it touch the floor.

32. Replace the foreskin in the male patient.

33. Tape the catheter or apply a Velcro leg strap to secure the catheter. Do not leave the room until the catheter is secured. The mechanical irritation caused by catheter movement can cause complications. The catheter in the female is secured to the upper thigh. The catheter in the male is secured to either the upper thigh or the abdomen.

34. Remove the drapes. Tear the center of the fenestrated drape to remove it over the catheter. Discard in the plastic bag.

35. Perform your procedure completion actions.

FIGURE 8-15 Hold the catheter in the center of the cup to collect a specimen.

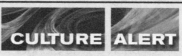

DIFFICULT PATIENT ALERT

Unless the patient is on fluid restriction or is NPO, encourage the catheterized patient to drink fluids each time you are in the room. If the patient does not like to drink water, offer fluids of choice, as permitted. The increased fluid prevents sediment formation and flushes the catheter. Check the level of urine in the drainage bag each time you are in the room. Empty it, if full. Place an I&O worksheet in the room when you insert a catheter, and document intake and output accurately. Check the worksheet each shift to make sure the fluid intake and urinary output reasonably balance. If not, inform the RN. (Do not forget, some fluid is eliminated through the skin, in respirations, and in the stool. Not all fluid taken in leaves the body in the urine.)

CULTURE ALERT

Some Koreans will not drink cold water or water with ice, believing it can cause disease. Some patients will refuse medications if offered with cold water. Others may have physician orders for no ice. Keep this in mind when encouraging fluids. Allowing the patient a choice of fluids is best.

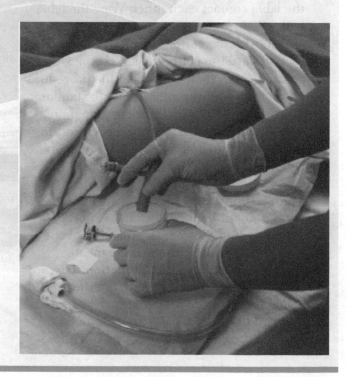

Special Considerations

Variations in catheter types and patient needs may make it necessary to adapt the catheterization procedure.

Methods of Filling the Balloon.

Indwelling catheters are available with several different types of balloons. One type is injected with air, then the end of the inflation port is folded over onto itself and secured with a clamp. Another type is self-inflating. The injection port is pierced with a needle, causing the balloon to inflate. Another similar type employs a clamp over the inflation port. When the clamp is removed, the balloon autoinflates. Familiarize yourself with the types of catheters used in your facility.

Methods of Positioning the Female Patient.

Medical problems may make it difficult or impossible for female patients to maintain the position necessary for catheterization. The catheter may be inserted with the patient positioned on her side. Position the patient in the lateral position, then draw the knees up toward the chest.

The Specimen Collection System.

In some situations, the physician will order a catheterized urine specimen. With incontinent patients, the only means of obtaining a urine specimen may involve catheterization. A special collection system is used in many health care facilities instead of a straight catheter. This product is called a specimen collection catheter, or Speci-Cath (Figure 8-16A and 8-16B). Several different brand names are available. Using this device is easier for staff and less traumatic for the patient. The closed system reduces the potential for accidental contamination.

The specimen collection system employs a tiny catheter attached to a test tube. This tiny catheter is much more comfortable for the patient than a full-sized catheter. The device comes packaged as a complete catheterization tray, or as an individual unit. If the individual unit is used by your facility, you must add the supplies to disinfect the perineum and the gloves. The procedure for performing the catheterization is essentially the same as for a straight catheter. However, the catheter remains attached to the test tube during the procedure. You may hold the test tube in your hand to insert the catheter in the female. After you have filled the test tube with urine, withdraw the catheter. After the catheter is withdrawn, pull it with your gloved hand. This will separate the catheter from the test tube. Discard the catheter in a plastic bag. Press on the spout of the test tube to seal it closed. The test tube is transported to the laboratory for testing. Label it with a biohazard label and transport it in a closed plastic bag.

For infection control purposes, the specimen collection tube is excellent for the laboratory. A urine specimen is normally transferred to a test tube by laboratory personnel. The tube is placed in a centrifuge as part of the routine urine testing procedure. The specimen collection test tube may be placed directly into the centrifuge, eliminating the

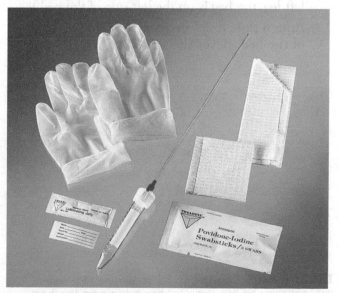

FIGURE 8-16(A) The female Speci-Cath insertion kit. (Courtesy of Medline Industries, Inc., Mundelein, IL; (800) MEDLINE)

FIGURE 8-16(B) The male Speci-Cath insertion kit. (Courtesy of Medline Industries, Inc., Mundelein, IL; (800) MEDLINE)

need to transfer the specimen to another container. The specimen collection device benefits the patient, nursing personnel, and laboratory personnel, and is commonly used by many facilities.

Caring for a Patient with a Catheter

When caring for a patient who has a catheter, you should:

- Secure the catheter with a strap at all times (**Figure 8-17**) to prevent inadvertent pulling and injury. Some facilities secure the catheter to the leg in women and to the abdomen, using tape, in men. When securing the catheter to the leg, position it on the top side. Avoid placing the catheter under the leg, which may pinch the tubing and obstruct the flow of urine. Know and follow your facility policy.

- Attach the tubing to the bed with a rubber band and plastic clip.

- Always wash your hands and apply gloves before handling the catheter and closed drainage system. Avoid environmental contamination with your gloves.

- Avoid opening the closed system, if possible.

- Use sterile technique if the catheter, bag, and tubing must be disconnected.

- Always keep the closed drainage system off the floor, as this contaminates the system.

- Position the drainage bag on the same side of the bed as the catheter. (If the catheter is on the left leg, the bag is on the left side of the bed.)

- Attach the closed drainage bag to the frame of the bed, never the side rail.

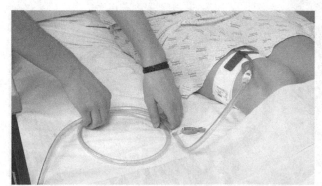

FIGURE 8-17 The Velcro strap is used to fasten the catheter to the leg. Coil the tubing on the bed. These measures prevent the catheter from moving and accidentally being pulled out during movement or transfers.

- Position the catheter on top of the leg when the patient is on his or her back.

- Position the catheter between the legs if the patient is positioned on his or her side. Make sure urine flow is not obstructed. Place the bag on the bed frame on the side the patient is facing. (For example, if the patient faces right, the bag hangs on the right side of the bed.)

- Carry the tubing and drainage bag below the level of the bladder when the patient is ambulating.

- Avoid elevating the urinary drainage bag and tubing above the level of the bladder. This causes a backflow of urine into the bladder, greatly increasing the risk of infection.

- Make sure the urine is draining freely through the system and there are no kinks or obstructions in the tubing.

- Use care when lifting, moving, turning, positioning, and transferring patients who have catheters to avoid accidentally dislodging the inflated catheter by pulling on the tubing.

- Move the bag first, then the patient when transferring the patient to a chair or wheelchair. Take care to avoid stepping on the tubing during the transfer.

- Attach the closed drainage bag to the frame of the chair or wheelchair.

- Monitor the level of urine in the drainage bag. Most people excrete about 50 to 80 mL of urine each hour. If the level of urine in the bag does not change, if the catheter is leaking, if no urine is present in the bag, or if the urine has an abnormal color, odor, or appearance, inform the RN.

- Wear a mask and protective eyewear when emptying the catheter bag, according to personal preference and facility policies. This procedure is a potential splash risk.

- Empty the catheter bag at the end of your shift and document the output. Use a graduate pitcher to empty the bag. Use the graduate for one patient only. Place a paper towel on the floor under the graduate (**Figure 8-18**). Remove the spout from the drainage bag. Avoid touching the tip with your fingers. Some facilities wipe the spout with alcohol after removing it. Others do not, believing that this manipulation increases the risk of contamination. Follow your facility policies. Center the spout over the graduate and open the clamp to empty the bag. Close the clamp when the bag is

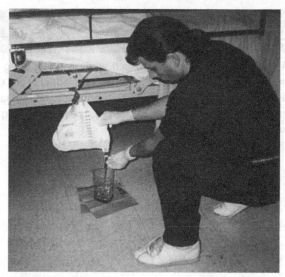

FIGURE 8-18 Center the graduate under the drainage spout. If the spout accidentally contacts your fingers or the edge of the graduate, wipe it with an alcohol sponge before returning it to the drainage bag.

empty and return the spout to the pocket in the drainage bag. Wipe with alcohol if the spout accidentally touches the sides of the graduate, or if this is your facility policy.

● Accurately document intake and output readings for all patients with catheters.

● Notify the RN if redness, irritation, drainage, crusting, or open areas are present at the catheter insertion site.

● Notify the RN if the patient complains of pain, burning, tenderness, or has other signs or symptoms of urinary tract infection.

● Inform the RN if the patient complains of feeling the urge to urinate after the catheter is inserted. This is due to the pressure of the balloon on the internal sphincter of the urethra. The pressure feels the same as the sensation of urine pressing on the sphincter.

● Follow your facility policy for measuring, recording, and documenting intake and output.

Guidelines for Opening a Closed Drainage System

● Always wash your hands and apply gloves before handling the catheter and closed drainage system. Avoid environmental contamination with your gloves. Use sterile technique.

● Position an incontinent pad under the connection between the catheter and drainage tube.

● Open the sterile package containing the catheter plug and cap (Figure 8-19A). Leave it open on the table, but avoid touching it. Disconnect the catheter and tubing. Hold both ends in your hand. Do not set them down. Insert the catheter plug into the end of the catheter (Figure 8-19B). Avoid touching the tip of the plug. Place the sterile cap

over the end of the drainage tube. After covering, both items may be put down.

● If accidental contamination occurs, wipe the ends well with an antiseptic wipe before placing the cap or inserting the plug.

● Empty the drainage bag, if necessary. Secure the tubing to the bed so it does not touch the floor.

● Reverse these steps to reconnect the catheter. If you find an unconnected, disconnected catheter, do not reconnect it. Inform the nurse at once.

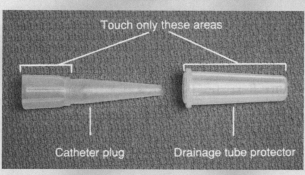

Touch only these areas

Catheter plug   Drainage tube protector

(A)

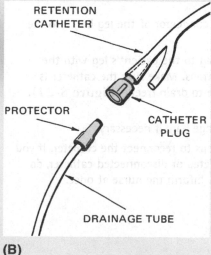

RETENTION CATHETER

PROTECTOR

CATHETER PLUG

DRAINAGE TUBE

(B)

FIGURE 8-19 (A) Sterile catheter plug and protective cap (B) Plug and protective cap in place.

Guidelines for Applying a Urinary Leg Bag

- Always wash your hands and apply gloves before handling the catheter and closed drainage system. Avoid environmental contamination with your gloves. Use sterile technique.

- Position an incontinent pad under the connection between the catheter and drainage tube.

- Open the sterile package containing the leg bag. Leave it open on the table, but avoid touching it.

- Open the sterile package containing the catheter plug and cap. Leave it open on the table, but avoid touching it. Disconnect the catheter and tubing. Hold both ends in your hand. Do not set them down. Insert the catheter plug into the end of the catheter (Figure 8-20). Avoid touching the tip of the plug. Place the sterile cap over the end of the drainage tube. After covering, both items may be put down.

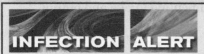

INFECTION ALERT

Avoid putting the patient to bed while wearing a leg bag. The urine may flow back into the bladder from the bag when the patient is in bed. Disconnect the leg bag and connect the catheter to the regular drainage bag when the patient is in bed.

- If accidental contamination occurs, wipe the ends well with an antiseptic wipe before placing the cap or inserting the plug.

- Secure the tubing to the bed so it does not touch the floor.

- Remove the catheter plug. Place it on the open, sterile package.

- Insert the upper connector of the leg bag into the catheter.

- Fasten the leg bag to the patient's leg with the Velcro or vinyl straps. Make sure the catheter is straight and able to drain freely (Figure 8-21). Check for leaks.

- Empty the drainage bag, if necessary.

- Reverse these steps to reconnect the catheter. If you find an unconnected or disconnected catheter, do not reconnect it. Inform the nurse at once.

- Avoid putting the patient to bed while wearing a leg bag. The urine may flow back into the bladder from the bag when the patient is in bed. Disconnect the leg bag and connect the catheter to the regular drainage bag when the patient is in bed.

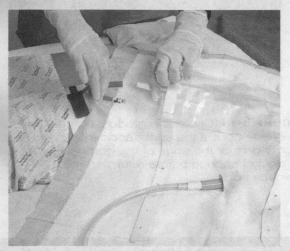

FIGURE 8-20 Carefully connect the catheter to the leg bag. Avoid touching anything against the end of the catheter. The drainage tubing on the bed bag is covered with a sterile cap that is left in place until it is reconnected to the catheter.

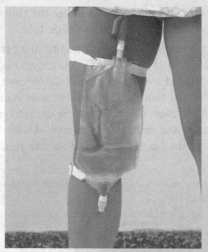

FIGURE 8-21 The leg bag is held in place by adjustable straps. The bag is smaller than a bed collection bag and must be emptied more often.

Guidelines for Drainage Bag Disinfection

Note: Using a new, sterile leg bag each day is the best method of preventing infection. However, some facilities have procedures for disinfecting the bags that markedly reduce the risk of infection. If this is the case, follow your facility policies and procedures. These disinfection guidelines apply only to those bags that are opened so that a leg bag can be attached. They do not apply to all drainage bags in the facility.

CAUTION: *Avoid contact of solution with eyes and skin. Irritation can occur. Metal bathroom fixtures can rust or corrosion can occur. Harmful fumes can arise from contact with other cleaning products. Follow facility policies for handling bleach solution. Be familiar with the information on the MSDS for the bleach.*

- Continuous drainage bags that are disconnected from the catheter and leg bags that are applied in their place must be decontaminated at least every 24 hours. The bags should be labeled with the patient's name and next date of change.
- Obtain a 500-mL plastic squeeze bottle. Label the bottle with the patient's name and next date of change. (The bottle should be changed each time the catheter bag is changed.) Fill the squeeze bottle with 480 mL of warm tap water. Pour 15 mL liquid bleach containing 5.25% sodium hypochlorite solution into a medicine cup.
- Wash your hands and apply gloves before handling the drainage system. Avoid environmental contamination with your gloves. Use sterile technique.
- Empty the bag.
- Using the squeeze bottle, empty one-half of the bottle of tap water into the top end of the leg bag or urinary drainage bag. Filling from the top end flushes bacteria out of the bag and away from the connection.
- Close the bag and shake vigorously for 15 seconds. Agitation is necessary to loosen bacteria.
- Empty the bag into the toilet. (For infection control purposes, avoid using the sink.)
- Repeat a second time with the remaining water and bleach solution in the bottle. Two rinses are necessary to flush bacteria from the bag.
- Fill the squeeze bottle half full with tap water. Pour 15 mL liquid bleach containing 5.25 percent sodium hypochlorite solution into a medicine cup. Add the bleach to the tap water in the bottle.
- Squirt 30 mL of the solution onto the outer surfaces of the drainage bag or leg bag spigot, bell, sleeve, and cap. These connections hold bacteria, so it is important to direct bleach to these sites.
- Squirt the remaining solution into the bag. Shake gently for at least 30 seconds. Make sure that the solution touches all surfaces inside the bag.
- Empty the solution into the toilet. (For infection control purposes, avoid using the sink.) Remove as much solution as possible. Bacteria are less likely to grow in a dry environment. Air-dried bags last longer than those stored with bleach solution trapped inside.
- Cover the open upper end with a cap, or use a clean gauze pad secured with a rubber band. Close the drainage port at the bottom of the bag.
- Hang the bag in the designated location in the soiled utility or patient bathroom.
- Discard the plastic medicine cup. Store the plastic squeeze bottle in a clear plastic bag according to facility policy.

SUPRAPUBIC CATHETERS

A **suprapubic catheter** (Figure 8-22) is inserted surgically through the abdominal wall directly into the bladder. This type of catheter is used for both temporary and permanent bladder catheterization. This type of catheter may also be called a *cystostomy tube*. It is commonly inserted after resection of a large prostate or after bladder repair surgery. It is attached to a regular drainage bag and may be used with a leg bag when the patient is ambulatory.

Complications of Suprapubic Catheter Use

Complications of suprapubic catheter use include:

- Urinary tract infections
- Systemic blood infections (septicemia)
- Urine leakage around the catheter
- Skin breakdown
- Bladder stones
- Blood in the urine (hematuria)

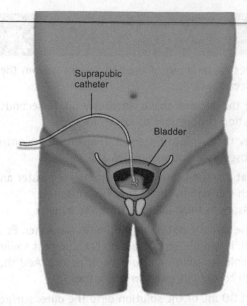

FIGURE 8-22 The suprapubic catheter is surgically inserted through the abdominal wall. The urethra is not functional.

Signs and symptoms of a plugged suprapubic catheter may include:

- Headache
- Profuse sweating
- Distended bladder
- Absent or inadequate urinary output
- Large amount of sediment in urine
- Autonomic dysreflexia

Caring for a Patient with a Suprapubic Catheter

General care of the patient with a suprapubic catheter is very similar to care for an indwelling urethral catheter, and includes:

- Using aseptic technique when caring for the catheter or opening the closed drainage system.
- Performing catheter care as ordered by the physician, or at the frequency specified by your facility policies.
- Careful cleansing of the tube insertion site, and proximal catheter.
- Maintaining a sterile closed drainage system.
- Anchoring the tube with tape or a Velcro strap to avoid tension and promote drainage.
- Scheduled changes of the catheter and drainage system according to physicians' orders and facility policy.

A few variations from regular indwelling catheter care are as follows:

- Hairs should be trimmed (not shaved) surrounding the stoma (insertion site) to reduce the risk of bacterial contamination.
- Monitor the skin around the catheter daily. A small amount of redness and clear drainage is normal. A large area of redness or colored or foul-smelling drainage should be reported to the RN.
- Place a sterile 4 × 4 pad around the stoma. Change daily or as ordered.
- Be gentle and careful when irrigating the catheter.
- You may be permitted to change the suprapubic catheter in an established tract. If this is the case, be aware that you may meet resistance due to spasticity. Avoid forcing the catheter. Wait until the spasticity subsides.

Note: In some states, PCTs may not be permitted to care for the suprapubic catheter. Your instructor will inform you if this is a PCT skill in your state. If not, you should not be offended. The laws in some states require licensed nurses to perform these treatments. Care for the suprapubic catheter only as permitted by state law and facility policies.

NEPHROSTOMY TUBES

Urine is produced in the kidneys, and drains downward into the bladder through tubes called the *ureters*. It is stored in the bladder until urination occurs. In some medical conditions, such as stones, infection, congenital malformation (abnormalities present at birth), tumors, swelling after kidney surgery, or trauma, urine cannot reach the bladder or cannot be eliminated from the bladder. A **nephrostomy tube** is surgically inserted through the skin and into the kidney (**Figure 8-23**). The tube drains urine directly from the kidney to the outside of the body. The nephrostomy tube is connected to a drainage bag. It drains urine continuously. Occasionally, the tube may become clogged, causing urine to stop draining. If this occurs, inform the RN promptly. He or she will flush the tube with a sterile solution.

Caring for a Patient with a Nephrostomy Tube

The nephrostomy tube is small and easily bent. Monitor it carefully to ensure that it does not kink or bend, which will cause a backflow of urine into

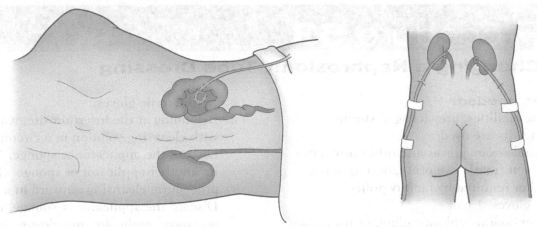

FIGURE 8-23 A nephrostomy tube is surgically inserted through the skin and into the kidney. The tube drains urine directly from the kidney to the outside of the body.

the kidney. The pressure from the urine could damage the kidney. In some situations, a plastic platform is placed at the insertion site to stabilize the tube. If this is the case, the RN will teach you how to care for this arrangement.

The physician will order the type of bathing permitted. A bedbath or partial bath may be ordered postoperatively. The patient may progress to a shower if a dressing covers the insertion site. The RN may instruct you to change the dressing immediately after the shower. A tub bath is usually prohibited.

Always keep the drainage system below the level of the bladder. Empty the drainage bag when it is half full. Avoid touching the spout to the graduate into which it is being drained. Avoid touching the spout with your hands. If a patient wears a leg bag, it will have to be emptied more frequently than the normal drainage bag. Change the drainage bag if it leaks, or appears dirty or foul-smelling. Inform the RN if changing the bag is necessary.

Observations to report to the RN are listed in the Observe & Report box.

Postoperative Care. During the immediate postoperative period:

- Monitor the patient for bleeding, swelling, bruising in the affected flank, decreased or no urine output, or abnormal vital signs.
- Maintain correct position of the tube. Make sure it is not kinked.
- Keep separate output records for right and left kidney. Anticipate bloody drainage to change to light pink within 48 hours.
- Measure output every hour for 4 hours; every 4 hours for 24 hours; then every 8 hours.
- Keep drainage below the level of the kidney.

Observe & Report

- The urine changes color, has a foul odor, or appears bloody.
- Urine leaks around the catheter and the dressing becomes wet.
- Your patient complains of pain in the back, sides, or abdomen.
- The patient has a fever.
- The patient complains of nausea or vomiting.
- Urine drainage stops or slows.
- The skin at the insertion site appears red, raw, or irritated, or develops a rash.
- The skin at the insertion site hurts.
- There is more than a tiny amount of yellow or green drainage at the tube site.

- Do not disconnect the tubing.
- Never attempt to reposition a dislodged tube. Notify the RN promptly.

Changing the Nephrostomy Tube Dressing. *Use strict aseptic technique* when caring for the nephrostomy tube, to prevent pathogens from entering the system. The direct route to the kidney makes the patient very vulnerable to infection. The dressing should be changed immediately if it becomes wet. It is routinely changed one to three times a week, or the frequency specified by the physician's orders.

Procedure 53

Changing a Nephrostomy Tube Dressing

Supplies needed:

▶ In some facilities, prepackaged sterile dressing kits are used

▶ Disposable exam gloves and other protective equipment (mask, eye protection, gown) as needed or required by facility policy

▶ Sterile gloves, 1 pair

▶ Povidone-iodine, chlorhexidine, or prescribed cleansing solution

▶ Sterile sponge or applicators for cleaning skin

▶ Sterile emesis basin or cup

▶ Precut 4 × 4 drain dressings and/or transparent film dressing

▶ Sterile drape

▶ Sterile forceps

▶ Incontinent pad

▶ Adhesive tape, if needed for dressing

1. Perform your beginning procedure actions.
2. Clean the overbed table. Disinfect the table, if soiled, or if required by facility policy.
3. Open the prepackaged tray or establish a sterile field.
4. Place the plastic bag for used supplies at the foot of the bed, or in a convenient location. Position the bag so that you do not have to cross over sterile supplies to discard soiled items.
5. Open the sterile packages on the sterile field, and arrange supplies as needed. Open several packages of gauze pads and place the pads in a sterile basin or cup. Pour cleansing solution over them or open the prepackaged cleansing sponge or applicators. If using a prepackaged tray, pour cleansing solution into a sterile cup or tray.
6. Position the incontinent pad under the patient's flank area and your workspace to keep the patient dry.
7. Apply exam gloves.
8. Carefully loosen tape and remove the dressing. Discard it in the plastic bag. Avoid crossing over the sterile field.
9. Remove your gloves and discard them in the bag.
10. Wash your hands or use an alcohol-based hand cleaner.

11. Apply sterile gloves.
12. Beginning at the insertion site, wipe the skin with cleansing solution in a circular motion. Discard the applicator or sponge. Next, pick up another applicator or sponge. Repeat the procedure, cleansing outward in a circle. Discard the applicator or sponge. Pick up one more applicator and cleanse in a circle beyond the second circle. When done, you should have cleansed a large area, approximately 3 to 4 inches in diameter. Discard the soiled supplies very carefully, to avoid contaminating your gloves.
13. Allow time for the cleansing solution to dry thoroughly. (Depending on the solution used, you may need to rinse it off with sterile normal saline, and pat the site dry.)
14. Pick up a slit 4 × 4 gauze pad and arrange it around the tube. If necessary, overlap two dressings.
15. Cover the 4 × 4s with transparent film, or tape them in place, according to facility policy (**Figure 8-24**).
16. Perform your procedure completion actions.

NOTE: *In some states, PCTs may not be permitted to care for the nephrostomy tube. Your instructor will inform you if this is a PCT skill in your state. If not, you should not be offended. The laws in some states require licensed nurses to perform these treatments. Care for the nephrostomy tube only as permitted by state law and facility policies.*

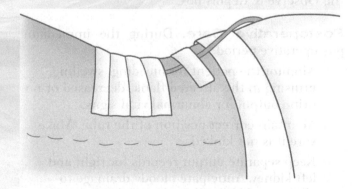

FIGURE 8-24 Cover the insertion site with 4 × 4 gauze pads and transparent film, or tape the pads securely in place.

BLADDER IRRIGATION

In some situations, the urinary catheter is irrigated to cleanse the bladder. This is common after surgery and other conditions in which blood clots are present. Bladder irrigation was once a common procedure. All patients with catheters received routine irrigations. It is now used only for conditions in which obstructions, such as blood clots, are present. Studies have shown that irrigation for other purposes increases the risk of infection.

Irrigation involves instilling fluid into the bladder. All of the fluid instilled should return. If less fluid returns than you instilled, notify the RN. Also notify the RN of abnormalities in the urine or returning irrigation solution, such as abnormal color, odor, or presence of clots, particles, or tissue.

Several methods of bladder irrigation are used. The open method of irrigation involves opening the closed drainage system, instilling solution, allowing it to drain out, and then reconnecting the closed system. In the closed method, a small amount of irrigant is injected through the injection port into the catheter. The closed system is not opened. The irrigation solution cannot be withdrawn with the needle and syringe. It drains into the urinary drainage bag. Continuous irrigation requires a three-way catheter (**Figure 8-25**). A large bag of irrigation solution, similar to an IV bag, hangs on an IV standard. This is connected to one port of the catheter, through which it enters. It drains from another

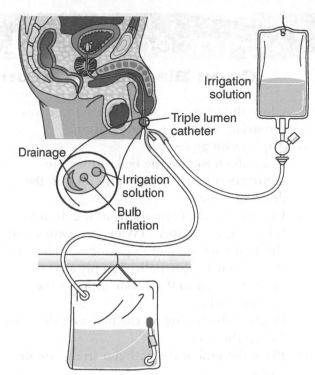

FIGURE 8-25 The continuous irrigation system

port. The closed system must be opened to change the bag of irrigation solution.

When instilling fluid into the bladder by one of the manual methods, always do so gently. Avoid forcing the solution. If you cannot instill the fluid with gentle pressure, notify the RN.

Procedure 54

Open Bladder Irrigation

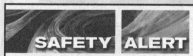

SAFETY | ALERT

Do not irrigate the catheter of a patient who has recently had prostate surgery. Check with the RN.

Supplies needed:
- Disposable exam gloves
- Sterile gloves
- Sterile irrigation set
- Sterile irrigation solution, as ordered by the physician
- Sterile basin (may be part of the irrigation set)
- Sterile protective cap for drainage tube
- Alcohol or povidone-iodine wipes
- Incontinent pad
- Plastic bag for used supplies

1. Perform your beginning procedure actions.
2. Place the incontinent pad under the connection between the catheter and the drainage tube.
3. Open the sterile irrigation set. Remove the lid of the container. Set it on the table with the inside facing up.
4. Open the irrigation solution and pour it into the irrigation set. The irrigation syringe is sterile. Avoid contaminating it during this part of the procedure.

(continues)

Procedure **54**, *continued*

Open Bladder Irrigation

5. Close the irrigation set. If the syringe was removed, return it to the solution.
6. Apply exam gloves.
7. Place the basin on the bed, under the connection between the catheter and the drainage tube.
8. Disconnect the catheter from the drainage tube (Figure 8-26A). (Wipe the connection site first with alcohol or povidone-iodine, if this is your facility policy.) Apply a sterile protective cap to the connection on the drainage tube.
9. Position the tubing on the bed so it does not fall on the floor.
10. Place the end of the catheter in the sterile basin.
11. Remove gloves and discard according to facility policy.
12. Wash your hands, or use alcohol-based hand cleaner.
13. Open package and apply sterile gloves.
14. Withdraw the specified amount of irrigation solution into the syringe.
15. Instill the correct amount of solution into the catheter (Figure 8-26B).

16. Pinch the catheter closed, then remove the syringe. Take care not to contaminate the tip. Insert the syringe into the irrigation solution container.
17. Hold the end of the catheter over the sterile basin and allow the fluid to drain into the basin. Center the catheter so it does not touch the sterile basin. Note the color, character, consistency, and amount of drainage.
18. Withdraw additional fluid, and repeat the procedure until the irrigation fluid returns clear and no blood clots are present.
19. Remove the cover from the connection on the drainage tube. Wipe the connection with alcohol or povidone-iodine, if this is your facility policy.
20. Securely connect the catheter to the drainage tubing.
21. Empty the basin.
22. Remove your gloves and discard them according to facility policy.
23. Secure the catheter to the patient's thigh with tape or a Velcro band, or tape the male patient's catheter to the abdomen.
24. Perform your procedure completion actions.

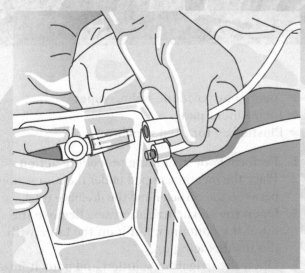

FIGURE 8-26(A) Disconnect the catheter and apply a sterile cap to the drainage tubing.

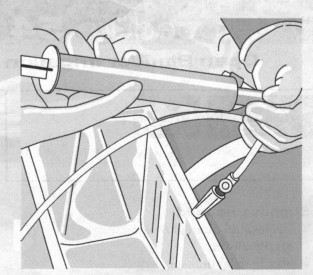

FIGURE 8-26(B) Insert the syringe into the catheter and slowly inject the solution. Avoid force.

Procedure 55

Closed Bladder Irrigation

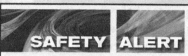

SAFETY ALERT

Do not irrigate the catheter of a patient who has recently had prostate surgery. Check with the RN.

Supplies needed:
- Disposable exam gloves
- Sterile irrigation set
- Sterile irrigation solution, as ordered by the physician
- Sterile 30-mL syringe
- Sterile 21-gauge needle
- Catheter clamp
- Alcohol or povidone-iodine wipes
- Incontinent pad
- Plastic bag for used supplies

1. Perform your beginning procedure actions.
2. Place the incontinent pad under the connection between the catheter and the drainage tube.
3. Open the sterile irrigation set. Remove the lid of the container. Set it on the table with the inside facing up.
4. Open the irrigation solution and pour it into the irrigation set. Avoid contaminating the irrigation syringe during this part of the procedure.
5. Draw up the amount of irrigation solution ordered, using the 30-mL syringe.
6. Open the needle and place it on the syringe.
7. Apply gloves.
8. Clamp the catheter, distal to the injection port.
9. Cleanse the injection port with alcohol or povidone-iodine. Allow to dry.
10. Insert the needle into the injection port. Slowly inject the solution into the port.
11. Withdraw the syringe from the port.
12. Remove the clamp.
13. Repeat the irrigation as ordered, or until the solution is clear with no blood clots. Clamp the catheter again each time you inject solution.
14. Remove gloves and discard according to facility policy.
15. Perform your procedure completion actions.

Procedure 56

Continuous Bladder Irrigation

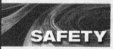

SAFETY ALERT

Do not irrigate the catheter of a patient who has recently had prostate surgery. Check with the RN.

Supplies needed:
- Disposable exam gloves
- Sterile irrigation solution, as ordered by the physician
- Sterile administration set for irrigation solution
- IV standard
- Alcohol or povidone-iodine wipes
- Incontinent pad
- Plastic bag for used supplies

1. Perform your beginning procedure actions.
2. Open the administration set package. Remove the cover from the spike. Avoid touching the spike, which is sterile. Insert the spike into the container of irrigation solution.
3. Hang the irrigation solution on the IV pole, 20 to 30 inches above the patient.
4. Fill the drip chamber halfway. Prime the tubing as you would for an IV.
5. Apply gloves.

(continues)

Procedure 56, *continued*

Continuous Bladder Irrigation

6. Using aseptic technique, remove the cover from the tubing. Attach it to the irrigation port in the three-way catheter.
7. Discard used supplies.
8. Remove your gloves and discard them according to facility policy.
9. Wash your hands, or use alcohol-based hand cleaner.

10. Adjust the drip rate of the irrigation solution, using the roller clamp.
11. Repeat the irrigation procedure, changing bags as ordered. Use aseptic technique to avoid contamination.
12. Perform your procedure completion actions.

REMOVING AN INDWELLING CATHETER

The indwelling catheter is removed as soon as possible to reduce the risk of infection. You may also have to remove the catheter if it is obstructed, or for a rou-tine change ordered by the physician. If you will not be reinserting the catheter, you must monitor the patient's voiding after catheter removal. Follow your facility policy for reporting to the RN. If the patient has not voided within 6 to 8 hours, or if he or she complains of abdominal pain, notify the RN.

Procedure 57

Removing an Indwelling Catheter

Supplies needed:
- Disposable exam gloves, 2 pair
- 10-mL syringe
- Incontinent pad
- Plastic bag for used supplies
- Washcloth
- Towel
- Washbasin
- Soap

1. Perform your beginning procedure actions.
2. Position the incontinent pad under the patient's buttocks.
3. Remove the tape or Velcro strap securing the catheter to the leg.
4. Manipulate the tubing so that any urine in the tubing flows into the drainage bag.
5. Open the syringe. Attach the syringe to the inflation port.
6. Withdraw the fluid from the balloon. The amount of fluid in the balloon may be marked on the catheter. Make sure you

withdraw this amount. Depending on the catheter used, the port may flatten when the fluid is withdrawn. Empty the fluid from the syringe, then reinsert the syringe and attempt to withdraw fluid again. When you are satisfied that the balloon is empty, proceed to the next step.
7. Gently pull the catheter. If you meet resistance, stop. The balloon may not be completely deflated. Repeat steps 5 and 6.
8. If no resistance is met, withdraw the catheter. Observe the tip for the presence of sediment, blood, or mucus. If present, inform the RN. He or she may request a culture.
9. Disconnect the catheter from the drainage tubing. Discard the catheter in the plastic bag, or according to facility policy.
   Some facilities culture the tip of the catheter after it is removed. If this will be done, you will need a sterile specimen cup and sterile scissors. After removing the catheter, hold the end over the open

(continues)

Procedure **57**, *continued*

Removing an Indwelling Catheter

specimen cup and clip it 3 inches from the tip. Cover the cup and discard the remainder of the catheter.

10. Remove your gloves and discard them in the plastic bag.

11. Wash your hands, or use alcohol-based hand cleaner.

12. Apply clean gloves.

13. Perform perineal care according to facility policy.

14. Empty the catheter bag, and measure and record output. Discard the empty bag in the plastic bag, or according to facility policy.

15. Perform your procedure completion actions.

After the catheter is removed, instruct the patient to drink fluids. Offer to take the patient to the bathroom, or offer the bedpan or urinal, in 2 to 4 hours. Inform the RN if the patient cannot void, or has complaints of urgency, pain, or burning.

CARE OF THE PATIENT WHO IS RECEIVING DIALYSIS

Some patients receive **dialysis** treatments. Dialysis is done to cleanse the blood of toxins and impurities when the kidneys have failed. It is usually a temporary measure while the patient awaits a kidney transplant. Patients receiving dialysis are served a special diet and have fluid restrictions. They are usually on strict intake and output. Most are weighed daily to monitor for fluid gains.

Hemodialysis

Patients receiving **hemodialysis** go out to a dialysis center several times a week for their dialysis treatment. This involves the use of a machine to clean wastes from the blood after the kidneys have failed. The blood travels through tubes to a dialyzer, a machine that removes wastes and extra fluid. The cleaned blood then goes back into the body. Patients are gone most of the day. Many facilities prepare a sack lunch to send with patients to the dialysis center.

Patients receiving hemodialysis have a **shunt,** or a connector to allow blood flow between two locations. Alternately, they may have a **graft** (Figure 8-27A) or **fistula** (Figure 8-27B) through which they receive treatment. A *graft* is a piece of plastic tubing that is surgically inserted and connects an artery to a vein. A *fistula* is the most desirable form of dialysis access. It involves connecting an artery to a vein in the arm. Over time, the vein enlarges,

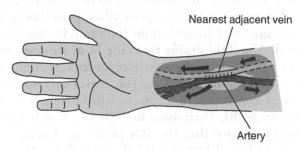

Nearest adjacent vein

Artery

(A) Edges of incision in artery and vein are sutured together to form a common opening.

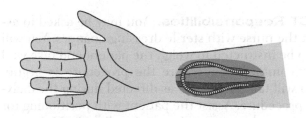

(B) Ends of natural or synthetic graft sutured into an artery and a vein.

FIGURE 8-27 (A) The arteriovenous graft (B) The arteriovenous fistula.

so it can readily accept the needles used to withdraw and replace blood during dialysis. It can last for many years. The dialysis solution is infused into one of these sites, which are commonly on the forearm or upper arm. Avoid taking the blood pressure or starting an IV in the arm used for dialysis.

When patients return from hemodialysis treatment, they may be weak. Monitor them closely when they ambulate. Watch for dizziness and syncope. Monitor the vital signs frequently after dialysis, or as directed by the RN. Usually, you will:

● Take the blood pressure immediately upon return, then every 2 to 4 hours for 8 hours.

● Take the TPR immediately upon return, then again in 4 hours.

You may also be asked to weigh the patient upon his or her return.

Peritoneal Dialysis

A type of dialysis procedure performed in the health care facility is called **peritoneal dialysis.** It involves inserting dialysis solution through a cannula into the patient's abdominal cavity. The dialysate is usually warmed in a basin of warm water for 20 to 30 minutes before use. The solution hangs on an IV pole and flows into the abdomen rapidly (within 5 to 10 minutes) to filter impurities. Once the solution infuses, the RN will clamp the tubing so the solution remains in the abdomen to filter impurities. It will remain there for a prescribed period of time (5 minutes to 4 hours), then the drain clamp is released. The fluid drains from the body through another tube. When the solution returns, it contains toxins and impurities. After the prescribed number of fluid exchanges, the system will be clamped off (**Figure 8-28**). Peritoneal dialysis is a highly technical procedure that the RN performs. Caring for the dialysis catheter is a sterile procedure. All personnel in the room must wear masks when the system is open or entered.

PCT Responsibilities. You may be asked to assist the nurse with sterile dressing changes. You will also be instructed to weigh the patient and take vital signs immediately before the procedure is begun. You will take vital signs as directed during the dialysis procedure. Assist the patient with positioning for maximum lung expansion during dialysis. Make sure the dialysis tubing is not kinked or obstructed. You may be instructed to assist the patient with deep breathing exercises to promote lung expansion. Inform the RN promptly if the patient experiences shortness of breath or signs of respiratory distress.

You may be instructed to empty the solution that flows from the body or to collect a sterile sample of the returning fluid for laboratory analysis. If these are your responsibilities, your instructor will teach you the facility procedures.

Continuous Ambulatory Peritoneal Dialysis

The type of dialysis used at the bedside in the subacute, long-term care, or skilled unit is usually **continuous ambulatory peritoneal dialysis (CAPD).** This is usually done for patients with endstage renal disease. The objective is to teach the pa-

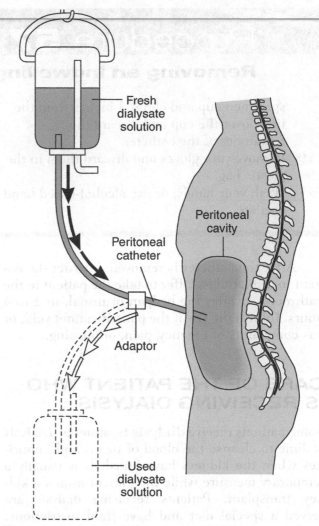

FIGURE 8-28 Waste products and excess fluid are removed as the dialysate flows out of the peritoneal cavity.

tient and family to perform the procedure so that they can do it at home. It usually takes several weeks to master this skill. Using CAPD gives the patient more independence and relieves him or her of the burden of spending several days a week at the hemodialysis facility.

Assisting with CAPD is also a highly sterile procedure. All personnel in the room must wear masks when the system is open or entered.

PCT Responsibilities. You may be asked to:

- Take vital signs and weight immediately before the procedure.
- Take vital signs periodically during the procedure.
- Warm the dialysate solution before the procedure.

● Make sure the tubing does not become kinked during the procedure.

● Assist the patient in opening and emptying the bag of fluid after the prescribed time has elapsed.

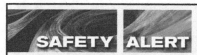

SAFETY ALERT

Assist the patient with positioning for maximum lung expansion during dialysis. Make sure the dialysis tubing is not kinked or obstructed. You may be instructed to assist the patient with deep breathing exercises to promote lung expansion. Inform the RN promptly if the patient experiences signs of respiratory distress.

Observations to Make for Peritoneal Dialysis and CAPD

Monitor the patient closely during and after dialysis. Observations to report to the RN are listed in the Observe & Report box.

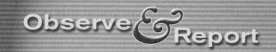

Observe & Report

● Returned dialysate that appears cloudy, bloody, or has blood clots in the solution
● Patient complains of abdominal pain or tenderness
● Wet or soiled dressing
● Fluid leaks around the insertion site
● Fever
● Shortness of breath or respiratory distress, difficulty breathing
● Involuntary twitching or spasticity
● Disconnected tubing or catheter
● Solution that is not running, or is running very slowly
● Drainage container is almost full
● Low blood pressure or dizziness
● Weakness or unsteadiness

Note: In some states, PCTs may not be permitted to assist with dialysis procedures. Your instructor will inform you if this is a PCT skill in your state. If not, you should not be offended. The laws in some states require licensed nurses to perform these treatments. Participate in patient care only to the extent permitted by state law and facility policies.

BOWEL ELIMINATION

Bowel elimination may be affected by illness, injury, immobility, and certain medications. Monitoring the patient's bowel movements (BMs) is an important responsibility. Follow your facility policies for recording BMs. If the patient does not have a bowel movement in three days, notify the RN.

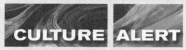

CULTURE ALERT

Patients from some cultures may be resistant to using a bedpan or urinal, or may refuse to use it entirely. A bedside commode may be much more acceptable, particularly when a treatment such as an enema or suppository is necessary. These cultures are Central American, Chinese American, Cuban, Filipino, Gypsy, Haitian, Iranian, Mexican American, Puerto Rican, and Samoan. Some individuals from these cultures may try to avoid having bowel movements while hospitalized, and will return home feeling very constipated. Monitor elimination carefully and report to the RN if the patient has not had a bowel movement in three days.

Members of these cultures are very modest. They will usually avoid discussing issues related to sex or sexuality. Male and females may prefer to wear underwear at all times. Males may refuse hospital gowns entirely, preferring to wear pajamas on the lower body. Most bathe and shampoo daily, but some will avoid bathing during illness.

Constipation can result in discomfort, including abdominal pain, a feeling of abdominal fullness, passing flatus (gas), constipation, and fecal impaction. Fecal impaction (**Figure 8-29**) is the most serious form of constipation. Unrelieved, it can be life-threatening, particularly in the elderly. In this condition, the feces become hard and the patient is unable to pass them. He or she may have loose stools, giving the impression of diarrhea. This is because the hard mass in the rectum prevents fecal matter above it from passing. Liquid stool seeps around the impaction. Pressure from the stool may cause more frequent urination. If the patient has a catheter, leakage may occur as a result of the increased pressure on the bladder.

The RN monitors patients' bowel elimination by reviewing the BM list, elimination record, or ADL log each day. If a patient does not have a bowel movement in three days, the nurse will administer a treatment to stimulate elimination, usually a laxative. Because of this, your documentation of patient bowel activity is a very important responsibility. You would not want the patient to receive a laxative or enema unnecessarily. This will result in loose stools,

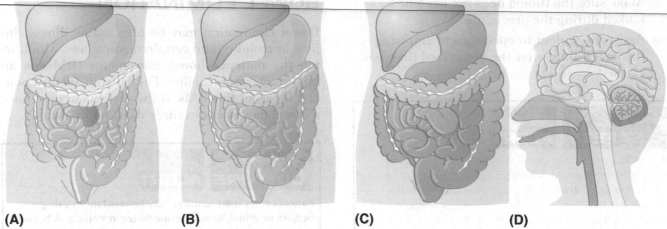

(A)   **(B)**   **(C)**   **(D)**

FIGURE 8-29 Progression of a fecal impaction, a life-threatening condition: (A) A fecal impaction blocks the rectum. The rectum and sigmoid colon become enlarged. (B) The colon continues to enlarge. (C) Fecal material fills the colon. Digested and undigested food back up into the small intestines and stomach. The patient has signs and symptoms of acute illness, including lethargy, distention, constipation, and pain that is dull and cramping. (D) The entire system is full, and the patient vomits fecal material. The feces are commonly aspirated into the lungs.

cramping, and patient discomfort. However, unrelieved constipation is also a serious, uncomfortable condition. The nurse depends on the accuracy of your documentation on the elimination record. He or she will use this record to contact the physician, and administer medications and other treatments related to bowel elimination.

Rectal Tube and Flatus Bag

The rectal tube is used to reduce and eliminate flatus (intestinal gas). Flatus can be very uncomfortable for the patient. It distends the intestines, stressing incisions in the abdomen. Placing a rectal tube in the rectum provides a passageway for the gas to escape. Accept the expulsion of gas as a normal body function. Do not contribute to the patient's embarrassment.

Your instructor will inform you if this is a PCT responsibility in your state. The disposable rectal tube is used once every 24 hours for no more than 20 minutes, if needed. Apply the principles of standard precautions for this procedure. Monitor the abdomen for the amount of distention (stretching). Relief may occur immediately when the tube is inserted. Upon completion of the procedure, question the patient about the degree of relief obtained.

Procedure 58

Inserting a Rectal Tube and Flatus Bag

Supplies needed:

▶ Disposable exam gloves, 2 pairs
▶ Disposable rectal tube and flatus bag
▶ Incontinent pad
▶ Water-soluble lubricant
▶ Tissue
▶ Hypoallergenic tape
▶ Paper towel
▶ Plastic bag
▶ Bath blanket, if needed
▶ Supplies for perineal care (peri care), if needed

1. Perform your beginning procedure actions.
2. Lower the head of the bed to the horizontal position and prop or position the patient, if needed. Assist the patient to turn on the left side with the right leg flexed.
3. Wash your hands, or use alcohol-based hand cleaner.
4. Apply gloves.
5. Place the incontinent pad under the patient's hips.
6. Adjust the bed linen to expose only the buttocks, or cover the patient with a bath blanket, exposing only the rectal area.

(continues)

Procedure 58, *continued*

Inserting a Rectal Tube and Flatus Bag

7. Lubricate the tip of the rectal tube.
8. Separate the buttocks. Ask the patient to bear down gently and take slow, deep breaths through the mouth.
9. Insert the lubricated tip of the rectal tube approximately 3 inches (2 to 4 inches).
10. Secure the tube in place with a small piece of tape (Figure 8-30).
11. Remove your gloves and discard them in the plastic bag.
12. Wash your hands, or use alcohol-based hand cleaner.
13. Adjust the bedding and make the patient comfortable. Make sure the call signal is in reach.
14. Return to the unit in 20 minutes.
15. Wash your hands, or use alcohol-based hand cleaner.
16. Apply gloves.
17. Gently remove the rectal tube and place it on a paper towel or in the plastic bag.
18. Clean the area around the anus, as needed.
19. Assist the patient with positioning, if needed.
20. Remove your gloves and discard them in the plastic bag.

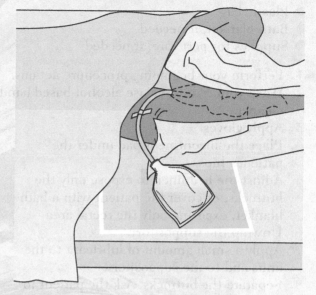

FIGURE 8-30 Secure the rectal tube, with flatus bag in place, using a small piece of hypoallergenic tape.

21. Wash your hands, or use alcohol-based hand cleaner.
22. Discard the bag according to facility policy.
23. Perform your procedure completion actions.

Rectal Suppositories

Rectal **suppositories** may be given to stimulate bowel elimination. Some medications are given in suppository form. Medicinal suppositories must be given by a nurse. In many states, a PCT can administer suppositories that soften the stool and promote elimination. Your instructor will inform you if this is a PCT responsibility in your state. Apply the principles of standard precautions for this procedure. To be effective, the rectal suppository must be positioned above the rectal sphincter and against the bowel wall. Body heat will cause the suppository to melt and stimulate bowel elimination and lubricate the rectum.

Procedure 59

Inserting a Rectal Suppository

Supplies needed:
- Disposable exam gloves, 2 pairs
- Incontinent pad
- Suppository, as ordered
- Water-soluble lubricant
- Toilet tissue
- Bedpan and cover, if needed

(continues)

Procedure **59**, *continued*

Inserting a Rectal Suppository

▶ Plastic bag
▶ Bath blanket, if needed
▶ Supplies for peri care, if needed

1. Perform your beginning procedure actions.
2. Wash your hands, or use alcohol-based hand cleaner.
3. Apply gloves.
4. Place the incontinent pad under the patient's hips.
5. Adjust the bed linen to expose only the buttocks, or cover the patient with a bath blanket, exposing only the rectal area.
6. Unwrap the suppository.
7. Apply a small amount of lubricant to the anus and to the suppository.
8. Separate the buttocks. Ask the patient to bear down gently and take slow, deep breaths through the mouth.
9. Insert the lubricated tip of the suppository approximately 2 to 3 inches (**Figure 8-31**).
10. Instruct the patient to relax, and take slow, deep breaths if uncomfortable, until the urge to defecate occurs. (This should take 5 to 20 minutes.)
11. Remove your gloves and discard them in the plastic bag.
12. Wash your hands, or use alcohol-based hand cleaner.
13. Adjust the bedding and make the patient comfortable. Make sure the call signal is in reach.
14. Return to the unit to check on the patient in 5 minutes.
15. Wash your hands, or use alcohol-based hand cleaner.
16. Apply gloves.
17. Assist the patient with the bedpan, commode, or toilet, as needed. Discard stool

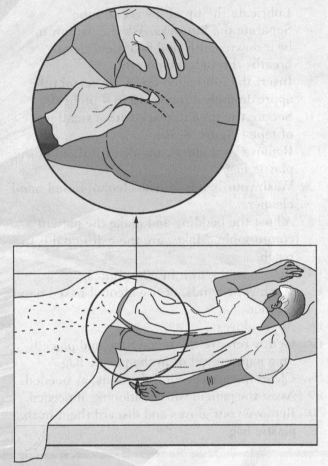

FIGURE 8-31 Lubricate the anus and insert the suppository beyond the sphincter muscle.

and soiled items, and clean the equipment, as needed. Observe the results of elimination and characteristics of the stool. If abnormal, save for the RN.
18. When the patient has finished, assist with hygiene, if needed. Cleanse hands and apply gloves intermittently, as needed.
19. Perform your procedure completion actions.

Enemas

An **enema** is the introduction of fluid into the lower bowel to cleanse the anus, rectum, and lower colon. The physician orders enemas. They are used to relieve constipation and empty the colon before some tests and surgeries. Occasion-ally enemas are given to relieve excessive flatu-lence. The physician always specifies the type of enema to give and the solution to use. The PCT is responsible for administering enemas in many health care facilities. Always apply the principles of standard precautions when you are performing this procedure. Avoid contaminating environmental surfaces with your gloves.

A **cleansing enema** removes fecal material from the rectum and lower bowel. It also stimulates peristalsis and softens the stool. A water-based solution is used in a cleansing enema. The cleansing enema is administered through a special enema bag or other container.

A **retention enema** may be given for constipation or fecal impaction. An oil-based solution, packaged in a small, commercial container, is used for the retention enema. The purpose of this enema is to soften hard stool and gently stimulate evacuation. The enema lubricates the rectum, making it easier to pass the stool.

Commercially prepared enemas (Figure 8-32) are administered in small, premeasured containers. Commercially prepared enemas are available with either cleansing or retention enema solutions.

The **Sims' position** (Figure 8-33) is a side-lying position used for giving enemas, rectal examinations, and other rectal treatments. This position promotes evacuation of the bowel. To assist a patient into the Sims' position, turn him or her onto the left side. Position the shoulder, arm, and hip for comfort. Bend the right leg at the knee and flex the leg forward slightly.

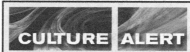

Some females prefer peri care with soap and water after toileting. Some patients will use toilet tissue; others prefer peri care instead of tissue. These cultures include all of those listed as being resistant to using the bedpan or urinal, plus Arab American, Korean, and Vietnamese.

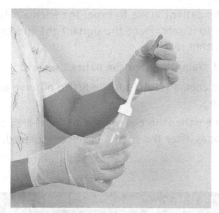

FIGURE 8-32 Remove the cover from the prelubricated tip of the container.

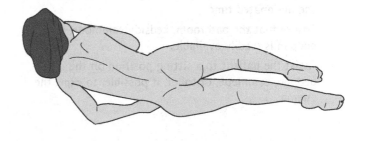

Sims' (left-lateral) Position

FIGURE 8-33 The Sims' (left lateral) position is used for enemas and rectal treatments.

Guidelines for Enema Administration

- Apply the principles of standard precautions. Avoid contaminating environmental surfaces with your gloves.

- Administer an enema only upon the direction of a licensed nurse.

- Consult the care plan or RN for the amount and type of solution to use, and any special instructions.

- Plan and organize your work. Avoid giving an enema within an hour after meals, because the increased peristalsis makes it difficult for the patient to retain the solution. Avoid administering an enema to a patient in a sitting position, such as on the toilet. The solution will not flow high into the colon when administered to a patient who is seated. It will cause the rectum to enlarge, causing rapid expulsion of the fluid.

- Provide privacy. Cover the patient with a bath blanket.

- Check the temperature of a water-based solution with a bath thermometer. The solution temperature should be 105°F.

- Commercially prepared enemas can be administered at room temperature, or warmed by placing the container in a basin of warm water.

- Lubricate the tip of the enema tubing well with a water-based lubricant before inserting it into the rectum. Most disposable units are prelubricated.

(continued)

Guidelines for Enema Administration (Continued)

However, if the tip appears dry, apply additional lubricant before inserting it into the rectum.

● Insert the enema tube gently into the rectum. The tube should be inserted 2 to 4 inches. If you meet resistance, do not force the tube. Remove it and consult the RN.

● An enema in a bag should be raised 12 to 16 inches above the rectum (**Figure 8-34**). Follow your facility policy.

● Administer the enema solution slowly. Instruct the patient to inhale and breathe in slowly through the nose and exhale through the mouth. If the patient complains of pain, stop the solution briefly before proceeding. If the pain is severe or persistent, stop the solution and notify the RN.

● Hold the enema tubing in place with your gloved hand when administering the solution.

● Instruct the patient to retain the enema solution for the designated time.

● Ensure that the bathroom, bedside commode, or bedpan is readily available.

● Assist the patient to a sitting position on the bedpan, commode, or toilet, if possible, to expel the enema.

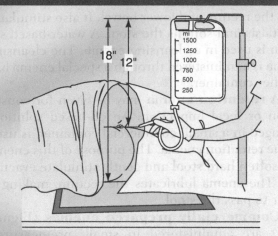

FIGURE 8-34 Elevate the container so the flow of fluid is unobstructed.

● Leave the patient alone to expel the enema solution, if doing so is safe. Place the signal light and toilet tissue within reach.

● Respond promptly when the patient signals.

● Save the enema results for the RN to observe before discarding.

● Assist the patient to cleanse the perineal area and wash hands after the enema has been expelled.

Procedure 60

Administering a Cleansing Enema

Supplies needed:
▶ Disposable exam gloves, 2 pairs
▶ Assembled enema kit
▶ Prescribed solution
▶ Water-soluble lubricant
▶ Bath blanket
▶ Bath thermometer
▶ Incontinent pad
▶ Bedpan
▶ Toilet tissue
▶ Washcloth
▶ Towel
▶ Washbasin
▶ Paper towel
▶ Plastic bag (1 or 2, as needed to discard used supplies)

1. Perform your beginning procedure actions.
2. Close the clamp on the enema container.
3. Prepare the enema solution in the bathroom or utility room, according to facility policy. Fill the enema container with water in the specified amount. This usually varies from 500 to 1,500 mL, but more or less solution can be used. Follow the RN's instructions. Check the water temperature with a bath thermometer (**Figure 8-35A**). It should be about 105°F.
4. If you are instructed to administer a soapsuds enema, empty the contents of the soap packet into the container *after* the water has been added (**Figure 8-35B**). Squeeze and agitate the bag slightly (or stir

(continues)

Procedure **60**, *continued*

Administering a Cleansing Enema

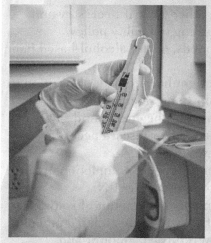

FIGURE 8-35(A) Use a bath thermometer to make sure the solution temperature is about 105°F.

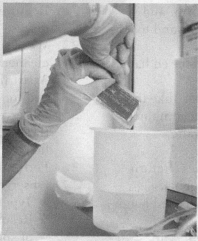

FIGURE 8-35(B) Add soap from the packet.

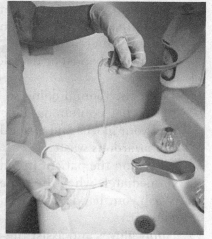

FIGURE 8-35(C) Run a small amount of water through the tubing to expel air.

gently with a tongue blade if a bucket-type container is used) to mix the solution.

5. Open the clamp on the tubing and allow the solution to flow through the tubing to the tip to prevent injection of air into the body (**Figure 8-35C**). Close the clamp when the solution begins to flow through the tip.

6. Take the solution to the bedside. Squeeze some water-soluble lubricant onto a paper towel or gauze sponge.

7. Wash your hands, or use alcohol-based hand cleaner.

8. Apply gloves.

9. Place the bed protector under the patient's buttocks. Cover the upper bedding with a bath blanket, then remove the linen from under the blanket without exposing the patient.

10. Assist the patient into the Sims' position and ensure that he or she is comfortable.

11. Expose the rectal area.

12. Remove the cap from the end of the tubing, and lubricate the tube if it is not prelubricated. If the tip appears dry, apply extra lubricant.

13. Separate the buttocks to expose the anal area.

14. Tell the patient you are going to insert the tube and ask him or her to take a deep breath, then exhale.

15. Gently insert the enema tubing 2 to 4 inches while the patient exhales.

16. Hold the solution 12 to 16 inches above the rectum, or according to facility policy.

17. Unclamp the tubing and allow the solution to flow into the rectum. Instruct the patient to try to relax and retain the solution.

18. Allow the desired amount of solution to flow into the rectum. When the fluid level reaches the bottom of the bag, clamp the tubing to avoid injecting air into the rectum.

19. Remove the tubing and insert the tip into the enema administration container.

20. Instruct the patient to retain the solution for the designated amount of time.

21. Place the enema container in a plastic bag.

22. Remove your gloves and place them in the plastic bag.

23. Assist the patient to the bathroom or commode, or place the bedpan. Instruct the patient not to flush the toilet after expelling the enema.

(continues)

Procedure 60, *continued*

Administering a Cleansing Enema

24. Make sure the patient is safe, warm, and comfortable. Leave the signal light and toilet tissue within reach.
25. Wash your hands, or use alcohol-based hand cleaner.
26. Leave the room if doing so is safe. Take the plastic bag containing the enema container and your gloves and discard it in the biohazardous waste.
27. Check on the patient in 5 minutes. Return immediately when the patient signals.
28. Wash your hands, or use alcohol-based hand cleaner.
29. Apply gloves and assist the patient with cleansing and perineal care, as needed.
30. Remove one glove or use a paper towel to turn on the faucet, and assist the patient with handwashing.
31. Remove the incontinent pad with the gloved hand, and discard according to facility policy. (You may use a second plastic bag to discard the disposable incontinent pad and gloves.)

32. Remove the other glove if necessary and discard according to facility policy.
33. Wash your hands, or use alcohol-based hand cleaner.
34. Assist the patient back to bed, or position in bed for comfort and safety.
35. Observe results of the enema and save for the RN, if needed, or discard according to facility policy.
36. Perform your procedure completion actions.
37. Observe and report to the RN:
    - Type of enema and amount of solution
    - Results of the enema, estimated amount of solution returned, amount and consistency of the stool
    - Unusual observations (if noted, save the returns for the RN to assess)
    - Presence of blood, mucus, undigested food (except corn and raisins), or parasites in the stool
    - The patient's response to the procedure

Procedure 61

Administering a Commercially Prepared Enema

Supplies needed:
- Disposable exam gloves, 2 pairs
- Commercial enema
- Water-soluble lubricant
- Bath blanket
- Incontinent pad
- Bedpan
- Toilet tissue
- Washcloth
- Towel
- Washbasin
- Paper towel
- Plastic bag (1 or 2, as needed to discard used supplies)

1. Perform your beginning procedure actions.
2. Warm the container of enema solution in a basin of warm water, if this is your facility policy. Dry the outside of the container.
3. Take the solution to the bedside.
4. Wash your hands, or use alcohol-based hand cleaner.
5. Apply gloves.
6. Place the incontinent pad under the patient's buttocks. Cover the upper bedding with a bath blanket, then remove the linen from under the blanket without exposing the patient.

(continues)

Procedure 61, *continued*

Administering a Commercially Prepared Enema

7. Assist the patient into the Sims' position and ensure that he or she is comfortable.
8. Expose only the rectal area.
9. Remove the cap from the end of the container, and lubricate the tip, if it is not prelubricated.
10. Separate the buttocks to expose the anal area.
11. Tell the patient you are going to insert the tube and ask him or her to take a deep breath, then exhale.
12. Gently insert the tip of the container while the patient exhales.
13. Gently squeeze and roll the container until the desired quantity of solution is administered (Figure 8-36). A small amount of solution will remain in the container. Avoid releasing pressure on the container, or the solution will return.
14. Instruct the patient to hold the breath, then gently remove the tip of the container.
15. Place the enema container in a plastic bag to avoid contamination.
16. Remove your gloves and place them in the plastic bag.
17. Assist the patient to the bathroom or commode, or place the bedpan. (Leave your gloves on if placing a bedpan.) Instruct the patient not to flush the toilet after expelling the enema.
18. Make sure the patient is safe, warm, and comfortable. Leave the signal light and toilet tissue within reach.
19. Remove your gloves and place them in the plastic bag.
20. Wash your hands, or use alcohol-based hand cleaner.
21. Leave the room if doing so is safe. Take the plastic bag containing the enema container and gloves and discard it in the biohazardous waste.
22. Check on the patient in 5 minutes. Return immediately when the patient signals.
23. Wash your hands, or use alcohol-based hand cleaner.

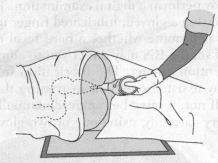

FIGURE 8-36 Squeeze the bottle from the bottom. A small amount of fluid will remain in the container.

24. Apply gloves and assist the patient with cleansing and perineal care, as needed.
25. Remove one glove or use a paper towel to turn on the faucet, and assist the patient with handwashing.
26. Remove the incontinent pad with the gloved hand, and discard according to facility policy. (You may use a second plastic bag to discard the disposable incontinent pad and gloves.)
27. Remove the other glove, if necessary and discard according to facility policy.
28. Wash your hands, or use alcohol-based hand cleaner.
29. Assist the patient back to bed, or position in bed for comfort and safety.
30. Observe the results of the enema and save for the RN, if needed, or discard according to facility policy.
31. Perform your procedure completion actions.
32. Observe and report to the RN:
    ▶ Type of enema
    ▶ Results of the enema, estimated amount of solution returned, amount and consistency of the stool
    ▶ Unusual observations (if noted, save the returns for the RN to assess)
    ▶ Presence of blood, mucus, undigested food (except corn and raisins), or parasites in the stool
    ▶ The patient's response to the procedure

Removing a Fecal Impaction

Elimination procedures are private, and you must handle them with sensitivity to prevent embarrassing the patient. If a fecal impaction is suspected, the RN may perform a digital examination. This involves inserting a gloved, lubricated finger into the rectum to determine whether a hard fecal mass is present. If so, the RN may direct you to administer an oil-retention enema. The lubrication from the enema may assist the patient in passing the fecal material. If not, it must be removed manually. This is done very carefully, using one or two gloved, lubricated fingers. The mass is broken up, removed from the rectum, and discarded appropriately. The procedure is uncomfortable for the patient. It is not without complications, particularly in patients with cardiac disease, or who have had recent pelvic or rectal surgery. In a patient with heart disease, removing a fecal impaction may stimulate the vagus nerve, causing the pulse to slow considerably. Stop the procedure and notify the RN if the patient experiences difficulty or complains of feeling faint, or if the pulse slows. In patients with these conditions, the RN may remove the fecal material. Know and follow your facility policies.

Procedure 62

Breaking Up and Removing a Fecal Impaction

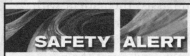

SAFETY ALERT

Do not remove a fecal impaction or perform rectal treatments on patients with known cardiac diagnoses. Check with the RN.

Supplies needed:

▶ Disposable exam gloves
▶ Water-soluble lubricant
▶ Bedpan
▶ Incontinent pad
▶ Toilet tissue
▶ Plastic bag for used supplies
▶ Washcloth
▶ Towel
▶ Washbasin
▶ Soap

1. Perform your beginning procedure actions.
2. Position the incontinent pad under the patient's buttocks.
3. Position the patient in the Sims' position. The patient should be on the left side, with the upper leg bent at the knee and positioned forward, over the lower leg.
4. Apply disposable gloves.
5. Position the bedpan, toilet paper, and plastic bag at the end of the bed, or in another convenient location where you can reach them.
6. Apply lubricant to your index finger.

7. Gently insert your index finger into the rectum. Instruct the patient to take slow, deep breaths. After the anus relaxes, two lubricated fingers can be inserted, if necessary.
8. Move your finger upward, probing for a hard fecal mass. If present, move your finger from side to side in the mass to break it up.
9. Continue to manipulate the stool, breaking it up into small pieces.
10. After the stool is broken into smaller pieces, bend your finger forward slightly and hook a piece of stool, pulling it downward and removing it from the rectum. Discard it in the bedpan.
11. Repeat the hooking action until all stool is removed.
12. Wipe the anus with toilet paper. Discard used paper in the bedpan.
13. Remove your gloves and discard them in the plastic bag.
14. Wash your hands, or use alcohol-based hand cleaner.
15. Fill the washbasin with warm water and carry it to the bedside.
16. Apply clean gloves.
17. Wash the patient's rectum, or provide perineal care, according to facility policy.
18. Discard the contents of the bedpan in the toilet, or according to facility policy.
19. Perform your procedure completion actions.

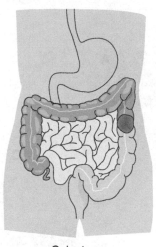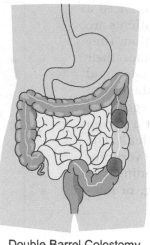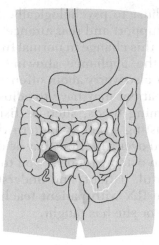

Colostomy   Double Barrel Colostomy   Ileostomy

FIGURE 8-37 Three common types of ostomies.

CARING FOR PATIENTS WITH OSTOMIES

An **ostomy** is a surgically created opening into the body. There are many types of ostomies (Figure 8-37). Some are performed for bowel elimination. These are usually done because of obstruction, cancer, bowel disease, or trauma. The opening to the outside of the body is called a **stoma** (Figure 8-38). An ostomy may be temporary or permanent. The location of the ostomy is determined by the part of the colon that is injured or diseased.

In some facilities, a licensed nurse will care for a newly created ostomy. However, in patients with well-established ostomies, the PCT is usually responsible for caring for the area. Know and follow your facility policy.

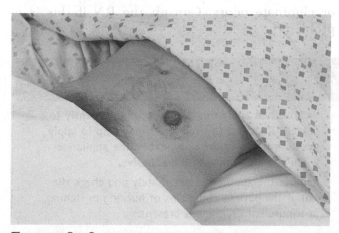

FIGURE 8-38 The colostomy stoma.

DIFFICULT PATIENT ALERT

Having an ostomy alters the way a patient eliminates waste. This alteration of body image can be very traumatic for the patient. Covering the pouch with an attractive cover (check with the enterostomal therapy nurse) may help the patient's self-esteem. The ostomy may have a profound effect on the patient's sex life. Be supportive and empathetic. Occasionally, a patient may become aroused or feel sexual pleasure when the ostomy is touched. Remain calm and professional and do not overreact. Avoid sending the patient mixed sexual messages, even in a joking manner. Inform the patient that sexual advances are not appropriate.

Colostomies

The **colostomy** is the most common type of ostomy. This ostomy is located between the colon and the abdomen. The intestines are brought to the outside of the body to create the stoma. A bag is attached to the stoma to collect fecal material. When the ostomy is first performed, the stool is loose and watery, but it becomes soft and formed over time. The amount of liquid in the stool is also determined by how much of the colon remains after surgery. If a large amount of colon is left, the colon will absorb water and the stools will be formed. If most of the colon has been removed, the body will be unable to absorb the water in the stool, so the stools in the ostomy are more liquid. Flatus is also passed through the stoma.

Many people live successfully for years with an ostomy, but this type of surgery is very difficult for patients to adjust to psychologically. They need a great deal of support and reassurance. Patients are often upset by this change in normal function. They worry about the appliance showing under their clothing. They also worry about offensive odors and sounds. The patient may have to adjust the diet to avoid gas-forming foods, such as fish, eggs, and broccoli. Adjusting a dietary pattern that a person has established over a lifetime may be difficult. The patient with an ostomy requires you to be very professional, tactful, patient, and understanding. You may assist the RN with patient teaching, or reinforce what he or she has taught.

The Ostomy Appliance

The ostomy **appliance** (Figure 8-39) is the plastic container into which the contents of the bowel are emptied. It is fastened to the body with a belt or a self-adhesive seal around the bag. Many different types of pouches are available. Some appliances are disposable; some are reusable. Some are self-adhesive; some require the use of separate adhesive. The two-piece system has an outer ring that snaps onto the pouch. The size of the ring in the pouch is very important. An improper fit can injure the stoma. It must seal the appliance around the stoma, but not fit so tightly that it squeezes the stoma. An improperly applied belt may also injure the stoma. Read the directions and make sure you understand how to use the type of device you are using.

Fecal material is very irritating to the skin. A new ostomy is sore and tender. The fecal material, particularly liquid stool, causes additional irritation. Even established ostomies become irritated from the combination of fecal material and adhesive on the skin. A special skin barrier product may also be used. Barrier products come in many forms, from liquid sprays to creams. Some of these products contain alcohol. Never use a barrier product with alcohol if the patient has raw, red, inflamed, or

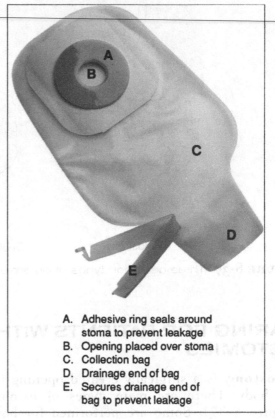

A. Adhesive ring seals around stoma to prevent leakage
B. Opening placed over stoma
C. Collection bag
D. Drainage end of bag
E. Secures drainage end of bag to prevent leakage

FIGURE 8-39 The colostomy appliance has an adhesive ring to prevent leaks.

open skin. The care plan or critical pathway will guide you in caring for the ostomy. Report redness or skin irritation to the RN. Always apply the principles of standard precautions when caring for the ostomy appliance.

Odors from ostomies are a particular problem. Good personal hygiene is essential. The skin around the stoma is washed and dried well each time the bag is removed. The used bag is discarded as biohazardous waste. Various deodorizing products are available to place inside the bag to reduce or eliminate odors. Consult the RN if this is a problem.

Guidelines for Caring for an Ostomy

- Apply the principles of standard precautions. Avoid environmental contamination from your gloves.
- Empty the appliance when it is 1/2 to 2/3 full. If a leak develops in the pouch, change the pouch immediately.
- The bowel is least active 2 to 4 hours after meals, so this is a good time to change the appliance.

- Remove and apply the ostomy appliance gently to prevent irritation to the skin. It may help to apply gentle traction to the skin next to the appliance when you are removing the adhesive.
- Remove the appliance immediately and check the skin if the patient complains of burning or itching, or if purulent drainage is present.

(continued)

Guidelines for Caring for an Ostomy (Continued)

- Empty the reusable bag and wash it thoroughly with soap and water after each bowel movement. Secure the clamp at the bottom of the bag to prevent leaking. Discard a disposable bag in the biohazardous waste container and replace it with a new bag.

- Observe the skin around the stoma for redness, irritation, and skin breakdown, and report to the RN.

- After the appliance has been removed, gently wipe the area surrounding the stoma with toilet tissue. Discard the tissue in the toilet or a plastic bag. If a plastic bag is used, discard it in the biohazardous waste container.

- Wash the skin around the stoma with mild soap when the appliance is removed. Rinse well and gently pat dry.

- Apply skin barriers, lubricants, or medicated creams to the area surrounding the stoma as stated on the care plan. Apply only a thin layer. Avoid caking the products on the skin.

- You may be required to cut an opening into the appliance before applying it to the skin. Cut the area about 1/8 inch larger than the size of the stoma.

- When reapplying a new appliance, seal the entire area surrounding the stoma, to prevent leaking. Holding your hands over the area for about a minute will help. The heat from your hands promotes a good seal.

- Observe the color, character, amount, and frequency of stools, and report abnormalities to the RN.

Procedure 63

Changing an Ostomy Appliance

Supplies needed:
- Disposable exam gloves, 2 pairs
- Bedpan
- Clean, drainable ostomy pouch
- Skin barrier product
- Gauze pads or disposable washcloths
- Washbasin of warm water
- Hand towel
- Toilet tissue
- Plastic bag for used supplies

1. Perform your beginning procedure actions.
2. Position the bedpan next to the patient, on the side with the stoma.
3. Position the end of the appliance in the bedpan. Remove the clip at the bottom and empty the device into the bedpan.
4. Gently lift the appliance to release the adhesive. Apply traction on the skin with one hand while slowly and gently lifting the pouch with the other.
5. Discard the pouch, or put it to the side for cleaning and reuse, according to the type of device.
6. Gently wash the skin surrounding the stoma with warm water. Pat dry with the hand towel.

If stool escapes during this procedure, remove it with toilet tissue. Monitor the skin for changes in the size, color, or presence of redness or skin breakdown. Report these changes to the RN.

7. Apply skin barrier product (Figure 8-40A).
8. Change your gloves, if soiled with stool.
9. Check the opening in the new pouch to ensure that it is large enough to fit the stoma. It should not fit tightly to the edges.

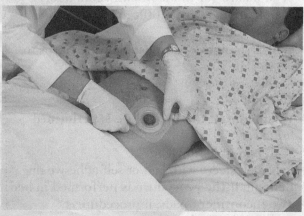

FIGURE 8-40(A) Apply the skin barrier.

(continues)

Procedure 63, *continued*

Changing an Ostomy Appliance

10. Remove the paper backing from the adhesive seal, or apply the skin barrier product, or moisten the ring, depending on the type of appliance used.

11. Center the ring in the pouch over the stoma, with the large part of the pouch down. Gently press it down over the skin (**Figure 8-40B**). Make sure the adhesive is wrinkle-free. Hold gentle pressure on the adhesive ring for a minute.

12. Check the end of the pouch to ensure that it is closed and clamped securely.

13. Perform your procedure completion actions.

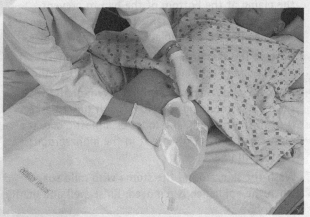

FIGURE 8-40(B) Center the pouch over the stoma, then press it into place.

Irrigating a Colostomy

Colostomy irrigation is done to regulate elimination. It is also done to cleanse the bowel before tests or procedures. For best results, the colostomy should be regulated at the same time each day. It may take 4 to 6 weeks before results are seen. In some facilities, the RN performs colostomy irrigation on newly created colostomies. Know and follow your facility policy. Prime the tubing before beginning the procedure. This eliminates air, which will cause painful cramps.

Procedure 64

Irrigating a Colostomy

Supplies needed:
▶ Disposable exam gloves, 2 pairs
▶ IV standard (or hook on bathroom door)
▶ Irrigation bag with 1,000 mL warm water (about 100°F)
▶ Gauze sponges or disposable washcloths to clean skin
▶ Mild soap
▶ Hand towel
▶ Washbasin, if the procedure is performed in bed
▶ Water-soluble lubricant
▶ Irrigation sleeve with belt or self-adhesive ring
▶ Bedpan, if the procedure is performed in bed
▶ Two incontinent pads, if procedure is performed in bed
▶ Plastic bag for used supplies

1. Perform your beginning procedure actions.

2. Assist the patient to the bathroom if the procedure will be done there. If it will be done in bed, position the incontinent pad to prevent soiling. Position a second underpad on a chair next to the bed, and place the bedpan on it (**Figure 8-41**).

3. Hang the irrigation bag approximately 20 inches above the patient. *The bottom of the bag should be at about the patient's shoulder level to prevent water from entering the bowel too quickly.*

4. Prime the irrigation tubing, if this was not done when you filled the bag.

5. Apply gloves.

(continues)

Procedure **64**, *continued*

Irrigating a Colostomy

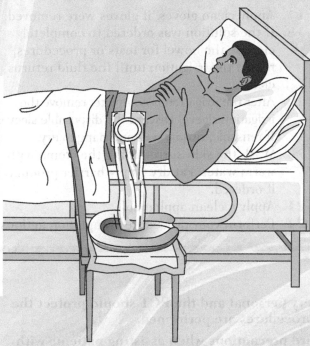

FIGURE 8-41 Place the bedpan on a chair next to the bed.

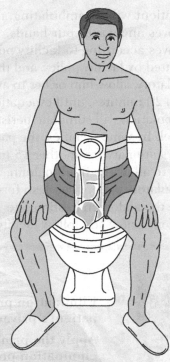

FIGURE 8-42 Cut the irrigation sleeve so it hangs just above water level.

6. Remove the colostomy bag and discard according to facility policy.

7. Apply the irrigation sleeve, securing it with the adhesive backing or an appliance belt.

8. Place the open end of the irrigation sleeve in the toilet or a bedpan on a chair next to the bed. If the procedure is done on the toilet, cut the bottom of the sleeve, if necessary, so that it hangs just above water level (**Figure 8-42**). If it hangs into the water, it may not drain. Avoid cutting it too short, as this increases the risk of splashing.

9. Lubricate the small finger of your gloved hand.

10. Gently insert your lubricated finger into the stoma. The stoma will tighten when you insert your finger, but will relax shortly. Determine the bowel angle with your finger. You will insert the irrigation cone at this angle.

11. Lubricate the cone on the irrigation set well.

12. Insert the cone gently, in the direction of the bowel. Although you must be gentle

when you insert the cone, it must fit securely.

13. Unclamp the tubing and allow the fluid to run in slowly. Adjust the rate of flow with the roller clamp, or pinch the tubing with your fingers to prevent the fluid from entering too fast. The bag of fluid should flow in over 10 to 15 minutes. If the patient complains of abdominal cramping, stop the flow of solution, leaving the cone in place. Cramping may occur if there is air in the tubing, if the flow is too rapid, if the water is too cold, or because the bowel is ready to empty. Troubleshoot the system, then begin the solution again. Advise the patient to take slow, deep breaths when the fluid is infusing.

14. When the bag is empty, remove the cone. Try to remove the cone when there is water in the tubing, to avoid injecting air. Close the tip of the sleeve if the patient will be ambulating.

(continues)

Procedure **64**, *continued*

Irrigating a Colostomy

15. If the patient will be ambulating, remove your gloves and wash your hands. Discard your gloves according to facility policy.

16. If permitted by facility policy, and the patient is ambulatory, allow him or her to ambulate for 15 to 20 minutes, until evacuation occurs. The ambulation will stimulate peristalsis in the bowel. In some facilities, the patient remains stationary for another 15 to 20 minutes to allow the fluid to drain. The nonambulatory patient can lean forward and massage the abdomen to stimulate evacuation. Know and follow facility policy.

17. Apply clean gloves, if gloves were removed.

18. If the solution was ordered to completely cleanse the bowel for tests or procedures, repeat the irrigation until the fluid returns clear.

19. After the irrigation is complete, remove the irrigation sleeve. Discard the disposable sleeve. If reusable, rinse it well and hang to dry.

20. Wash the skin surrounding the stoma with warm water. Pat dry. Apply barrier product, if ordered.

21. Apply a clean appliance.

22. Perform your procedure completion actions.

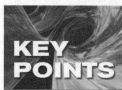

KEY POINTS

▶ Elimination procedures are very personal and the PCT should protect the patient's privacy when these procedures are performed.

▶ Apply the principles of standard precautions when assisting patients with elimination procedures.

▶ Reagents are chemicals that react in a certain way when they contact the patient's body fluids. They are used for performing certain tests on the nursing units.

▶ Measuring the pH provides information about the acidity or alkalinity of a substance.

▶ Some reagent strips perform multiple tests. These strips must be held horizontally when processing so the chemicals do not run together.

▶ Glucose testing should be done using a fresh urine specimen, whenever possible.

▶ Specific gravity provides information about how well the kidneys concentrate urine.

▶ High levels of glucose and protein in the urine elevate the specific gravity.

▶ Urine should be at room temperature when tested.

▶ The instrument used to measure specific gravity is a urinometer.

▶ A catheter drains urine from the bladder. An indwelling catheter remains in the bladder to drain urine continuously. A straight catheter is inserted to empty the bladder, and is then removed.

▶ The presence of a catheter increases the risk of infection.

▶ An indwelling catheter is not a treatment for incontinence.

▶ Catheterization requires a physician's order.

▶ The prostate gland surrounds the urethra just below the bladder in males. It often enlarges with age, causing dribbling, difficulty in urinating, or inability to urinate.

(continues)

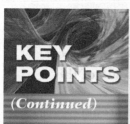

KEY POINTS
(Continued)

▶ A specimen collection system is a small catheter attached to a test tube. Its use benefits the patient, nursing personnel, and laboratory personnel.

▶ A suprapubic catheter may also be called a *cystostomy tube*. It is inserted surgically through the abdominal wall directly into the bladder. It may be for temporary or permanent bladder catheterization.

▶ A nephrostomy tube is surgically inserted through the skin and into the kidney. It drains urine continuously, directly from the kidney to the outside of the body.

▶ Hemodialysis is done at a dialysis center and involves the use of a machine to clean wastes from the blood after the kidneys have failed.

▶ Peritoneal dialysis may be done in the hospital, and involves inserting dialysis solution through a cannula into the patient's abdominal cavity.

▶ Continuous ambulatory peritoneal dialysis is usually done for patients with end-stage renal disease. The patient and family are taught to perform the procedure so that they can do it at home. This eliminates the need to go to the dialysis center several times a week.

▶ Catheter irrigation is a sterile procedure done to cleanse the bladder to remove blood clots.

▶ Bladder irrigation can be done by the open method, closed method, or continuous irrigation.

▶ Notify the RN if the patient has not voided within 6 to 8 hours following catheter removal.

▶ The rectal tube is used to reduce and eliminate flatus (intestinal gas).

▶ Rectal suppositories soften the stool and stimulate bowel elimination.

▶ An enema is the introduction of fluid into the lower bowel to cleanse the anus, rectum, and lower colon.

▶ A cleansing enema removes fecal material from the rectum and lower bowel. It also stimulates peristalsis and softens the stool.

▶ A retention enema may be given for constipation or fecal impaction. An oil-based solution, packaged in a small, commercial container, is used to soften hard stool, lubricate the rectum, and gently stimulate evacuation.

▶ Commercially prepared enemas are administered in small, premeasured containers. They are available with either cleansing or retention enema solutions.

▶ The Sims' position is a side-lying position used for giving enemas, rectal examinations, and other rectal treatments. The patient is turned onto the left side with the right leg bent at the knee and flexed forward slightly.

▶ Loose stools may be an indication of fecal impaction.

▶ Fecal impaction may be life-threatening in the elderly.

▶ In a patient with heart disease, removing a fecal impaction may stimulate the vagus nerve, slowing the heart rate.

▶ An ostomy is a surgically created opening for elimination that is performed for obstruction, cancer, bowel disease, or trauma.

▶ The stoma is the opening of the ostomy to the outside of the body, through which stool is eliminated.

▶ A colostomy is the most common type of ostomy.

▶ The amount of liquid in the stool is determined by the amount of bowel remaining after surgery. When a large amount of bowel is left, the stool is more solid; when most of the colon is removed, the stool is liquid.

(continues)

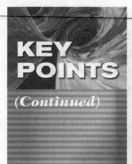

KEY POINTS
(Continued)

▶ Having a new ostomy is a difficult adjustment for the patient to make and he or she will have many concerns. The PCT must provide emotional support.

▶ The ostomy appliance is the container into which the contents of the bowel are eliminated.

▶ Fecal material is very irritating to the skin surrounding the stoma.

▶ Colostomy irrigation is done to regulate elimination; this may take 4 to 6 weeks.

CLINICAL APPLICATIONS

1. You are assigned to test Mr. White's urine for sugar and ketones. You have him void, then instruct him to drink water, telling him you will return in an hour to collect another urine specimen. When you return, the patient tells you he is unable to void. What action should you take?

2. You are assigned to test Mrs. Herrera's urine specific gravity. The patient has a fever of 103°F. Describe what action you will take.

3. You are inserting an indwelling catheter in Miss Petermann. As you begin to insert the catheter, the patient moves her leg. You are not sure if she touched the catheter or not. What action should you take?

4. You are removing Miss Petermann's indwelling catheter. You withdraw fluid from the balloon and gently pull on the catheter. The patient complains of discomfort. How will you proceed?

5. Mr. Hitchcock, a cognitively impaired, elderly patient, is admitted to your unit. He is lethargic, has a fever, and is having loose stools. The patient is passing gas. Occasionally, he grimaces and appears to be bearing down. Sometimes loose stool passes during this activity. What could be causing this problem? What action will you take?

CHAPTER REVIEW

Multiple-Choice Questions

Select the one best answer.

1. Reagents are commonly used:
   a. in the operating room during surgical procedures.
   b. for diagnostic testing.
   c. by licensed personnel only.
   d. to stimulate bowel elimination.

2. pH is a measure of:
   a. glucose in the urine.
   b. protein in the urine.
   c. acidity or alkalinity.
   d. ketones in the blood.

3. Specific gravity is a measure of:
   a. the ability of the kidneys to concentrate urine.
   b. acidity or alkalinity of a substance.
   c. protein in the urine.
   d. glucose in the blood.

4. A straight catheter is used for:
   a. irrigating the bladder.
   b. patients with prostate problems when an indwelling catheter cannot be inserted.

c. medication administration.
d. obtaining a sterile urine specimen.

5. The purpose of bladder irrigation is to:
   a. prevent infection.
   b. remove blood clots.
   c. cleanse the catheter.
   d. stimulate urination.

6. Signs and symptoms of fecal impaction include:
   a. indigestion.
   b. heartburn.
   c. fever over 103°F.
   d. passing liquid stools.

7. You are assigned to remove a fecal impaction. Supplies you will bring to the room include:
   a. disposable exam gloves.
   b. rectal tube.
   c. enema bag.
   d. rectal suppository.

8. When irrigating a colostomy, position the IV standard:
   a. 36 inches above the patient's head.
   b. so the bottom of the bag is even with the patient's shoulder.

c. at the level of the heart.

d. 42 inches above the bed.

9. When changing an ostomy bag, cut the hole for the stoma:

a. so it fits tightly around the stoma.

b. 1 inch larger than the stoma.

c. 1/8 inch larger than the stoma.

d. 2 inches larger than the stoma.

10. After removing the Keto-Diastix from the urine, hold it:

a. vertically.

b. with the chemical pads facing down.

c. by the chemical pads.

d. horizontally.

11. When a patient uses a urinary leg bag, you should:

a. leave the bag in place 24 hours a day.

b. disinfect the leg bag and bed bag at least once a day.

c. irrigate the bladder every 4 hours.

d. empty the bag at least once every 24 hours.

12. Complications of suprapubic catheter use include:

a. urinary tract infections.

b. loose stools.

c. fecal impaction.

d. renal failure.

13. When caring for a suprapubic catheter, you should:

a. change the drainage bag daily.

b. use clean technique.

c. use aseptic technique.

d. apply antibiotic cream to the insertion site.

14. A nephrostomy tube:

a. drains urine from the kidney to the outside of the body.

b. is surgically inserted directly into the bladder.

c. must be drained and irrigated manually once every shift.

d. is cared for using clean technique.

15. When caring for a patient with a nephrostomy tube, report to the RN if:

a. urine is amber in color.

b. urine is clear.

c. urine drains into the tube continuously, so the bag must be emptied frequently.

d. there is copious yellow drainage at the insertion site.

16. The patient with a nephrostomy should take a:

a. tub bath.

b. whirlpool bath.

c. shower.

d. sitz bath.

17. The purpose of dialysis is to:

a. cleanse impurities from the blood.

b. restore kidney function to normal.

c. add extra fluid to the body.

d. improve and restore fluid balance.

18. Peritoneal dialysis:

a. is a clean procedure.

b. must be done in the operating room.

c. must be done at a dialysis center.

d. requires strict sterile technique.

19. The rectal tube:

a. relieves constipation.

b. provides a passageway for flatus to escape.

c. is used to stimulate elimination and relieve impaction.

d. increases abdominal distention.

20. When administering rectal treatments, you should position the patient in the:

a. Sims' position.

b. right lateral position.

c. Trendelenberg position.

d. Fowler's position.

E X P L O R I N G   T H E   W E B

A to Z Guide to Dialysis	http://www.kidney.org
American College of Gastroenterology	http://www.acg.gi.org
CAPD Articles, Reviews, and Guidelines Concerning This Specialty	http://www.irontherapy.org
Catheterization Basics	http://www.nursingceu.com
The Client with Alterations in Bowel Elimination	http://www.camden.rutgers.edu
Combined Health Information Database	http://chid.nih.gov
Continent Ostomy Centers	http://www.ostomy.com
Digital Urology Journal	http://www.duj.com

Discovery Health	http://health.discovery.com
Dr. Greenson's Gastrointestinal and Liver Pathology	http://www.pds.med.umich.edu
EnemaBag.com	http://www.enemabag.com
Enhanced Texas Department of Health Curriculum for Dialysis Technician Training	http://www.nephron.com
Family Practice Notebook—Urinary Catheter	http://www.fpnotebook.com
Female Urinary Catheter Care Suggestions	http://www.urologyclinicofhouston.com
International Ostomy Association	http://www.ostomyinternational.org
Internet Pathology Laboratory—Urinalysis	http://medlib.med.utah.edu
Johns Hopkins Gastroenterology and Heptology Resource Center	http://hopkins-gi.org
Lab and Pathology Topics Index	http://www.palpath.com
LabTestsOnline	http://www.labtestsonline.org
Loyola University Department of Urology	http://www.luhs.org
Medline Plus Constipation	http://www.nlm.nih.gov
Medline Plus Fecal Impaction	http://www.nlm.nih.gov
National Institute of Diabetes, Digestive, & Kidney Diseases	http://www.niddk.nih.gov
Nephron Information Center	http://www.nephron.com
Peritoneal Dialysis	http://www.kidneyoptions.com
Peritoneal Dialysis: Its Indications and Contraindications	http://www.eneph.com
Rotherham Clinical Policies and Procedures	http://www.rotherhampct.nhs.uk
Society of Gastroenterology Nurses and Associates	http://www.sgna.org
Society of Urologic Nurses and Associates	http://suna.inurse.com
Stanford Department of Urology	http://www.med.stanford.edu
Suprapubic Urinary Catheter Suggestions	http://www.urologyclinicofhouston.com
UCLA Department of Urology	http://www.urology.medsch.ucla.edu
United Ostomy Association	http://www.uoa.org
University of Michigan Department of Urology	http://www.um-urology.com
University of Virginia Urology	http://www.healthsystem.virginia.edu
Urinary Catheter Care Instructions	http://www.chclibrary.org
Urinary Indwelling Catheter	http://www.nmh.org
Urology at Hopkins	http://urology.jhu.edu
Urology Nurses Online	http://www.duj.com
UrologyChannel	http://www.urologychannel.com
Wound, Ostomy, & Continence Nurses Society	http://www.wocn.org
Yahoo Health	http://health.yahoo.com

CHAPTER 9

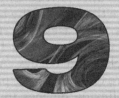

Enteral Nutrition

OBJECTIVES:

After reading this chapter, you should be able to:

- Spell and define key terms.
- State the difference between a nasogastric tube and a gastrostomy tube.
- List five reasons for enteral tube insertion.
- Demonstrate nasogastric tube insertion and care.
- List the reasons for checking for proper tube placement.
- State the purpose of checking for residual feeding in the stomach.
- Describe and demonstrate how to administer tube feeding by the bolus and pump methods.
- Describe insertion site skin care for a patient with a gastrostomy tube.
- List precautions to take when handling tube-feeding formula to prevent complications.
- State what to do when an equipment alarm sounds.

TUBE FEEDING

Feeding tubes may be inserted for many reasons. They may be inserted before surgery, or in preparation for certain tests. A **nasogastric tube (NG tube)** is inserted through the nose and threaded through the esophagus to the stomach. A **gastrostomy tube (G-tube)** (Figure 9-1) is surgically inserted through the abdominal wall into the stomach. The **jejunostomy tube (J-tube)** is a long, small-bore tube that is threaded through the gastrointestinal (GI) tract until the tip reaches the small intestine. These tubes may be placed through the nose (nasojejunostomy), or surgically through an incision in the abdominal skin. Surgical insertion is most common. This is considered a long-term tube. Jejunostomy tubes are used for patients who do not have a stomach, and those in whom recurrent formula aspiration is a problem. You will not insert this type of tube, but you may care for patients who have J-tubes in place. All three types of tubes are called *enteral tubes*.

A nasogastric tube is usually used when it is anticipated that the patient will require the tube for a

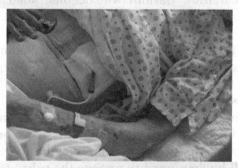

FIGURE 9-1 A gastrostomy tube is surgically inserted through the abdominal wall.

short period of time, usually seven days or less. A gastrostomy tube is used for long-term or permanent use. The patient is fed liquid nutritional formula through the tube. Feedings are commonly administered at a slow rate over a long period of time. However, they can be given intermittently every few hours by a bolus or drip method of feeding. Tube insertion, formula type, amount, type of administration (bolus, drip, or continuous), and feeding frequency must be ordered by the physician. The registered dietitian will closely follow all patients who are using enteral tubes.

Reasons for Tube Feeding

Many patients receive tube feeding during acute illness, when they cannot take food and fluids normally. This type of tube will be removed when the patient recovers. Reasons for inserting feeding tubes include:

- To withdraw samples of gastric contents for tests
- To wash the stomach in certain medical conditions
- Surgical procedures
- Unconscious patients
- When patients cannot eat normally
- Inability to swallow
- To prevent or treat weight loss

Some patients receive tube feedings because of swallowing disorders. Their condition causes **aspiration** of food and fluids. Aspiration is a serious condition in which food or liquid enters the lungs. Patients who aspirate may be permanently fed by tube. The speech therapist will assess their ability to swallow and make recommendations. Sometimes a **modified barium swallow** is ordered by the physician. This study shows the patient's potential for aspiration on an X-ray. After this procedure, push fluids, unless the patient is NPO. Monitor the patient's bowel movements carefully. Barium will become solid in the colon, causing obstruction and other serious complications. Monitoring fluid intake and bowel movements is important. The nurse may administer laxatives to assist in removing the barium. Report to the RN if the patient is not taking fluids, or if he or she does not have a bowel movement daily.

Some patients receive tube feedings because of weight loss. Some of these patients can consume food orally. A gastrostomy tube may be inserted. A plan will be developed to remove the tube at a later time. The patient is served a tray at each meal and also receives tube feedings during the night. This is because the tube-feeding solution fills the stomach. If it is given during the day, it suppresses the appetite, so the patient does not eat. You may be assigned to work with the patient so that he or she does not lose the ability to self-feed.

Basic Care of Patients Being Tube-Fed

Keep the head of the bed elevated at least 30 to 45 degrees while the tube feeding is being administered. This reduces the risk of aspiration of formula. The head should remain elevated for 30 to 60 minutes, or according to facility policy, after the feeding is completed. Patients receiving continuous feedings must have the head of the bed elevated at all times. This decreases the risk of aspiration, but increases the risk of skin breakdown on the hips, buttocks, and coccyx. Anticipate this and plan your care to position the patient correctly. Use pressure-relieving devices to avoid breakdown.

Patients receiving tube feedings require frequent mouth care. The mucous membranes in the mouth dry out when the patient does not take liquids orally. The mouth should be cleansed routinely every 2 hours, or according to facility policy. If the patient has a nasogastric tube, the nostrils must be cleansed and lubricated regularly. Lubricate the lips as needed.

When moving a patient in bed, know the location of the tube at all times and avoid pulling on it. Serious complications can result if a feeding tube is dislodged. The skin around the feeding tube must be kept clean and dry. Sometimes the skin around a gastrostomy tube is covered with gauze. If the patient has a nasogastric tube, it may be clipped to the gown or clothing to prevent pulling.

DIFFICULT PATIENT ALERT

The NG tube must be fastened securely. Most facilities tape the tube to the nose and face with hypoallergenic tape. Some fasten it by using a Velcro strap, such as a catheter strap, around the forehead. Monitor the nostrils frequently. Pressure from the tube promotes skin breakdown and erosion of the side of the nostril. If this occurs, the tube is usually moved to the other nostril, or a gastrostomy tube is inserted.

Many of the procedures in this chapter involve using a syringe. Always use a syringe that holds 30 mL or more. A syringe smaller than 30 mL increases the internal pressure exerted on the tube and stomach. Larger syringes exert less pressure. The risk of complications is greatly reduced when 30-mL to 60-mL syringes are used.

NASOGASTRIC TUBE INSERTION AND CARE

You may be asked to insert a nasogastric tube. The tube is most commonly placed for feeding. It may also be used to irrigate and suction the stomach contents. This is sometimes necessary in cases of bleeding from the stomach, or when the patient has ingested a caustic or poisonous substance.

Nasogastric tubes use the French size scale, like catheters. In adults, the most common sizes are 12, 14, 16, and 18 French. The RN will tell you which size to use. The most common tubes are called Levin tubes. These tubes have a single lumen. The Salem tube has two lumens. In most facilities, an RN or physician will insert this tube. A triple-lumen tube, called the Moss tube, is usually inserted surgically.

Position the patient in a sitting or high Fowler's position to insert a nasogastric tube. This position reduces the risk of complications. Drape the towel or disposable underpad around the patient's shoulders, under the chin. Place an emesis basin and tissues within the patient's reach. Instruct the patient to face forward, with the neck in a neutral position. Avoid positioning the neck forward or backward. When you are explaining the procedure to the patient, agree on a signal the patient will use, such as raising the hand, if he or she needs you to stop the procedure momentarily.

Inserting the nasogastric tube correctly is important. The tube is inserted blindly. You cannot tell where the tip will end up. Because the stomach and the lungs share the internal structures in the back of the throat, a tube may be inserted into the lungs. Serious complications will result if liquids are administered. Monitor the patient for signs of respiratory distress while you are inserting the tube. If the tube is inserted into the lungs, the patient may begin coughing, choking, or become cyanotic. If these occur, withdraw the tube.

Check the tube carefully for proper placement after it is inserted. The tube may slip from its original position, so the patient requires close observation. Periodic checks of tube placement are also necessary. Most tubes have a radiopaque strip down the side, or at the tip, so that tube placement can be determined by x-ray. Most facilities routinely x-ray the tube after insertion, before any feeding is administered.

Procedure 65

Inserting a Nasogastric Tube

Supplies needed:

▶ Disposable exam gloves
▶ Nasogastric tube, size determined by the RN
▶ Water-soluble lubricant
▶ Towel or disposable underpad
▶ Emesis basin
▶ Tissues
▶ 1-inch tape
▶ Rubber band
▶ Safety pin
▶ Emesis basin
▶ Stethoscope
▶ 30-mL to 60-mL catheter tip or bulb syringe
▶ Glass of water and straw, if appropriate
▶ Tongue blade
▶ Flashlight
▶ Plug for end of tube, or setup for tube feeding or suction
▶ Plastic bag for used supplies

1. Perform your beginning procedure actions.
2. Visually inspect the tube for rough spots, cracks, or leaks. If the tube is stiff, coil it around your hand and hold it under warm, running water. If the tube is limp, place it in a basin of ice.
3. Measure the distance of the tube from the nose to the stomach. Do this by holding the internal tip of the tube at the tip of the nose. Draw the tube to the tip of the earlobe (**Figure 9-2**). You may wish to mark the tube here, using a piece of tape that can be quickly and easily removed. Next, draw the tube down from the tip of the ear to the tip of the sternum, or xiphoid process (**Figure 9-3**). Mark this location on the tube with a piece of tape, or according to facility policy. In some facilities, you may be instructed to add 2 to 5 centimeters (1 to 2 inches) to this measurement, to ensure that the tip of the tube enters the stomach. This is especially important with tall patients. Your instructor will guide you on which method to use for measuring tube length. Bend the end of the tube forward so it is curved slightly.

(continues)

Procedure 65, *continued*

Inserting a Nasogastric Tube

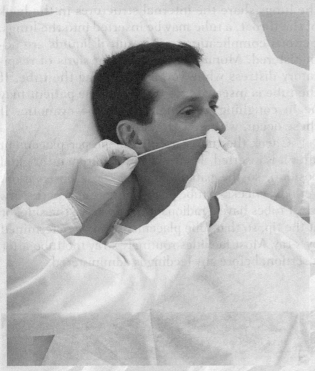

FIGURE 9-2 Measure from the tip of the nose to the tip of the earlobe.

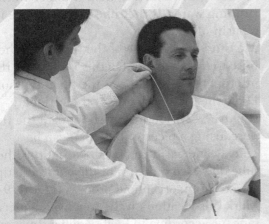

FIGURE 9-3 Measure from the tip of the earlobe to the tip of the sternum.

NOTE: An alternate method of checking tube length used by some facilities is to measure from the tip of the earlobe to the tip of the nose, then from the tip of the nose to the tip of the sternum. Follow your facility policies and your instructor's recommendations.

4. Place water-soluble lubricant on a tissue or gauze sponge. Lubricate the first three inches of the internal tip of the tube.

5. Gently insert the tube into the patient's nostril. Aim the tube downward and thread it slowly and gently toward the patient's ear.

6. You will feel slight resistance when the tube enters the nasopharynx. Instruct the patient to sip water from a straw, if possible. If the patient is NPO, instruct him or her to swallow. This helps to advance the tube. If you have marked the placement with tape, quickly remove the tape. Instructing the patient to bend the head forward before advancing the tube further will decrease the risk of the tube entering the lungs.

7. Continue threading the tube slowly while the patient sips water. Stop advancing the tube when you reach the mark on the tube.

8. With a tongue blade and flashlight, look in the patient's mouth and the back of the throat. Make sure the tube is not coiled in this area.

9. Attach the catheter tip or bulb syringe to the end of the tube. Withdraw stomach contents through the syringe by pulling back on the plunger. If you are using a bulb syringe, depress the bulb before inserting it into the tube, to avoid injecting air into the stomach. If you do not withdraw secretions, position the patient on the left side. This will move gastric secretions near the tip of the tube. Attempt to withdraw secretions again. If you withdraw gastric secretions, return them to the stomach.
Note: Some facilities check the pH of gastric contents with a reagent strip or pH meter. Know and follow your facility policy.

10. If you are unable to withdraw gastric secretions in the syringe, advance the tube another inch. With the syringe, inject 10 mL of air into the tube, while simultaneously listening over the stomach with a stethoscope. You should hear air movement in the stomach through the stethoscope.

(continues)

Procedure **65**, *continued*

Inserting a Nasogastric Tube

11. If these actions do not confirm tube placement, consult the RN. Do not administer feeding solution or water through the tube until placement has been confirmed. *Note: Most facilities x-ray all tubes to confirm placement. If this is the case, complete the procedure and notify the RN, who will order the x-ray.*

12. Secure the tube to the patient's nose with tape (Figure 9-4). Cut a 3- to 4-inch section of 1-inch tape. Split the tape lengthwise, up the center, approximately 1½ inches. Fold over the ends of the split sections slightly, forming tabs. Place the uncut part of the tape on the patient's nose. The split in the tape should begin about 1 inch from the tip. Wrap the split ends of the tape around the tube by crisscrossing them over each other. Apply another piece of tape across the nose to secure the tube. A commercial product is available to hold tubes in place. Use this instead of tape, if available.
    Note: Some facilities measure the length of the tube from the tip of the nostril to the free end of the tube immediately after insertion. This measurement is recorded in a convenient location. The tube is measured again each time tube placement is checked. The measurement should be the same.

13. Insert the plug into the open end of the tube, or fasten to the tube-feeding solution administration set or suction, as ordered.

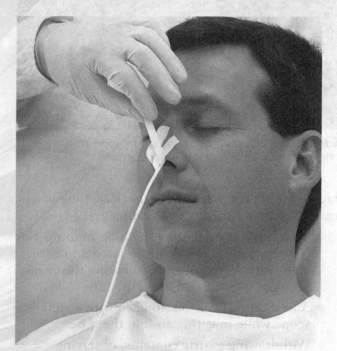

FIGURE 9-4 Tape the tube securely in place.

14. Wrap a rubber band around the tube, about 6 inches below the patient's chin. Loop one end of the rubber band inside the other. Secure it to the patient's gown with a safety pin. An alternative is to wrap a piece of tape around the tube, securing this to the gown with a safety pin. This reduces the risk of accidentally dislodging the tube.

15. Perform your procedure completion actions.

CHECKING NASOGASTRIC TUBE PLACEMENT

The position of the nasogastric tube must be checked periodically. The interval for checking is determined by facility policy. Always check for tube placement before adding feeding solution, water, or medication to the tube. Patient movement, pulling on the tube, violent coughing, vomiting, dry heaves, and tracheal suctioning may cause the tube to migrate to another location. Performing this check is very important to prevent aspiration and other complications.

Methods of Checking Nasogastric Tube Placement

The most accurate method of checking placement is by x-ray. However, it is not realistic to use this method each time tube placement has to be checked. For many years, nurses checked tube placement by placing the end of the tube in a glass of water and checking for the presence of bubbles. We now know that this method is inaccurate and should never be used. Placement may be confirmed by several methods. Using two methods confirms the accuracy of the check. Follow your

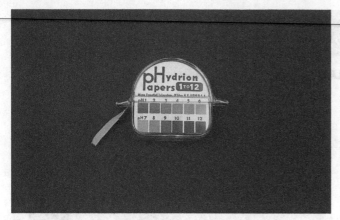

FIGURE 9-5 Use reagent strips or tape to measure the pH of abdominal contents.

facility policy for methods of checking tube placement. Common methods of testing are:

- Measuring the length of the tube from the tip of the nostril to the tip of the tube immediately after insertion and comparing this measurement with the length of the tube
- Auscultating over the stomach with a stethoscope while injecting air into the tube
- Withdrawing gastric contents, observing them, then returning them to the stomach
- Checking the pH of gastric secretions with a reagent strip or tape (**Figure 9-5**), litmus paper, or a pH meter

SAFETY ALERT

In the recent past, blue food coloring was added to tube feedings to help personnel identify vomitus and oral secretions. Occasionally, patients developed blue discoloration of the skin, urine, feces, or serum. The blue color was associated with serious complications such as hypotension, metabolic acidosis, and death. Besides the possibility of systemic toxicity, tinted enteral feedings interfered with some diagnostic examinations, such as the hemoccult test. Seriously ill patients and patients with sepsis may be at greater risk for complications. Because there may be a causal relationship between blue food coloring in the enteral feeding and serious or life-threatening outcomes, the FDA issued an alert in 2003 recommending that the practice of adding food coloring to enteral feedings be discontinued. Do not add food coloring to an enteral formula. This is no longer considered safe.

Of the methods listed, the last two are the most accurate. Allow at least an hour after medication administration before checking the appearance of

the gastric contents. Medication will also alter the color of the fluid. Stomach fluid varies slightly in color from one patient to the next. It is typically green or off-white, cloudy, or colorless. Fluid from the intestines is yellow or brownish. Fluid from the lungs is usually tan, off-white, clear, or pale yellow.

pH Method of Checking Tube Placement. Checking the pH of the fluid is a very accurate method of testing. The pH of body fluids is listed in **Table 9-1**. In some facilities, these conditions must be present before doing pH testing:

- No feedings within the past 2 to 4 hours
- No antacids within the previous 4 hours
- No medications within the past hour
- Patient does not receive acid-inhibiting medications
- Tube must be flushed with 20 to 30 mL of air before aspiration of fluid for pH testing

If it is not possible to meet these conditions, another method of testing should be used.

pH testing may be done with a reagent strip or tape, litmus paper, or a pH meter. Avoid using reagent strips manufactured for urine testing. The upper reading on these strips may not be high enough for checking stomach and intestinal contents.

Before removing the stomach contents, inject 20 mL of air into the nasogastric tube. Next, withdraw stomach contents with the syringe. If you are unable to aspirate stomach contents, inject another 20 mL of air. If this does not work, turn the patient on the left side, wait a few minutes, inject 20 mL of air, and try

Table 9-1 pH of Body Fluids	
Body Fluid	**pH**
Stomach contents	0 to 5, most commonly 1 to 4
Intestinal contents	6 to 8, most commonly 7.5 to 8
Respiratory secretions	usually 7 or higher, can be as low as 6

The safest method of checking is to confirm placement with an X-ray if the pH is 6 or higher.

again. If you are still unable to aspirate fluid, inform the RN, and follow his or her instructions.

Before you add any fluid, formula, or water to the tube, you must be certain that the tip of the tube is in the stomach, based on the checks you have done. If you have any doubt, ask the RN to verify placement.

Procedure 66

Checking Nasogastric Tube Placement

Supplies needed:
- Disposable exam gloves
- Towel or disposable underpad
- 30- to 60-mL syringe, depending on procedure
- Cap or plug for administration set tubing
- Stethoscope, if this is your facility policy
- Litmus paper, reagent strip, or pH meter, if this is your facility policy
- Plastic medication cup for stomach aspirate, if pH method is used
- Plastic bag for used supplies

1. Perform your beginning procedure actions.
2. Disconnect the nasogastric tube from the administration set. Cap the administration set tubing.
3. Insert the syringe into the nasogastric tube.
4. Follow the procedure used by your facility:
   a. Inject 10 mL of air into the tube, while simultaneously listening over the stomach with a stethoscope (**Figure 9–6**); if the patient burps after air is injected, suspect esophageal placement instead of stomach.
   b. Inject 20 mL of air into the stomach. Pull back on the syringe to aspirate stomach contents. Observe the appearance of the returns to identify gastric fluid. Return the aspirate to the stomach.
   c. Inject 20 mL of air into the stomach. Pull back on the syringe to aspirate

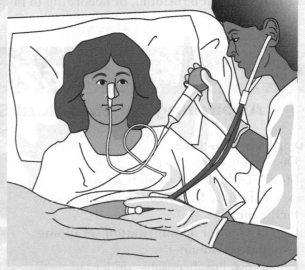

FIGURE 9-6 Inject air into the stomach while listening over the stomach with a stethoscope.

stomach contents. Follow your facility policy for checking the contents with a reagent product or pH meter. Return the fluid to the stomach.

The amount of air used in this procedure varies from one facility to the next, with amounts varying from 10 mL to 30 mL. Your instructor will guide you on the total amount of air to use. Learn and follow your facility policies.

5. Perform your procedure completion actions.

DETERMINING RESIDUAL STOMACH CONTENTS

Most health care facilities have policies and procedures for checking residual stomach contents before beginning a new feeding or adding formula to the continuous tube feeding. This is done to prevent overfilling the stomach, and other complications of tube feeding. Some facilities check the residual stomach contents every 2 to 4 hours. Follow your facility policy and the physician's orders for this procedure. Elevate the head of the bed 30 to 45 degrees when withdrawing stomach contents.

When checking residual, you will withdraw formula from the stomach, check the amount, then return the formula to the stomach. The feeding is withheld if the amount withdrawn exceeds 100 mL or 1 1/2 times the amount delivered in 1 hour by continuous administration. Thus, if the patient receives 100 mL of formula per hour, the next feeding is withheld if he or she has 150 mL or more feeding residual remaining in the stomach. If a patient is receiving a continuous feeding, stop the feeding 15 minutes before checking for stomach residual, or according to facility policy. Notify the RN if the amount of residual exceeds the amount specified in your facility policy. He or she will notify the physician. Do not administer another feeding until you receive directions from the RN.

Repeatedly checking the nasogastric tube for residual increases the risk of plugging the tube. In many facilities, the tube is routinely irrigated with a small amount of fluid after the stomach contents are replaced. Because the jejunostomy tube is not in the stomach, you cannot check for residual. Doing so increases the risk of complications.

Procedure 67

Aspirating for Residual Stomach Contents

Supplies needed:

▶ Disposable exam gloves
▶ 60-mL catheter-tip or bulb syringe
▶ Normal saline for irrigation, if this is your facility policy
▶ Cap or plug for administration set tubing
▶ Graduated container
▶ Clean towel or disposable underpad
▶ Plastic bag for used supplies

1. Perform your beginning procedure actions.
2. Disconnect the nasogastric tube from the administration set. Cap the administration set tubing.
3. Insert the syringe into the nasogastric tube.
4. Gently withdraw the stomach contents. When no longer able to withdraw stomach contents, measure the contents. Use the graduated container if the amount is more than a graduated syringe can hold.
5. Expel air from the syringe.
6. Replace the stomach contents.
7. Perform your procedure completion actions.

IRRIGATING A NASOGASTRIC TUBE

Sometimes the formula in the nasogastric tube coagulates and adheres to the inside of the tube. Tube irrigation usually requires a physician order. The PCT should not irrigate a tube without specific instruction from the RN. Sometimes a nasogastric tube must be irrigated to prevent the tube from plugging. Irrigation may also be necessary in patients with some medical conditions, such as bleeding in the stomach. However, it is contraindicated in some conditions.

The solution for irrigation varies with facility policy and the purpose of the irrigation. Most facilities use water or normal saline. However, some use cola or cranberry juice, particularly if the tube is plugged. If the patient is bleeding, normal saline or iced normal saline is used. Iced normal saline has been used for years to reduce or stop stomach bleeding. Over the last few years, however, this practice has fallen out of favor, and is somewhat controversial. Physicians are now ordering room-temperature normal saline instead. Cola and other products are not used for stomach irrigation if bleeding is known or suspected. Elevate the head of the bed 30 to 45 degrees when irrigating the tube.

Procedure **68**

Irrigating a Nasogastric Tube

Supplies needed:

▶ Disposable exam gloves
▶ Irrigation solution ordered by physician, or according to facility policy
▶ 30- to 60-mL catheter-tip syringe
▶ Cap or plug for administration set tubing
▶ Emesis basin
▶ Clean towel or disposable underpad
▶ Plastic bag for used supplies

1. Perform your beginning procedure actions.
2. Check for tube placement according to facility policy.
3. Draw up 30 mL of irrigation solution, or the amount ordered by the physician, in the syringe.
4. Insert the syringe into the nasogastric tube.

5. Slowly inject the irrigation solution into the tube with the syringe, or allow it to flow in by gravity, according to facility policy. Gravity may be used for irrigation if the tube is not plugged. A bulb syringe may be used for gravity irrigation. Follow your facility policy. Avoid forcing the solution.
6. Withdraw the irrigation solution. Subtract the amount instilled from the amount withdrawn. Record the difference on the intake and output record.
7. Draw up fresh irrigation solution and repeat the procedure at least twice, or according to facility policy and physician orders. If the tube is plugged, irrigating once may not be sufficient to clear it.
8. Perform your procedure completion actions.

REMOVING A NASOGASTRIC TUBE

A nasogastric tube is removed when it is no longer needed, or when the tube must be changed. Elevate the head of the bed 30 to 45 degrees when removing the tube. Take care to avoid aspiration of fluid during tube removal.

Procedure **69**

Removing a Nasogastric Tube

Supplies needed:

▶ Disposable exam gloves
▶ Towel or disposable underpad
▶ Clamp or Kelly
▶ Washcloth
▶ Towel
▶ Supplies for oral hygiene
▶ Plastic bag for used supplies

1. Perform your beginning procedure actions.
2. Clamp the tube. Disconnect from the feeding administration set.

3. Loosen the tape on the patient's nose.
4. Pinch the tube near the nostril, and in one continuous, steady pull, remove the tube gradually.
5. Discard the tube in the plastic bag.
6. Assist the patient to wash his or her face, particularly around the nostrils and top of the nose. Remove adhesive from the skin.
7. Offer oral hygiene and lubricant for lips and nostrils. Assist as necessary.
8. Perform your procedure completion actions.

CARING FOR A PATIENT WITH A GASTROSTOMY

Several different procedures are used to insert a gastrostomy tube. A **percutaneous endoscopic gastrostomy (PEG)** is surgically inserted by the physician by threading the tube through the patient's mouth and into the stomach. The tube is pulled out through an incision in the patient's abdomen. A gastrostomy tube is inserted directly into the stomach through an incision in the abdominal wall. Until the incision in the abdomen has healed, the operative site must be observed at least once each shift. If this is your responsibility, you will check for redness, irritation, drainage, **induration** or swelling, and other skin problems. A small amount of clear drainage is normal in the first few weeks after insertion. Change the dressing as often as necessary during this time. Select an absorbent dressing to prevent skin irritation.

Immediately after surgery, the insertion site will be covered with a dressing. After the incision has healed, no dressing is necessary. In fact, some authorities state that the risk of infection is increased if a dressing is present. Upon return from surgery, measure the length of the tube from the tip to the abdominal wall. Record this measurement according to facility policy. This important first step provides a baseline with which to compare subsequent measurements. Some facility policies require measurement of the length of the gastrostomy tube each time site care is performed.

G-Tube Alternative. A gastrostomy feeding button is an alternative feeding device used for some ambulatory patients who are receiving long-term enteral feedings. The buttons may be used to replace a gastrostomy tube if necessary. The gastrostomy button has a mushroom-shaped dome at one end and two wing tabs with a flexible, plastic safety plug at the other. The button is almost level with the skin, with only part of the safety plug visible. This device is easily managed, reduces the risk of skin irritation and breakdown, and is less likely to migrate or become dislodged compared with an ordinary gastrostomy tube. It may be inserted into an established tract in place of a G-tube. A one-way, antireflux valve inside the button dome prevents leakage of gastric contents. The device may require replacement every 3 to 4 months, because the antireflux valve wears out. Occasionally, it will pop out, such as when the patient coughs or retches forcefully. If this occurs, a new button is reinserted.

Stabilizing the Gastrostomy Tube

Take care, when moving the patient, to avoid pulling on the tube. This increases the risk of injury and accidental dislodgement. The tube must be kept stabilized to prevent leakage, migration, and other problems. Intervene promptly if you observe a patient tugging at the tube, and notify the RN.

For many years, an indwelling Foley catheter was used in place of a gastrostomy tube. This is no longer done. We now know that the gastric secretions damage the catheter and the balloon that holds it in place. This increases the risk of balloon rupture and requires more frequent changes. Special gastrostomy tubes are used that can better withstand the action of stomach acids. These tubes have an external disk on the outside of the abdominal wall. This disk stabilizes the tube, helping prevent migration inward. Avoid placing a dressing between the disk and the abdominal skin. After the site has healed and sutures have been removed, the disk must be rotated 90 degrees at least once a day to prevent pressure and irritation.

Gastrostomy Tube Care

Meticulous care to the skin around the gastrostomy tube is done as ordered by the physician until healed, then at least daily. The RN will provide instructions about the type of dressing to use and the frequency of dressing changes. The dressing for a new PEG tube usually remains in place for 48 hours. After that, it is changed daily, or as ordered. A split dressing, such as that used for a tracheostomy tube, is used in some facilities. Take care not to move the disk in a newly inserted PEG. Secretions tend to cake around the insertion site. These must be gently removed. Inform the RN if you observe redness, drainage, swelling, a rash, irritation, or other signs of problems at the insertion site.

The RN will advise you regarding the cleansing solution to use for gastrostomy tube care. When cleansing a newly inserted PEG tube, half-strength hydrogen peroxide and normal saline may be used to remove secretions. However, some physicians prefer other solutions, as hydrogen peroxide can be harmful to healing tissue.

When cleansing the insertion site, work outward in progressively larger circles. Make sure to rinse the skin well to remove the cleansing solution. After the site has healed, it may be cleansed with normal saline or soap and water. Follow your facility policy, the RN's instructions, and physician's orders for the cleansing solution.

Procedure 70

Gastrostomy Tube Care

Supplies needed:

- Disposable exam gloves, 2 pairs
- Cleansing solution as ordered by the physician, or according to facility policy
- Normal saline
- Two plastic medicine cups for cleansing solution and normal saline
- Absorbent dressing, if site has not healed
- 1-inch tape, if dressing is used
- Sterile applicators
- 2 × 2 gauze sponges
- Plastic bag for used supplies

1. Perform your beginning procedure actions.
2. Remove the dressing, if present, and discard it in the plastic bag.
3. Cleanse the site with normal saline or the prescribed cleansing solution:
   a. Beginning at the insertion site, wipe around the insertion site in a circular motion with a sterile applicator moistened in cleansing solution. Discard the applicator in the plastic bag.
   b. With a second applicator, wipe around the area you cleansed first, extending the clean area outward. Discard the applicator in the plastic bag.
   c. Repeat with a third applicator until a site 3 inches in diameter is cleansed, or according to facility policy.
   d. Rinse the cleanser with applicators moistened with normal saline, unless a no-rinse product was used. Follow the same pattern as you did for cleansing the site. Use a new applicator with each circle.
4. Dry the skin thoroughly with gauze or sterile applicators. Discard used materials in the plastic bag.
5. If the site has healed, perform your procedure completion actions. If the site has not healed, remove your gloves and discard them in the plastic bag.
6. Wash your hands.
7. Apply clean exam gloves.
8. Apply a sterile dressing around the tube and fasten with tape.
9. Perform your procedure completion actions.

Inserting a Gastrostomy Tube into an Established Tract

Replacing a PEG tube is a surgical procedure that must be done by the physician. In some facilities, qualified nursing service personnel may replace the gastrostomy tube into a well-established tract. This is a stoma that has been used for a period of time and is well healed. The individual changing the tube must have successfully completed a course designed specifically for gastrostomy tube replacement, overall patient evaluation, and evaluation of the gastrostomy site. A registered nurse or a physician must provide supervision during the learning process. The individual changing the tube must demonstrate competency in the procedure. Whether the patient's tract meets the "established tract" definition is determined only by an RN or physician.

Gastrostomy tubes are not routinely changed. Occasionally, the tube will plug or a balloon will leak, creating a need to replace the gastrostomy tube. When changing a gastrostomy tube, use only a tube made specifically for this purpose. Never use a Foley catheter, which may migrate and cause serious complications, including **peritonitis,** a very serious inflammation of the peritoneum, the membrane that lines the abdominal cavity. This condition often develops as a complication of intestinal perforation from a tube, and may become life-threatening. The outcome is often poor, and may result in serious complications, including death.

Note: In some states, gastrostomy-tube replacement may be done only by licensed nurses who are qualified to perform the procedure. Your instructor will inform you if PCTs in your state may perform this skill. Never change or replace a gastrostomy tube that has been recently placed. Replace an established gastrostomy tube only if you are permitted to do so by state law, facility policies, and RN (or physician) assessment of the stoma.

Procedure 71

Inserting a Gastrostomy Tube into an Established Tract

Supplies needed:

- Disposable exam gloves
- 10-mL syringe, or larger if needed to deflate the balloon
- Foley catheter insertion tray without catheter
- Sterile gastrostomy tube
- 50-mL or 60-mL catheter-tip syringe, or irrigation set to check tube placement
- Litmus paper to check pH of stomach contents
- Sterile plug, clamp, or cap for tube, according to facility policy
- Absorbent dressing, if needed
- 1-inch tape, if dressing is used
- Plastic bag for used supplies

1. Perform your beginning procedure actions.
2. Clean the overbed table. Disinfect the table, if soiled, or if required by facility policy.
3. Apply gloves. Attach the syringe to the inflation port on the tube. Gently withdraw the fluid.
4. After all fluid is withdrawn, gently pull on the tube to remove it. If you meet resistance and cannot remove the tube, reattach the syringe and attempt to withdraw more fluid. If you still cannot remove the tube easily, call the RN.
5. Open the catheterization tray and establish a sterile field.
6. Open the gastrostomy tube and place it on the sterile field.
7. Place the plastic bag for used supplies at the foot of the bed, or in a convenient location. Position the bag so that you do not have to cross over sterile supplies to discard soiled items.
8. Remove your gloves and discard them in the plastic bag.
9. Wash your hands, or use alcohol-based hand cleaner.
10. Apply sterile gloves.
11. Open the sterile packages on the sterile field, and arrange supplies as needed.
12. Inspect the new gastrostomy tube for cracks or rough spots. If found, replace the tube.

13. Attach the syringe filled with sterile water or saline to the inflation port on the gastrostomy tube. Inject the fluid into the tube to check the balloon for leaks. If the balloon will not inflate, or if leaks are present, replace the gastrostomy tube. Pull back on the plunger of the syringe to deflate the balloon.
14. Open the package of povidone-iodine or other antiseptic solution. Carefully pour the solution over the cotton balls or applicators.
15. With the forceps in the tray, pick up a cotton ball moistened with disinfectant solution. Cleanse the patient in a circular motion, beginning at the stoma and working outward. Discard the cotton ball. Pick up another cotton ball and repeat the procedure. Discard the cotton ball. Pick up another cotton ball and cleanse the area again, progressively working outward. The circle should extend at least 4 inches in diameter. Discard the cotton ball and forceps.
16. Pick up the **fenestrated drape** (the sterile drape with the hole in the center). Stand away from the bed and hold the drape away from your body, allowing it to unfold.
17. Fold the drape back, over your gloves.
18. Position the hole in the center of the drape over the gastrostomy stoma.
19. Open the package of lubricant.
20. Lubricate the tip of the gastrostomy tube. The lubricant should cover the proximal end of the gastrostomy tube for approximately 2 inches.
21. Pick up the gastrostomy tube. Hold it approximately 1 to 2 inches from the tip.
22. Insert the gastrostomy tube into the stoma: Visualize the stoma. Tell the patient you will be inserting the gastrostomy tube now. Instruct the patient to cough, bear down, or whistle. *Never force a gastrostomy tube. If you meet resistance and are unable to advance the tube, stop the procedure and notify the RN.*

(continues)

Procedure **71**, *continued*
Inserting a Gastrostomy Tube into an Established Tract

23. Pick up the syringe and attach it to the inflation port in the gastrostomy tube. Slowly push the plunger to inflate the balloon with the designated amount of sterile fluid. *Very gently* pull the tube back to ensure that it is near the stomach wall. The tube should be near the wall, but not tightly. Take care not to pull the inflated balloon through the incision.
24. Verify tube placement by aspirating stomach secretions with a syringe and checking the pH. Return stomach contents.

25. Clamp or plug the gastrostomy tube, if this was not done previously.
26. Apply a dressing to the insertion site, if ordered.
27. Remove the drapes. Tear the center of the fenestrated drape to remove it over the tube. Discard in the plastic bag.
28. Perform your procedure completion actions.

NOTE: Do not insert formula, water, or any other substance into the tube until placement has been verified by X-ray.

FEEDING PATIENTS WITH AN ENTERAL TUBE

An **enteral tube** is a catheter, stoma, or tube such as a nasogastric, gastrostomy, or jejunostomy tube used to provide nutrition and deliver nutrients to the gastrointestinal tract, distal to the oral cavity. The tubes may also be called *enteral access devices.*

Patients with an enteral tube can be fed by several different methods:

- Bolus method—pouring formula into the tube through a syringe (remove the plunger or bulb first and allow the formula to flow in by gravity)
- Intermittent or continuous drip—formula drips into the tube by gravity from an administration set that hangs on an intravenous standard next to the bed
- Pump method—continuous feeding that is regulated by an electronic pump

Formula for Tube Feeding

Many different types of tube-feeding formulas are available commercially. Like a therapeutic diet, many are designed to be used for patients with specific medical problems. Special types of formulas are available to meet the patient's medical needs. For example, one formula is recommended for patients with pressure ulcers. Another type is recommended for patients with COPD. Yet another contains 2 calories per mL of fluid and is often administered to patients who have problems with weight loss. The type of formula is ordered by the physician. The registered dietitian closely follows patients who receive tube feedings. He or she evaluates their caloric needs, medical diagnoses, laboratory reports, and other factors. The dietitian makes recommendations about the patient's dietary needs. This team member is invaluable in the care of patients receiving enteral feedings.

Nutritional Adequacy of Enteral-Feeding Formula. Most enteral formulas deliver 1 calorie per milliliter. With most formula preparations, the patient must receive 1,600 to 1,800 calories a day to receive all of the vitamins and nutrients recommended for a balanced diet. Thus, for an 1,800-calorie diet, the continuous tube feeding on a pump or continuous drip infusion will run at a rate of 75 mL an hour. When the enteral feeding begins, the physician may order half-strength formula. This is half water and half formula. With this solution, the patient receives 900 calories a day. This is done to ensure that the patient will tolerate the feeding solution, which may cause side effects when first administered. The formula is advanced to three-quarter strength, and then full strength, over several days. Diluted formulas are not for long-term use because they are not adequate calorically.

Preparing and Hanging an Enteral Feeding

The principles of tube-feeding and handling formula are the same regardless of which technique is used for administering the formula. When preparing a tube feeding, use good aseptic technique. The bolus method of tube-feeding is an open system. The continuous infusion drip and the pump methods may be closed systems, but are commonly open systems. Any open-system method of tube feeding is subject to contamination if poor technique is used. Avoid contamination of the formula or system, which increases the risk of foodborne illness. Use clean supplies and wash your hands well each time you manipulate or work with the tube feeding. If contamination is suspected at any time, notify the RN. He or she may instruct you to discard the administration set, formula, and tubing, and replace them with new items.

Check the expiration date on the formula before opening the can. Never administer formula that is past its expiration date. Always shake the can of formula well before opening it to mix the contents. Formula is administered at room temperature. If you use a partial can of formula, cover it, and refrigerate. Mark the container with the date and time. This container should be used at the next feeding, or discarded within 24 hours. When removing tube-feeding formula from the refrigerator, warm it to room temperature in water. Avoid overheating it. The formula should not be hot when administered.

Administering Water. The physician may order water in addition to the formula feeding. Water is also used to flush the tube before and after medication administration. Some tube-feeding pumps are set to routinely deliver water once an hour. Water may also be administered by bolus injection into the tube, or may be infused through the administration set and pump. Patients with tube feedings can and do become dehydrated. Enteral formulas are partially solid, so the entire amount is not considered free liquid. Most formulas contain about 15 percent solids. The physician will order water flushes in addition to the formula. The dietitian will calculate the patient's daily fluid needs. Take your responsibility for water administration very seriously. Know and follow your facility policies for administering water.

Patients who are receiving tube feedings will be on intake and output. Record all liquids administered through the tube accurately. Accurately record each irrigation, the type and amount of solution used, and the character and volume of aspirate, according to facility policy. Nursing personnel must make sure the patient's individualized minimum daily fluid needs are met, and carefully record, monitor, and evaluate the data on the I&O sheet to ensure that water intake is adequate.

Caring for a Patient with a Jejunostomy Tube

The small intestine is approximately 12 feet long. Food passes from the stomach through the small intestine, where digestion and absorption of nutrients take place. A *jejunostomy* is a surgical opening into the jejunum (small intestine). It is usually placed through an incision in the surface of the abdomen. The J-tube is a small, flexible catheter. It remains in place at all times, and may be clamped between feedings to prevent leakage of intestinal contents. The J-tube is used to administer food and fluids directly into the jejunum. The J-tube is surgically placed low on the abdomen, and is at high risk of becoming dislodged. Secure the tube as ordered. Monitor tube location carefully, and make sure that the end of the tube is never tucked into the patient's pants.

Jejunostomy tubes are used for patients who do not have a stomach and for those in whom aspiration is a problem. These tubes have a smaller diameter than the other tubes and will become plugged more easily. A jejunostomy feeding tube usually requires a very slow infusion of formula, because there is no reservoir to accept a large amount of liquid, and the small intestine cannot buffer the solution as effectively as the stomach. The formula may be diluted, because the GI tract will pull water into the lumen of the tube to dilute the formula. Because of this, patients receiving jejunostomy feeding often have an increased incidence of loose stools and diarrhea. The patient's weight, caloric intake, and I&O must be accurately monitored to reduce the risk of complications.

Care for a patient with a jejunostomy is similar to care of other tube-fed patients, except where noted. The tube bypasses the protective mechanisms of the stomach, so the risk of infection is slightly higher. You may be instructed to alter your procedures and use sterile water and other sterile equipment to reduce the risk of infection.

Because the tip of the tube is in the small intestine, you cannot check for residual stomach contents. However, before administering formula or water into the tube, you must make sure that the tube is correctly situated in the jejunum. Tube position can be checked by:

- Measuring the length of the tube from the exit site to the cap and verifying that it is the same each time.
- Checking the pH of any fluid that flows back from the tube for acidity; it should be alkaline. Aspirated contents should be golden-yellow in color, with a pH of 6 or above. If

you cannot remove fluid, the pH is more than 6, or no sounds are heard over the right lower quadrant when air is injected in the tube, do not administer the feeding. Inform the RN.

- Injecting 2 to 5 mL of air into the tube, while holding a stethoscope over the right lower quadrant of the abdomen. If the tube is properly positioned, you will hear a crackling or swishing sound.

- Ensuring that the tube irrigates freely with sterile water; it is flushed with sterile water two or more times each day, and after each feeding.

Complications of Tube-Feeding

Remember to elevate the head of the bed 30 to 45 degrees or higher when the feeding is being administered, and for 1 hour thereafter. If you observe the patient coughing, vomiting, choking, gagging, burping, or having difficulty breathing, stay in the room and call for immediate assistance. Stop the feeding.

Sometimes patients receiving tube feedings will develop diarrhea or constipation. Always notify the RN if these conditions occur, and follow his or her instructions. Never force the tube-feeding formula or irrigation water into the feeding tube. If the liquid will not enter the tube by gravity, notify the RN.

Monitor the patient carefully for skin breakdown of the buttocks, hips, and coccyx. Also monitor the insertion site in the nostril. The tube may cause erosion of the skin in the nose. Lubricating the nostril with water-soluble ointment decreases crusting of secretions and reduces the risk of skin breakdown. Report problems to the RN. The patient may need special skin care. You may be instructed to move the tube to the other nostril. Frequently assess the tape holding the tube to the nostril. If the patient is diaphoretic, you may have to change it frequently.

Monitor the drip rate for the tube feeding, or the preset rate on the pump, each time you are in the room, or according to facility policy. Troubleshooting and complications of nasogastric tube feeding are listed in **Table 9-2**. Troubleshooting gastrostomy tube problems is listed in **Table 9-3**. Correct the problem only if you are permitted to do so. Although you may troubleshoot and correct certain complications, always inform the RN of the problem. Follow his or her instructions.

Table 9-2 Troubleshooting Nasogastric Tube-Feeding Problems	
Problem	**Potential Care**
Nausea and vomiting	Improper positioning/head not elevated 30° to 45°. (If vomiting persists after other potential causes are ruled out, position patient on his or her right side.)
	Tube placement incorrect
	Infusion rate too fast
	Total volume is too great
	Too much residual formula in stomach
	Feeding tube is incorrect size or type
	Formula intolerance
	High-fat formula
	Fecal impaction
Aspiration	Improper positioning/head not elevated 30° to 45°
	Tube placement incorrect/tube has migrated or become dislodged

(continues)

Table 9-2 Troubleshooting Nasogastric Tube-Feeding Problems (Continued)

Problem	Potential Care
	Absent or depressed gag reflex
	Vomiting, gastric reflux
	Feeding tube is incorrect size or type
	Too much residual formula in stomach
Diarrhea or irritable bowel	Formula intolerance
	Infusion rate too fast
	Formula too cold
	Bacterial contamination in system, formula, or infusion set
	Inadequate free water administered in addition to formula
	Malnutrition
	Inadequate fiber in formula
	Intolerance to lactose
	Sorbitol or other sugar alcohols in formula
	Illness, flu, infection
	Some medications, such as antibiotics and antacids
Constipation	Inadequate free water in addition to formula
	Dehydration
	Inadequate fiber in formula
	Side effect of medication
	Inactivity/immobility
	GI obstruction
Dehydration	Inadequate free water administered in addition to formula
	Excessive output, including urine and perspiration
	Fever
	Infection

(continues)

| Table 9-2 Troubleshooting Nasogastric Tube-Feeding Problems (Continued) ||
Problem	**Potential Care**
	Age-related changes in urinary tract
	High blood sugar
	High-protein formulas
Plugged tube	Medication sticks in tube
	Inadequate water flushes/tube irrigation
	Acid precipitation of formula

| Table 9-3 Troubleshooting Complications of Gastrostomy Tubes ||
Complication	**Possible Cause(s)**
Fluid leakage around external gastrostomy tube	Improper positioning/head not elevated 30° to 45°
	Tube migration outward
	Tube migration inward
	Fecal impaction
Tube blockage	Tube is dislodged
	Inadequate flushes/tube irrigation
	Undissolved medication
	Walls of tube are caked with formula
	Backup of gastric contents into tube, resulting in curdling of formula and gastric contents
	High-protein formula
	Slow formula administration
	Formula administered too warm
Skin irritation around insertion site	Tube migration outward
	Allergy to ointment or soap used around insertion site
	Unhealed insertion tract
	Leakage of gastric fluids to skin surface

(continues)

Table 9-3 Troubleshooting Complications of Gastrostomy Tubes (Continued)

Complication	Possible Cause(s)
Aspiration	Tube dislodged
	Head of bed not elevated during feedings
	Absent or depressed gag reflex
	Reflux of feedings into esophagus or mouth
	Vomiting
Diarrhea	New tube feeding
	Certain medications, such as antibiotics and antacids
	Rapid formula administration
	Formula too cold
	Bacterial contamination of formula, infusion set, or system
	Lactose intolerance
	Sorbitol or other sugar alcohols in formula
	Dumping related to rapid transit time
Constipation	Side effect of medication
	Inadequate fiber
	Inadequate fluid intake
	GI obstruction
Distention, gas, bloating, cramping	Slow gastric emptying
	Changes in small intestine related to malnutrition
	Nutrient malabsorption
	Lactose intolerance
	Rapid formula administration; intermittent administration of cold formula; formula too hot
	Tube migration from stomach to small intestine

(continues)

Table 9-3 Troubleshooting Complications of Gastrostomy Tubes (Continued)

Complication	Possible Cause(s)
Nausea and vomiting	Air in tube
	Prolonged antibiotic therapy
	Rapid formula administration
	Total volume too great
	Gastric retention
	High-fat formula
	Bowel obstruction
Dehydration	Inadequate fluid intake or excessive fluid loss

A serious problem associated with PEG tubes is **buried bumper syndrome.** This is an ulceration of the tissue at the feeding-tube exit site or the internal mucosal layer of the gastric wall. This syndrome may develop if the tubes used have internal and external retention bumpers that hold the tube in place. Excessive tension between the internal and external bumpers promotes ulceration and migration of the tube into the muscular layer of the stomach, with the potential for very serious complications. The strain on the tube may be caused by excessive traction at the time of tube insertion, maintenance of a very tight skin disk, or failure to pull back and rotate the disk daily. Other common causes are failure to loosen the external bumper after weight gain and excessive dressings under the external bumper. Unrecognized and untreated, this condition can lead to peritonitis, gastrointestinal bleeding, and death. Signs and symptoms of this condition should be reported to the RN promptly, and include:

- Bleeding from the stoma
- Formula leakage
- Leakage of gastric secretions
- Sudden onset of intolerance to formula that the patient tolerated previously

Reduce the risk for this potential problem by paying close attention to the tension between the external and internal bumpers. Leave a small amount of space between the bumper and skin level.

Infection Control

Enteral nutrition is a potential source of infection. Problems with infection are commonly traced to the formula, substandard handling of nutrient solutions, contamination of the dispensing system, or faulty administration. Tube feeding has been implicated in the transmission and development of pneumonia, bacterial infections, *Clostridium difficile* (*C. diff.*) diarrhea, and other diarrheal illnesses.

The length of time the solution hangs is one consideration in the development of infection. Formula manufacturers have recommendations for maximum hang time of solution. The total hang time is partially determined by the type of delivery system being used. Instructions may be found on the can or bottle, package insert, or the manufacturer's Web site. Never exceed the manufacturer's maximum recommendations. Your facility will have policies and procedures for infection control of the enteral feeding systems. Always follow your facility guidelines. Additional infection control considerations are listed in **Figure 9-7.**

- Use good handwashing and aseptic technique.
- Use gloves for preparing and hanging tube feedings, according to facility policy.
- Avoid contacting the sink area with your hands, and all parts of the tube-feeding system and tubing. The sink is a very contaminated area, and you may inadvertently pick up a pathogen.
- Prepare the tube feeding on a clean work surface. Avoid the sink area.
- Most facilities use tap water in enteral feedings. In some facilities, only sterile water is used for tube feeding, irrigations, and flushes. (This is because Legionnaire's disease has been implicated in several hospitals as a result of tube feeding. Immunocompromised patients may contract other diseases from tap water.) Know and follow your facility policies for the type of water to be used.
- The system used should require minimal handling to assemble, and be compatible with the patient's enteral feeding tube.
- Use a no-touch technique when assembling the system and spiking the formula.
- Avoid contacting the patient's clothing or bedding when attaching the administration set to the feeding tube.
- Feeding bags must be filled with no more than 4 hours' worth of formula.
- Prepackaged (closed-system) containers of formula may hang for up to 24 hours, or according to the manufacturer's recommendation. Change the tubing every 24 hours or when the formula bottle is changed.
- Use undiluted (canned or prefilled) formula whenever possible.
- If powdered formula is used, mix it using cooled boiled water or freshly opened sterile water. Use a no-touch technique. Refrigerate the solution with the date and time on the container label. Use or discard within 24 hours of mixing.

- Formula left in the bag for more than 4 hours encourages bacterial growth.
- Discard any formula left in the bag at the end of 4 hours (then rinse the bag).
- Never add fresh formula to "top off" formula remaining in the feeding bag. This helps prevent bacterial growth.
- Rinse the feeding bag well with tap water every 4 hours, or before adding fresh formula.
- Discard the feeding bag and tubing every 24 hours. Hang a new bag and tubing.
- Bulb or piston syringes are commonly used for bolus feedings, checking tube placement, and irrigation. A catheter irrigation set works well for this purpose. Rinse the syringe well after each use. Keep it covered or in the irrigation setup when not in use. Date the unit when opened, and discard after 24 hours, or according to facility policy.
- When changing the feeding bag, ensure that the bag is labeled with the date, time, and type of formula, additives, and rate of administration. Remember that permanent marker will bleed through plastic. Affix a label or write on a piece of tape.
- Administer enteral formula at room temperature. Commercial formulas may be stored at room temperature until opened.
- If you use a partial can of formula for a feeding, cover the remaining formula. Write the date, time, and your initials on the can. Refrigerate. Use this can for the next feeding (warm to room temperature in hot water; do not serve cold), or discard after 24 hours.
- Wipe the top of the can before opening.
- Cover the tip of the feeding tube with a sterile cap or plug when the tube is not in use.
- Wipe or clean the IV standard, pump, and other permanent equipment used for enteral feeding.

FIGURE 9-7 Infection control considerations in enteral nutrition.

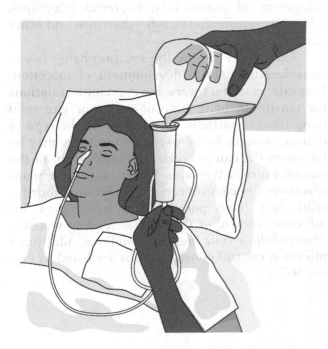

FIGURE 9-8 When using the bolus method of tube feeding, formula enters the stomach by gravity.

Bolus Enteral Feeding

Bolus feeding is an intermittent method of feeding with a syringe. The formula is allowed to flow into the tube by gravity (**Figure 9-8**). Avoid forcing the solution through the tube with the syringe plunger or bulb. After all formula is administered, the tube is flushed with water and clamped. Avoid allowing air into the tube, as it can cause discomfort. Add formula to the syringe before it empties completely. The rate of flow is determined by the height of the syringe. Raising the syringe increases the rate. Lowering the syringe slows the rate.

Procedure 72

Bolus Enteral Feeding

Supplies needed:
- Disposable exam gloves
- 50-mL or 60-mL catheter-tip syringe or irrigation set
- Formula ordered by physician
- Water
- Graduated container
- Clamp, if desired
- Cap or plug for open end of tube
- Plastic bag for used supplies

1. Perform your beginning procedure actions.
2. Verify tube placement.
3. Check for residual. If more than 100 mL, notify the RN before beginning the procedure. Return stomach contents.
4. Shake the formula well. Wipe the top of the can.
5. Remove the plunger or bulb from the catheter-tip syringe.
6. Remove the plunger or bulb from the syringe.
7. Clamp or pinch the feeding tube.
8. Remove the cap or plug from the feeding tube and insert the catheter-tip syringe. Keep the tube clamped or pinched.
9. Fill the syringe with formula.
10. Release the clamp or remove your fingers, allowing the formula to flow in by gravity.
11. Add formula to the syringe when it is ¼ full. Do not allow the syringe to empty.
12. Administer the prescribed amount of formula, then flush the tubing with 30 mL of water, or the amount ordered by the physician.
13. Cap the tube immediately after the water flows through, to prevent air from entering.
14. Perform your procedure completion actions.

Continuous Enteral Tube-Feeding with a Pump

A pump is commonly used to deliver formula to the enteral tube (**Figure 9-9**). The pump delivers a consistent amount of feeding every hour. The solution is usually administered 24 hours a day. Many different pumps are used in health care facilities. The directions for use vary with the type of pump used in your facility.

Drip and pump feedings are administered through an administration set. This set must be primed with formula (**Figure 9-10**). Avoid injecting air into the patient's stomach. The feeding tube is connected directly to the administration set for feeding. A PEG tube is plugged into an adapter, which is connected to the administration set. Make sure the adapter is secure before connecting the administration set. If the adapter is loose, formula will leak into the bed. Another type of gastrostomy tube has a button that sits flat against the skin surface.

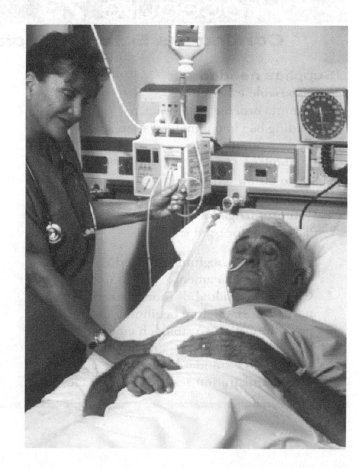

FIGURE 9-9 Tube feedings are commonly delivered through a continuous feeding pump. (Photo used with permission of Ross Products Division, Abbott Laboratories, Columbus, OH)

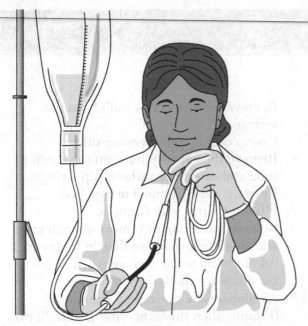

FIGURE 9-10 Prime the tubing with formula before connecting it to the feeding tube.

A special adapter and feeding catheter are used with this type of device.

When you hang a tube feeding, follow your facility policy for marking the date and time on the bag or other container. Like IV solutions, write on a label and affix it to the container. Do not write directly on the plastic. Pathogen growth is possible if formula hangs too long. Formula should not hang for more than 4 hours, or according to facility policy and the manufacturer's recommendations. Never pour new formula on top of formula that is already in the bag used for drip or pump feedings. Rinse the administration set well with water each time formula is added. Change the administration set and tubing every 24 hours. A closed-system feeding set can hang for 24 hours, or longer as recommended by the manufacturer. Closed-system feedings are sterile. If the closed system is used, the formula and administration set are changed at the same time. This system is prepackaged as a single unit, and is not opened to add formula. When the bottle is empty, the unit is discarded and replaced with a new one.

Procedure 73

Continuous Enteral Feeding with a Pump

Supplies needed:

- Disposable exam gloves
- Formula ordered by physician
- Feeding bag and administration set
- Feeding pump
- IV standard
- 30- to 60-mL syringe
- Graduate container
- Water for irrigation
- Plastic bag for used supplies

1. Perform your beginning procedure actions.
2. Verify tube placement.
3. Check for residual. If more than 100 mL, notify the RN before beginning the procedure. Return stomach contents.
4. Attach the feeding bag and administration set to the IV standard. Check the clamp on the administration set. It should be closed.
5. Shake the formula well.
6. Lower the IV standard, if necessary, to a height that you can reach to fill the bag with formula. After filling the bag with the designated amount, elevate it.
7. Open the clamp and prime the tubing for the administration set.
8. Thread the tubing through the pump according to the manufacturer's directions.
9. Attach the primed tubing to the enteral tube.
10. Set the pump to the prescribed rate and turn it on.
11. Stay with the patient for a minute to ensure that he or she is not having problems with the feeding. Make sure the head is elevated 30° to 45° or higher.
12. Perform your procedure completion actions.

EQUIPMENT ALARMS

The tube-feeding pump, as well as many other pieces of equipment used in the health care facility, has a built-in alarm. Some alarms are used as restraint alternatives. With these, the alarm sounds if the patient tries to get up without assistance. Alarms sound when something is wrong. This could be something simple, like an empty formula bag. The alarm may also indicate something more serious, such as an equipment malfunction or a patient in distress.

Always follow facility policies. These vary regarding PCT responsibilities for equipment alarms. Before correcting an equipment alarm, make sure that you are permitted to perform the procedure and that you have been taught to use the equipment. Always notify the RN of the corrective action taken.

Generally speaking, go to the patient's room immediately if you hear an alarm. If the problem is something you can correct, do so. If not, notify the RN of the alarm immediately. Do not turn the alarm off and walk away. If you turn the alarm off, remain in the room until the RN arrives.

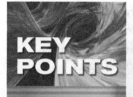

KEY POINTS

▶ A nasogastric tube is inserted through the nose and threaded through the esophagus to the stomach.

▶ A gastrostomy tube is surgically inserted through the abdominal wall into the stomach.

▶ A PEG tube is surgically inserted by the physician, using an endoscope. The tube is threaded down the esophagus and exits through an incision in the abdomen over the stomach.

▶ The jejunostomy tube (J-tube) is threaded through the GI tract until the tip reaches the small intestine. It is used for patients who do not have a stomach and for those in whom aspiration is a problem.

▶ A gastrostomy feeding button is an alternative feeding device used for some ambulatory patients who are receiving long-term enteral feedings.

▶ An enteral tube is a catheter, stoma, or tube such as a nasogastric, gastrostomy, or jejunostomy tube used to provide nutrition and deliver nutrients to the gastrointestinal tract, distal to the oral cavity. The tubes may also be called enteral access devices.

▶ Peritonitis is a very serious inflammation of the peritoneum. It may develop as a complication of intestinal perforation from a tube, and may become life-threatening. The outcome is often poor, and the condition may result in serious complications, including death.

▶ Buried bumper syndrome is an ulceration of the tissue at the feeding tube exit site or the internal mucosal layer of the gastric wall. This syndrome may develop if the tubes used have internal and external retention bumpers that hold the tube in place. Tension between the internal and external bumpers promotes ulceration and migration of the tube into the muscular layer of the stomach, with the potential for very serious complications.

▶ Feeding tubes are inserted to withdraw samples of gastric contents for tests, to wash the stomach in certain medical conditions, because of surgical procedures, when patients cannot eat normally, when patients are unconscious, for patients who are unable to swallow, and to prevent or treat weight loss.

▶ The head of the bed must be elevated at least 30° to 45° when the feeding is administered, and for an hour after meals. This position increases the risk of pressure ulcers, so preventive measures must be employed.

(continues)

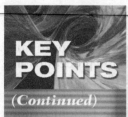

KEY POINTS

(Continued)

▶ Patients receiving tube feedings need frequent mouth care.

▶ For enteral tube procedures, use a syringe at least 30 mL or larger, to prevent complications.

▶ The position of the nasogastric tube must be checked carefully upon insertion and before feeding to ensure that the tube is not in the lungs.

▶ Observing gastric contents and checking the pH are the most accurate bedside methods of checking enteral tube placement.

▶ Tube feeding should be withheld if 100 mL of formula, or 1½ times the hourly amount, remain in the stomach.

▶ Stomach contents are replaced after checking the pH or determining feeding residual.

▶ Observe the gastrostomy tube insertion site for redness, drainage, irritation, and induration.

▶ Change the dressing over the gastrostomy tube insertion site as often as necessary until the site is healed; after it has healed, no dressing is necessary.

▶ Avoid dislodging the feeding tube when moving the patient.

▶ A Foley catheter is not used in place of a gastrostomy tube; the stomach acids erode the catheter.

▶ Half-strength peroxide is used to remove secretions around the gastrostomy tube insertion site; rinse the solution well.

▶ Tube-feeding formula may be administered by the bolus, continuous or intermittent drip, or pump methods.

▶ Patients with tube feedings can and do become dehydrated.

▶ Enteral formulas contain approximately 15 percent solids.

▶ Most tube-feeding formulas deliver 1 calorie per mL.

▶ Tube-feeding formulas address specific nutritional problems.

▶ The dietitian will follow patients who are receiving tube feedings, and will make recommendations for their care.

▶ Enteral nutrition is a potential source of infection. Infection is commonly traced to the formula, substandard handling of nutrient solutions, contamination of the dispensing system, or faulty administration. Tube feeding has been implicated in the transmission and development of pneumonia, bacterial infections, *Clostridium difficile* diarrhea, and other diarrheal illnesses.

▶ Use good aseptic technique when administering tube feedings and handling feeding equipment.

▶ Formula should not hang for more than 4 hours, or according to the manufacturer's recommendation, unless a closed system is used.

▶ Administer formula at room temperature.

▶ Label the continuous tube-feeding administration set with the date and time that formula was added.

▶ The length of time the solution hangs is one consideration in the development of infection. Follow manufacturers' recommendations and facility guidelines for formula hang time and changing the various components of the tube-feeding system.

(continues)

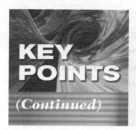

▶ If the patient is coughing, vomiting, choking, gagging, burping, or having difficulty breathing, stop the formula, stay in the room, and call for immediate assistance.

▶ Go to the patient's room immediately if you hear an equipment alarm. Correct the problem, if permitted, and notify the RN of the situation.

CLINICAL APPLICATIONS

1. You are inserting a nasogastric tube in Mrs. Elam. She begins coughing and choking when you pass the tube through her throat. What should you do?

2. Mrs. Elam's nasogastric tube has been inserted successfully. She is receiving full-strength formula. When you reposition the patient, she vomits. What action will you take?

3. Mr. Strong is being fed by a gastrostomy tube attached to a pump. You enter Mr. Strong's room. The tube feeding is running. The patient is positioned on his left side. The head of the bed is flat. Mr. Strong is sleeping and is in no distress. What action will you take?

4. Late in the shift, the alarm sounds on Mr. Strong's tube-feeding pump. When you enter the room, you notice that the bag of tube-feeding solution is empty. What action will you take?

5. You are assigned to check Miss Haley's feeding residual, then add 2 cans of formula to her continuous drip tube-feeding infusion. You must also verify tube placement, using the pH method. The pH of the fluid aspirated from the tube is 5.0. You aspirate 200 mL of solution from the tube. Approximately 100 mL remains in the bag of feeding solution. What action will you take?

CHAPTER REVIEW

Multiple-Choice Questions

Select the one best answer.

1. A gastrostomy tube is:
   a. threaded through the nose into the esophagus.
   b. threaded through the nose into the stomach.
   c. surgically inserted through the abdominal wall.
   d. surgically threaded through the esophagus.

2. Enteral tubes are used for all of the following *except*:
   a. to treat weight loss.
   b. to obtain specimens for laboratory analysis.
   c. to wash the stomach in some medical conditions.
   d. patients who are combative at mealtime.

3. The most accurate bedside method of checking for enteral tube placement is:
   a. placing the end of the tube in a glass of water and checking for bubbles.
   b. checking the pH of fluid aspirated from the tube.
   c. auscultating over the stomach while injecting air into the tube.
   d. aspirating a small amount of fluid and checking the appearance.

4. The pH of fluid aspirated from the stomach is usually:
   a. 0 to 5.
   b. 2 to 7.
   c. 7 to 8.
   d. 8 to 12.

5. You withdraw fluid from the gastrostomy tube to check residual before hanging the next feeding. 60 mL are withdrawn. The feeding runs at 75 mL per hour. The bag is empty. You should:
   a. withhold the feeding and promptly notify the RN.
   b. discard the fluid removed from the stomach and notify the RN.
   c. return the fluid to the stomach and hang the feeding immediately.
   d. return the fluid to the stomach, rinse the bag, and hang the feeding.

6. You are administering a gastrostomy tube feeding by the bolus method. You should:
   a. inject the fluid with a bulb syringe.
   b. allow the fluid to flow in by gravity, adding fluid before the syringe empties.
   c. allow the fluid to flow in by gravity, adding fluid after the syringe empties.
   d. administer the fluid by connecting an administration set and adaptor to the gastrostomy tube.

7. Mrs. Roosevelt's gastrostomy tube was inserted three days ago. You must cleanse the insertion site. You will:
   a. use aseptic technique.
   b. lift the disk before beginning.
   c. wash the area well with soap and water.
   d. scrub well, using a side-to-side motion.

8. You have half a can of formula remaining after administering a bolus tube feeding. You should:
   a. discard the formula.
   b. cover, label, and date the can and refrigerate it.
   c. administer the remainder of the formula.
   d. ask the RN what to do.

9. Tube-feeding formula in an open-system bag should hang for:
   a. 2 hours or less.
   b. no more than 4 hours.
   c. no more than 8 hours.
   d. no more than 24 hours.

10. The alarm on a patient's tube-feeding pump sounds. You should:
    a. ignore it if you are not assigned to the patient.
    b. tell the RN that the alarm is sounding.
    c. turn off the alarm until the RN checks the patient on rounds.
    d. go to the room and troubleshoot the cause of the problem.

11. A nasogastric tube is usually inserted in patients who require tube feeding:
    a. for approximately seven days or less.
    b. for a year or more.
    c. once a day.
    d. permanently, for the remainder of the patient's life.

12. The gastrostomy tube button is most commonly used for:
    a. dependent, bedfast patients.
    b. alert patients.
    c. ambulatory patients.
    d. cooperative patients.

13. Gastrostomy tubes are:
    a. changed once a month.
    b. not routinely changed.
    c. changed weekly.
    d. never changed.

14. Peritonitis is:
    a. an ulceration of the esophagus.
    b. blockage of the lower intestine.
    c. not a serious condition, except in children.
    d. inflammation of the peritoneum.

15. A fenestrated drape:
    a. is always sterile.
    b. is never sterile.
    c. has a hole in the center.
    d. is folded in half when used.

16. An enteral tube:
    a. conducts nutrients and fluids into the GI tract.
    b. is used only for patients who are at risk of choking.
    c. provides total nutrition through the venous system.
    d. is used only for confused patients.

17. Enteral formulas are:
    a. comparable to milk.
    b. about 20 percent liquid.
    c. for oral consumption.
    d. about 15 percent solid.

18. The buried bumper syndrome:
    a. may be caused by excessive dressings under the external bumper.
    b. is an inflammation of the esophagus caused by excessive vomiting.
    c. is an ulceration caused by undue tension on the PEG tube bumpers.
    d. is a common complication of peritonitis.

19. Always prepare the enteral feeding solution:
    a. at the sink.
    b. on a clean workspace.
    c. in the bathroom.
    d. in a sterile area.

20. Wipe or clean the IV standard, pump, and other permanent equipment used for enteral feeding:
    a. weekly.
    b. daily.
    c. every three days.
    d. hourly.

EXPLORING THE WEB

All about Tubes: Your Guide to Enteral Feeding Devices. Nursing 2000	http://www.findarticles.com
ASPEN Standards of Practice for Nutrition Support Nurses	http://www.clinnutr.org
DADS Medical Quality Assurance Vision for Tube Feeding	http://mqa.dhs.state.tx.us
Enteral and Parenteral Nutrition: Evidence-Based Approach	http://www.cabi-publishing.org
Enteral Nutrition	http://healthlinks.washington.edu
Enteral Nutrition in the Critically Ill Adult—Practice Guidelines	http://www.criticalcarenutrition.com
Enteral Nutrition—Problem Solving Guide	http://www.criticalcarenutrition.com
Gastrostomy	http://atoz.iqhealth.com
Gastrostomy	http://www.chclibrary.org
Medical Position Statement: Guidelines for the Use of Enteral Nutrition	http://www3.us.elsevierhealth.com
Percutaneous Endoscopic Gastrostomy: Clinical Applications	http://www.medscape.com
Role of Percutaneous Endoscopic Gastrostomy	http://www.sages.org
Rotherham Clinical Policies and Procedures	http://www.rotherhampct.nhs.uk
Vanderbilt University Policies Gastrostomy Care & Management	http://vumcpolicies.mc.vanderbilt.edu

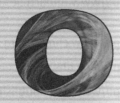

CHAPTER 10

Specimen Collection

OBJECTIVES:

After reading this chapter, you should be able to:

- Spell and define key terms.
- List the guidelines for specimen collection.
- Describe patient preparation for specimen collection.
- State the purpose of culture and sensitivity testing.
- Identify common complications of Group A Strep infection and state why identifying this pathogen quickly is important.
- State the purpose of obtaining a swab specimen from a wound bed, and describe how this is done.
- Define sputum, and describe where this body fluid is located.
- State the purpose of gastric analysis.
- State the purpose of collecting a 24-hour urine specimen.
- Describe the monitoring and nursing care for a patient with renal calculi.
- Describe how to collect a urine specimen from a child who does not have bladder control.
- State the purpose of performing the Hemoccult test on stool.
- Explain how to collect a stool specimen and rectal swab specimen for culture and sensitivity testing.
- List the normal blood sugar range.
- List at least 15 infection control precautions for blood glucose monitoring, and state why using good technique is important for this procedure.
- State the purpose of testing for glycated hemoglobin.

SPECIMEN COLLECTION

You may be responsible for collecting specimens. Bedside testing is done on some blood samples. Others are sent to the laboratory for analysis. The physician will use the information gathered to aid in diagnosis and treatment of the patient. Collecting specimens accurately is an important responsibility. The collection container must be labeled with the patient's name and other information required by your health care facility. A laboratory requisition is completed and attached to each specimen. The req-

uisition contains identifying patient information and specifies the type of test to be done. Specimens are biohazardous materials. They must be labeled as such, and transported and discarded according to facility policy. Follow your facility policy for labeling the specimen collection container and completing the laboratory requisition form.

The three enemies of specimen collection are:

- Time (in terms of transporting the specimen)
- Temperature (avoid extremes)
- Desiccation (do not let the specimen dry out)

Guidelines for Collecting a Specimen

- Apply the principles of standard precautions. Avoid environmental contamination from your gloves.
- Make sure to collect a sufficient quantity of the specimen material.
- Regard each specimen as irreplaceable.
- Check your facility infection control or laboratory manual to become familiar with the policies and procedures for the sample you are obtaining.
- If you must remove the lid to a specimen collection container, always place it top side down on the table, so that the clean inner side faces up.
- Avoid touching the inside of the collection container or lid with your hands.
- Some specimens, such as urine or feces, must be transferred into another container. Pour or transfer

the specimen carefully to avoid splashing and contamination. If you will be placing the container on a counter or other flat surface, place a paper towel under it.

- After you have collected the specimen, put the lid on the container and place it in a sealed transport bag labeled with a biohazardous waste emblem. The **transport bag** is a plastic bag that can be sealed tightly to prevent leaking.
- If the specimen cannot be transported to the lab immediately, it can be stored in a designated refrigerator or cooler for lab specimens. Follow the storage directions for the specimen you have collected. The refrigerator must be marked with the biohazard emblem. Avoid storing laboratory specimens in a refrigerator with food, beverages, or medications.

Preparing the Patient

The patient may feel anxious about specimen collection. Always explain the procedure to the patient and allow him or her to ask questions. Describe what the patient can expect. For example, when collecting a throat culture, the patient may experience a gagging sensation. When collecting blood for a fingerstick blood sugar, the patient will feel the needlestick. Inform him or her in advance. If the patient asks a question and you do not know the answer, check with the RN. If the patient refuses to have the test done, stop the procedure and notify the RN.

If the patient must collect the specimen, such as a urine sample, make sure that he or she understands the directions. When explaining the procedure, always describe container handling. Describe how to place the lid on the table, with the sterile, inner side facing up. Instruct the patient not to touch the inside of the collection device with the fingers. Handling the inside of the container or lid will contaminate the specimen. Get feedback by asking the patient to repeat the instructions.

Sometimes special measures must be taken before a specimen can be collected. For example, the patient may require a special diet before testing. For many lab tests, the patient must be fasting, or NPO, for a period of time before the specimen is collected. Make certain the patient understands food and fluid restrictions. After you have collected the specimen, inform the RN, who will release fluid, food, and medication restrictions.

Personal Protective Equipment

Specimens for laboratory analysis are always infectious. The information gathered by analyzing blood, body fluids, secretions, and excretions provides important information about how the body is functioning. Because specimen collection always involves handling biohazardous materials, apply the principles of standard precautions. Select the personal protective equipment you will need during the procedure, and bring it to the room before beginning.

CULTURE AND SENSITIVITY TESTING

Culture and sensitivity testing is done to look for the presence of pathogens in exudate in body fluids, secretions, excretions, and from body cavities and wounds. The culture component of the test determines if a pathogen is present, and, if so, whether the pathogen growth is heavy or light. The culture identifies the specific pathogen that is causing the infection. The sensitivity part of the test shows which antibiotics will best eradicate the pathogen. The physician uses this information to treat the infection. From the time the test is collected, it takes approximately three days to get the complete results, although preliminary results of the culture are available every 24 hours. Cultures are always collected in sterile containers. Avoiding external contamination is very important when collecting culture and sensitivity tests. Send the specimen to the laboratory immediately after collection.

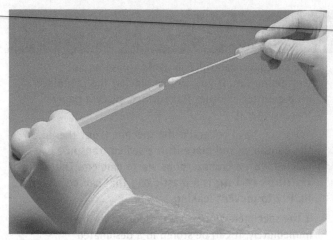

FIGURE 10-1 The swab is inserted into the plastic container. After the container is tightly sealed, squeeze the bottom to crush the ampule of transport medium to preserve the specimen.

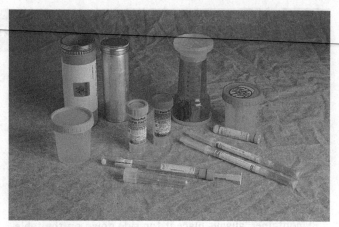

FIGURE 10-2 Cultures are always collected in sterile containers. Various containers are used, depending on the type of specimen being collected.

Swab Cultures

A culturette is used for collecting swab cultures. The device looks like a sterile applicator in a plastic tube. After the specimen is collected, the applicator is inserted into the tube (**Figure 10-1**), which must be closed tightly. The bottom of the tube contains a special transport medium in an ampule. This medium preserves the specimen properly. Squeeze the bottom of the outer plastic tube to break the ampule, if the swab is being used for culture and sensitivity testing. Push the applicator down, well into the medium, to keep it moist. Sometimes a swab specimen is collected for a test called *Gram stain*. If this is the case, *do not break the ampule* in the bottom of the culturette. The culture medium in the ampule may interfere with the Gram stain test. Transport the tube to the laboratory immediately after collection, with the proper label and requisition form.

Secretion, Excretion, and Body Fluid Cultures

Specimens collected for body fluid cultures are collected in various types of sterile containers (**Figure 10-2**). If you are unsure about which type of container to use, check with the RN or the laboratory

procedure manual. Some procedures require special patient preparation, such as cleansing the perineal area before collecting a urine culture.

Collecting Culture and Sensitivity Tests

Proper collection of laboratory specimens is essential to good patient care. The physician and others depend on laboratory results to guide treatment of patients. A poorly collected or transported specimen may cause inaccurate test results or diagnostic testing of normal flora, leading to improper patient treatment. It may also result in failure to isolate the causative microorganism. The laboratory must provide complete guidelines for collection and transport of specimens to ensure quality patient care. In most facilities, a laboratory manual is available that describes safety considerations, procedures for proper specimen collection, special patient preparation (such as NPO), special handling requirements for the specimen, and so forth. The diagnostic information received from the laboratory depends on the technique used in specimen collection and the quality of the specimen received.

When collecting a specimen, follow the guidelines in the accompanying box.

Guidelines for Collecting Culture and Sensitivity Specimens

- Apply the principles of standard precautions.
- Select the PPE necessary to do the task, including protective eyewear, face masks, or hoods, if necessary.

- Treat all specimens as biohazardous substances.
- Take care to avoid contaminating the work surface, the outside of the collection container, the laboratory requisition, and other paperwork.

(continues)

Guidelines for Collecting Culture and Sensitivity Specimens (Continued)

- Make sure the specimen is properly labeled with the patient's name, unit identification number, and specimen type.

- Minimize direct handling during transportation of specimens to the lab. Use a sealable transport bag or container that is properly labeled. The transport bag should have a separate pouch for the lab requisition slip.

- Most specimens obtained by needle (butterfly) aspiration should be transferred to a sterile tube or anaerobic transport vial before the specimen is sent to the laboratory. Dispose of the needle and syringe properly.

- Collect culture and sensitivity specimens before antibiotics are administered, if possible. If this causes a prolonged delay, check with the RN.

- Use good technique to avoid picking up normal body flora and environmental contaminants.

- Use the proper collection device. Use a sturdy, screw-cap, leakproof container with a lid that does not create an aerosol when opened. Always use sterile equipment and aseptic technique.

- Collect an adequate amount of specimen. An inadequate amount of specimen may yield false negative results.

- Mark the requisition or follow facility policy to inform the laboratory when unusual pathogens are suspected or if the physician orders a "rule-out" test.

- Identify the specimen source and specific body collection site so that the laboratory staff can select the proper culture media.

- If a specimen must be collected through intact skin, cleanse the skin well, such as by using 70 percent alcohol or povidone–iodine. (Make sure the patient does not have an iodine allergy.) Cleanse excess iodine from the skin after the specimen is collected.

- Some specimens may be refrigerated, if necessary, but the best practice is to transport the specimen to the laboratory promptly. If you anticipate a transportation delay, check the lab procedure manual for instructions on storing and preserving the specimen.

- If a pneumatic tube transport system is used for lab specimens, check the laboratory manual or pneumatic tube manual for specific instructions on sending specimens through this system.

THROAT CULTURE

The throat culture is a swab culture. Position the patient in a sitting position. Remind him or her that the procedure may cause slight gagging, but that it will be over quickly. When you are ready to collect the specimen, ask the patient to tip the head back. Depress the tongue with a tongue blade. If the patient begins to gag, remove the tongue blade for a moment. When you reinsert the tongue blade, place it closer to the front of the tongue than you did previously. While holding the tongue down, use a flashlight to look at the throat. Look for inflamed areas or white pustular areas. Make sure you swab these when you begin the culture.

To collect the specimen, depress the tongue once again with the tongue depressor. Collect the swab from the back of the throat (**Figure 10-3**). Wipe the tonsil area from side to side with the applicator (**Figure 10-4**). Swab all areas. Avoid touching the tongue with the applicator. Touching the tongue contaminates the specimen with the bacteria in the mouth.

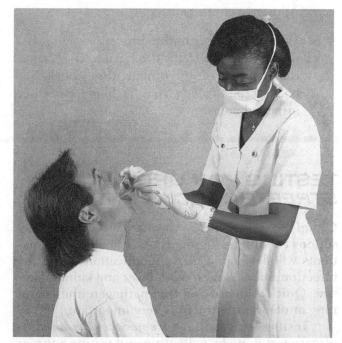

FIGURE 10-3 Depress the tongue with the tongue blade, then carefully insert the swab. Avoid touching the tongue.

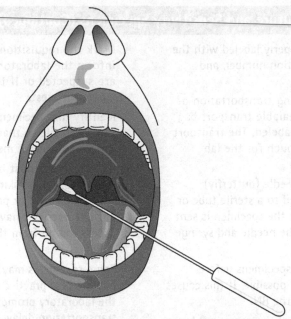

FIGURE 10-4 Swab the back of the throat from side to side.

Procedure 74

Collecting a Throat Culture

Supplies needed:
▶ Disposable exam gloves
▶ Surgical mask
▶ Tongue blade
▶ Flashlight or penlight
▶ Culturette container

1. Perform your beginning procedure actions.
2. Ask the patient to tilt the head back. Place a tongue blade on the tongue, then check the back of the throat with a flashlight for red or inflamed areas.

3. Remove the tongue blade and flashlight.
4. Remove the culturette from the plastic tube.
5. Depress the tongue with the tongue blade, using your nondominant hand.
6. With your dominant hand, swab the throat from side to side with the culturette. Avoid the tongue.
7. Remove the culturette and insert it in the plastic tube. Crush the ampule of transport medium in the bottom of the tube. Push the swab down into the medium.
8. Perform your procedure completion actions.

TESTING FOR GROUP A *STREPTOCOCCUS* ANTIGEN

Group A *Streptococcus pyogenes* causes many very serious conditions. If not properly treated, some patients will develop serious complications from this infection, such as rheumatic fever and kidney damage. Quickly identifying this pathogen and beginning antibiotic treatment is very important.

Testing for group A *Streptococcus* is a point-of-care test done by collecting and testing a throat swab. Many different kits are available for per-forming this test, and the instructions vary for each. Facility policies also vary. In some facilities, you will be expected to use the test kit to test the results of the swab. False negative results sometimes occur. Because of this, the laboratory will verify the test results. In other facilities, nursing department staff collect the specimen and all testing is done by the laboratory. Know and follow your facility policies. If you are testing the sample, you must follow the manufacturer's directions for the kit you are using exactly. There is no margin of error with this test.

The physician may order both a throat culture and a test for group A *Streptococcus* antigen. It is a good idea to collect two swabs. The swab used for the Strep A testing must be dacron, not cotton. Make sure you have the proper equipment to collect the specimen. The culturettes used in your facility probably meet the requirement for Strep A testing, but verify that the swab is dacron before you collect a specimen.

Poor throat sampling technique may miss the group A *Streptococci* in the patient's pharynx, resulting in false negative testing. Take care to use good technique to collect a swab specimen from the tonsils and posterior pharynx. If you see inflamed areas, vesicles, and pustular tonsils, make sure to swab these areas. Avoid the tongue, inner cheeks, teeth, and gums. Withdraw the swab and insert it into the culture tube. Crush the ampule of culture medium at the bottom of the tube, and then push the swab down into the medium to keep it moist. Maintain the swab at room temperature, and transport it to the lab promptly.

WOUND INFECTION

Many factors affect wound healing. One of these is the presence of infection. Pathogens in the wound compete for the substances needed for healing. If the patient's ability to heal is already compromised, the presence of pathogens in the wound bed may tip the scales toward not healing. Signs of infection commonly include:

- Increased pain.
- Erythema or increasing abnormal redness and inflammation due to capillary congestion and dilation.
- Discoloration of formerly healthy tissue in the wound bed, such as changing from bright red to a pale grey or deep red color.
- Tissue in the wound bed becoming more fragile.
- Increased bleeding.
- Increased drainage that may be watery or serous in appearance. However, it may also be cloudy, puslike, or have an abnormal color, such as yellow or green.
- Wound or drainage that develops a foul odor.
- Fever.
- Wound that stops healing or shows signs of worsening.

All Stage II, III, and IV pressure ulcers become colonized with bacteria. Because of this, we do not routinely culture all wounds until we suspect infection. **Colonization** is the multiplication of a microbe after it has invaded the wound. When a wound is colonized, the microbe has successfully reproduced. The bacteria are present on the surface or in the deeper tissue without signs or symptoms of infection. Usually, using standard precautions and good technique for cleansing and wound care prevents bacterial colonization from progressing to the point of infection. Treated properly, a colonized ulcer will heal. An infected wound will not heal until the infection has been eliminated. Effective cleansing will remove the debris that supports bacterial growth and delays wound healing. The longer a wound remains in a nonhealing state, the more likely it is to become infected, and the less likely it is to heal. For example, a clean, Stage II pressure ulcer should show signs of healing within several weeks.

By definition, wound infection implies that pathogens in the wound are harming the host. Wound infection occurs when pathogens within the wound negatively affect the patient. Signs and symptoms may be subtle if the patient is otherwise in good health. If the infection progresses untreated, it will become systemic. A **systemic infection** spreads throughout the body, affecting many systems or organs. It is not confined to one spot area. This infection is serious and often becomes life-threatening.

If wound healing does not occur, the RN must evaluate the entire treatment plan. Inform the RN promptly if signs of infection are present. The RN may also request the assistance of other members of the interdisciplinary team, such as the dietitian and infection control nurse. Using the team approach improves the chances of successful wound healing. Nursing personnel must always be alert to signs of infection and act promptly if they occur. To reduce the risk of spreading the organisms, drainage must be controlled. Monitor infected wounds daily. The RN will take weekly measurements and assess the color and exudate of the wound. If the wound improves or worsens, inform the RN promptly. Do not wait for his or her weekly evaluation. Monitoring progress, being aware of the factors affecting healing and the phases of healing, and being able to identify abnormalities mean that problematic wounds can be identified and treated promptly.

Wound Cultures

Obtaining a wound culture is a simple procedure, but careful technique is essential. The technique used for culturing wounds is an area of great controversy, and requires further study. We have practiced the technique of using a swab for culture sampling for more than 100 years. Although other techniques have been recommended, in many facilities, a regular swab culture is done to identify the presence of pathogens in a wound in which infection is suspected.

Procedure 75

Obtaining a Swab Culture from a Wound

Supplies needed:
▶ Disposable exam gloves
▶ Sterile gloves
▶ Sterile culturette
▶ Sterile normal saline
▶ 4 gauze 4 × 4 sponges
▶ Sterile dressing materials
▶ Plastic bag for used supplies

1. Perform your beginning procedure actions.
2. Open packages. Maintain sterility of the contents. Position these so that you do not cross over sterile supplies when discarding used items.
3. Loosen tape and remove the soiled dressing. Discard tape and dressing in the plastic bag.
4. Cleanse the wound using 4 × 4 sponges and sterile saline. Moisten one sponge. Wipe across the wound in one direction, then discard the sponge in the plastic bag. Repeat until you have cleansed the entire wound. If excessive debris remains on the surface, repeat the procedure.
5. Remove gloves.
6. Wash your hands, or use alcohol-based hand cleaner.
7. Apply sterile gloves.
8. Hold the culturette in one hand. With the other hand, remove the cap and attached sterile applicator.
9. Follow facility policy for swabbing the wound. Avoid areas of eschar. Do not touch the skin surrounding the wound. Swab only the open wound bed. Common techniques are:
   ▶ First, cleanse the skin surrounding the wound.
   ▶ Roll the applicator over once (Figure 10-5A). Ensure that the entire applicator has contacted the wound bed.
   ▶ Swab the wound gently. Press the wound edges gently, if necessary, to obtain discharge on the applicator.

Culturing Technique

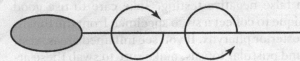

FIGURE 10-5(A) Roll the applicator over once to ensure that the entire applicator has contacted the wound bed.

   ▶ Swab the wound using a zigzag motion (Figure 10-5B).
   ▶ If the wound is deep, insert a swab into the deepest part, and rotate it to obtain drainage.
   ▶ If the wound is dry, check with the RN. In some facilities the transport medium in the culturette is crushed to moisten the swab. The swab is removed, then the sample is obtained using the moistened applicator. Rotate the swab in the wound surface.
10. Carefully return the applicator to the tube and cap the tube. Avoid touching your glove or other surfaces with the applicator.

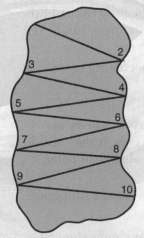

• Thoroughly rinse wound with sterile saline before culturing

• Do not use pus to culture

• Do not swab over hard eschar

• Use sterile Ca Alginate swab or rayon (not cotton) swab

• Rotate swab

• Swab wound edges and 10-pt coverage

FIGURE 10-5(B) Swab the wound using a zigzag motion, working from top to bottom.

(continues)

Procedure 75, *continued*

Obtaining a Swab Culture from a Wound

11. Crush the ampule of transport medium and push the swab down into the liquid if a culture and sensitivity test has been ordered. Do not break the inner capsule if a Gram stain has been ordered.
12. Apply new dressings to the wound.
13. Discard all trash in the plastic bag. Tie the bag for disposal in the biohazardous waste.
14. Perform your procedure completion actions.

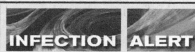
INFECTION ALERT

To reduce the risk of skin contamination, cleanse the area surrounding the wound with chlorhexidine or an alcohol or povidone–iodine sponge, and allow to dry before collecting the culture. Take care to avoid red, open, or macerated areas, as the product may cause burning. Never use alcohol on the perineal area. Make sure the alcohol or povidone-iodine does not enter the wound.

SPUTUM CULTURE

Sputum is a secretion from the mucous membranes lining the trachea and lungs. A sputum culture is collected to identify pathogens in the respiratory tract. This specimen is collected by the patient. You will provide the sputum collection container and give very specific instructions. The patient must understand that the fluid collected must be from the lungs, not saliva from the mouth.

A sputum specimen is best collected early in the morning, if possible. This will capture secretions that have accumulated overnight. If the patient wears dentures, it is best to remove them, so they are not accidentally coughed out during specimen collection. If possible, instruct the patient to rinse the mouth with water before collecting the specimen. This reduces contamination from microbes in the mouth. Avoid using mouthwash or toothpaste, which contain alcohol, or other antimicrobial products. The patient should be in a sitting position when he or she produces a sputum specimen. If possible, obtain 15 mL of fluid. Follow your facility policies for labeling the container. Transport the specimen to the laboratory immediately.

Procedure 76

Collecting A Sputum Specimen

Supplies needed:
- Disposable exam gloves
- Surgical mask
- Gown, mask, goggles, if needed, or according to facility policy
- Emesis basin
- Sputum collection container
- Alcohol or other disinfectant

1. Perform your beginning procedure actions.
2. Instruct the patient to rinse the mouth with water, then spit it into the emesis basin.

3. Advise the patient to take several deep breaths, then **expectorate** sputum from the lungs into the collection device. To *expectorate* means to spit or eject fluid from the mouth. After the patient's sample is in the collection device, cap the device securely.
4. After the specimen is obtained, handle the container with gloves. Disinfect the outside of the container with alcohol or facility-approved disinfectant solution before affixing the label or handling the container with your hands.
5. Perform your procedure completion actions.

GASTRIC SPECIMEN

Occasionally, the physician may order a test called **gastric analysis** to check for the presence of acid in the stomach. To perform this test, a nasogastric tube must be inserted (see Procedure 65). The patient must be fasting when the speci-mens are collected. Collecting fluid for gastric analysis is a multistep procedure that is done over several hours.

Position the head of the bed in the semi-Fowler's position for this procedure. In some facilities, this procedure must be performed by an RN, and you will assist. Know and follow your facility policy.

Procedure 77

Collecting a Specimen for Gastric Analysis

Supplies needed:
- Disposable exam gloves
- Supplies for nasogastric tube insertion
- Sterile irrigation kit, or bulb syringe and medium-size basin
- 12 sterile specimen collection containers with lids, labeled #1 through #12

1. Perform your beginning procedure actions.
2. Insert a nasogastric tube, if not already in place (Procedure 65).
3. Tape the nasogastric tube securely to the patient's nose, according to facility policy.
4. Attach the bulb syringe to the nasogastric tube. Withdraw the gastric contents. Discard in the basin.
5. Wait 15 minutes.
6. Collect 4 additional gastric specimens, each 15 minutes apart. Place each specimen in a separate container, using the containers labeled #1 through #4.
7. Inform the RN when the last specimen has been collected. He or she will administer an injection to stimulate acid production in the stomach.
8. Wait 15 to 30 minutes, or the time designated by facility policy.
9. Collect 8 additional gastric fluid specimens, each 15 minutes apart. Place these in the specimen collection containers labeled #5 through #12.
10. Obtain instructions from the RN on whether to leave the nasogastric tube in place or remove the tube.
11. Perform your procedure completion actions.

URINE SPECIMEN COLLECTION

Many different tests are done on urine samples. Special collection techniques are necessary for certain tests. Following the directions for specimen collection is important to ensure accurate results.

Midstream Urine Specimen

A **midstream (clean-catch) urine specimen** is collected to learn if an infection is present. The sample is collected from the middle of the urinary stream and is as sterile as possible. The cup in which the specimen is collected is sterile. Urine in the bladder is normally sterile. Precautions are taken to avoid contamination when obtaining the specimen.

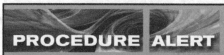

PROCEDURE ALERT

The first morning void is preferred for a midstream specimen. A minimum of 10 to 15 mL of urine is necessary.

The perineum is washed before collecting the specimen to eliminate microbes on the skin. The patient starts to void into the toilet or other container. Voiding washes additional microbes off the skin. The sterile specimen collection container is then placed under the urethra, and the patient voids into the container until an adequate amount of urine is obtained. The cup is removed and the patient finishes the elimination in the toilet.

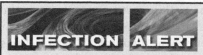

INFECTION ALERT

Perineal care is one of the most important procedures the PCT will perform. Always apply the principles of standard precautions. Remember that there are mucous membranes in the genital area, so if you are wearing gloves, change them before beginning perineal care. Proper technique is critical because of the high risk of contamination and infection. Avoid scrubbing back and forth. Always wipe from clean to dirty with a single wipe, then turn or discard the cloth, according to facility policy. Guidelines for female perineal care vary with the institution. In some facilities, you will be instructed to clean the center first, then each side. In others, you will clean the sides of the genitalia first, then the center. Know and follow your facility policies. Discard your gloves properly and avoid contaminating environmental surfaces with your used gloves.

Procedure 78

Collecting a Midstream Urine Sample

NOTE: The guidelines and sequence for this procedure vary slightly from state to state and from one facility to the next. Your instructor will inform you if the sequence in your state or facility differs from the procedure listed here. Know and follow the required sequence for your state requirements and facility policies.

Supplies needed:

▶ Disposable exam gloves
▶ Bedpan, urinal, commode, or toilet
▶ Paper towel
▶ Midstream urine collection kit OR
  —Washbasin of water
  —Soap or facility-approved cleansing solution
  —Towel
  —3 sterile 4 × 4 gauze sponges
  —Sterile specimen collection cup with lid
  —Transport bag with biohazard label
  —Plastic bag for used supplies

1. Perform your beginning procedure actions.
2. Cleanse the labia in the female with soap and water or a facility-approved cleansing solution.
   a. Separate the labia with the thumb and forefinger.
   b. Wipe down the center of the inner labia from front to back; wipe only once. Discard the gauze sponge.
   c. Wipe down the far side of the inner labia from front to back; wipe only once. Discard the gauze sponge.
   d. Wipe down the near side of the inner labia from front to back; wipe only once. Discard the gauze sponge.

   Cleanse the penis in the male patient with soap and water or a facility-approved cleansing solution.
   a. Retract the foreskin.
   b. Cleanse the penis in a circular motion, beginning at the urethra; wipe only once. Discard the gauze sponge.
   c. Cleanse the penis in another circle, extending to a larger area than the first; wipe only once. Discard the gauze sponge.
   d. Cleanse the penis in another circle, extending to a larger area; wipe only once. Discard the gauze sponge.
3. Instruct the female patient to hold the labia apart after cleansing, or hold them apart with your gloved hand.
   Instruct the male patient to keep the foreskin retracted until after voiding, or hold it with your gloved hand.
4. Instruct the patient to begin voiding in the bedpan, urinal, toilet, or commode.
5. Without stopping the flow of urine, place the specimen collection cup under the urine stream. Collect an adequate amount of urine in the cup: 30 mL to 50 mL, or according to facility policy.
6. Remove the specimen cup, cap it, and place it on a paper towel. Allow the patient to finish voiding in the toilet.
7. Instruct the patient to wash hands. Assist, if necessary.
8. Perform your procedure completion actions.

24-Hour Urine Collection

The human body secretes hormones, electrolytes, and proteins in the urine over a 24-hour period. To test for these substances, a 24-hour urine sample is collected. All urine excreted by the patient is collected for 24 hours. The physician may also order timed specimens for other intervals. Sometimes timed specimens are collected after certain medications are administered by the RN. The specimen collection period starts when the patient has an empty bladder. While the specimen is being collected, instruct the patient that all urine must be stored in the collection bottle. If a specimen is accidentally discarded, the test is discontinued. Collection must be-

gin again. Advise the patient not to contaminate the specimen with toilet tissue. Provide a plastic bag or other receptacle for tissue disposal. Most facilities place a sign in the patient's room or bathroom to alert staff to the test. Follow your facility policy for posting signs. Make sure the collection container is properly labeled. Transport the specimen to the laboratory immediately upon test completion.

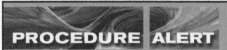

PROCEDURE ALERT

Encourage fluids before and during the test, if permitted, to ensure adequate urine flow. Document I&O, if ordered.

Procedure 79

Collecting a 24-Hour Urine Specimen

Supplies needed:
- Disposable exam gloves, box
- 4-liter collection bottle with lid, or special container used by facility (**Figure 10-6**)
- Bedpan, urinal, commode, or specimen collection device (**Figure 10-7**)
- Graduated container for measuring and transferring urine
- Refrigerator or basin of ice to store collection container
- Plastic bag for toilet tissue and used supplies

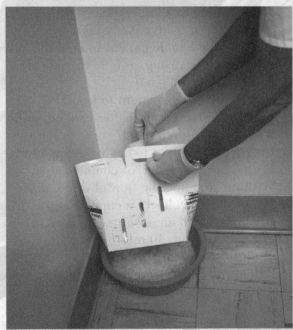

FIGURE 10-6 The 24-hour urine is collected in a plastic bottle or other specimen container; it must be refrigerated or kept on ice.

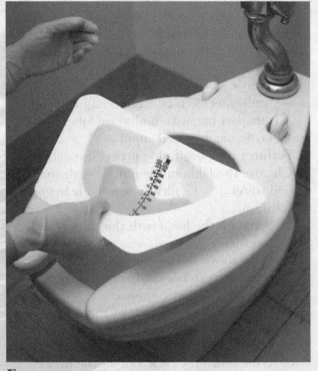

FIGURE 10-7 The specimen collection device may also be called a "nun's hat."

(continues)

Procedure **79**, *continued*

Collecting a 24-Hour Urine Specimen

1. Perform your beginning procedure actions.
2. Ask the patient to void. Discard this urine.
3. Begin timing the specimen collection.
4. Each time the patient voids, record intake and output, if ordered. Transfer the specimen to the collection container. Refill ice in the storage container as often as necessary.
5. At the end of 24 hours, stop the collection. Ask the patient if he or she needs to void, and add this sample to the container.
6. Perform your procedure completion actions.

Collecting a Sterile Urine Specimen from an Indwelling Catheter

You have learned that the inside of the closed catheter system is sterile. The system is not opened when a urine specimen is collected. The catheter is clamped to collect urine for 10 to 15 minutes. Urine is withdrawn from a collection port on the catheter using a needle and syringe.

Procedure **80**

Collecting a Sterile Urine Specimen from an Indwelling Catheter

Supplies needed:
- Disposable exam gloves
- Catheter clamp or rubber band
- Sterile specimen collection container
- Alcohol sponge
- 20-mL to 30-mL syringe with 25-gauge needle
- Incontinent pad
- Sharps container
- Paper towel
- Plastic bag for used supplies

1. Clamp the catheter below the collection port for 10 or 15 minutes.
2. Perform your beginning procedure actions.
3. Remove the lid from the sterile specimen cup. Place the cup on a paper towel. Place the lid with the inside up on the table.
4. Wipe the collection port with the alcohol sponge. Allow the alcohol to dry.
5. Remove the cap from the needle. Turn the bevel of the needle facing up. Insert the needle into the collection port at a 30- or 45-degree angle.
6. Gently pull back the plunger, withdrawing the urine sample (Figure 10-8). Collect at

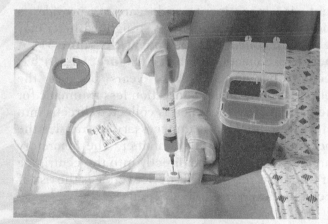

FIGURE 10-8 Withdraw the urine from the collection port.

least 10 mL of urine, or follow your facility policy. Remove the needle from the collection port.
7. Remove the clamp or rubber band from the catheter.
8. Transfer the urine into the collection cup (Figure 10-9). Depress the plunger gently to avoid splashing.

(continues)

Procedure **80**, *continued*

Collecting a Sterile Urine Specimen from an Indwelling Catheter

9. Do not recap the needle. Discard the needle and syringe in the sharps container.

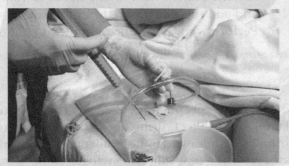

FIGURE 10-9 Carefully transfer the urine to the sterile cup without splashing.

10. Perform your procedure completion actions.

OSHA ALERT

Hospitals purchase many different types of equipment. A urine sample may be obtained from some indwelling catheters by attaching the syringe only (without a needle, or by using a needleless adapter) to the sampling port. When inserting a catheter, select the needleless method, if possible, as it reduces the risk of injury. Modify the procedure written here if the needleless system is used.

Catheterized Urine Specimens

The physician may order a catheterized urine specimen when a sterile specimen is required, or the patient is incontinent and cannot provide a midstream urine specimen. A straight catheter may be used to collect this specimen (Procedure 51). A specimen collection catheter (**Figure 10-10**) has become popular in recent years because the catheter is tiny, making insertion less traumatic for the patient. The specimen is collected directly into a test tube, making it unnecessary to transfer the specimen to a separate container. The laboratory can place this test tube directly into the centrifuge for urinalysis testing. This device reduces the risk of accidental exposure to body fluids.

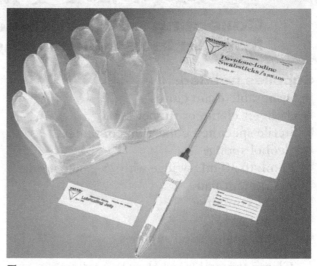

FIGURE 10-10 The female Speci-Cath collection device is less traumatic for the patient, and presents a lower infection control risk for staff than the straight catheter. (Courtesy of Medline Industries, Inc., Mundelein, IL; (800) MEDLINE)

Procedure **81**

Obtaining a Urine Specimen Using the Speci-Cath Collection Device

Supplies needed:
- Disposable exam gloves
- Washcloth

- Towel
- Bath blanket
- Washbasin

(continues)

Procedure **81**, *continued*

Obtaining a Urine Specimen Using the Speci-Cath Collection Device

▶ Soap and water
▶ Incontinent pad
▶ Male, female, or pediatric Speci-Cath collection kit containing:
   —8 Fr. vinyl catheter attached to test tube, with cap and label
   —Sterile gloves
   —3 povidone-iodine swabsticks
   —Fenestrated drape
   —Sterile packet of water-soluble lubricant
▶ Plastic bag for used supplies

1. Perform your beginning procedure actions.
2. Place the incontinent pad under the patient's buttocks.
3. Position and drape the patient for perineal care.
4. Apply gloves.
5. Provide perineal care.
6. Discard used supplies.
7. Wash your hands, or use alcohol-based hand cleaner.
8. Adjust or position the lighting, if necessary.
9. Clean the overbed table. Disinfect the table, if soiled, or if required by facility policy.
10. Open the Speci-Cath kit and establish a sterile field.
11. Place the plastic bag for used supplies at the foot of the bed, or in another convenient location. Position the bag so that you do not have to cross over sterile supplies to discard soiled items.
12. Apply sterile gloves.
13. Open the sterile packages on the sterile field and arrange supplies as needed.
14. Open the package of povidone-iodine swabsticks.
15. Open the package of lubricant.
16. Lubricate the tip of the catheter. The lubricant should cover the catheter for approximately 2 inches for a female and 4 to 5 inches for a male.
17. Pick up the fenestrated drape. Stand away from the bed and hold the drape away from your body, allowing it to unfold.

18. Fold the drape back, over your gloves.
19. Position the hole in the center of the drape over the perineum. If it is necessary to lift the penis to position the drape, use your nondominant hand. This hand will be contaminated after touching the patient's skin and cannot be used to contact sterile supplies.
20. Use the swabsticks to cleanse the genitals:
   Female patient: Separate the labia with the nondominant hand. This hand is now contaminated. Wipe the swabstick across the center of the labia from top to bottom. Use one stroke, then discard the swabstick. Pick up another swabstick and repeat the procedure on the labia opposite where you are standing. Discard the swabstick. Pick the last swabstick and cleanse the labia closest to you from top to bottom. Discard the swabstick. Keep the labia separated throughout the procedure. Do not let go after cleansing.
   Male patient: Pick up the penis with the nondominant hand. This hand is now contaminated. Retract the foreskin of the penis. Beginning at the urinary meatus, wipe the penis with a swabstick in a circular motion. Discard the swabstick. Pick up another swabstick and repeat the procedure, cleansing outward from the meatus in a circle. Discard the swabstick. Pick up the last swabstick and cleanse in a circle beyond the second circle. When done, you should have cleansed a large area. Discard the swabstick.
21. Pick up the test tube.
22. Insert the catheter:
   Female patient: Visualize the urinary meatus. Tell the patient you will be inserting the catheter now. Instruct the patient to cough. This will help relax the urinary sphincter. Insert the catheter into the urethra, threading it into the bladder (about 2½ or 3 inches) until urine flows. If urine

(continues)

Procedure **81**, *continued*

Obtaining a Urine Specimen Using the Speci-Cath Collection Device

does not flow immediately, hold the catheter in place until urine drains. If no urine flows, the catheter may be in the vagina. Leave it in place. You must get another Speci-Cath and repeat the procedure. Leaving it in place will make it easier to find the urethra the next time. Remove it after the catheterization is successful. If an assistant is helping you, continue to hold the labia apart, and send him or her for another Speci-Cath. When he or she returns, have the assistant open the Speci-Cath. Grasp it with your sterile hand and repeat the procedure.

Male patient: Hold the penis upright with your nondominant hand. Insert the catheter into the meatus. Tell the patient you will be inserting the catheter now. Instruct the patient to cough while you are inserting the

catheter. The patient may also bear down, as if to urinate. Encourage him to continue throughout the procedure. Advance the catheter until urine flows.
Never force a catheter. If you meet resistance and are unable to advance the catheter, stop the procedure and notify the RN.

23. Fill the test tube completely, then withdraw the catheter slowly.
24. Pull the end of the catheter. This will remove it from the top of the test tube. Discard the catheter in the plastic bag. Snap the top of the test tube down, sealing the tube.
25. Replace the foreskin in the male patient.
26. Remove the drape. Discard it in the plastic bag.
27. Perform your procedure completion actions.

Straining Urine for Renal Calculi

Renal calculi, or kidney stones, may develop anywhere in the urinary tract. They are formed from mineral salts collecting around bacteria, blood clots, or other particles. Calculi are a complication of immobility, but there are other causes, such as excess calcium in the diet, inadequate intake of fluids, dehydration, and heredity. The stones appear tiny, but are very painful for the patient. The size ranges from microscopic to several centimeters. They may be excreted with the urine. Sometimes they become lodged in the urinary tract. Signs and symptoms of renal calculi include:

● Hematuria.
● Urinary frequency and/or urgency.
● Painful elimination.
● Urinary retention.
● **Renal colic,** or flank pain caused by obstruction to the flow of urine, such as from a stone. The pain is commonly sharp and severe in the lower back, just above the waist, and radiates around the body into the groin and testicles.

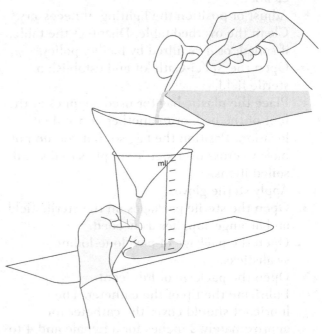

FIGURE 10-11 When a physician writes an order to strain urine, each voiding is poured through filter paper to retrieve kidney stones.

- Nausea, vomiting, and/or abdominal pain.
- Fever, chills.

To test for kidney stones, nursing personnel must carefully strain all of the patient's urine through a fine-mesh gauze pad, filter paper, or fine-mesh strainer (Figure 10-11). If a substance is found in the urine, it is sent to the laboratory for further evaluation. Renal calculi may be various colors, each of which has diagnostic value. If renal calculi are suspected, the urine is strained until all stones are passed or removed surgically. If the patient has an indwelling catheter, strain all urine each time the drainage bag is emptied.

Procedure 82

Straining the Urine for Renal Calculi

Supplies needed:
- Disposable exam gloves
- 4 × 4 gauze pad, fine-mesh sieve, filter paper, or a commercial strainer used by your facility
- Bedpan, urinal, bedside commode, or specimen collection "hat"
- Graduated measuring device
- Specimen collection container (leave in room in case calculi are found)
- Rubber bands
- Plastic bag for used supplies

1. Perform your beginning procedure actions.
2. Post a sign in the bathroom, stating to "Strain All Urine," only if permitted by facility policy. Post signs in other designated areas, such as over the bed and on the collection container, as required. Follow facility privacy policies when posting signs.
3. Inform the patient to notify you after each voiding.
4. After the patient urinates, place the commercial strainer, filter paper, or unfolded 4 × 4 gauze pad over the top of the graduated measuring device. Secure with a rubber band, if necessary.
5. Apply gloves, if you have not done this previously.
6. Carefully pour the specimen from the urinal into the measuring device.
7. Carefully examine the strainer for calculi. If residue is found, or if the appearance of the filter is questionable, place the filtered substance into the specimen cup, close the lid, and send it to the laboratory.
8. If there are no particles in the strainer, discard it or rinse it for reuse, according to the device being used.
9. Rinse and disinfect the graduate and specimen collection device.
10. Perform your procedure completion actions. Inform the RN if the patient complained of pain during voiding.

Pediatric Urine Specimen Collection

Collection of a urine specimen from a child who does not have bladder control requires a variation from the usual urine collection procedure. The pediatric urine collection bag is an excellent alternative for collecting a urine specimen, and eliminates the need for catheterization. However, the pediatric collection device is fastened to the perineum by means of a self-adhesive surface. It should not be used for children with diaper rash, inflamed, or excoriated skin. If this is the case, or if the child is allergic to adhesive tape, check with the RN before proceeding. If using the pediatric collection bag is not possible, try applying a disposable diaper inside out. After the child voids, remove the diaper carefully. Pour the urine from the plastic outer surface (which is facing inside) into a specimen collection cup or test tube.

Procedure 83

Collecting a Pediatric Urine Specimen

Supplies needed:

▶ Midstream (clean-catch) urinalysis kit, according to facility policy, or the following:
▶ Disposable exam gloves, 2 pairs
▶ Pediatric urine specimen collection bag
▶ Two disposable diapers
▶ Bandage scissors
▶ Washcloth
▶ Towel
▶ Soap
▶ Washbasin
▶ Incontinent pad
▶ Specimen collection cup with lid
▶ Plastic specimen transport bag
▶ Plastic bag for used supplies

1. Perform your beginning procedure actions.
2. Perform peri care, rinse well, and pat dry gently, to avoid stimulating urination.
3. Cut a 2-inch slit in a diaper, from the center point toward one of the shorter edges. Set aside.
4. Position the child in the frog position, with the legs separated and knees flexed. Ask an assistant or a parent to help hold the child, if necessary.
5. Remove the adhesive coverings from the adhesive flaps on the bag.
6. For the female patient, separate the labia. Gently and carefully press the lower rim of the bag against the perineum. Work upward toward the pubis, attaching the remaining adhesive inside the labia majora.
7. For the male patient, position the bag over the penis and scrotum. Carefully press the adhesive edge to the skin.

8. Gently pull the collection bag through the slit in the diaper. This reduces the risk that the diaper will compress the bag and enables you to visualize the specimen immediately after the child voids.
9. Fasten the diaper on the child.
10. Remove your gloves and discard them in the plastic bag.
11. Wash your hands, or use alcohol-based hand cleaner.
12. Leave the room, but return periodically to check on the specimen.
13. When you can see urine in the bag, wash your hands (or use alcohol-based hand cleaner), and apply gloves.
14. Gently unfasten the tape on the sides of the diaper.
15. Gently break the adhesive seal on the bag.
16. Hold the bottom port of the bag over the specimen.
17. Remove the tab from the bottom port and allow urine to flow into the specimen cup.
18. Measure and document output, if the patient is on I&O.
19. Discard the soiled diaper and specimen collection bag in the plastic bag.
20. Provide perineal care, making sure to wash the remaining adhesive from the skin.
21. Check the perineum. If it appears excoriated from the collection device, apply barrier cream or the ordered product. Inform the RN.
22. Apply a clean diaper.
23. Perform your procedure completion actions.

STOOL SPECIMEN

Stool is usually collected in a single specimen, but multiple specimens are collected for certain tests. Ask the patient to void before having a bowel movement. Accidental contamination with urine may cause inaccurate test results. Do not discard toilet tissue in the specimen. Provide a plastic bag or other device for tissue collection. Some tests are performed in the laboratory, whereas others are performed on the nursing unit. If the specimen must be analyzed by the laboratory, transport it immediately after collection.

Procedure 84

Collecting a Stool Specimen

Supplies needed:
- Disposable exam gloves, 2 pairs
- Bedpan and cover, commode, or specimen collection pan
- Toilet tissue
- Paper towels
- Specimen container with lid
- Tongue blade
- Transport bag
- Plastic bag for used supplies

1. Perform your beginning procedure actions.
2. Complete the label and put it on the container.
3. Ask the patient to defecate into the designated collection device. Instruct him or her not to discard toilet tissue into the collection device. Provide a plastic bag for this purpose.
4. Provide privacy and make sure the call signal and toilet tissue are within reach.
5. Remove your gloves and discard them in the plastic bag.
6. Wash your hands, or use alcohol-based hand cleaner.
7. Return immediately when the patient signals.
8. Wash your hands, or use alcohol-based hand cleaner.
9. Apply gloves and remove the stool specimen collection container.
10. Provide a clean container or bedpan for urination, if necessary. Allow the patient to urinate. Provide privacy.
11. Cover the specimen collection container and assist the patient with cleansing, returning to bed, or positioning. Wear gloves and apply the principles of standard precautions if appropriate to the activity.
12. Cover the container and take the collection device to the bathroom or other designated location, according to facility policy. Avoid contaminating environmental surfaces with your gloves. Remove one glove or place a paper towel in your gloved hand to open doors, turn on faucets, and so on, as necessary.
13. Place the container with the specimen on paper towels.

14. Place the specimen collection cup on paper towels. Open the lid. Place it on the counter, with the clean inner side up (top side down).
15. Uncover the specimen collection container. Use the tongue blade to remove feces from the collection device and place the sample in the sterile specimen container. About two tablespoons of stool are necessary. Taking a small sample from each part of the stool is best (Figure 10-12). Collect any color or substance that appears abnormal. Discard the tongue blade in the plastic bag.

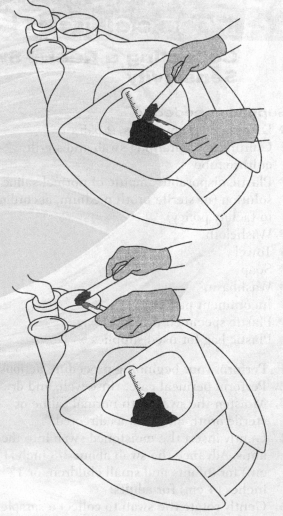

FIGURE 10-12 Collect a specimen from each part of the stool. Use a tongue blade to transfer the specimen from the collection device to the specimen cup.

(continues)

Procedure 84, *continued*

Collecting a Stool Specimen

16. Put the lid on the specimen container. Place the container on a paper towel on the counter.
17. Rinse and disinfect the bedpan or collection container according to facility policy.
18. Remove one glove and place the specimen collection container into the transport bag with your gloved hand. Avoid touching the outside of the bag with your glove. Handle the transport bag with your ungloved hand.

19. Remove the other glove and discard according to facility policy.
20. Wash your hands, or use alcohol-based hand cleaner.
21. Perform your procedure completion actions.
22. Take the specimen to the designated location.
23. Discard the plastic bag containing the waste in the biohazardous waste container.
24. Report collection of the specimen and any abnormalities to the RN.

Procedure 85

Collecting a Rectal Swab Specimen for Culture and Sensitivity

Supplies needed:
- Disposable exam gloves, 2 pairs
- Culturette, containing swab and sterile culture tube
- Plastic disposable ampule of normal saline solution (or sterile broth medium, according to facility policy)
- Washcloth
- Towel
- Soap
- Washbasin
- Incontinent pad
- Plastic specimen transport bag
- Plastic bag for used supplies

1. Perform your beginning procedure actions.
2. Perform perineal care, rinse well, and dry.
3. Moisten the swab with normal saline or sterile broth medium, as directed.
4. Gently insert the moistened swab into the anus. Advance the swab about 3/8 inch (1 cm) for infants and small children, or 1½ inches (4 cm) for adults.
5. Gently rotate the swab to collect a sample from the walls of the rectal mucosa.
6. Carefully withdraw the swab.

7. Place the swab in the sterile culture tube and crush the ampule of transport medium.
8. Cleanse the rectal area as needed.
9. Perform your procedure completion actions.

PROCEDURE ALERT

Insert the swab 1½ inches into the rectum. Do not advance it farther than 2 inches. Avoid water-soluble lubricants, which will destroy the specimen. Moisturize the swab with normal saline only. Gently rotate the swab against the walls of the rectum while withdrawing it to obtain a sample from the rectal mucosa.

HEALTH CARE ALERT

Sometimes the physician will order three stool specimens (X3) for ova and parasites (O&P). Unless otherwise ordered, these specimens should be collected 24 hours apart. A 12-hour minimum may be acceptable, depending on the circumstances. Check with the RN before discarding a specimen. Do not collect an O&P specimen after a lower GI series (barium enema), after the administration of a prep for lower colon X-rays, or after the administration of other laxatives or suppositories. Normal saline enema specimens are acceptable, but must be labeled as "saline enema specimen." If in doubt about the preparation for the specimen, check with the RN or the lab.

Bleeding in the stool suggests the presence of tumors, cancer, and some other conditions. A stool specimen may be tested for the presence of blood. If the results are positive, additional testing is done.

The Hemoccult or guaiac test (Figure 10-13) is a bedside test done to check for the presence of occult blood in the stool. If blood is found, the physician will order further diagnostic tests.

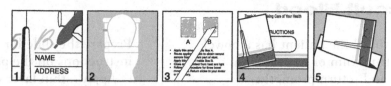

1. Remove slide from paper dispensing envelope. Using a ball-point pen, write your name, age, and address on the front of the slide. **Do not tear the sections apart.**
2. Fill in sample collection date on section 1 before a bowel movement. Flush toilet and allow to refill. You may use any clean, dry container to collect your sample. Collect sample before it contacts the toilet bowl water. Let stool fall into collection container.
3. Open front of section 1. Use one stick to collect a small sample. Apply a thin smear covering Box A. Collect second sample from different part of stool with same stick. Apply a thin smear covering Box B. Discard stick in a waste container. **DO NOT FLUSH STICK.**
4. Close and secure front flap of section 1 by inserting it under tab. Store slide in any paper envelope until the next day. **Important: This allows the sample to "air dry."**
5. Repeat steps 2-4 for the next two days, using sections 2 and 3. After completing the last section, store the slide overnight in any paper envelope to air dry.

The next day, remove slide from the paper envelope and place in the Mailing Pouch, if provided. Seal pouch carefully and **immediately return to your doctor or laboratory.**

Note: Current U.S. Postal Regulations prohibit mailing completed slides in any standard paper envelope.

IMPORTANT NOTE: Follow the procedure exactly as outlined above. Always develop the test, read the results, interpret them and make a decision as to whether the fecal specimen is positive or negative for occult blood BEFORE you develop the Performance Monitors®. Do not apply Developer to Performance Monitors® before interpreting test results. Any blue originating from the Performance Monitors® should be ignored in the reading of the specimen test results.

READING AND INTERPRETATION OF THE HEMOCCULT® TEST
the world's leading test for fecal occult blood

Negative Smears*

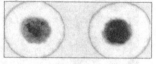

Sample report: negative
No detectable blue on or at the edge of the smears indicates the test is negative for occult blood.
(See **LIMITATIONS OF PROCEDURE.**)

Negative and Positive Smears*

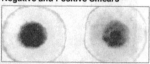

Positive Smears*

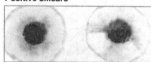

Sample report: positive
Any trace of blue on or at the edge of one or more of the smears indicates the test is positive for occult blood.

FIGURE 10-13 The Hemoccult Sensa test (Courtesy of Beckman Coulter, Inc.)

Procedure 86

Collecting and Testing a Stool Specimen for Occult Blood

Supplies needed:
- Disposable exam gloves, 2 pairs
- Bedpan, commode, or specimen collection device
- Tongue blade
- Hemoccult test kit, or other brand of guaiac test
- Guaiac developing solution
- Plastic bag for used supplies

1. Perform your beginning procedure actions.
2. Assist the patient with the bedpan or commode, or position the specimen collection device in the toilet.

(continues)

Procedure **86**, *continued*

Collecting and Testing a Stool Specimen for Occult Blood

3. Provide privacy until the patient has a bowel movement. Instruct him or her to signal when finished, and return promptly.
4. Apply gloves.
5. Assist the patient with cleaning the perineum, handwashing, and returning to bed, as necessary.
6. Using the tongue blade, collect a small amount of stool.

7. Prepare the slide for testing according to the instructions on the package:
   a. Apply a thin layer of stool on panel one.
   b. Obtain a second small specimen from a different part of the stool. Apply a thin layer to panel two (**Figure 10-14A**).
   c. Turn the package over.
   d. Lift the flap.
   e. Apply 2 drops of developing solution on each panel of stool, and to the control at the bottom of the slide (**Figure 10-14B**).
   f. Within 60 seconds, compare the results with the color changes described on the package. If the sample turns blue, this suggests the presence of blood.
8. Perform your procedure completion actions.

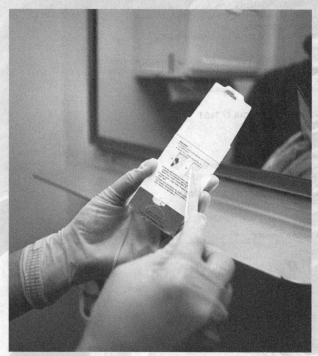

FIGURE 10-14(A) Smear a small amount of stool onto the slide.

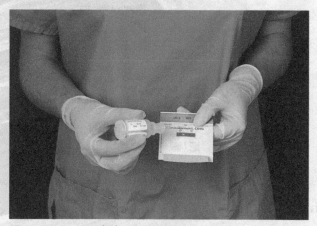

FIGURE 10-14(B) Drop the developing solution onto the sample.

MEASURING BLOOD GLUCOSE

Bedside glucose testing has become very common in the management of patients with diabetes. Many individuals perform this testing at home several times each day. The antidiabetic medication is adjusted by the doctor according to the patient's blood sugar.

The physician will order specific times for blood sugar testing. The specimen may be collected at a fixed interval, such as before meals. The RN may administer insulin to the patient based on the blood sugar. The physician may also order fasting blood sugar or **two-hour postprandial blood sugars (PPBS)**. A postprandial blood sugar is collected exactly two hours after the patient finishes eating. After meals, the blood sugar becomes elevated. Within two hours, it should return to normal. Collect the capillary sample exactly as ordered. Specimens that are not collected at the proper time can cause misinterpretation of the results. Always report the value to the RN.

If the RN suspects that a patient is having complications related to diabetes, he or she may ask you to obtain a stat blood sugar. This test must be performed immediately. Report the results immediately, as well.

Fingerstick Blood Sugar

Fingerstick blood sugar (FSBS) is checked by collecting a sample of capillary blood with a lancet. This is transferred to a reagent strip or other test strip. For most reagent strips, you must place a hanging drop of blood onto the reagent pad. Avoid smearing the strip against the finger. The Multistix (Figure 10-15) and Chemstrip BG can be read visually, by comparing the color on the reagent strip with the color key on the bottle. The Chemstrip BG may also be used in the Accucheck blood glucose meter. After making the fingerstick, a drop of blood is transferred to the test strip, which is inserted into the meter before beginning. The Glucometer Elite does not use a reagent strip. It works like a capillary tube, drawing blood to the inside. This feature works well for patients from whom obtaining a hanging drop of blood is difficult. An audible beep informs you when the tube has collected enough blood.

Many different blood glucose meters are available. All are accurate and simple to use. Each meter has its own reagent or test strip. For accuracy, make sure the strip is compatible with the meter you are using (Figure 10-16). Also, check the expiration date on the bottle. Do not use the strips beyond the expiration date. Follow the directions for the meter and reagent strips you are using. All are slightly different.

Many different lancets are also available for performing blood glucose checks. The type of lancet used is similar to that used for capillary blood sticks. Many health care workers prefer retractable lancets,

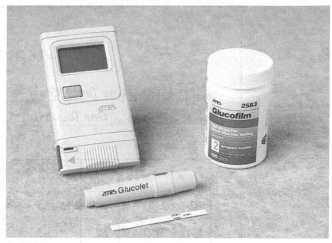

FIGURE 10-16 The reagent strips must be compatible with the glucose meter.

which are spring-loaded. The needle withdraws after the finger has been punctured, reducing the incidence of needlestick injuries. Discard lancets into the puncture-resistant sharps container. Many health care workers have been injured by lancets that were inadvertently dropped in the bed or on the floor.

Health care facilities vary as to what are considered normal blood sugar values. The normal range in most facilities is somewhere between 65 and 120, with the normal value commonly being 70 to 110. Values below 70 suggest hypoglycemia. Values above 110 suggest hyperglycemia. Learn the normal values for your facility. Values that are well above or below the normal range suggest serious diabetic problems. Signs and symptoms of diabetic complications are listed in the Observe & Report box. Notify the RN immediately of abnormal blood sugar values or other signs and symptoms of blood sugar problems.

Some blood glucose meters do not have a large range. Typically, handheld blood glucose meters will read a blood sugar value as low as 40. A few measure blood sugars as low as 20. For values below the lowest meter reading, the screen will display the word "low." On the high end, most meters do not read values above 400 or 500. If the fingerstick blood sugar exceeds the meter high reading, the display will read "high." If the screen displays the word *low* or *high*, the patient has the potential for serious complications. His or her condition may deteriorate quickly. Inform the RN immediately. He or she may ask you to collect a venous sample of blood (Procedure 30) for the laboratory to analyze.

Meter Calibration. Blood glucose meters must be calibrated daily, or as often as required by facility policy. Calibration is done to ensure that the meter

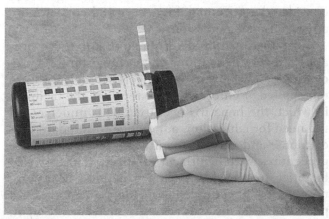

FIGURE 10-15 Multistix are used for many different tests.

QUALITY CONTROL LOG SHEET

Test or Procedure: <u>One Touch Glucose</u>   Lot Number of Control Product: <u>503853A</u>

Instrument or Device: <u>One Touch II</u>   Control Product: <u>Normal Glucose Control</u>

Date	Time	Control Value	Acceptable Range	Accept/Reject	Corrective Action	Performed by
10/1	7:30 AM	87	85-120 mg/dl	Accept	–	NJ
10/2	7:40 AM	90	"	Accept	–	NJ
10/3	7:20 AM	91	"	Accept	–	NJ
10/4	7:30 AM	93	"	Accept	–	JB
10/7	7:25 AM	89	"	Accept	–	JB
10/8	7:10 AM	91	"	Accept	–	JB
10/9	7:15 AM	83	"	Reject	Opened Fresh Package of Control	NJ
10/9	7:30 AM	89	"	Accept	–	NJ

FIGURE 10-17 Calibrate the glucose meter according to facility policy, and record the results on a log.

is accurate. Depending on the type of meter used, calibration is done by running a test using a special test strip or a liquid control solution. If the reading obtained during the calibration procedure is not within the acceptable range for the product you are using, inform the RN. Do not use the meter until the problem has been corrected. The results of daily calibrations must be recorded on a log (Figure 10-17).

Infection Control. Regular monitoring of blood glucose levels is an important part of routine diabetes care. Capillary blood is sampled with a fingerstick device and tested with a portable meter. The CDC and Food and Drug Administration (FDA) have recommended since 1990 that fingerstick devices be restricted to individual use. However, most health care facilities have used community meters, and have depended on their personnel to apply the proper precautions and cleansing techniques to prevent the spread of infection. In 2005, the CDC reported three incidences of nosocomial infection with hepatitis B that developed in long-term care facili-

ties. These were attributed to shared devices and other breaks in infection control practices related to blood glucose monitoring. A **nosocomial infection** is a hospital-acquired infection, or a new infection that developed in, or is associated with being treated in, a health care facility. An infection is generally considered nosocomial if it occurs 48 hours or more after a hospital admission.

An investigation determined that in these situations, recommendations concerning standard precautions and the reuse of fingerstick devices were not applied or enforced consistently in the facilities in which the hepatitis occurred. This underscored the need for education, adherence to standard precautions, and careful monitoring of diabetes-care procedures in all health care settings. It also caused facilities to reevaluate their practices. Many are now issuing a new, individual glucose meter to each patient. He or she may take the meter home upon discharge. It is discarded if left at the hospital.

In one of the facilities implicated in the hepatitis infection, the spring-loaded barrel of a fingerstick device was used for all patients. This device was believed to be the source of infection. The CDC also noted that it is possible that used lancets were accidentally returned to the clean lancet supply, and were accidentally reused. In another facility, investigators suspected the infection was transmitted because nursing personnel did not routinely wear gloves when performing fingerstick procedures. They also suspected inadequate hand hygiene.

Similar indirect transmission of HBV has occurred in health care facilities through contaminated environmental surfaces or inadequately disinfected equipment. Other diseases may also be spread in a similar manner, such as hepatitis C infection (HCV) and human immunodeficiency virus (HIV), the virus that causes AIDS. These viruses are stable on environmental surfaces at room temperature, and infected patients are often asymptomatic, despite having high concentrations of virus in their blood and body fluids. Because of this, the

virus may be passed easily to workers and other patients if improper techniques are used. CDC recommends that health care workers avoid carrying supplies from patient to patient and avoid sharing devices, including blood glucose meters, among patients. Other CDC infection control recommendations are listed in **Figure 10-18.**

AGE-APPROPRIATE CARE — ALERT

When doing a fingerstick capillary test on a child or adult, instruct the patient to wash his or her hands under warm, running water. This reduces the risk of infection and increases blood flow to the hand. After piercing the skin with the lancet, squeeze lightly to stimulate blood flow. Avoid prolonged pressure, as this may cause incorrect results by introducing tissue fluids. The fingerstick should be deep enough so that hard pressure is not required. If gentle pressure is not effective to start blood flow, repeat the puncture.

- Never reuse needles, syringes, or lancets.
- Avoid recapping needles, syringes, and lancets. Place them in the sharps disposal container immediately after use.
- Use single-use lancets that retract immediately after puncturing the skin.
- Discard lancets and other sharps at the point of use.
- Assign separate glucose meters to each patient. If a single device is used for community use, it should be properly cleaned and disinfected before and after each use.
- Any other environmental surface that has been contaminated or potentially contaminated by blood and/or body fluid should be promptly cleaned and disinfected.
- Store individual supplies, such as meters and lancets, in patient rooms whenever possible.
- Health care workers should avoid carrying patient care supplies in their pockets.

- Keep trays or carts used for carrying medications, treatments, and other supplies in the hallway, whenever possible. Avoid taking them into patient rooms if this can be avoided.
- Unused supplies taken to a patient's bedside should not be used in the care of another patient.
- Wear gloves for fingerstick blood sugar monitoring, as well as for other procedures in which there is a risk of contact with blood or body fluids.
- Change gloves between patient contacts and after every procedure (in the care of the same patient) that involves potential contact with blood, body fluids, secretions, excretions, mucous membranes, or nonintact skin.
- Discard used gloves in the proper receptacle.
- Perform hand hygiene with soap and water or alcohol-based hand cleaner immediately after removing gloves and before touching other medical supplies or environmental surfaces.

FIGURE 10-18 Recommended practices for prevention of viral transmission.

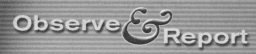

Important Observations of Diabetic Patients

Inadequate food intake
Eating food not allowed on diet
Refusal of meals, supplements, or snacks
Nausea, vomiting, or diarrhea
Inadequate fluid intake
Excessive activity
Complaints of dizziness, shakiness, racing heart
Blood sugar values outside of normal reporting range for your facility

(continues)

Observe & Report (Continued)

SIGNS AND SYMPTOMS OF HYPERGLYCEMIA	SIGNS AND SYMPTOMS OF HYPOGLYCEMIA
Nausea, vomiting Weakness Headache Full, bounding pulse Fruity smell to breath Hot, dry, flushed skin Labored respirations Drowsiness Mental confusion Unconsciousness Sugar in the urine High blood sugar as measured by FSBS	Complaints of hunger, weakness, dizziness, shakiness Skin cold, moist, clammy, pale Rapid, shallow respirations Nervousness and excitement Rapid pulse Unconsciousness No sugar in urine Low blood sugar as measured by FSBS

Procedure 87

Obtaining a Fingerstick Blood Sugar

NOTE: This procedure is generic and applies the principles used for most blood glucose meters. Follow the directions for the meter and strip you are using. The operating directions are slightly different for each.

Supplies needed:
- Disposable exam gloves
- Alcohol sponge
- Lancet
- Blood glucose meter
- Reagent strip or test strip for the blood glucose meter being used
- Sharps container
- Plastic bag for used supplies

1. Perform your beginning procedure actions.
2. Wipe the patient's finger with the alcohol sponge. Allow the alcohol to dry.
3. Pierce the side of the middle or ring finger using the lancet.
4. Discard the lancet in the sharps container.
5. Squeeze the sides of the finger gently to obtain a drop of blood.
6. Hold the puncture site directly over the reagent strip and place a hanging drop of blood onto the reagent pad. If using a device with a capillary-type strip, place the test strip next to the puncture site and allow the test strip to withdraw the blood into the center tube.
7. Insert the strip into the meter, if this was not done previously.
8. Wipe the patient's finger with the alcohol sponge and allow to dry. Apply pressure until bleeding stops. Apply a bandage, if necessary.
9. Wait the designated period of time for the meter you are using. An audible beep will indicate when the value is displayed on the screen.
10. Perform your procedure completion actions.

MEASURING GLYCATED HEMOGLOBIN

Glycated hemoglobin is a term used to describe a series of stable minor hemoglobin components formed from hemoglobin and glucose. Glycated hemoglobin may also called Ghb, glycohemoglobin, glycosylated hemoglobin, HbA1c, HbA1, or %A1C. It is commonly called "A1C," which is the abbreviation we use here. Simply put, this test is a measurement of glucose levels in the blood over a prolonged period of time. It differs from the fingerstick blood sugar because it provides a snapshot of the patient's diabetic control over the past two to three months. The percentage of A1C in whole blood is approximately:

- 50 percent from the most recent 30 days
- 25 percent from the previous 30 to 60 days
- 25 percent from the previous 60 to 90 days

A1C Blood Glucose Values

In persons without diabetes, the normal A1C value is approximately 5.0 percent. The ADA recommends that the goal of therapy should be a value of less than 7 percent. The physician, RN, diabetes educator, and dietitian will evaluate the patient and address values above this level. In some facilities, all patients with values over 6.5 percent are further evaluated, and may have additional diagnostic tests done to rule out complications. The approximate blood glucose equivalent values are listed in Table 10–1.

Having the A1C profile information enables the physician to evaluate the patient's control at home; order additional diagnostic tests, if necessary; regulate medications; and establish a monitoring routine. Patient teaching is a very important part of the care given to persons who have diabetes. Knowing the degree of diabetic control enables the RN and certified diabetes educator to plan and provide specific patient teaching targeted toward normalizing the blood sugar and maintaining good control. The information helps the dietitian to assist the patient with diet management, food preparation, and methods of meeting the patient's individual dietary wants and needs.

The handheld meter used for A1C testing is very expensive (approximately $3,100). Using it at the bedside carries the same risks of accidental blood contamination and viral transmission as the blood glucose meter, which is less expensive (approximately $25 to $50). Because of this, single-use, disposable meters are commonly used for A1C testing. The A1C test is not a screening test. It is used only for testing ongoing glucose control in persons who have been diagnosed with diabetes. If testing is done regularly, it helps predict and control the risk for development of many serious, chronic complications. The American Diabetes Association (ADA) recommends hemoglobin A1C testing twice a year for patients who are meeting treatment goals, and four times a year for patients who are not meeting treatment goals, or those who need more intensive monitoring. Home testing kits are now available. The single-use, disposable kits are also being used in physicians' offices, and as a point-of-care bedside test in hospitals and long-term care facilities.

A1C Testing

No special preparation is necessary for an A1C test, and the patient does not have to be fasting. You may wish to do this test when you obtain the fingerstick blood sugar. The test is sensitive to temperature extremes. Room temperature should be between 64°F and 82°F. Avoid doing the test in direct sunlight, or in an environment that is very hot or cold, or on a surface that is hot or cold to the touch. The kit should be at room temperature when the test is done. Do not unwrap the kit or open packages until you are ready to do the test.

The single-use, disposable meters used for A1C testing are all similar. Follow the instructions for the unit you are using. These meters are used once and then are discarded. Discard the used lancet in the sharps container. The outer packages may be discarded in the wastebasket. The other items that have had contact with the patient's blood must be discarded in the biohazardous waste.

Table 10–1 Blood Glucose Equivalent Values	
Hemoglobin A1C	**Average Daily Blood Glucose**
12.0%	345 mg/dL
11.0%	310 mg/dL
10.0%	275 mg/dL
9.0%	240 mg/dL
8.0%	205 mg/dL
7.0%	170 mg/dL
6.0%	135 mg/dL
5.0%	100 mg/dL
4.0%	65 mg/dL

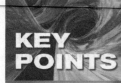

KEY POINTS

▶ The container holding laboratory specimens must be labeled with the patient's name and other identifying information, according to facility policy.

▶ A laboratory requisition is completed and accompanies each specimen to the laboratory.

▶ Laboratory specimens are transported in a plastic transport bag with a biohazard label.

▶ Apply the principles of standard precautions when collecting laboratory specimens.

▶ Specimens are not refrigerated in the same refrigerator with food, beverages, or medications.

▶ Explain the specimen collection procedure to the patient before beginning.

▶ Culture testing is done to identify pathogens. Sensitivity testing is done to identify antibiotics that will eliminate the pathogen.

▶ Swab cultures are collected using a culturette.

▶ Group A *Streptococcus pyogenes* causes many very serious conditions. It must be promptly identified and properly treated to prevent serious complications, such as rheumatic fever and kidney damage.

▶ An infected wound will not heal until the infection is resolved.

▶ All Stage II, III, and IV pressure ulcers become colonized with bacteria.

▶ Wounds are cultured only if infection is suspected.

▶ Treated properly, a colonized wound will heal.

▶ Wound infection occurs when pathogens within the wound adversely affect the patient.

▶ A systemic infection spreads throughout the body, affecting many systems and organs. It may become life-threatening.

▶ Erythema is increasing, abnormal redness and inflammation due to capillary congestion and dilation.

▶ Specimens for culture testing are always collected in sterile containers.

▶ A sputum specimen is collected to analyze mucus from the lungs, not saliva from the mouth.

▶ The gastric analysis checks for the presence of acid in the stomach.

▶ A midstream urine sample is collected from the middle of the urinary stream.

▶ The 24-hour urine test checks for hormones, electrolytes, and proteins in the urine secreted over a 24-hour period.

▶ When a patient has a catheter, the urine specimen is collected by withdrawing urine from a port on the catheter, using a needle and syringe.

▶ The specimen collection catheter (Speci-Cath) is tiny, making catheterization less traumatic for the patient. Using this catheter also reduces exposure to bloodborne pathogens because the unit eliminates the need to transfer urine from one container to another.

(continues)

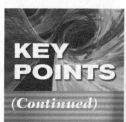

KEY POINTS

(Continued)

▶ Renal calculi, or kidney stones, may develop anywhere in the urinary tract when mineral salts collect around bacteria, blood clots, or other particles. They may be caused by immobility, excess calcium in the diet, inadequate intake of fluids, dehydration, and heredity.

▶ Renal calculi appear tiny, but are very painful for the patient.

▶ If renal calculi are suspected, the patient's urine is strained until all stones are passed or are surgically removed.

▶ Attaching an adhesive collection bag to the perineum is the method most commonly used for collecting a urine specimen from a child who does not have bladder control.

▶ If a pediatric urine specimen cannot be collected using an adhesive collection bag, an alternative is to apply a disposable diaper inside out. Pour the urine from the plastic outer surface into a specimen collection cup or test tube.

▶ Blood is present in the stool if the reagent in the Hemoccult test turns blue.

▶ Always apply the principles of standard precautions when collecting specimens.

▶ When collecting a urine or stool specimen, ask the patient not to discard toilet tissue into the collection device. Provide a plastic bag for this purpose.

▶ The 2-hour postprandial blood sugar is collected 2 hours after a meal; the blood sugar should have returned to normal by this time.

▶ A nosocomial infection is a hospital-acquired infection, or a new infection that developed in, or is associated with being treated in, a health care facility. An infection is generally considered nosocomial if it occurs 48 hours or more after a hospital admission.

▶ Because of the risk of spreading infections during blood glucose testing, many hospitals issue a new, individual glucose meter to each patient. The patient takes the meter home upon discharge.

▶ The CDC recommends that each patient's blood testing supplies be stored in the individual patient's room whenever possible.

▶ The normal blood sugar value ranges between 65 and 120; in most facilities the value is 70 to 110.

▶ Blood sugar values below 70 suggest hypoglycemia. Blood sugar values above 110 suggest hyperglycemia.

▶ The reagent or test strip used for blood sugar testing must be compatible with the blood glucose meter.

▶ Glycated hemoglobin is commonly called A1C. This is a measurement of glucose levels in the blood over a three-month period.

▶ In persons without diabetes, the normal A1C value is approximately 5.0 percent. According to the American Diabetes Association, the goal of diabetes therapy should be a value of less than 7 percent.

▶ Patient teaching is a very important part of care for persons with diabetes.

▶ Single-use, disposable meters may be used for bedside A1C testing. The meter is discarded after one test.

CLINICAL APPLICATIONS

1. You have collected a midstream urine specimen from Mrs. Lange. The patient picks up the lid with her fingers and hands it to you. Her fingers touched the inside of the lid. What action, if any, will you take?

2. Mr. Stanislaus has a sore throat. The RN instructs you to collect a throat culture. When you inspect the patient's throat, you observe that it is very red, with pustules. Mr. Stanislaus gags and starts to cough when you depress his tongue with the tongue blade. What personal protective equipment should you wear when collecting this specimen? Describe how to collect the specimen.

3. Miss Palu-ay is on a 24-hour urine collection. Another PCT confides in you that she accidentally discarded a urine specimen. What will you tell the PCT? Should you inform the RN?

4. You have completed a Hemoccult test on Mr. Tucker. The reagent changed color, indicating the presence of blood in the stool. Mr. Tucker is very anxious and asks you what the results of the test were. What will you tell him?

5. Mrs. Martinez's fingerstick blood sugar is 350. What does this value suggest? What action will you take?

CHAPTER REVIEW

Multiple-Choice Questions

Select the one best answer.

1. Specimens for culture testing are always collected in:
   a. latex containers.
   b. sterile containers.
   c. glass containers.
   d. clean containers.

2. The purpose of culture testing is to identify:
   a. the antibiotic that will eliminate the pathogen.
   b. pathogens in the specimen.
   c. blood in the specimen.
   d. pus in the specimen.

3. When collecting a throat culture, swab the:
   a. back of the throat from side to side.
   b. base of the tongue.
   c. inside of the cheeks.
   d. pustules in the throat only.

4. Sputum is produced by the:
   a. mouth.
   b. sinuses.
   c. nose.
   d. lungs.

5. Before collecting a sputum specimen, have the patient:
   a. rinse the mouth with mouthwash.
   b. brush the teeth.
   c. rinse the mouth with water.
   d. drink a hot beverage.

6. When collecting specimens for gastric analysis, you should collect:
   a. 8 specimens, each 30 minutes apart.
   b. 10 specimens, each 15 minutes apart.
   c. 12 specimens, each 15 minutes apart.
   d. 16 specimens, each 5 minutes apart.

7. When the patient has an indwelling catheter, collect the urine specimen by:
   a. withdrawing urine from the port with a syringe.
   b. separating the catheter from the drainage tubing.
   c. emptying urine from the catheter bag.
   d. withdrawing fluid from the catheter balloon.

8. Blood in the stool will turn the Hemoccult developing solution:
   a. red.
   b. blue.
   c. green.
   d. gray.

9. A 2-hour postprandial blood sugar is collected:
   a. while the patient is NPO.
   b. 2 hours before meals.
   c. 2 hours after meals.
   d. every 15 minutes for 2 hours.

10. The normal blood sugar range is:
    a. 90–150.
    b. 40–100.
    c. 60–140.
    d. 65–120.

11. The swab used for Strep A testing must be:
    a. nylon.
    b. gauze.
    c. cotton.
    d. dacron.

12. When collecting a specimen for Strep A testing, you should swab the patient's:
    a. teeth and tongue.
    b. cheeks and gums.
    c. tonsils and posterior pharynx.
    d. gums and mucous membranes.

13. Signs and symptoms of renal calculi include:
    a. hematuria.
    b. clear urine.
    c. green tinge to the urine.
    d. low blood pressure.

14. Renal colic is:
    a. caused by kidney stones in the urethra.
    b. flank pain from obstructed urine flow.
    c. not a painful condition.
    d. an indication of kidney failure.

15. To test for renal calculi, you should:
    a. strain all of the patient's urine.
    b. perform various reagent tests.
    c. check vital signs hourly.
    d. insert a Foley catheter.

16. To collect a urine specimen from a child who does not have bladder control, you should:
    a. apply gloves and squeeze the wet diaper over a wide-mouth specimen cup.
    b. insert a Foley catheter.
    c. tape a test tube to the child's urethral area; check it hourly.
    d. apply a self-adhesive collection bag to the child's perineum.

17. When collecting a stool specimen, you should:
    a. use a tongue blade to collect 2 tablespoons from each part of the stool.
    b. instruct the patient to defecate in a stool specimen cup.
    c. have the patient defecate in a bedpan; then you will transfer the entire specimen.
    d. apply sterile gloves and use a sterile tongue blade to obtain stool from the bottom of the sample.

18. When collecting a rectal swab specimen for culture and sensitivity:
    a. use a dry sterile swab.
    b. dip the culturette in water-soluble lubricant.
    c. moisten the swab with normal saline.
    d. insert the swab at least 3 inches into the anus.

19. The three enemies of specimen collection include all of the following *except*:
    a. desiccation.
    b. sterilization.
    c. temperature.
    d. time.

20. Signs of wound infection include all of the following *except*:
    a. increased pain in the wound bed.
    b. wound tissue that becomes more fragile.
    c. a wound that stops draining serous fluid.
    d. a wound that stops healing or worsens.

21. A wound that is colonized:
    a. is infected.
    b. contains drug-resistant pathogens.
    c. should always be cultured.
    d. contains microbes that have reproduced.

22. To reduce the risk of spreading microbes, wound drainage should be:
    a. managed and contained.
    b. suctioned out at least once each shift.
    c. collected in a drainage bag.
    d. disinfected with alcohol or peroxide.

23. When collecting fingerstick blood sugars, the CDC recommends:
    a. using a separate meter for each patient.
    b. sharing the meter between two roommates only.
    c. disinfecting the meter at least once a week.
    d. using the same meter for all patients on the unit.

24. Glycated hemoglobin is a measurement of:
    a. daily blood sugar.
    b. the amount of oxygen in the blood.
    c. the blood sugar over a 30-day period of time.
    d. the blood sugar over a 90-day period of time.

25. When doing A1C testing, you should use:
    a. a reagent strip.
    b. a single-use, disposable meter.
    c. the glucometer.
    d. the same meter for all patients on the unit.

EXPLORING THE WEB

About Diabetes	http://diabetes.about.com
American Association of Clinical Endocrinologists	http://www.aace.com
American Association of Diabetes Educators	http://www.aadenet.org
American Diabetes Association	http://www.diabetes.org
Ask Noah	http://www.noah-health.org
The Basics of Specimen Collection and Handling of Urine Testing	http://www.bd.com
Canadian Diabetes Association	http://www.diabetes.ca
Check Your A1C at Home	http://www.mendosa.com
Collection Instructions for Urine and Feces	http://www.mgh.org
Collection of 24-Hour Urine Specimen	http://www.mdsdx.com
Combined Health Information Database	http://chid.nih.gov
Dartmouth-Hitchcock Medical Center Laboratory Procedures Manual	http://labhandbook.hitchcock.org:591
Diabetes Mall	http://www.diabetesnet.com
Diabetes Monitor	http://www.diabetesmonitor.com
Diabetes Public Health Resources	http://www.cdc.gov
Directory of Diabetic Organizations	http://www.niddk.nih.gov
Doctors' Guide to Diabetes	http://www.docguide.com
Eisenhower Army Medical Center Stool Specimen Collections	http://www.ddeamc.amedd.army.mil
Ensuring Prompt, Accurate Sputum Testing	http://dhfs.wisconsin.gov
Gastric Analysis	http://www.nhhn.org
General Specimen Collection, Handling, & Transportation	http://referencelab.clevelandclinic.org
Guideline for the Collection and Storage of Bacteriology Specimens for Testing	http://www.oaml.com
Guidelines for Stool Specimen Collection in an Outbreak (adapted from CDC guidelines)	http://www.epi.state.nc.us
International Diabetes Federation	http://www.idf.org
LSUHCS-Shreveport, Specimen Collection: Midstream Clean-Catch Urine	http://www.sh.lsuhsc.edu
Medline Plus	http://www.nlm.nih.gov
MedWeb Plus	http://www.medwebplus.com
Merck Manual	http://www.merck.com
Midstream Specimen Collection	http://www.emro.who.int
National Diabetes Education Program	http://ndep.nih.gov

National Diabetes Fact Sheets	http://www.cdc.gov
National Institute of Diabetes	http://www.niddk.nih.gov
Ova and Parasites—Stool	http://referencelab.clevelandclinic.org
Preferred Specimen Collection/Transport Guide for Enteric Orders	http://www.legacyhealth.org
Preventive Health Center	http://www.md-phc.com
Procedure-Specific Precautions for Patients with Known or Suspected Active Tuberculosis	http://info.med.yale.edu
Routine Sputum Culture	http://health.ucsd.edu
Specimen Collection and Handling	http://www.mgh.org
Specimen Collection Guide	http://depts.washington.edu
Specimen Collection Manual	http://www.crlcorp.com
Specimen Collection Urine and Feces	http://www.mgh.org
Specimen Preparation	http://www.bioreference.com
Sputum AFB Culture	http://health.ucsd.edu
Stool Collection and Fixation	http://www.practicalscience.com
Strep A Test	http://www.genzymediagnostics.com
Swab Specimen Collection	http://www.edu.rcsed.ac.uk
Throat Cultures	http://www.dcss.cs.amedd.army.mil
Throat Cultures and Strep Testing	http://www.troybio.com
Urinalysis	http://www.pathguy.com
Urine Collection	http://www.rnceus.com
Urine Culture	http://www.chclibrary.org
Urine Culture—Catheterized Specimen	http://www.umm.edu
Urine Culture, Comprehensive	http://www.labcorp.com
Urine Culture, Routine	http://www.labcorp.com
UTHCPC Procedures—Specimen Collection from a Wound for Culture	http://www.uth.tmc.edu
Wound AFB Culture	http://health.ucsd.edu
Wound or Drainage Culture	http://health.ucsd.edu
Wound Swabbing	http://www.rdns.net.au
Wounds/Tissues/Aspirates Culture Manual	http://microbiology.mtsinai.on.ca
Yahoo Health	http://dir.yahoo.com

Perioperative Care

OBJECTIVES:

After reading this chapter, you should be able to:

- Spell and define key terms.
- Define perioperative care, list at least 10 qualities that are essential for perioperative nursing personnel, and identify the primary concerns for workers in the operating area.
- Identify methods of preventing infection used by perioperative personnel.
- Explain why preoperative shaving may not be ordered by the physician.
- List precautions and considerations for removing hair preoperatively.
- List the guidelines for postoperative incision care.
- State the purpose of coughing and deep breathing exercises.
- Describe the purpose for and use of the incentive spirometer.
- State the purpose of using antiembolism hosiery, list the guidelines for applying the hosiery, and identify complications for which to monitor.
- State the purpose of pneumatic compression cuffs.
- List contraindications in using pneumatic compression cuffs.
- Describe the care of patients who have fractures and other orthopedic injuries and conditions.
- Describe the care of patients who have casts, including ongoing monitoring of the casted extremity.
- Describe the care of patients who have hip fracture, surgical hip repair, and joint replacement surgery.
- List at least 12 precautions to consider when caring for a patient who has had hip replacement or repair surgery.
- State the purpose of continuous passive motion, and list the contraindications and precautions associated with this procedure.
- Describe compartment syndrome, and list the signs and symptoms of this condition.
- State the purpose of traction, and differentiate skin traction from skeletal traction.

PERIOPERATIVE NURSING CARE

The term **perioperative nursing** describes the care given in the hospital surgical department(s), day-surgery units (also called ambulatory surgery units), clinics, and physicians' offices. Perioperative care is provided before, during, and after surgery and other invasive procedures. Some perioperative staff specialize in the care of patients who need specific procedures, such as cardiac, orthopedic, or neurologic surgeries. The operating room is a high-technology area in which change is a constant. Lasers, robotics, video equipment, and computers are standard equipment in the operating department. New technology is constantly needed as scientific and medical research advance. The personnel providing perioperative care must:

- Have good problem-solving skills
- Have good communication skills
- Interact well with many different kinds of people in stressful situations
- Accept responsibility
- Be emotionally stable
- Use good judgment
- Work well with others as contributing team members
- Have a solid knowledge base in sterile technique and procedures
- Be proficient in the use of a computer
- Be competent to perform the skills needed in the operating area
- Have the physical stamina for prolonged standing, lifting, and moving of patients and heavy objects

The perioperative staff works closely with surgical patients, their families, physicians, and other health care professionals. As you can see, this can be a demanding area in which to work, but it is very rewarding.

Working in Perioperative Care

Infection control and prevention are primary concerns in the operating area. Personnel must wear scrub suits while at work, instead of uniforms. These clothes are usually provided, laundered, and maintained by the hospital. Personnel put them on when they arrive at work, and change into street clothes before leaving. If a worker must leave the operating suites during the shift, his or her scrubs must be covered with a lab coat, which is removed immediately upon return to the department.

Hand and Forearm Antisepsis. Staff working in the operative suite may be required to scrub their hands and forearms with a sponge or brush at the beginning of the shift (**Figure 11-1**), and periodically after that. Additional special measures are required for staff who assist with op-

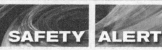

SAFETY ALERT

Have you ever heard the expression, "When your feet hurt, you hurt all over?" Most experienced health care workers will tell you this old adage is true. Buying a sturdy pair of athletic shoes or duty shoes is one of the best investments you will make in your uniform. Make sure that the bottoms are appropriate for the floor surface in your facility. In most cases, this means having a nonslip sole. The operating room floor is not carpeted, so athletic or nursing shoes work best. Having supportive footwear will make you feel better and reduce your risk of falls and injuries.

Electrostatic sparks that do not cause problems in your daily life have the potential to cause serious problems in the presence of some anesthetic gases, which are explosive and flammable. Conductive shoes are effective measures for preventing such problems. Shoes with conductive panels on the soles may be purchased from a uniform store, or you may use disposable shoe covers with a conductive strip that is inserted into the shoe, and runs the length of the foot. If you will be working in an area with potentially harmful gases, you will be instructed to wear conductive footwear. Because the health care facility is a source of many serious pathogens, consider leaving your duty shoes at work. Remove them, wash your hands, and put on another pair of shoes at the end of your shift.

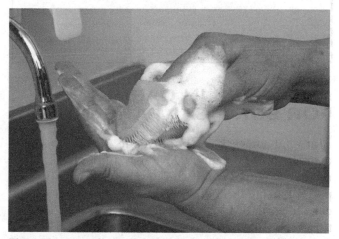

FIGURE 11-1 Staff working in the operative suite must scrub their hands and forearms with a sponge or brush at the beginning of the shift, and periodically throughout the day.

erations. To reduce the risk of infection, perioperative personnel should:

- Keep hands and fingernails short; nails should not extend more than one-quarter inch beyond the fingertip.
- Avoid artificial nails, including acrylic nails, tips, and sculpted nails; many facilities prohibit direct care workers from using any type of artificial nail.

- Avoid nail polish.
- Keep fingernails clean.
- Scrub the hands and forearms for at least 2 to 5 minutes using an appropriate antiseptic upon arrival at work. Scrub the hands and forearms up to the elbows. Use the brush or sponge to clean under and around fingernails.
- Avoid hand and arm jewelry.

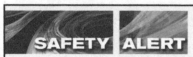

All personnel involved in the perioperative care of the patient must be alert to make sure that the correct surgical procedure is done on the correct patient, and that the surgery is done on the correct site. This may involve marking the site of the surgery with a marker. Various forms and checklists are used to verify the patient and surgical site. Take your responsibilities for identifying the patient and operative site seriously. This is an area of nursing practice where there is no room for error.

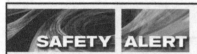

Remove dentures from a comatose patient to prevent accidental airway obstruction. Remove dentures from patients preoperatively to prevent potential damage to the dentures and accidental airway obstruction in surgery.

ADVANCES IN CARING FOR SURGICAL PATIENTS

Many advances have been made in surgical care over the past 25 years. Previously, patients were admitted to the hospital the day before surgery. The patient became acquainted with staff who would care for him or her postoperatively. Various laboratory tests were completed. The patient's skin was prepared with surgical scrubs. Body hair in the operative area was shaved. The patient was sent to the operating room from the nursing unit. He or she returned to the same room after surgery.

Today, most patients complete their laboratory testing on an outpatient basis before surgery. Patients remain at home until they are admitted for surgery. They are advised not to eat or drink anything after midnight on the evening before their scheduled surgery. They are often instructed to shower with a special antibacterial soap before coming to the hospital early in the morning, on the day of surgery. After they are admitted, a nurse or PCT completes the skin preparation. The patient

then goes right to surgery. Many surgeries are performed on an outpatient basis. The patients go home, or return to a long-term care or subacute care facility, after they have recovered from the anesthesia. If the patient experiences complications, he or she will be admitted to the hospital. Many patients are first admitted to the nursing unit after surgery, so they are not familiar with the staff.

Previously, preoperative teaching was done on the nursing unit the evening before surgery. Now, because most patients are not admitted until after surgery, patient teaching may be done later. Patient teaching is also done in the physician's office before surgery. The office may mail instructions to the patient before hospital admission. Some physicians hold informational classes. Personnel in the operating room may also do some patient teaching, but you must reinforce it on the nursing unit. You will be assisting the RN in teaching the patient how to move and turn, do coughing and deep breathing, perform foot and leg exercises, manage pain, and other aspects of care.

PREOPERATIVE SKIN CARE

Before some surgical procedures, the skin is scrubbed and shaved. Years ago, patients were shaved routinely for all procedures, including childbirth. Studies have shown that shaving causes nicks and cuts in the skin. These may be visible, but they may also be very tiny and difficult to see. These nicks and cuts increase the risk of infection, so some physicians may order a skin scrub, but no shave. The Association of Operating Room Nurses (AORN) recommends that hair not be removed unless it is thick enough to interfere with the surgery. In most facilities, a physician's order is required for preoperative hair removal. Follow the physician's orders and your facility policy.

Shaving the Operative Site

If you will be doing the skin preparation, take care to avoid nicking or cutting the patient, as well as to avoid causing abrasions with the razor. Use only a sterile disposable or reusable razor. Perform this procedure as close to the time of surgery as possible. This provides less time for microbes to proliferate on the skin. If the razor becomes dull, get another. The texture of some patients' body hair makes it difficult to remove, and a dull razor increases the risk of injury. If you observe a cut, rash, redness, irritation, or other break in the skin near the operative site, notify the RN.

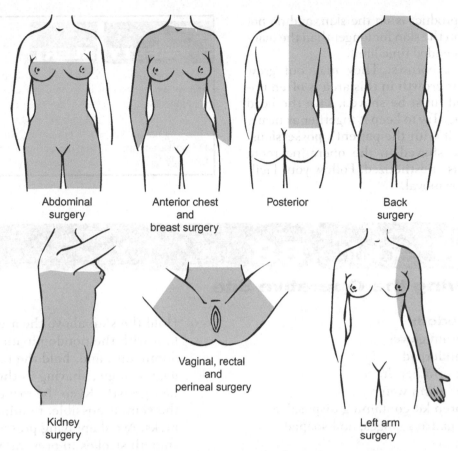

Abdominal surgery

Anterior chest and breast surgery

Posterior

Back surgery

Kidney surgery

Vaginal, rectal and perineal surgery

Left arm surgery

FIGURE 11-2 The shaded areas indicate areas that may be shaved preoperatively.

When preparing the operative area, you will scrub and/or shave the actual site of the surgical incision, and the skin surrounding the area (**Figure 11-2**). Use warm water for washing the area. This facilitates removal of body oil, soil, and hair. Change the water and use warm, clear water for rinsing.

If you will be shaving the operative area, clipping the hair with scissors first will prevent pulling if the hair is long and thick. If you are using a disposable or reusable razor with a sharp blade to shave a patient, *always wear gloves*, because of the high probability of contact with blood during this procedure. In some facilities, electric clippers with disposable heads are used to remove hair preoperatively. Some studies have shown that using clippers is associated with a lower risk of infection. Avoid shaving neck and facial hair on women and children, if possible.

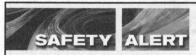

SAFETY ALERT

When shaving the patient, remember to hold the razor at a 45-degree angle. Maintain contact with the skin. Try to avoid lifting the razor and then putting it down again. Doing this increases the risk of nicks and cuts.

OSHA ALERT

Handle needles, razors, and other sharp objects with care. Needles are never cut, bent, broken, or recapped by hand. After using a sharp object, dispose of it in a puncture-resistant sharps container. Avoid overfilling the sharps container. Seal the cap when the container is three-quarters full. The cap is designed so it cannot be snapped back off after it is closed. The sealed sharps container is stored until it can be picked up with the biohazardous waste. The biohazardous waste disposal area is used for discarding items contaminated with blood or body fluids. Special precautions are taken to contain waste in this area.

If a cognitively impaired adult or pediatric patient will not sit still, consider using depilatory cream. However, realize that depilatories can be very irritating to the skin of some people, causing redness, burning, skin breakdown, and rash. Always test a small area first to determine whether the patient will have a skin reaction to the depilatory product. If the patient does not react adversely to the test area, apply the product to the operative site and surrounding skin. Read product instructions carefully, remain in the room with the patient when the product is on the skin, and do not leave the product on the skin for longer than the manufacturer's recommended time limit.

Never shave eyebrows. They may not grow back, and new hair growth in this area is often unsightly. If the head must be shaved, save the head hair in a plastic bag. Try to keep it together as neatly as possible. Store it with the patient's possessions. The head may be shaved in the operating room while the patient is anesthetized. Follow your facility policy for hair removal.

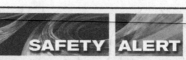

SAFETY ALERT

The anesthesiologist often orders an injection of analgesic and relaxing medication to be given within an hour of the scheduled surgery time. Always keep the side rails up after the patient receives this injection. Make sure the call signal is within reach. Never allow a patient to get up and go to the bathroom alone after the perioperative medication has been given.

Procedure 88

Shaving the Operative Site

Supplies needed:
- Disposable exam gloves
- Disposable underpad
- Bath blanket or other drape
- Washbasin of warm water
- Disposable prep kit containing disposable drape, razor, gauze sponges, and soaped scrub sponge
- Washcloth
- Towel
- Plastic bag for used supplies

1. Perform your beginning procedure actions.
2. Position the disposable underpad under the area to be shaved.
3. Open the disposable prep kit. Remove the drape and position it over the operative area.
4. Wet the sponge in the basin. Squeeze it so it is moist but not dripping.
5. Apply the sponge to the area to be scrubbed. Begin scrubbing in a circular motion in the center of the area, working outward. Work up a good lather on the skin.

6. Hold the skin above the area to be shaved taut with the nondominant hand. With the dominant hand, hold the razor at a 45-degree angle, shaving in the direction of hair growth. Keep the razor in contact with the skin, if possible, to minimize cuts and nicks. Avoid applying pressure, and use smooth strokes to prevent abrasions. Remove hair from the razor as often as necessary with the gauze sponges. Rinse the razor as often as necessary. Apply more soap to the skin as needed to keep the skin soapy and wet.
7. Empty the basin and rinse it well. Refill it with clean warm water.
8. Rinse the skin with a washcloth and pat dry with the towel.
9. Ask the RN to check the prep. You may be instructed to perform a 10-minute surgical scrub to the area.
10. Perform your procedure completion actions.

DURING THE OPERATIVE PERIOD

While the patient is in the operating room, you will prepare the room for the patient's return:

- Prepare a surgical bed by making the bed with fresh linen. Fanfold the upper bed linen to the far side of the bed (**Figure 11-3**).

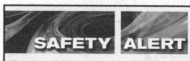

SAFETY ALERT

Be alert when removing bed linen. Look carefully for items that are a potential source of injury, such as lancets and needles. Make sure the patient's personal items (such as dentures, hearing aids, and eyeglasses) are not accidentally sent to the laundry with the bed linen.

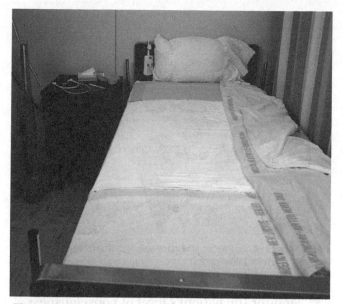

FIGURE 11-3 Fanfold the linen to the side of the bed to receive the patient.

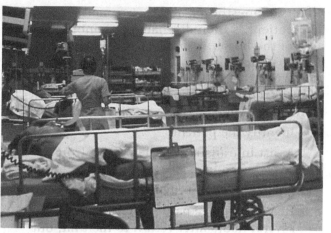

FIGURE 11-4 The postanesthesia care unit (PACU) is where the patient is monitored and wakes up after surgery. (Courtesy of Memorial Medical Center of Long Beach, CA)

- Tie a waterproof pillow to the headboard of the bed with gauze bandage, or position it according to the facility policy.
- Apply a disposable underpad to the center of the bed, and at the head of the bed if the surgery was done in the head and neck area, or according to facility policy.
- Make sure the bed has side rails. Check them to make sure they lock in the raised position.
- Arrange the room so there is adequate room to bring the stretcher in and position it next to the bed. Leave the bed locked in position at stretcher height.
- Anticipate positioning needs when the patient returns. Bring extra pillows and other items that will be needed to the room.
- Make sure an intravenous standard, oxygen, suction, drainage bags, and other necessary equipment are brought to the room.
- Remove everything from the top of the bedside stand except the emesis basin, tissues, tongue depressor, and equipment to check vital signs.
- Check with the RN for any special instructions.
- Watch for the patient's return when carrying out your other duties. When the patient returns, immediately go to the room to help transfer and position the patient.

POSTOPERATIVE CARE

During the immediate postoperative period, the patient recovers from anesthesia. For this period, he or she will be transferred to the recovery (recovering) room (**Figure 11-4**). The recovery room is next to the operating room and is sometimes called the *postanesthesia care unit* (PACU). The PACU is the area where patients are monitored and cared for until they have recovered from the

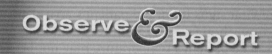

Postoperative Observation and Reporting

Decreased responsiveness or unresponsiveness
Change in the level of responsiveness
Increased restlessness accompanied by complaints of thirst
Changes in blood pressure
Weak, rapid, or irregular pulse
Changes in temperature
Changes in respiratory rate
Difficulty breathing; labored or noisy respirations
Nausea or vomiting
Complaints of pain
Increased drainage, wet or saturated dressings
Active bleeding
Coughing or choking

effects of anesthesia, and their condition is stable. The patient is then discharged to another unit or area of the hospital, or to home, depending on the circumstances.

When the patient's condition has stabilized, he or she is returned to the unit. Upon the patient's return, you should:

- Identify the patient.
- Assist in transferring the patient from stretcher to bed.
- Never leave the unconscious patient alone.
- Realize that the patient may be drowsy for several hours after return to the unit, but should respond to stimulation.
- Prevent heat loss, Have extra blankets available. Anesthesia reduces body temperature. Many patients complain of feeling very cold.
- Notify the RN if the patient's body temperature is below 97°F.

Always follow the protocol for vital signs used by your facility. The vital sign schedule may be altered by the RN if the patient's condition warrants. The physician may also order vital signs at a designated frequency. The following are routine instructions that should be followed unless otherwise ordered:

- Always wear gloves and use standard precautions when contact with blood, body fluids, mucous membranes, or nonintact skin is likely.
- Take vital signs upon the patient's arrival on the unit, then every 15 minutes for 4 readings. The patient's temperature may not be taken each time. Follow facility policies and the RN's instructions.
- When taking postoperative vital signs, count the pulse and respirations for one full minute. Most facilities have policies for taking postoperative vital signs at specified frequencies that decrease if the vital signs are stable (approximately the same), such as:
  - every 15 minutes for 1 hour
  - if stable, every 30 minutes for 1 hour
  - if stable, every hour for 2 hours
  - if stable, every 4 hours for 24 hours
- Check the pulses distal to the operative site. Compare the pulse in the operative extremity to the pulse in the other extremity. Inform the RN of abnormalities, or if pulses are weak or cannot be felt.

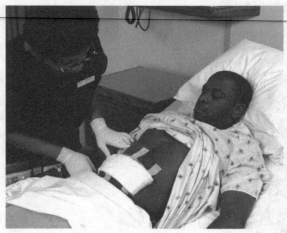

FIGURE 11-5 Check the dressings frequently for drainage and bleeding.

- Monitor the patient's level of consciousness (drowsy, unresponsive, alert) each time you check the vital signs.
- Many facilities consider pain to be the fifth vital sign. You should ask the patient if he or she is having pain each time you check vital signs. Use a pain scale, if this is permitted by your facility. Inform the nurse if pain is present.
- Check dressings for the amount and type of drainage (**Figure 11-5**). Inform the RN, who may instruct you to reinforce the dressings, if necessary.
- Reinforcing a dressing means placing an additional dressing on top of the existing dressing.
- Never remove the dressing that covers a fresh surgical incision unless the RN specifically instructs you to do so.
- Check the IV solution for flow rate. Check the insertion site for signs of infiltration. Never let an IV bag run dry.

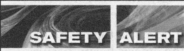

SAFETY ALERT

Remember that when they undergo surgery, most patients receive many drugs that have the potential to alter their mental status. The drugs are excreted from the body slowly. The patient may sleep soundly upon return to the unit. Keep the side rails up and follow all safety precautions until the patient is fully awake and the RN instructs you that side rails are no longer necessary. Do not leave liquids at the bedside until the RN instructs you that doing so is safe. Check on the patient regularly.

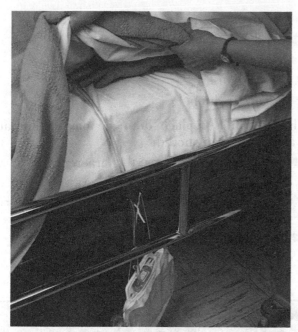

FIGURE 11-6 Monitor drainage tubes to make sure they are draining properly, and are not twisted, kinked, or obstructed.

- Check the pulse oximeter to ensure that the alarm is on and set at the ordered limit each time you are in the room.
- Encourage the patient to cough, deep breathe, and move in bed. Assist the patient to reposition at least every 2 hours.
- Turn the patient's head to one side and support it if he or she is vomiting. Have an emesis basin and tissues ready. You may also need a wet washcloth and towel. If the patient is conscious, allow him or her to rinse the mouth after vomiting. Note the type and amount of vomitus and record on the output worksheet. Report the vomiting to the RN.
- Make sure that all drainage tubes have been connected and are draining properly. Check for kinks and obstructions each time you are in the room (**Figure 11-6**). If a tube is clamped shut, check with the RN before connecting.
- Measure and document the first postoperative voiding. Inform the RN.
- If the patient was given a spinal anesthetic:
  - Give extra care in turning frequently and maintaining good alignment.
  - Remember that the patient will not be able to move independently until sensation and motor function return. Calm the patient's fears about this.

- Some physicians require the patient to remain flat on the back, without a pillow, for 8 to 12 hours following spinal anesthesia, to avoid headaches.
- Inform the RN if the patient complains of a headache.
- Provide extra blankets if the patient complains of feeling cold.

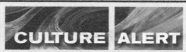

CULTURE ALERT

After surgery, you will assist the patient to resume drinking fluids and eating a progressive diet, beginning with liquids and progressing to regular solid foods. Be aware that many people from India, and those of the Hindu faith, will usually not eat until they have bathed. Allow time to assist the patient with toileting, bathing, and comfort measures before the meal tray arrives.

Pain Management

Most patients have pain after surgery. All patients have the right to pain relief. Report complaints of pain to the RN, who will assess the patient and implement measures to relieve the pain. Pain interferes with the patient's optimal level of function and rehabilitation.

Some patients have a device called a PCA pump connected to their IV. **Patient-controlled analgesia (PCA)** is a method of enabling patients to self-administer their own pain medications (**Figure 11-7**). The dosage is controlled to prevent the risk of an accidental overdose. The PCA system

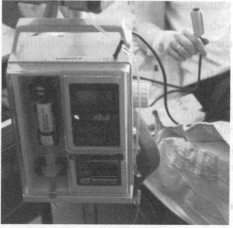

FIGURE 11-7 The patient pushes a button connected to the PCA pump to self-administer pain medication. The patient is the only person who is legally authorized to press the button to dispense medication.

uses a pump containing a medication. It is programmed by the RN to deliver either measured amounts of the medication or a continuous infusion, or both, through an intravenous line. Only the patient should push the button to dispense medications. The patient's family members should not push the buttons, nor should hospital staff. Inform the RN if this occurs. Monitor the patient for excessive sleepiness or shallow respirations, and notify the RN if present.

After the Patient Has Recovered from Anesthesia

When the patient has responded sufficiently and vital signs are stable, he or she may be refreshed by:

- Washing the hands and face
- Straightening or changing the linen
- Being given a light backrub

The patient is now ready to participate more actively in recovery. Exercises taught in the preoperative period should be practiced, including:

- Deep breathing and coughing
- Leg exercises

Deep breathing and coughing clear the air passages. This helps to prevent postoperative respiratory complications, such as pneumonia and **atelectasis,** which is the inability to expand the lungs due to collapse of the alveolar air sacs. This may be an uncomfortable task when the patient has a new incision and feels fatigued. You can best assist the patient by:

- Explaining the importance of the exercise and encouraging the patient to do the procedure.
- Scheduling these activities according to pain medication administration. Coordinate the exercises to be done approximately 45 minutes after pain medication is given.
- Learning from the RN how many deep breaths and coughs should be attempted. The usual number is 5 to 10 breaths and 2 to 3 coughs.
- Using a pillow or binder to support the incision during the procedure.

Drainage

When a body cavity is the operative site, it may be necessary to drain fluid from it, such as blood, pus, serous drainage, or gastric contents, before or after surgery. Always wear gloves if contact with drainage is likely. The drainage outlet may be a:

- Catheter
- T-tube
- Jackson-Pratt (J-P) or Hemovac drain
- Penrose drain
- Cigarette drain

When a drain is in place, drainage may accumulate in a dressing. You should:

- Monitor the amount and character of drainage.
- Check with the RN before changing or reinforcing a dressing.
- Use sterile technique whenever you manipulate or empty a tube or drain or change a dressing.

DIFFICULT PATIENT | ALERT

A closed wound drain and vacuum system are placed when the surgeon anticipates substantial wound drainage. The tubing exit site is considered a surgical incision, and the drain is often sutured to the skin. Some patients will have more than one closed drain. Having a drain in place prevents swelling and promotes wound healing. It reduces the risk of infection and skin breakdown. Fewer dressing changes are necessary. Fasten the vacuum unit for the drain to the bed or patient's gown, if he or she is ambulatory. Make sure the vacuum unit remains below the level of the wound. Avoid traction on the tubing. You must empty the drain and record the output at the end of each shift, and more often if the drain is full. A full drain applies less suction to the wound, and the additional fluid accumulation under the skin will strain the suture line. If the patient has multiple drains, you should number them and record the output from each separately. Follow the procedure guidelines in Chapter 5 when caring for the drain.

At times, the withdrawal of fluids is controlled by attaching the drainage tube to a connecting tube, then to a suction apparatus. The drainage accumulates in a container. The container must be emptied at the end of each shift, and whenever full. Wear a mask and eye protection during this procedure to prevent accidental splashes. Document the amount of drainage on the output record accurately. Measure the drainage in a graduate or specimen collection cup. Do not estimate the quantity. The Jackson-Pratt and Hemovac drains are closed drainage systems. The drains are placed directly in a wound, and drainage goes into an expandable container. A record of the amount and character of drainage is entered in both the output record and the nursing notes. It is your responsibility to:

- Select and apply the correct protective apparel for the procedure, to prevent potential personal exposure to bloodborne pathogens.
- Report either heavy or light drainage.
- Report a change in the appearance, amount, or character of drainage.
- Make sure that the flow of drainage is not blocked.

Never assume the responsibility for emptying chest tube bottles. This is the nurse's responsibility, unless you have been taught to do it correctly and are permitted to perform this procedure in your facility.

Careful preoperative preparation and postoperative care can help limit the patient's postoperative discomfort and complications. The patient must be closely observed, especially during the first 24 hours. Some guidelines for postoperative monitoring are listed in the Observe & Report box. Postoperative complications and PCT actions are listed in Table 11-1.

Table 11-1 Postoperative Complications and PCT Actions

Discomfort	Patient Complaint/ PCT Observation	PCT Action
Thirst	Dryness of lips, mouth, skin	Carefully check I&O. Give ice chips or increase fluid by mouth, as ordered. Give mouth care. Check blood pressure and pulse. Monitor for signs of shock and hemorrhage.
Singultus (hiccups)— intermittent spasms of the diaphragm	Hiccups	Allow the patient to rest. Hiccups can be tiring. Support the incisional area with a pillow. Assist the patient to breathe into a paper bag. Have the patient swallow air and belch.
Pain	Location, intensity, type	Inform the RN. Monitor for effectiveness of pain medication. Use nursing comfort measures, such as changing position, supporting the patient's body with pillows, giving a backrub, adjusting room temperature for patient comfort.
Distention, gas in bowel	Distention, complaints of gas pain	Increase mobility. Insert a rectal tube, if ordered.
Nausea, vomiting	Nausea, character of vomitus	Keep an emesis basin and tissues at the bedside. Monitor IV fluids that are substituted for oral fluids. Limit fluids by mouth. Give oral care. Encourage the patient to breathe deeply.
Urinary retention	Amount and time of first voiding, distention, restlessness, imbalance between I&O	Monitor I&O carefully. Check for bladder distention. Assist with toileting. Catheterize, if so ordered. Do an ultrasound bladder scan, if permitted by facility policies and if unit is available.
Hemorrhage, excessive blood loss	Decreased blood pressure; cool, moist skin; weak, rapid pulse; restlessness; pallor or cyanosis; thirst; condition of dressing	Report to RN immediately. Keep NPO. Monitor pulse oximeter and vital signs. Keep the patient as quiet as possible. Increase the IV fluids, if ordered. Obtain blood from blood bank and monitor blood transfusion.

(continues)

Table 11-1 Postoperative Complications and PCT Actions (Continued)

Discomfort	Patient Complaint/ PCT Observation	PCT Action
Shock	Decreased blood pressure; cool, moist skin; weak, rapid pulse; restlessness; apprehension; pallor or cyanosis; thirst	Report to RN immediately. Keep NPO. Monitor pulse oximeter and vital signs. Keep the patient as quiet as possible. Increase the IV fluids, if ordered.
Hypoxemia	Restlessness, crowing respirations, pounding pulse, perspiration	Report to RN immediately. Administer oxygen as ordered. Monitor pulse oximeter and vital signs.
Atelectasis	Dyspnea, cyanosis, pallor	Report to RN immediately. Administer oxygen as ordered. Monitor pulse oximeter and vital signs.
Wound infection	Increased pain in incisional area, fever, chills, anorexia, increased drainage, pus or other abnormal drainage	Report to RN immediately. Obtain culture and sensitivity, as ordered. Monitor regularly, and change or reinforce dressings as needed.
Wound dehiscence or disruption	Splitting, separating, or gaping open of suture line. Pinkish drainage. Complaints of "feeling open," "broken," "given way."	Report to RN immediately. Support the area. Keep the patient quiet.
Pulmonary emboli	Anxiety, dyspnea, shortness of breath, heaviness in chest, cyanosis, chest pain	Report to RN immediately. Administer oxygen as ordered. Monitor pulse oximeter and vital signs. Elevate head of bed.

Leg Exercises

Leg exercises following surgery encourage steady circulation. This helps to prevent postoperative blood clots. A blood clot or **deep vein thrombosis (DVT)** could develop in the venous system and block the essential blood flow. A small clot could travel through the vascular system and lodge in the lungs. A specific order must be written for leg exercises when surgery has been done on the legs. Otherwise, leg exercises may be routinely done by the patient. If he or she is weak, you will assist.

Guidelines for Leg Exercises

- Remind the patient to do leg exercises when you assist with position changes.
- Have the patient brace the incisional area with laced hands.

- Curl the toes down and up (Figure 11-8A). Repeat.
- Rotate each ankle by drawing imaginary circles with the toes (Figure 11-8B).

(continued)

Guidelines for Leg Exercises (Continued)

- Dorsiflex (draw the toes up toward the knee) and plantar flex (point toes and foot down) each ankle.
- Flex and extend each knee by sliding the leg up and down in bed (Figure 11-8C). Monitor this action and teach the patient to relieve pressure on the heel to prevent a friction or shearing injury. If this is not possible, consider applying a heel protector.

- Flex and extend each hip.
- Repeat each exercise 3 to 5 times every 1 to 2 hours. Assist as needed.
- Apply or reapply antiembolism hose after exercises are done.

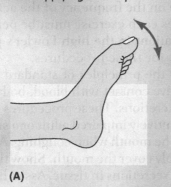
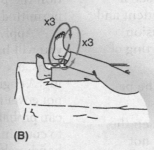
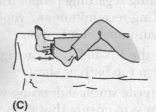

(A) (B) (C)

FIGURE 11-8 Help the patient perform leg exercises to encourage circulation. (A) Curl the toes down and up. Repeat 5 times. (B) Make circles with the feet clockwise 3 times and counterclockwise 3 times. Repeat 5 times. (C) Slide one leg up and down in bed. Do the same with the other leg. Repeat 5 times.

Initial Ambulation

Early ambulation is always a goal of postoperative care. Getting patients up and moving quickly stimulates circulation, promotes healing, improves their sense of well-being, and reduces the risk of complications. Many patients are permitted to be up in the chair at the bedside, or to ambulate in the room, after the effects of the anesthesia have worn off. The first ambulation is usually short. The patient should dangle at the bedside for a few minutes. If he or she tolerates this well, you may assist the patient with ambulation. If the patient has had abdominal or chest surgery, do not wrap a gait belt around the operative area. Remain with the patient. Assist with drainage tubes and IVs as needed (Figure 11-9). Take the patient's pulse before and after standing. If there is a difference of more than 10 points, return the patient to bed and inform the RN.

SAFETY ALERT

Remain next to the patient during the first dangling and ambulation. For patient safety, do not turn your back or leave the bedside. These precautions will probably not be necessary as the patient recovers and gains strength. Use common sense; follow the care plan and the RN's instructions.

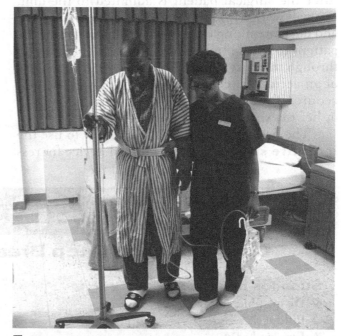

FIGURE 11-9 Drainage tubes and intravenous lines may be in place after surgery. Carefully move these with the patient.

Postoperative Incision Care

When caring for postoperative wounds, use the procedures in Chapter 5. The CDC lists some additional infection control precautions for caring for postoperative wounds:

- Apply a sterile dressing for at least 24 to 48 hours postoperatively, or as ordered.
- Apply the principles of standard precautions and careful handwashing before and after dressing changes and contact with the surgical site.
- Always use sterile technique when changing the dressing over a surgical incision.
- Check with the RN and care plan to see if you will be expected to assist with patient and family teaching regarding proper incision care, including recognition and reporting of signs and symptoms of infection.
- Check with the RN before allowing the patient to take a tub bath or shower.
- Cover the sterile surgical dressing when the patient bathes, to ensure that it does not become wet.

RESPIRATORY EXERCISES

After the surgical patient is admitted to the unit, you will work with him or her to perform coughing and deep breathing exercises. When instructing the patient to inhale, make sure he or she breathes in through the nose, if possible. This reduces the risk of an accidental cough during this part of the procedure. If the patient has lung disease, advise him or her to exhale slowly through puckered lips.

The patient may also have an order to use the **incentive spirometer,** a handheld device for respiratory exercises. Coughing, deep breathing, and using the incentive spirometer are done to inflate the lungs and remove mucus, preventing pneumonia and other complications. Personnel in the surgical department may teach the patient these procedures before surgery. Do not assume that he or she remembers them. Stay with the patient to ensure that he or she performs the activity correctly. The RN or respiratory care professional will advise you on the frequency of the activity, and how many times each exercise must be performed. Position the patient in the high Fowler's position, or as permitted, for these procedures.

Apply the principles of standard precautions if you will have contact with blood, body fluids, secretions, or excretions. These procedures induce coughing. A cognitively impaired adult or a small child may not cover the mouth when coughing. An alert patient can probably cover the mouth. Show the patient how to contain secretions in tissue. Assist him or her with handwashing after the activity. Wear eye protection and a surgical mask if this is your facility policy, or if you anticipate contact with secretions from the patient's coughing. Report frequency of deep breathing, cough, and any complaints to the RN.

Contraindications for Coughing and Deep Breathing. Although we routinely encourage postoperative patients to cough and deep breathe, you must be aware of a few exceptions. Avoid this procedure with patients who have had eye, nose, rectal, or neurologic surgery. Coughing and deep breathing will increase pressure, causing complications in these patients. Check with the RN if you are unsure of what action to take.

Procedure 89

Coughing and Deep Breathing Exercises

Supplies needed:
- Disposable exam gloves
- Pillow (if needed)
- Emesis basin
- Tissues
- Mouthwash
- Cup
- Straw
- Plastic bag for soiled items

1. Perform your beginning procedure actions.
2. Instruct the patient to hold a pillow across the abdomen or chest to splint the incision, if he or she had recent abdominal or chest surgery. He or she may also place one hand on either side of the rib cage, or place the hands over the operative site (Figure 11-10A).
3. Tell the patient to hold the pillow across the surgical site and inhale slowly through the nose, then hold his or her breath.

(continues)

Procedure **89**, *continued*

Coughing and Deep Breathing Exercises

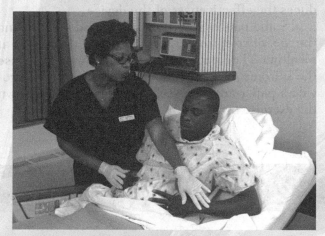

FIGURE II-10(A) Encourage the patient to perform deep breathing exercises.

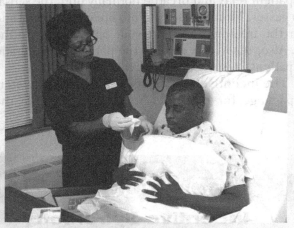

FIGURE II-10(B) A pillow helps support the abdomen and splint the incision during coughing and deep breathing.

4. Hold the breath for 3 seconds, then slowly exhale through the mouth. If the patient has lung disease, advise him or her to exhale slowly through puckered lips. Make sure the hand on the pillow rises on inhalation.
5. Tell the patient to take another slow, deep breath through the nose. Have the patient hold the breath for 3 seconds, then cough two or three times in a row during

exhalation while squeezing the pillow over the surgical site (**Figure 11-10B**).
6. Make sure you are wearing gloves to assist with tissues and the emesis basin to remove secretions, if necessary.
7. Repeat this exercise 5 to 10 times, or as ordered.
8. After the procedure, offer mouthwash to rinse the mouth.
9. Perform your procedure completion actions.

Incentive Spirometry

Incentive spirometry is a form of goal-directed respiratory therapy. The purpose is deep breathing. The goals for incentive spirometry are individualized for the patient. The respiratory therapist will develop the goals and specify the frequency of spirometer use. The goals will be achievable for the patient, but only with some effort. The incentive is for the patient to visualize how much air he or she is taking in with each inhalation (**Figure 11-11**). This is accomplished by inhaling from the spirometer. The patient watches the position of the ping-pong balls inside. Apply the principles of standard precautions when assisting with this procedure.

The incentive spirometer is usually left at the bedside. In addition to helping to prevent pneumonia, it also improves blood flow and increases lung volume.

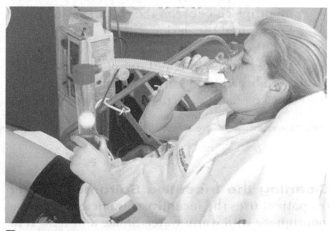

FIGURE II-II The incentive spirometer improves blood flow, increases lung volume, and prevents pneumonia.

The patient will be prompted to use it hourly throughout the day. He or she is instructed to take a designated number of slow, deep breaths using the spirometer. If the patient becomes dizzy or complains of tingling in the fingers, he or she may be breathing too fast. Have the patient relax and breathe normally until the sensation passes. Monitor the patient's breathing before and after the treatment. Report your observations to the RN. Also, report the volume the patient reached and the patient's response to the treatment.

The incentive spirometer is packaged in a sterile package for first use. You must assemble the pieces. Remove the flow tube and mouthpiece. Connect them and then connect the tube to the spirometer. Set the volume goal indicator at the designated level. The spirometer should be upright on a flat surface when the patient uses it. Tilting reduces the effectiveness of the device.

Some patients become nauseated when using the incentive spirometer. Avoid using the device at mealtime. The patient may be encouraged to use the spirometer independently in a day or two. Provide a paper and pen so he or she can write down the exercise times.

Procedure 90

Incentive Spirometry

Supplies needed:
- Disposable exam gloves
- Incentive spirometer
- Tissue
- Emesis basin
- Mouthwash
- Cup
- Straw
- Plastic bag for soiled items

1. Perform your beginning procedure actions.
2. Assist the patient to sit in the high Fowler's position.
3. Instruct the patient to exhale slowly, emptying the lungs as much as possible.
4. Have the patient place the spirometer mouthpiece between the teeth, closing the lips around the device.
5. Tell the patient to take a slow, deep breath, using the diaphragm. Prompt the patient to keep breathing in until the indicator on the device reaches the highest level possible.

The patient should work toward the goal each time he or she uses the incentive spirometer. (If the patient achieves the goal, notify the appropriate person. The goal may be advanced.)
6. Instruct the patient to hold the breath for 3 to 5 seconds.
7. Tell the patient to exhale normally. Encourage the patient to cough to loosen secretions. Instruct the patient to take several normal breaths before using the spirometer again. The patient should take 5 to 10 breaths each time, or as ordered.
8. Provide the emesis basin and tissues if the patient coughs up secretions. Assist as necessary. Make sure you are wearing gloves.
9. Instruct the patient to rest briefly between breaths, then repeat the procedure.
10. Offer the patient mouthwash to rinse the mouth. Assist as necessary.
11. Perform your procedure completion actions.

Cleaning the Incentive Spirometer. After the patient uses the incentive spirometer, clean the mouthpiece with warm water. Shake it or hang it to dry, according to facility policy. Store the device in a plastic or paper bag, labeled with the patient's name, after use. Wear gloves when cleaning the incentive spirometer.

SUPPORT HOSIERY

Support hosiery are commonly called **antiembolism stockings,** or are referred to by the brand name, such as TED or Jobst hose. They may also be called *graduated compression stockings (GCS)*. This refers to the graduation of pressure. The stockings are tightest at the ankle, and become looser as they move up the leg. The hosiery are used for patients who have circulation problems or high-risk conditions. They are commonly used during and after surgery to prevent deep vein thrombosis (DVT) and other complications. Deep vein thrombosis is a blood clot that most commonly occurs in the deep veins of the legs. The major complications are pulmonary emboli. Surgery and immobility are the most important risk factors. Although there is a risk with all general surgical procedures, the risk is greatest with orthopedic procedures, such as hip surgery and knee replacement. Immobility during the postoperative recovery period adds to these risks. Without prophylaxis, the risk of DVT ranges from 25 percent to 30 percent for general surgical patients and up to 70 percent following some orthopedic procedures.

Elastic stockings have been used in the treatment of varicose veins for more than 150 years. They may also be used to prevent edema. The stockings are made of stretchable elastic and fit tightly. They may be knee length or thigh length, covering most of the leg. The stockings apply pressure to the legs, which increases the blood flow. Several different types of antiembolism hose are used. Some have closed toes, but most have an opening near the toe end. The hole is positioned on the top or the bottom of the foot, just proximal to the toes, depending on the type of hosiery used by your facility. The hole may be called the *inspection toe*. Check the heel placement on the stocking. By using the heel as a landmark, you will see where to position the hole in the stocking.

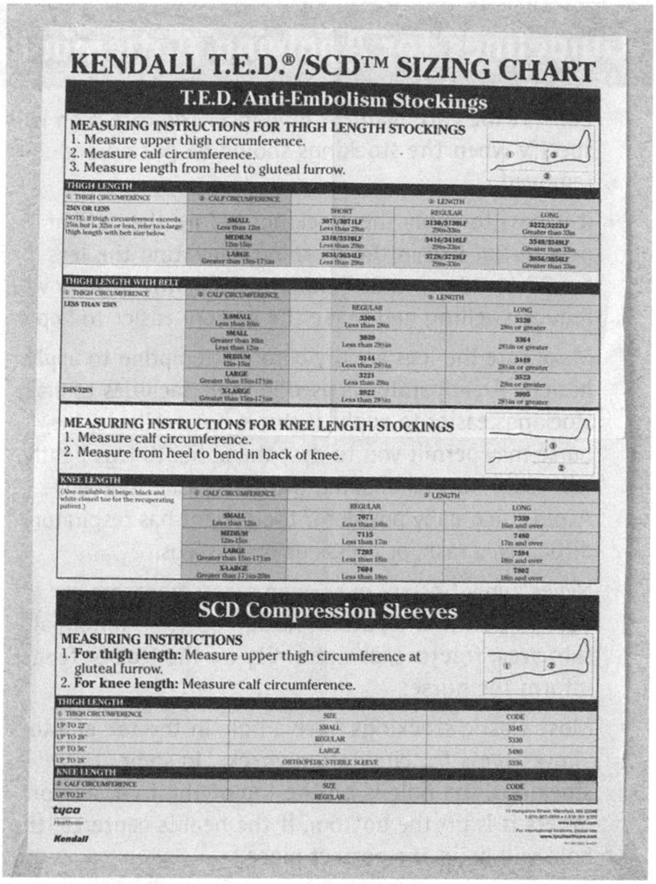

Preventing Complications

A physician's order is needed to apply special hosiery. The ordering physician will specify if knee-high or thigh-high hose should be used. Antiembolism hosiery are available in various grades of pressure, ranging from 8 mm Hg through 46 mm Hg. Become familiar with the criteria used by your facility to establish what constitutes light, medium, and firm compression. Make sure you apply the correct hosiery, according to the original order and facility policies.

The risk of complications with antiembolism hosiery is low. However, they are not risk-free. The greatest risk is a reduction in blood flow from pressure. This leads to decreased oxygen in the tissues and the potential for blood clots. Patients with diabetes and certain circulatory conditions are at high risk. Other reported complications are pressure ulcers, gangrene, and arterial occlusion. These often occurred when the patient sat for a prolonged period without moving. In another case, the tourniquet effect created by

FIGURE 11-12 Measure the patient's leg with the disposable paper tape measure, then compare the measurements to the manufacturer's chart to determine the correct size hosiery.

bunched-up layers of elastic hose, combined with swelling of the leg, caused serious skin breakdown, leading to amputation. The tourniquet effect of stockings that do not fit properly may also increase the risk of blood clots and occlusion of blood flow.

Follow your facility procedure manual and the product package for applying antiembolism hosiery. Never guess at the size. Always use a tape measure to ensure that the size is accurate. Ill-fitting hosiery is the most common cause of complications, so nursing personnel must:

- Measure legs with a tape measure to ensure correct hosiery fit. Compare the measurements with the size chart (**Figure 11-12**), then select the correct size.
- Follow the schedule for applying and removing the hosiery. Remove the hosiery for patient bathing each day. Evaluate the appearance of the feet and legs regularly, at least several times each day.
- Promptly inform the RN of abnormalities or complications. Intervene early if complications occur.

Guidelines for Applying Antiembolism Stockings

- Consult the care plan for guidance. The care plan will specify when the stockings should be put on and removed.

- It is best to apply the stockings before the patient gets out of bed in the morning. Elevating the legs for 20 to 30 minutes before applying the hosiery will reduce swelling and make the hosiery easier to apply.

- Make sure the legs are dry before attempting to apply hosiery. An apparatus is used in some facilities to make stockings easier to apply. If this is not available, the nurse may permit you to dust the patient's legs lightly with baby powder, making the hose easier to apply. Avoid using baby powder if the patient has respiratory difficulty, a rash, or dressings on the legs.

- Never apply hosiery over open areas, fractures, or deformities. If the patient has an open or abnormal skin area, fracture, or deformity on the legs or feet, inform the nurse.

- Most elastic stockings have a hole in the toe end to allow access for circulation checks. In some stockings, the hole is on the top of the foot, and on others it is on the bottom. If the heel is centered, the hole will be in the correct place.

- Make sure the stockings are applied smoothly with no wrinkles.

- Check the stockings every few hours to be sure the tops have not rolled or turned down. Keep the fabric straight.

- The care plan will specify the wearing schedule for the stockings, according to physician orders and facility policies. For most patients, the hosiery is applied during the day and removed at bedtime.

- Monitor circulation in the patient's toes every 2 to 4 hours, or as specified on the care plan. Note color, sensation, swelling, temperature, and ability to move. Report abnormalities to the RN. Document that you have done regular skin and circulation checks.

- Follow your facility policy for washing antiembolism stockings. These must be hand-washed and drip-dried. The stockings are damaged by the commercial washers and dryers used in a health care facility. Because of this, your facility may issue two pairs to each patient.

- To preserve the life of the stockings, avoid contact with lotions, ointments, or oils containing lanolin or petroleum products. These products deteriorate the elastic.

Procedure 91

Applying Antiembolism Stockings (Graduated Compression Hosiery)

Supplies Needed:
- Disposable tape measure
- Antiembolism hosiery, correct size and length

1. Perform your beginning procedure actions.
2. Follow the instructions on the back of the package or chart showing where and how to measure the legs. Proper fit is needed for positive outcomes. Never guess at the size. Measure both legs when the patient is in bed and edema is least. A slight difference in leg size is normal. Some patients have legs of vastly different size, such as those with postpolio syndrome and other neuromuscular diseases. If this is the case, two different sizes may be necessary.

    For knee-high stockings, measure:

- The narrowest part of the ankle, about 2.5 cm above the medial malleolus
- The base of the heel to just below the knee
- The widest part of the calf

For thigh-high stockings, measure:

- The narrowest part of the ankle, above the ankle bone
- The base of the heel to just below the knee
- The widest part of the calf
- The widest part of the thigh
- The distance between the base of the heel and the gluteal fold

3. Document the measurements according to facility policy.
4. Obtain hosiery in the correct size, length, and pressure (light, medium, or firm compression, as ordered). Do not guess at size!

(continues)

Procedure **91**, *continued*

Applying Antiembolism Stockings (Graduated Compression Hosiery)

5. Expose one leg.
6. Insert one hand into stocking as far as the heel pocket. Holding the heel pocket, turn the stocking inside out.
7. Carefully position the stocking over the foot and heel (**Figure 11-13A**).
8. Place the index and middle fingers of both hands into the stocking foot.
9. Face the patient and ease the stocking up over the foot, stretching sideways as you go. Center the heel pocket (**Figure 11-13B**). An acceptable alternative is to face the foot, then pull the stocking up, similar to the manner in which you apply your own socks.

10. Continue pulling the stocking up over the ankle and calf, smoothing and stretching the elastic (**Figure 11-13C**). The top of a knee-high stocking should be 1 to 2 inches below the knee. The top of a thigh-high stocking should be 1 to 3 inches below the groin.
11. Check the fit to be sure the stocking is even and free of wrinkles. Pull up slightly on the toes to ensure that the stocking is not too tight (**Figure 11-13D**).
12. Expose the patient's other leg.
13. Repeat the procedure.
14. Perform your procedure completion actions. Follow facility policies and physician orders for doing circulation checks and removing the hosiery.

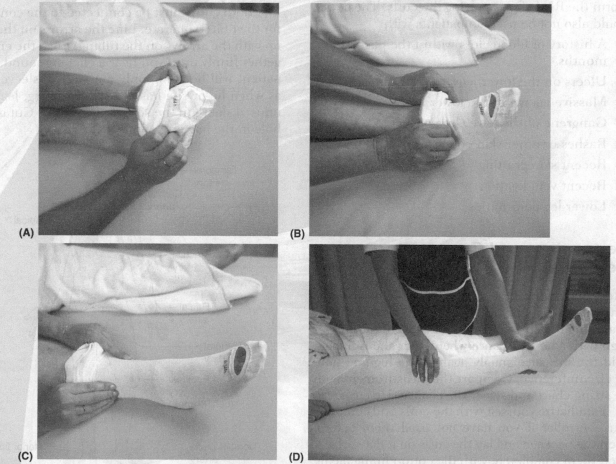

(A)

(B)

(C)

(D)

FIGURE 11-13 (A) Gather the stocking and slip it over the patient's toes. (B) Position the opening on the top of the foot, at the base of the toes. (C) Draw the stocking smoothly up to knee. (D) Check to make sure the stocking is free of wrinkles.

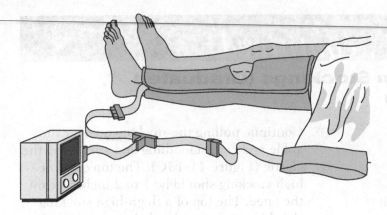

FIGURE 11-14 Pneumatic compression cuffs prevent blood clots and improve circulation.

PNEUMATIC CUFFS

Pneumatic cuffs may also be called a **sequential compression device.** This garment prevents blood clots in surgical patients. It promotes blood flow by massaging the legs in a wavelike motion. Pneumatic cuffs (**Figure 11-14**) inflate and deflate rhythmically. This device is contraindicated in patients with arterial disease. Shiny, hairless skin is an indication of this condition. If you observe any hard nodules, red areas, or warm areas on the patient's lower legs, inform the RN before applying the cuffs. The device should also not be used on patients with:

- A history of blood clots within the past six months
- Ulcers on the lower legs
- Massive edema of the lower legs
- Gangrene of the lower legs or feet
- Rashes or other skin conditions
- Recent skin grafting
- Recent vein ligation
- Lower leg deformities

Measuring and Connecting the Cuffs

Before beginning this procedure, you must determine the proper size cuffs for the patient. Do this by measuring the circumference of the patient's upper thigh with a tape measure when he or she is in bed. Hold the measure snugly against the leg and note the circumference. Compare the measurement with the sizing chart and select the proper size cuffs.

Familiarize yourself with the cuffs and compression controller if you have not used them before. Open the package and lay the cuffs on a flat surface. Open them completely, with the cotton lining facing up. Inside you will notice markings for the ankle and knee. When you apply the garment to the patient's

leg, it must be lined up exactly with these landmarks. Next, familiarize yourself with the compression controller. The device may have a cooling adjustment. This is used to cool the patient. It is turned off during routine use. Follow your facility policy and the RN's instructions for activating this feature. The controller also has arrows to adjust the pressure inside the cuffs. It should be set at 35 mm Hg to 55 mm Hg. The unit may automatically set at 45 mm Hg, the midway point. The RN will instruct you on the setting to use.

Both cuffs must be connected to the controller for the unit to operate. Line the arrows on the cuffs up with the arrows on the tubing. Push the ends together firmly until you hear a clicking sound. If the patient will be using only one cuff or sleeve, such as when he or she has a cast on one leg, leave the unused sleeve in the sealed plastic bag. Cut a small hole in the bag and connect the tubing.

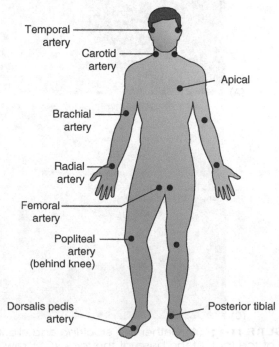

FIGURE 11-15 Pulse locations.

Using Pneumatic Cuffs

Before applying the cuffs, palpate the pedal and posterior tibial pulses (Figure 11-15). Compare the movement, sensation, and color in both feet. If abnormalities are noted, consult the RN before continuing. Document your findings. The RN will assess the patient's legs and check for contraindications. Follow his or her instructions.

Pneumatic cuffs are worn 24 hours a day until the patient is completely ambulatory. They are used when the patient is lying down. The cuffs may be removed for bathing and ambulation, then reapplied immediately upon completion of the activity. The RN may instruct the patient to perform certain leg exercises while the device is being used. Pneumatic cuffs may be applied over antiembolism hosiery. However, the hosiery must be smooth and wrinkle-free, to reduce the risk of skin breakdown.

Procedure 92

Applying the Pneumatic Compression Device

Supplies needed:
- Cuffs of proper size
- Compression controller

1. Perform your beginning procedure actions.
2. Open the cuffs, laying them flat on the bed with the markings opposite the knee and ankle.
3. Lift the patient's leg, sliding the cuff under it. Begin on the side of the leg opposite the plastic tubing. Wrap the sleeve around the leg with the opening in front, over the knee.
4. Beginning at the ankle, fasten the Velcro fasteners securely. Next, secure the ankle and calf, then the thigh.
5. Check the fit by inserting two fingers between the cuff and the patient's leg. The fit should feel snug, but not tight.
6. Wrap the other leg, beginning on the side opposite the plastic tubing. After wrapping the leg, check the fit.
7. Attach the plastic tubing on each leg to the compression controller by lining up the arrows on the tubing.
8. Plug the controller in and turn on the power.
9. Remain with the patient for one complete cycle to ensure that he or she tolerates the procedure.
10. Perform your procedure completion actions.

Caring for the Patient Who Is Wearing Pneumatic Cuffs

The compression controller has a visual display that lists which chamber is inflated at any given time. When the chambers decompress, the unit will say "vent." The unit has an audible alarm, which is controlled with a key on some devices. Make sure that the alarm is turned on and the key is removed. If the alarm sounds, the panel will display a message code. A card in a slot in the top of the unit will display the numerical message code with the nature of the problem. Follow the directions on the card to correct the problem. The cuffs will deflate when the alarm sounds.

Every 4 hours, turn the power off on the unit and remove the cuffs. Observe the skin under the device and provide skin care as ordered. Avoid massaging the legs. Massage may dislodge a blood clot, which will quickly migrate to the lungs. Inform the RN when you will be removing the device so that he or she can assess the patient's legs.

The cuffs will be discontinued when the patient is fully ambulatory. The unit is not disposable. Clean and store the unit after use.

Documentation

Follow your facility policy for documenting use of pneumatic compression cuffs. You may be asked to document the procedure, the patient's response, and the settings, including use of the alarm and the cooling settings.

CARING FOR PATIENTS WHO HAVE ORTHOPEDIC DISORDERS

As a PCT, you will be responsible for caring for patients who have orthopedic disorders. **Orthopedics** is the branch of medicine that deals with the prevention or correction of injuries or disorders of the skeletal system and associated structures. Originally, this specialty was concerned with the correction of childhood deformities, but has expanded to include the study and treatment of muscles, ligaments, tendons, bones, and related soft tissues. Orthopedics is also the specialty that deals with treatment of patients needing amputations and the fitting of artificial limbs.

Caring for Patients Who Have Fractures

Fractures, or broken bones, are the most common orthopedic injury. You will care for patients who are being treated for fractures. A new fracture is usually treated in the hospital emergency department. Admission for surgical correction of the fracture may be necessary. The immediate goals of care are to:

- Control pain
- Prevent complications of immobility
- Prevent or reduce edema
- Keep the fracture in good alignment
- Keep the fractured extremity immobile

Fractures are treated by keeping the injured area immobilized in proper position until healing occurs. Injured bones take from several weeks to several months to heal. Immobilization is achieved through use of:

- Pins
- Screws
- Splints
- Bone plates
- Casting
- Traction

Treatment for patients with fractures begins soon after admission. The type of treatment is determined by the location and type of fracture, and the method of fracture reduction. Patients who have fractures will be evaluated by the physical and occupational therapists. Therapists will design rehabilitation programs to meet the patient's needs and help him or her to regain as much mobility as possible.

Special Beds. Special beds and attachments may be necessary to make nursing care easier and improve patient comfort and safety. Be sure you know how to operate each bed and attachment before giving care. Some devices, such as a **CircOlectric bed** (Figure 11-16) or Stryker frame, require two people to operate it, for safety. Most CircOlectric beds are operated electronically, but some hospitals have manual models. The bed can be rotated to reposition the patient between the back and abdomen. The patient is secured to the inner frame before the bed is moved. The entire inner frame is rotated forward. This allows a position change without causing stress on the patient.

The Stryker frame may also be called a *spinal bed* or *wedge bed*. This turning frame serves the same purpose as the CircOlectric bed, but is manually operated. Once the patient is secured by placement of the upper frame, a crank is used to turn the entire frame and patient. The patient lies on the frame until being turned again. When using the Stryker frame, always turn the patient in the direction of the narrow wedge, to reduce the risk of falls. Turn the frame quickly and smoothly. Close the locks and replace the pins after the patient has been turned. If the perineal section of the frame must be removed for patient elimination, remember to replace it promptly.

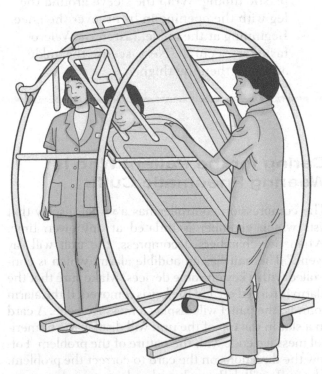

FIGURE 11-16 CircOlectric beds may be operated manually or electronically. Two people should be present when the patient is turned.

These special turning beds may be very frightening for the patient. You must be confident in your ability to operate them correctly, and to reassure the patient. Use special beds only if you have been taught to use them properly and are permitted to use them. In most facilities, two or more staff must be present when a patient is turned on a special bed. Make sure to follow the manufacturer's directions for use of the bed, and ensure that all safety straps are fastened properly before moving the patient. Know and follow your facility policies.

Care of Patients Who Have Casts. Two types of casting materials are commonly used:

1. Plaster of Paris, which can take up to 48 hours to dry completely
2. Fiberglass, which dries very rapidly

Cast material is wet when it is applied. During the drying period, the cast gives off heat. Special care for the newly casted patient includes:

- Supporting the cast and body in good alignment with pillows covered by cloth pillowcases, and keeping the cast uncovered.
- Elevating the casted extremity on a pillow. When positioning a patient with a leg cast, elevate the foot higher than the hip. The fingers should be higher than the elbow. Avoid placing the cast on a flat surface. Avoid placing anything plastic under a wet cast. Check the skin distal to the cast frequently for signs of poor circulation.
- Turning the patient frequently to promote cast drying. Turning promotes air circulation to all parts of the cast. Maintain support. *Use the palms of your hands, not your fingers, to move the cast.*
- Not positioning any part of the cast against the side rail or footboard, which may dent the cast and increase pressure on the skin and internal structures. If the patient is cold, cover the cast with a sheet. Avoid tucking the sheet under the mattress. A bed cradle may be used, if necessary. The greatest area of heat loss is the head. Covering the upper body, back, and top of the head with a blanket may help keep the patient warm. Another alternative may be to fashion a cap or sock to cover the fingers or toes using stockinette.
- Closely observe the uncasted areas of the extremities, such as the fingers and toes, for signs of decreased circulation. Report coldness, cyanosis, edema, increased pain, numbness, or tingling immediately.
- Closely observing the skin around the cast edges for signs of irritation. Cover rough edges with strips of adhesive tape.
- Recall the following key reportables when checking the patient:
  - C = color
  - M = motion
  - E = edema
  - T = temperature

Special Care after the Cast Is Completely Dry. After a cast has completely dried:

- Turn the patient to the noncasted side. This is particularly important for patients with body casts, because turning to the casted side may crack the cast.
- Always support the cast when moving the patient. Two staff members may be needed.
- Teach the patient to use the trapeze to assist with moving, and to become independent with moving.
- Tape the edges of the cast to prevent abrasion and irritation, if necessary.
- Use plastic to protect the edges of the cast near the perineum during elimination.
- With the RN's permission, cover the cast with a plastic bag to enable the patient to shower. A shower stool or chair may be needed so the patient can sit to bathe.

A fiberglass cast dries immediately. A plaster arm or leg cast will take 24 to 48 hours to dry completely. A plaster body or spica cast will take 48 to 72 hours to dry. Proper positioning of the cast is essential during the drying period to prevent depressions that can cause pressure and edema. Never use a table or hard object to support the cast during the drying period. Avoid rubber or plastic pillows, which increase heat under the cast. *Always remember to use the palms of your hands, not your fingers, to move the cast until it is completely dry.* Dents in the case promote breakdown, ulceration, and infection of the skin under the cast. When the cast is dry, it will look white and shiny. It will not appear soft or damp.

After the cast dries, odor from the cast and drainage through the cast suggest infection or ulceration under the cast. Inform the RN of these complications promptly. You may be instructed to

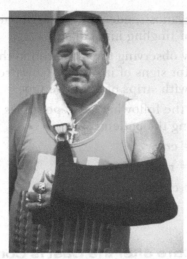

FIGURE 11-17 A sling may be ordered to elevate the hand and wrist.

trace the edges of the drainage with a marker on the cast. This helps the RN to visualize if the area is getting larger, indicating that drainage is increasing.

The care plan may instruct you to keep the casted extremity elevated to prevent edema. A sling (**Figure 11-17**) may be used to elevate an arm cast when the patient is out of bed. A wheelchair with an elevated leg rest is used for patients who have leg casts. You will probably have to place a pillow on the elevated leg rest, and position the leg carefully so it will not slip off.

Keep small objects from getting inside the cast. The patient may complain of an itching sensation under the cast. Discourage him or her from placing objects down the cast to scratch. Inform the RN if the patient complains of itching.

Procedure 93

Applying an Arm Sling

Supplies needed:
▶ Arm sling or triangular bandage
▶ Padding for neck, if needed

1. Perform your beginning procedure actions.
2. Position the affected arm at a 90-degree angle.
3. Apply the sling:
   ▶ If a triangular bandage is used, place one end of the triangle over the unaffected shoulder. Position the point of the triangle under the affected elbow. Bring the other end of the triangle over the shoulder on the affected side, covering the arm. Adjust the bandage so the fingers are elevated, and tie the ends of the bandage in back. Position the knot slightly to the side so it is not directly over the spine. Pad the skin under the knot to prevent pressure and irritation. Fold the extra fabric over at the elbow. Secure it on the inside with pins or tape.
   ▶ If a commercial sling is used, support the affected arm. Guide the sling up over the hand until the elbow is covered and the fingers are exposed. Wrap the strap around the patient's neck, then fasten it to the buckle on the sling. Adjust the

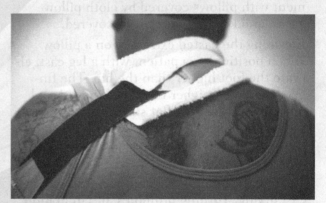

FIGURE 11-18 Pad the neck of the sling to prevent pressure and irritation from the weight of the cast.

strap so the fingers are elevated. Pad the strap under the neck (**Figure 11-18**) to prevent pressure and irritation.
4. Perform your procedure completion actions.

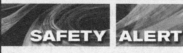
SAFETY ALERT

If the patient has an arm sling, monitor the skin at the back of the neck for irritation and breakdown from the strap. Monitor the skin under the arm daily for redness and breakdown. Make every effort to keep the underarm area clean and dry.

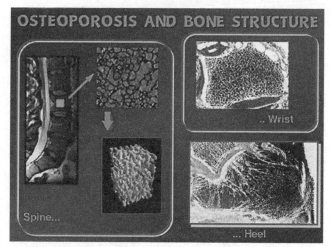

FIGURE 11-19 Bone loss from osteoporosis causes painful, disabling fractures in both sexes. About 40 percent of women and 13 percent of men will suffer a bone fracture due to osteoporosis in their lifetime. (Courtesy of Sharmila Majumdar, Ph.D., Professor, University of California, San Francisco)

Hip Fractures

Hip fractures are seen in patients of all ages. They are the most common type of fracture in elderly persons. It is not unusual for an elderly patient to be admitted to the hospital for treatment of another problem, then fall and break a hip. The most common cause of hip fractures is falls, but fractures may also occur because of osteoporosis. **Osteoporosis (Figure 11-19)** is a decrease in bone mass that leads to fractures with minimal trauma. In this case, the patient may hear a popping sound in the bone, then fall. An x-ray will reveal a fracture. The term "hip fracture" really is not accurate. This term refers to a fracture anywhere in the upper third or head of the femur.

Signs and Symptoms of Hip Fracture. A patient with a fractured hip is usually found on the floor. He or she will be unable to get up or move the injured leg. The leg on the affected side may be shortened and in a position of external rotation. In this position, the toes point outward. The shortening and rotation occur because the strong muscles in the upper leg contract. This causes the bone ends to override each other. The patient will complain of severe pain in the hip. The pain of a hip fracture is usually localized in the hip. Some patients complain of pain in the knee. This may be confusing or misleading. Edema and ecchymosis may be present in the hip, thigh, groin, or lower pelvic area.

Emergency Care. Avoid moving the patient until you are instructed to do so by an RN. You will use a sheet, backboard, or other device to move the patient. Avoid excessive movement, which can worsen the injury. Moving a patient with a hip fracture requires four or five individuals. The patient is log-rolled onto the lifting device. The device is lifted to the bed or stretcher. You may be assigned to monitor the patient's vital signs and check for signs of shock. Some patients are treated with Buck's traction.

Open Reduction Internal Fixation. The most common treatment for a fractured hip is a surgical procedure called **open reduction internal fixation (ORIF).** In this procedure, the surgeon makes an incision, manipulates the fractured bone into alignment, then inserts a nail, pin, or rod to hold the fractured bone in place. When caring for a patient who has had this surgery, you must:

- Know how to position the patient in bed. You must avoid adduction, internal and external rotation of the affected hip.
- Know the correct procedure if the patient is allowed to ambulate. The patient may not be permitted to bear weight on the affected extremity for a few weeks after surgery.

DIFFICULT PATIENT ALERT

A patient who has had hip surgery will probably have physician orders for antiembolism hosiery and an incentive spirometer. A pressure-relieving mattress may also be ordered. Following hip surgery, the patient will be at very high risk for pressure ulcer development, particularly on the heels. Take active measures to prevent pressure. Remember, heel protectors prevent friction and shearing. They do not relieve pressure. Keeping the heels off the surface of the bed works best. Follow the care plan. Check the skin regularly for redness, irritation, and breakdown.

Total Joint Replacement

Sometimes joints must be completely replaced because of arthritis or severe damage to the joint. The goal of joint replacement surgery is to relieve pain, which is often so severe that the patient avoids using the joint as much as possible. This weakens the muscles and worsens the problem. Hip and knee replacements are the most common, but joint replacement surgery can be done on the ankle, foot, shoulder, elbow, and fingers. Postoperative care will vary with the surgical procedure. General care for joint replacement surgery includes:

- Prevention of infection
- Prevention of blood clots; the patient may receive a medicine to thin the blood, and so is at increased risk of bruising and bleeding
- Application of antiembolism hosiery
- Exercises to increase blood flow in the surrounding muscles, if not contraindicated
- Exercises to maintain range of motion in nonoperative joints
- Sequential compression therapy

Total Hip Arthroplasty

Total hip arthroplasty (THA) involves removal of a portion of the pelvic bone and femur, and insertion of a prosthesis (artificial body part). This procedure may be done because:

- The patient has fractured a hip, and it cannot be repaired by other methods
- The patient has degenerative arthritis and the hip joint has deteriorated and is very painful

The hip joint is surgically removed and a metal or synthetic ball and socket (**Figure 11-20**) are inserted. The physician will specify how long the patient must avoid weight bearing after surgery. The physical and occupational therapists will work with the patient to restore function. Some patients can ambulate shortly after surgery. A walker is commonly used for a period of time. Some patients are not permitted to bear full weight on the operative leg for up to six weeks after surgery. Your immediate goal of care is to prevent complications of immobility. You will do range-of-motion exercises on unaffected joints and assist with coughing, deep breathing, and use of the incentive spirometer. Pay close attention to positioning and pressure relief, particularly on the heels. Use pillows, props, and foam to support nonoperative extremities, if needed. Check the patient's skin daily for signs of red or open areas. Report them promptly to the RN, if noted.

Caring for the Patient Who Has Had Hip Surgery. After hip surgery, the following general procedures are commonly ordered:

- A trapeze is attached to the bed to assist with movement. The patient is instructed not to press down on the foot of the affected leg when using the trapeze.

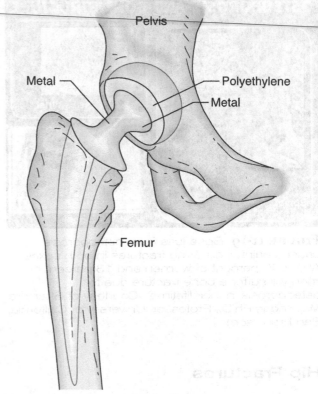

FIGURE 11-20 A hip prosthesis replaces the ball of the femur and the socket when the patient has a total hip arthroplasty.

- Antiembolism stockings are applied.
- A fracture bedpan or urinal is used initially for elimination. When the patient can use the toilet, an elevated toilet seat is used.
- The head of the bed is not elevated more than 45 degrees without a specific order.
- Avoid acute flexion of the hip and legs. The physician will give directions for positioning and the degree of flexion permitted.
- Patients who have had hip replacement surgery will usually have a special pillow, called an **abduction pillow,** to keep the legs apart (**Figure 11-21**). This is particularly important when the patient is turned on the side. The patient will be instructed to avoid crossing the legs, which can cause a dislocation.

The physician will specify how long the patient must avoid weight bearing after surgery. The physical therapist will work with the patient to restore mobility. Some patients can ambulate soon after surgery. Some physicians do not permit full weight bearing for as long as four to six weeks. Initially, you will assist with procedures to prevent the complications of im-

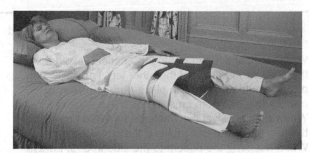

Figure 11-21 An abduction pillow is commonly used after hip surgery to keep the hips and knees apart, to avoid adducting or crossing at the ankles.

mobility. These include range-of-motion exercises of the unaffected extremities, turning and repositioning, and coughing and deep breathing exercises. Patients with hip surgery are at very high risk of developing heel pressure ulcers. Follow the care plan and get specific instructions from the RN for positions and techniques to use for turning and repositioning the patient. Relieve pressure from the heels and check the patient's skin carefully each day for signs of red or open areas.

Hip Precautions

Dislocation of a hip prosthesis is uncommon, but may occur during the first 90 days following hip replacement surgery. Hip precautions are usually ordered by the physician and physical therapist. Patients who have had hip repair or replacement surgery may need special hip precautions for a minimum of six to eight weeks, or until the operative site has fully healed. If hip precautions are ordered, follow the care plan and the specific instructions listed in the nursing procedure manual. Hip precautions are listed in **Figure 11-22**.

Continuous Passive Motion

Continuous passive motion (CPM) therapy (Figure 11-23) may be ordered following joint replacement and other orthopedic procedures. Moving a joint is painful for most patients postoperatively. If the patient fails to move the joint, stiffness and limited range of motion will occur. Months of physical therapy will be necessary for the patient to recover fully. CPM therapy prevents stiffness by delivering a form of passive range-of-motion exercise so the joint is moved without the patient's muscles being used. CPM therapy is effortless for the patient. A machine moves the affected joint through a prescribed range of motion for an extended period of time. The goals of CPM therapy are to:

- Enhance circulation, which lowers the risk of blood clots
- Reduce edema
- Promote collagen formation within the joint, which enhances healing
- Reduce scarring
- Decrease stiffness
- Improve range of motion (which decreases postoperatively without movement)
- Reduce the risk of complications in the joint, such as contractures and adhesions
- Help relieve pain

Many orthopedic surgeons prescribe CPM therapy following knee replacement and other surgical procedures. CPM devices are available for the knee, ankle, toes, jaw, shoulder, elbow, wrist, and hand. Indications for using CPM therapy are:

- Crush injuries of the hand without fractures or dislocations
- Burn injuries
- Stable fractures
- Joint and tendon repair
- Surgical release of contractures
- Knee or hip replacement
- Reconstructive surgery on bone, cartilage, tendons, and ligaments
- Prolonged joint immobilization

The physician prescribes how the CPM unit should be used. He or she orders the settings on the CPM unit that control the speed, duration of use, range of motion, pause settings, hours of use per day, and rate of increase of motion. The directions for use will vary slightly depending on the body area being treated, the type of CPM machine used, and the physician's orders. In some facilities, this procedure is done only by licensed RNs. In others, the PCT can set up the unit, but the RN must check the settings for accuracy. This is a key step. Improper settings can damage reconstructive work in the joint. Follow your facility policies and procedures (refer to Procedure 94).

Contraindications for CPM therapy include:

- Untreated infections
- Unstable fractures
- Known or suspected blood clots (deep vein thrombosis)
- Hemorrhage
- Spastic paralysis

Hip precautions may be ordered by the physician after hip fracture repair or hip replacement surgery. They should be listed on the care plan.

- Patients who have had hip replacement surgery may need an abduction pillow to keep the legs apart. Keep the pillow in place at all times when the patient is in bed. It is particularly important when the patient is turned on the side.
- Apply a trapeze to the bed frame to assist with patient movement. Remind the patient not to press down on the foot on the operative side when using the trapeze.
- Apply antiembolism stockings. Remove the socks one or more times each shift to check circulation, signs of skin breakdown, and presence of pedal pulses. Remove the hosiery daily for bathing.
- Assist the patient with continuous passive motion exercises, as ordered.
- Provide a fracture bedpan or urinal for elimination. As mobility increases, furnish an elevated toilet seat or commode for toileting. This is an essential procedure because toileting greatly increases the risk for prosthesis dislocation. When the patient can use the toilet, provide an elevated toilet seat. *This is essential during the first six weeks following hip replacement surgery, because of the risk for prosthesis dislocation.*
- Never elevate the head of the bed more than 45 degrees without first checking with the RN. A specific physician order may be needed.
- Keep the operative leg in good alignment, without internal or external rotation. Support the legs with pillows or trochanter rolls, if necessary to provide support and prevent external rotation when in bed.
- The therapist will provide instructions for positioning and the degree of flexion permitted. The patient must avoid acute flexion of the hip and legs. This means to avoid flexion beyond 90 degrees.

- When positioning and turning the patient, avoid rolling the operative leg toward the other leg. The abduction pillow should always be in place during turning to prevent the legs from crossing.
- When sitting, swivel the whole body. Avoid turning or twisting the upper body toward the operative hip.
- When assisting the patient to the side in bed, always support the operative leg.
- Instruct the patient to:
  - Avoid sleeping on the stomach or operative side.
  - Avoid crossing the legs, which may cause hip dislocation.
  - Avoid sitting on low chairs or couches. He or she should use only chairs with arms where the knees remain lower than the hips.
  - Avoid leaning forward while sitting.
  - Avoid picking up items from the floor or bending to put on shoes and socks.
  - Avoid flexing the hips more than 80 degrees or rotating the foot and leg inward.
  - Avoid raising the knee higher than the hip on the operative side.
  - Keep the legs at least 3 to 6 inches apart when sitting, or use the abduction pillow.
  - Avoid stretching the operative hip back.
  - Avoid kneeling on one knee.
  - Avoid turning the foot outward on the operative side.
  - Avoid twisting the body away from the operative hip.
  - Avoid standing with the toes pointed outward; keep the toes of the operative leg pointed forward when standing, sitting, or walking.
  - Avoid swinging the operative leg outward away from the body.
  - Not assume a straddling position.

FIGURE 11-22 Hip Precautions

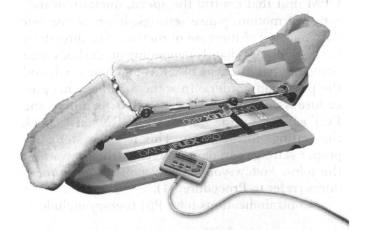

FIGURE 11-23 The continuous passive motion machine performs passive range-of-motion exercises on the affected joint without straining the patient's muscles. (Courtesy of OrthoRehab, Inc.)

If the patient develops any of the following signs or symptoms upon using the device, stop the unit and inform the RN promptly:

- Fever
- Increasing redness or irritation
- Increasing warmth
- Edema
- Bleeding
- Increased or persistent pain

Do not continue with treatment until the RN informs you that the physician has approved continued use of the device.

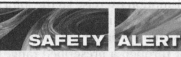

SAFETY ALERT

Make sure the side rail is up on the side where the CPM unit is placed. Position the edge of the tibia sling slightly above the support bar.

Procedure 94

Continuous Passive Motion Therapy

NOTE: In some states, PCTs are not permitted to perform this procedure. Additionally, the policies of some facilities state that only licensed nurses may perform this procedure. Your instructor will inform you if this is a PCT procedure in your state and facility. Perform this procedure only if you are permitted to do so by state law and facility policies.

NOTE: These instructions are generic and are not device-specific. The person(s) setting up the device should be educated in the use of the device being used, and have an operating manual available.

Supplies needed:
▶ CPM unit
▶ Soft goods kit, if available, or gather:
  ▶ Sheepskin foot pad
  ▶ Tibia/femur sling
  ▶ Hip pad
  ▶ Velcro fasteners

1. Perform your beginning procedure actions. Apply the principles of standard precautions during this procedure if contact with wound drainage or nonintact skin is likely.
2. Check the unit for safety and stability. Make sure that the attachments are tight, the frame is stable, and the electric controls work. Have the RN adjust the settings according to the physician's orders, or follow facility policy for setting the speed and degree of flexion. (In some facilities, assistants are permitted to adjust the settings. If this is the case, have the RN check the settings before proceeding.) Stop the machine in full extension.
3. Raise the side rail on the side of the bed where you will be placing the unit.
4. Position the CPM unit on the bed and secure the attachment, depending on the type of device being used.
5. Fasten the foot pad to the foot plate with a Velcro fastener.
6. Attach the tibia/femur sling (wide section toward the footrest). Fasten the Velcro closures under the sling.
7. Apply the hip pad to the hinge area of the adjustment bar. Position the femur sling

straps over the hinges, then fasten underneath with Velcro.
8. Fit the CPM machine to the patient's leg length by lengthening or shortening the frame.
9. Align the knee joint with the knee hinge, then position the knee approximately 1 inch below the knee joint line (**Figure 11-24A**).
10. Center the leg on the unit. Avoid pressure on the side and middle of the knee joint.
11. Adjust the foot pad so the patient's foot is comfortable and well supported (**Figure 11-24B**). The leg should be lifted at the thigh with no pressure on the foot. Secure the Velcro straps across the thigh and top of the foot (**Figure 11-24C**).

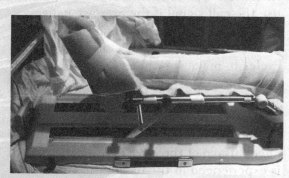

FIGURE 11-24(A) Position the leg straight, with the toes upright. Line the knee up with the marking at the hinge.

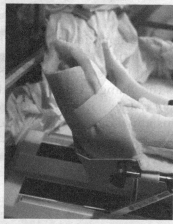

FIGURE 11-24(B) Make sure the foot is comfortable and well supported. Add padding, if needed, for patient comfort.

(continues)

Procedure 94, *continued*

Continuous Passive Motion Therapy

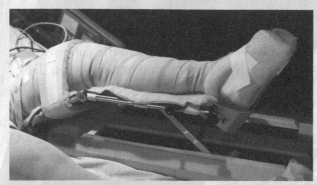

FIGURE 11-24(C) Secure the straps across the leg and foot. Make sure the strap is not too tight.

12. When the leg is in the proper position, give the patient the control (Figure 11-24D). Instruct the patient to start the unit. Instruct the patient to turn the unit off and use the call signal if the exercise causes extreme pain, or the unit malfunctions.
13. Stay with the patient for at least two full cycles to make sure he or she tolerates the procedure.
14. Return to check on the patient frequently when the unit is in use. Some devices have compliance monitors that allow you to check usage of the device. After the patient is experienced in the use of the CPM machine, he or she may be instructed to keep a record of the times the unit is used,

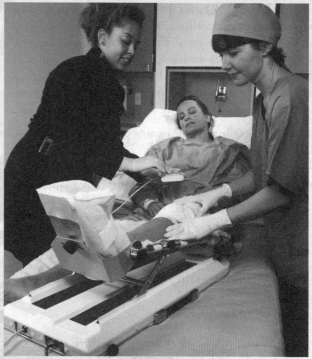

FIGURE 11-24(D) Show the patient how to turn the unit on, then give her the switch. Stay in the room until the machine goes through at least two cycles if the unit is being used for the first time. (Courtesy of OrthoRehab, Inc.)

or you may be required to document this information.
15. Perform your procedure completion actions.

Check the patient periodically when using a CPM machine. Each time the settings are changed, stay with the patient for several cycles to be sure he or she tolerates the change. Check the skin every 2 hours for signs of redness, irritation, or breakdown. Report problems and abnormalities to the RN.

HEALTH CARE ALERT

You may remove the CPM sleeves when the patient is walking, bathing, or leaving the room for any reason. Reapply them immediately upon his or her return to bed. To disconnect the sleeves, press the latch on each side of the connectors, then pull the connectors apart.

Compartment Syndrome

Compartment syndrome is a very painful condition that occurs when pressure within the muscles builds up, preventing blood and oxygen from reaching muscles and nerves. This is a very serious complication that may develop following an injury or surgical procedure. It may also occur following athletic injuries, burns, snake bites, IV infiltration, frostbite, and musculoskeletal conditions in which there is no fracture. Patients of all ages can be affected. The most common location of compartment syndrome in adults is in a fractured tibia. The most common location of compartment syndrome in children is the humerus.

Compartment syndrome is usually seen after a traumatic injury, such as a long-bone fracture. It may develop if an injury or surgical site swells after a cast has been applied. A tough membrane, called *fascia*, surrounds the muscles in the arms and legs. The fascia does not expand readily. Compartment syndrome develops gradually over several hours. Bleeding or swelling occurs in the muscle tissue, under the fascia. Occasionally, pressure from a cast or compression device also increases the pressure from the outside. If the swelling is not relieved, pressure on the muscles and nerves builds. Eventually, the pressure inside the fascia compartment will exceed the blood pressure, causing the capillaries to collapse. Blood flow to the muscles and nerves stops. If it is not restored promptly, tissue death begins.

Signs and Symptoms. The most common symptom of acute compartment syndrome is severe pain, especially when the muscle is moved. The pain may seem out of proportion to the injury. The patient may also complain of:

- Severe pain when the muscle is gently stretched
- Tenderness when the area is touched gently
- Pain on deep breathing
- Tingling
- Burning
- Numbness
- Feeling tight or full in the affected muscle
- Abnormal sensations in the affected area
- Weakness or inability to use the muscle

Observations by the PCT include:

- The color of the extremity may appear pale, cyanotic, or red.
- The skin of an extremity with no cast may feel warm to the touch.
- The fingers or toes of a casted extremity may feel cool to the touch.
- There may be edema (swelling).

Loss of the pulse in the extremity is a late sign. Rapid identification and treatment of this condition is necessary.

PCT Responsibilities. Follow the care plan and do frequent monitorings of patients who have musculoskeletal injuries and casts. Monitor for changes in the affected extremity. Check the color and temperature of the extremity distal to a cast.

Notify the RN if the color is abnormal. Ask the patient if he or she can move fingers or toes. Notify the RN promptly of any unusual findings. If the patient complains of severe pain, or if the pain is not relieved after the patient receives pain medication, notify the RN promptly. This condition is frightening for the patient. Provide emotional support.

Compartment syndrome is a surgical emergency. The RN will assess the patient and notify the physician of the findings. If compartment syndrome is suspected, the patient will be taken to surgery quickly to relieve the pressure. Follow facility policies and the RN's instructions to prepare the patient for surgery.

Caring for Patients in Traction

Traction may be used to treat fractures, dislocations, muscle spasms, and other musculoskeletal conditions. It is commonly used as a treatment for fractures of the long bones. The bone ends are pulled into place with ropes and weights. The patient's body weight stabilizes the upper part of the bone. A bag of water, sandbags, or metal disks are attached to pull on the opposite end of the fracture. This stabilizes the lower part of the bone, bringing it into good alignment. **Skin traction** (Figure 11-25) involves applying a halter or belt of foam rubber, a boot, or other device to the injured extremity. The belt is attached to ropes and weights. **Skeletal traction** (Figure 11-26) involves surgically placing a wire, pin, or tongs into or through the fractured bone. The pin protrudes through the skin, where ropes and weights are attached. Traction may be used as a temporary measure until the fracture is surgically repaired. It may be used until the fracture completely heals in patients who are not good candidates for surgery. Placement of the straps and the amount of weight used for traction are prescribed by the physician. When caring for patients in traction, you should:

- Review the correct placement of straps and weights with the RN.
- Avoid moving, dropping, or releasing the weights. They should not touch the bed, swing freely, or rest upon any object or surface. The weights hang still at the end of the bed.
- Make sure the ropes are correctly positioned in the pulley tracks.
- Position the patient in the center of the bed in good body alignment. The feet should not rest against the end of the bed.

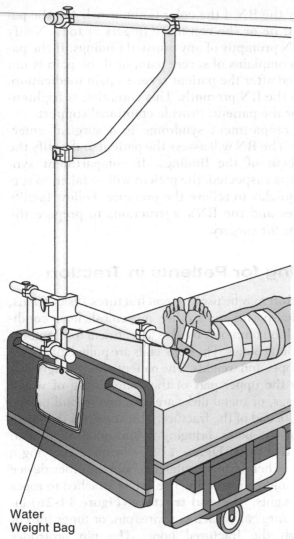

Water
Weight Bag

FIGURE 11-25 Buck's traction is a type of skin traction that may be used for temporary treatment or nonsurgical treatment of a hip fracture.

- Get instructions for moving the patient up in bed and turning to the sides, as ordered.

- Keep the traction straps smooth and free from wrinkles. Monitor the position of the straps each time you are in the room.

- Monitor the skin under the straps for signs of irritation or breakdown.

Disc problems in the back and some other conditions may be treated with traction (**Figure 11-27**). This is an older form of treatment. In recent years the use of traction for disc problems has decreased. In these conditions, the traction may be used intermittently. You will manage the traction in the same manner as if the patient had a fracture. The RN will provide specific directions.

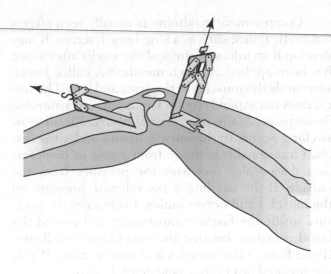

FIGURE 11-26 Skeletal traction.

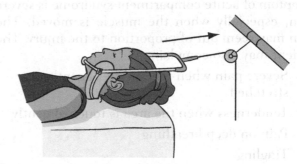

FIGURE 11-27 Cervical traction.

The patient's traction is connected to a frame on the bed. The type of frame used is determined largely by the design of the bed. Various types of frames are pictured in **Figure 11-28**. The most common type is the claw frame. With this device, claw attachments connect the frame to the headboard and footboard of the bed. The directions for setting up the traction vary with the type of device used. Your central services department should have the designated devices available, with the proper pieces sorted together. You should not have to ask for each section individually.

When attaching the traction to the bed frame, position the patient safely in the center of the bed. Ask several assistants to help you. If the patient is in the emergency department or operating room, set the traction up in an empty bed, before the patient arrives.

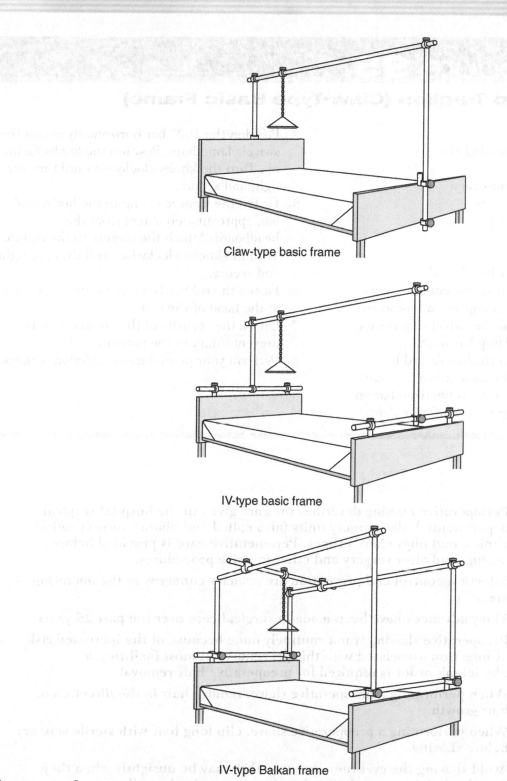

Claw-type basic frame

IV-type basic frame

IV-type Balkan frame

FIGURE 11-28 Traction is used for many different purposes.

Procedure 95

Setting up Traction (Claw-Type Basic Frame)

Supplies needed:

▶ Claw-type frame consisting of:
— 102" plain bar
— Two 66" swivel clamp bars
— Two headboard clamps
— Two footboard clamps
— Trapeze
— Clamp for trapeze
— Rubber bumper for headboard

1. Perform your beginning procedure actions.
2. Attach a headboard clamp and a footboard clamp to each end of the swivel clamp bars.
3. Fasten one swivel clamp bar to the footboard and one to the headboard by turning the knobs clockwise until they are tight and secure. Pull the rubberized bar on the headboard clamp back until it is tight.
4. Position the 102" bar horizontally across the swivel clamp bars. Position the knobs facing up. Turn the knobs clockwise until they are tight and secure.
5. Fasten the trapeze clamp to the horizontal bar, approximately 2 feet from the headboard. Attach the trapeze to the clamp. Turn the knobs clockwise until they are tight and secure.
6. Fasten the rubber bumper to the vertical bar at the head of the bed.
7. Check the security of the connections to prevent injury to the patient.
8. Perform your procedure completion actions.

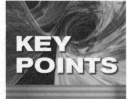

KEY POINTS

▶ Perioperative nursing describes the care given in the hospital surgical department(s), day-surgery units (also called ambulatory surgery units), clinics, and physicians' offices. Perioperative care is provided before, during, and after surgery and other invasive procedures.

▶ Infection control and prevention are primary concerns in the operating area.

▶ Many advances have been made in surgical care over the past 25 years.

▶ Preoperative shaving is not routinely done because of the increased risk of infection associated with this procedure. In most facilities, a physician's order is required for preoperative hair removal.

▶ When performing a preoperative shave, remove hair in the direction of hair growth.

▶ When performing a preoperative shave, clip long hair with sterile scissors before shaving.

▶ Avoid shaving the eyebrows, because they may be unsightly when they grow back; in some patients, they do not grow back at all.

▶ Always use a sterile razor for the preoperative shave.

▶ When caring for a postoperative patient, report these changes to the RN:

  ▶ Decreased responsiveness or unresponsiveness

  ▶ Change in the level of responsiveness

  ▶ Increased restlessness accompanied by complaints of thirst

  ▶ Changes in blood pressure

(continues)

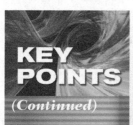

KEY POINTS

(Continued)

> ▶ Weak, rapid, or irregular pulse
> ▶ Changes in temperature
> ▶ Changes in respiratory rate
> ▶ Difficulty breathing; labored or noisy respirations
> ▶ Nausea or vomiting
> ▶ Complaints of pain
> ▶ Increased drainage; wet or saturated dressings
> ▶ Active bleeding
> ▶ Coughing or choking

▶ Sterile dressings and sterile technique must be used on new postoperative incisions.

▶ Patient-controlled analgesia is a method of enabling patients to self-administer their own pain medications. The dosage is controlled to prevent the risk of accidental overdosage.

▶ Coughing and deep breathing exercises should not be done on patients who have had neurologic, eye, or nasal surgery, because these exercises increase the pressure inside the head.

▶ Coughing and deep breathing exercises and use of the incentive spirometer expand the lungs and help loosen secretions, preventing pneumonia.

▶ When assisting with coughing and deep breathing exercises, splint the patient's abdomen with a pillow if he or she has had abdominal surgery.

▶ Antiembolism stockings are used during and after surgery to prevent deep vein thrombosis, which is a blood clot that most commonly occurs in the deep veins of the legs. The major complication of DVT is pulmonary embolus.

▶ Complications of antiembolism stockings are pressure ulcers, gangrene, and arterial occlusion.

▶ Pneumatic cuffs are used to prevent blood clots in postoperative patients.

▶ Pneumatic cuffs are contraindicated in patients who have:
> ▶ A history of blood clots within the past six months
> ▶ Ulcers on the lower legs
> ▶ Massive edema of the lower legs
> ▶ Gangrene of the lower legs or feet
> ▶ Rashes or other skin conditions
> ▶ Recent skin grafting
> ▶ Recent vein ligation
> ▶ Lower leg deformities

▶ Palpate the pedal and posterior tibial pulses before applying pneumatic cuffs.

▶ Check the patient's skin under the pneumatic compression cuffs every 4 hours.

▶ Orthopedics is the branch of medicine that deals with the prevention or correction of injuries or disorders of the skeletal system and associated structures.

(continues)

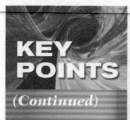

KEY POINTS
(Continued)

▶ Fractures are broken bones. The immediate goals of fracture care are to:
  ▶ Control pain
  ▶ Prevent complications of immobility
  ▶ Prevent or reduce edema
  ▶ Keep the fracture in good alignment
  ▶ Keep the fractured extremity immobile

▶ Two types of casting materials are commonly used. Plaster of Paris may take up to 48 hours to dry completely. A fiberglass cast dries very rapidly.

▶ The key reportables for a patient with a cast are:
  ▶ C = color
  ▶ M = motion
  ▶ E = edema
  ▶ T = temperature

▶ Handle a fresh cast with the palms of your hands, not your fingertips.

▶ Hip fractures are the most common type of fracture in elderly persons.

▶ Osteoporosis is a decrease in bone mass that leads to fractures with minimal trauma. A patient with osteoporosis may develop a spontaneous fracture.

▶ The term "hip fracture" refers to a fracture anywhere in the upper third or head of the femur.

▶ When a patient sustains a hip fracture, the leg on the affected side is commonly shortened and externally rotated.

▶ An open reduction internal fixation is a surgical procedure in which the surgeon manipulates the fractured bone into alignment, then inserts a nail, pin, or rod to hold the fractured bone in place.

▶ The goal of joint replacement surgery is usually to relieve pain. Joint replacement may also be done when a fractured bone cannot be repaired.

▶ General care for joint replacement surgery includes:
  ▶ Prevention of infection
  ▶ Prevention of blood clots
  ▶ Application of antiembolism hosiery
  ▶ Exercises to increase blood flow in the surrounding muscles, if not contraindicated
  ▶ Exercises to maintain range of motion in nonoperative joints
  ▶ Sequential compression therapy

▶ Total hip arthroplasty involves removal of part of the pelvic bone and femur, and insertion of a prosthesis (artificial body part).

▶ Patients who have had hip surgery are at very high risk of pressure ulcers, particularly on the heels.

▶ Routine postoperative care for patients with hip surgery includes:
  ▶ Attaching a trapeze to the bed to assist with movement, and showing the patient how to use it and/or assisting as needed
  ▶ Applying antiembolism stockings

(continues)

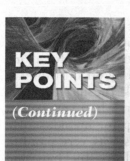

KEY POINTS
(Continued)

▶ Using a fracture bedpan or urinal for elimination, then progressing to an elevated toilet seat

▶ Elevating the head of the bed no more than 45 degrees

▶ Avoiding acute flexion of the hip and legs

▶ Using an abduction pillow to keep the legs apart

▶ Hip precautions are routinely used after hip joint replacement to prevent dislocation of the prosthesis.

▶ Continuous passive motion therapy may be ordered following joint replacement and other orthopedic procedures. CPM therapy prevents stiffness by delivering a form of passive range of motion so the joint is moved without the patient's muscles being used.

▶ The goals of CPM therapy are to:

　▶ Enhance circulation, which lowers the risk of blood clots

　▶ Reduce edema

　▶ Promote collagen formation within the joint, which enhances healing

　▶ Reduce scarring

　▶ Decrease stiffness

　▶ Improve range of motion (which decreases postoperatively without movement)

　▶ Reduce the risk of complications in the joint, such as contractures and adhesions

　▶ Help relieve pain

▶ Compartment syndrome is a very serious complication that may develop following an injury or surgical procedure. It is very painful, and occurs when pressure within the muscles builds up, preventing blood and oxygen from reaching muscles and nerves.

▶ Compartment syndrome is a surgical emergency. If this condition is suspected, the patient will be taken to surgery quickly to relieve the pressure.

▶ Traction is used to treat fractures, dislocations, muscle spasms, and other musculoskeletal conditions.

▶ Skin traction involves applying a halter or belt of foam rubber, a boot, or other device to the injured extremity; the belt is attached to ropes and weights.

▶ Skeletal traction involves surgically placing a wire, pin, or tongs into or through the fractured bone; the pin protrudes through the skin, where ropes and weights are attached.

▶ Traction is connected to a frame on the bed; the type of frame used is determined largely by the design of the bed.

CLINICAL APPLICATIONS

1. You are assigned to shave Mr. Long's operative area, which includes part of the chest, then do a 10-minute surgical scrub. The hair on his chest is very long and coarse. Describe how you

will remove the hair without cutting or injuring the patient.

2. After Mr. Long's surgery, you will assist him with coughing and deep breathing exercises and use of the incentive spirometer. You explained these procedures to the patient preoperatively, but he does

~~not remember. Explain how you will teach this pa-~~
tient to perform these procedures correctly.

3. Mr. Long has a large abdominal incision. He tells you he cannot do the deep breathing exercises because he is afraid the incision will pop open. How can you help this patient?

4. The physician has ordered pneumatic cuffs for Mr. Long. When you apply them, you notice two round, healed scars on his left lower leg. When you ask him about them, he says he had ulcers on the leg in the past. Mr. Long tells you he was treated for a blood clot six months ago. What action will you take, if any? Explain the reason for your decision.

5. James Lefferdink was transferred to your facility Friday afternoon from another hospital. The patient had previously had hip surgery in another facility, and has transferred to your hospital to be closer to home. He has a history of diabetes and peripheral vascular disease. He had antiembolism hosiery in place upon admission to your unit. The physician's orders specify that the stockings are to be removed every shift for a circulation check, then reapplied. Mr. Lefferdink arrived at the end of your shift, and you put him to bed but did not re-

move the hosiery. You took his vital signs, put his belongings away, and completed the admission, then went off duty. You were off for a long weekend, with a personal day off on Monday. When you returned to work Tuesday, Mr. Lefferdink screamed with pain when you moved his right foot to sit him up for breakfast. He said that touching his toes was very painful. You remove the antiembolism stockings and find that the toes are purple-black, with necrosis. He also has a dark purple spot on the top of the foot. Another PCT told you the unit had been short of staff over the past few days, and that the patient's hosiery had not been removed as ordered. What action will you take? Should you have done anything different at the time of admission? List some measures you will use in the care of this patient.

6. You are assigned to change a postoperative dressing on a new surgical incision that is approximately 2 inches long. There is minimal bloody drainage. The patient worries that his clothing will rub against the incision and irritate it. What type of dressing will you use to cover this wound? What advice will you give the patient to allay his fears?

CHAPTER REVIEW

Multiple-Choice Questions

Select the one best answer.

1. Shaving the operative area is not commonly recommended because:
   a. it embarrasses the patient.
   b. it increases the risk of infection.
   c. patients are admitted immediately before surgery.
   d. the hair is unsightly when it grows back.

2. Precautions to take when shaving a patient before surgery include:
   a. use a clean razor.
   b. never shave the eyebrows.
   c. shave in the opposite direction of hair growth.
   d. use plenty of shaving cream.

3. When assisting a patient with coughing and deep breathing exercises, teach him or her to:
   a. inhale through the nose.
   b. inhale through the mouth.
   c. exhale through the nose.
   d. keep the hands behind the neck to expand the lungs fully.

4. When using the incentive spirometer, the patient should:
   a. take a deep breath, then exhale into the mouthpiece.
   b. take a shallow breath, then exhale into the mouthpiece.
   c. breathe in through the mouthpiece.
   d. breathe in and out through the mouthpiece.

5. The main purpose of coughing and deep breathing, and using the incentive spirometer, is to prevent:
   a. pneumonia.
   b. dizziness.
   c. pain.
   d. anxiety.

6. The main purpose of pneumatic compression hosiery is to prevent:
   a. edema.
   b. pneumonia.
   c. blood clots.
   d. contractures.

7. Pneumatic cuffs are contraindicated in all of the following *except:*
   a. arterial disease.
   b. if the patient has a history of blood clots.
   c. if a rash is present on the lower legs.
   d. if the patient has diabetes or other risk factors for skin breakdown.

8. Skeletal traction is used to treat:
   a. dislocations.
   b. muscle spasms.
   c. fractures.
   d. bulging discs.

9. Primary concerns in the operating area include:
   a. the cost of new technology.
   b. infection control and prevention.
   c. shortage of qualified personnel.
   d. teaching staff to work as team players.

10. When working in the operating area, you should:
    a. change to street clothes before going on lunch break.
    b. pin a name badge to your scrubs before leaving.
    c. cover your scrubs with a lab coat when leaving the department.
    d. never leave the department for breaks or lunch.

11. Contraindications for coughing and deep breathing include:
    a. patients with asthma and allergies.
    b. COPD, diabetes, and arthritis.
    c. eye, nose, or neurologic surgery.
    d. orthopedic and hip surgery.

12. Deep vein thrombosis is:
    a. a blood clot in the deep veins of the legs.
    b. a clot that travels through the bloodstream.
    c. a blood clot in the heart muscle.
    d. a clot that cannot move through the small vessels in the brain.

13. When applying antiembolism hosiery to a patient for the first time, you should:
    a. check with the RN to find out which size to use.
    b. select the size that matches the patient's weight.
    c. check the length of the legs with a ruler.
    d. measure the legs with a tape measure.

14. The PCA pump enables the patient to:
    a. administer pain medication.
    b. do passive range-of-motion exercises.
    c. turn over in bed independently.
    d. improve circulation in the legs to prevent clots.

15. When caring for a patient who wears antiembolism stockings, you should:
    a. center the hole in the foot over the heel.
    b. monitor circulation in the patient's toes every 2 to 4 hours.
    c. remove the hosiery when using the pneumatic compression garment.
    d. cover the stockings with plastic bags when the patient showers.

16. Treatment for patients who have fractures begins:
    a. after the bone is well healed.
    b. soon after admission.
    c. when the physical therapist gives permission.
    d. immediately before discharge.

17. When positioning a patient who has a left leg cast, you should:
    a. support the foot against the footboard of the bed.
    b. position the leg near the side rail to maintain alignment.
    c. keep the toes warm by covering them with a sheet and blanket.
    d. elevate the left foot so it is higher than the left hip.

18. When positioning a patient who is postoperative ORIF, you should:
    a. avoid adduction and internal and external rotation of the affected hip.
    b. avoid abduction and internal and external rotation of the affected hip.
    c. assist the patient to maintain the high Fowler's position.
    d. not turn the patient, as this is the RN's responsibility.

19. Patients who have had hip surgery are at very high risk of developing:
    a. COPD.
    b. diabetes.
    c. heel ulcers.
    d. skin infections.

20. After hip replacement surgery, keep the patient's legs apart by using a/an:
    a. adduction pillow.
    b. abduction pillow.
    c. sandbag.
    d. foam wedge.

21. When repositioning a patient on his or her side following hip replacement surgery, you should:
    a. remove the special foam pillow when turning.
    b. avoid crossing the patient's legs when turning.
    c. roll the operative leg over the unaffected leg.
    d. have the patient push with the operative foot.

22. CPM therapy is used to:
    a. rotate joints to prevent clots.
    b. flex joints to relieve pain.
    c. stretch joints to reduce spasms.
    d. move joints effortlessly.

23. Contraindications for CPM therapy include:
    a. blood clots.
    b. hip surgery.
    c. tendon repair.
    d. burn injuries.

24. The most common location of compartment syndrome in adults is:
    a. a fractured humerus.
    b. a snake bite.
    c. a fractured tibia.
    d. an infiltrated IV.

25. Signs and symptoms of compartment syndrome include:
    a. pain out of proportion to the injury.
    b. fever and high blood pressure.
    c. cough and congestion.
    d. fingers of a casted arm that feel warm to the touch.

E X P L O R I N G   T H E   W E B

Articles on Preoperative and Postoperative Infection Control	http://www.infectioncontroltoday.com
Asepsis and Aseptic Practices	http://www.infectioncontroltoday.com
Aseptic Technique: The ABCs of Infection Control	http://www.iceinstitute.com
Association of Perioperative Registered Nurses	http://www.aorn.org
Best Practice: Impact of Preoperative Hair Removal on Surgical Site Infection	http://www.joannabriggs.edu.au
Best Practice: Knowledge Retention from Preoperative Patient Information	http://www.joannabriggs.edu.au
Compression Hosiery in the Prevention and Treatment of Venous Leg Ulcers	http://www.worldwidewounds.com
Continuous Passive Motion	http://www.arthroscopy.com
Deep Vein Thrombosis Full-Text Article Links	http://www.ctcdvt.com
Deep Venous Thrombosis Prophylaxis: Drugs, Leg Pumps, Foot Pumps	http://www.venous-info.com
Deep Venous Thrombosis Prophylaxis in the Surgical or Trauma Patient	http://www.surgicalcriticalcare.net
Graduated Compression Stockings for the Prevention of Post-operative Venous Thromboembolism	http://www.joannabriggs.edu.au
Graduated Compression Stockings: Updating Practice, Improving Compliance	http://www.ctcdvt.com
A Guide to Bed Safety	http://www.patientsafety.com
Guidelines for Preventing Surgical Site Infection	http://www.nailm.com
Hill-Rom Beds	http://www.hill-rom.com
Hospital Bed and Bedrail Safety Advice	http://www.ecri.org
Hospital Bed Safety	http://www.fda.gov/cdrh
Nursing Specialties Perioperative Nursing	http://allnurses.com

Nutrition & the Surgical Patient	http://www.facs.org
Perioperative Nursing Slides	http://www.indstate.edu
Postoperative Care of Children	http://www.musckids.com
PowerPoint Slides—Perioperative Care	http://www.nursing.uaa.alaska.edu
Prevention and Management of Hip Fracture in Older People	http://www.sign.ac.uk
Prevention of Perioperative Deep Venous Thrombosis and Pulmonary Embolism	http://www.dcmsonline.org
Principles of Sterile Technique	http://www.free-ed.net
Principles of Sterile Technique for the OR	http://www.lhsc.on.ca
Procedure for Transferring Patient to the OR	http://www.cc.nih.gov
Pulse Oximetry	http://www.utmb.edu
Stryker Corporation	http://www.strykercorp.com
Stryker Medical	http://www.med.strykercorp.com

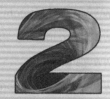

CHAPTER 12

Heat and Cold Applications

OBJECTIVES

After reading this chapter, you should be able to:

- Spell and define key terms.
- State the purpose, benefits, indications, and contraindications of heat and cold treatments.
- Describe safety factors to consider when using heat and cold applications.
- Differentiate the purpose of moist heat and cold treatments from dry treatments.
- Identify an aquathermia pad and a hydrocollator and state the purpose of each.
- List the benefits of applying a warmed blanket to geriatric patients.
- Define hydrotherapy and state the guidelines for giving a whirlpool bath.
- State the purpose of a sitz bath.
- State the purpose of therapeutic baths.
- State the purpose of applying warm and cool eye compresses, and describe how to perform this treatment.
- Differentiate primary hypothermia, secondary hypothermia, and perioperative hypothermia.
- Differentiate heat stroke from heat exhaustion.
- State the purpose of the hypothermia-hyperthermia blanket and list observations to report to the RN when the patient is using this device.

HEAT AND COLD TREATMENTS

Heat treatments (**thermotherapy,** or **diathermy**) and cold treatments (**cryotherapy**) are commonly used to treat musculoskeletal conditions. Cold is often applied immediately after an injury. Heat may be used later. Many types of applications are used. Moist applications can be hot or cold. These applications penetrate deeper than dry applications. Water touches the skin during a moist application. Dry applications are those in which no water touches the skin. Some dry applications, such as a hot wa-

ter bottle, have water inside, but the outside of the application stays dry. Moist applications conduct heat or cold better than dry applications. Dry applications may be used to maintain the temperature of moist applications.

A **localized application** delivers heat or cold to a specific area. An ice bag to a sprained ankle is an example of this type of application. A **generalized application** delivers heat or cold to the entire body. A cooling bath or hypothermia blanket to reduce a fever is a generalized application. Heat **dilates** or enlarges blood vessels, bringing oxygen and nutrients to the area. This action relieves pain

Table 12-1 Warm and Cold Applications

Dry Warm Applications	Dry Cold Applications	Moist Warm Applications	Moist Cold Applications
Hot water bottle	Ice cap, ice collar	Warm soaks	Cool compresses
Electric heating pad	Ice bag	Aquathermia pad (Aquamatic K-Pad)	Hypothermia blanket
		Tub baths	Cool soaks
Gel warm pack	Gel cold pack	Sitz baths	Cold packs
Disposable (chemical) warm pack	Disposable (chemical) cold pack	Tepid sponge baths	Aquathermia pad (Aquamatic K-Pad)
		Whirlpool bath Hyperthermia blanket Hydrocollator packs	

and speeds healing. Local cold applications relieve pain and prevent or relieve edema. Cold applications are also used to control bleeding. Cooling reduces the blood flow to the area and **constricts** blood vessels, making them smaller. Table 12-1 summarizes types of heat and cold applications.

Principles of Using Heat and Cold Applications

Follow your facility policies and state rules for using heat and cold. Localized heat and cold applications that contact the skin must be covered. This protects the skin from frostbite and burns. Covers are usually made of flannel. Pillowcases, towels, or a thin layer of foam are also used. If the device has a metal cap, face it away from the patient. The metal conducts heat or cold, which can injure the patient. When doing heat and cold treatments, assist the patient into a comfortable position. He or she must be comfortable and able to maintain the position for the duration of the treatment. Expose only the part of the body that you will be treating.

Guidelines for Using Heat and Cold Applications

Before using a heat or cold application, you should know the:

- Type of application
- Area of the patient's body to be treated
- Length of time the application is to remain in place
- Proper temperature of the application
- Safety precautions to use
- Side effects to watch for

Other precautions:

- Apply the principles of standard precautions if your hands will contact blood, moist body fluids (except sweat), secretions, excretions, nonintact skin, or mucous membranes.

- If the patient has a dressing covering the area to be treated, consult the RN for directions.
- Check the temperature of the solution with a thermometer. You may need to add more liquid during the treatment to maintain the temperature. Avoid pouring hot or cold liquid directly over the patient.
- Avoid using heat treatments with temperatures over 105°F, unless instructed by the RN. Use the average low and high temperature guidelines in this chapter to learn whether the ordered temperature range is reasonable and safe for the patient. Temperatures higher than this can cause burns, especially in infants and elderly patients.

(continued)

Guidelines for Using Heat and Cold Applications (Continued)

- Remove all metal jewelry, buttons, or zippers that could conduct heat or cold and thus injure the skin.
- Always cover applications before using them.
- Check the skin under the application every 10 minutes, or according to facility policy. If the skin under a heat application appears red, or a dark area appears, stop the treatment. Notify the nurse immediately. Stop a cold application and notify the RN if the patient's skin appears cyanotic, pale, white, or bright red; if the patient complains of numbness; or if the patient is shivering. Cover the patient with a blanket.
- Avoid using heat in the first 48 hours after an injury.
- Heat and cold applications are usually not left in place longer than 20 minutes, according to the purpose and type of treatment. Follow the care plan and nurse's instructions.
- Discard chemical packs after one use, or when the temperature changes. Never attempt to refreeze or reheat a chemical pack.
- Make sure the patient can tolerate the weight of the application without increased pain.
- After the treatment, pat the skin dry. Make the patient comfortable. Clean and store used equipment. Remove gloves, if worn, and dispose of them according to facility policy. Wash your hands. Report to the RN that the procedure was completed and the patient's reaction.
- Follow all safety rules to prevent spills and falls.

Infants and elderly patients are very sensitive to heat and cold. Patients with paralysis, impaired sensation, or fragile skin may be injured by a treatment that is too hot or cold. Some areas of the body, such as scar tissue and stomas, may be more sensitive to the effects of heat. Check with the RN if you have any doubts about the safety of the treatment considering the patient's medical condition. Sensitive and fragile skin begins to burn at about 115°F, but in some patients this figure could be a little more or less. Prolonged contact with cold may cause frostbite and other injuries.

HEAT TREATMENTS

Heat is used to relieve muscle spasms, pain, and inflammation. It may be ordered to increase drainage from an infected wound. Heat increases circulation and speeds healing. It increases tissue metabolism, reduces pain, and decreases congestion of blood vessels and internal organs. *Heat should not be used if bleeding or edema is present.* The heat application should feel comfortably warm to the patient, not uncomfortably hot. If you will be applying a pack or pad, touch the device to your forearm to check the temperature immediately before applying it. If the patient complains of burning, remove the application and consult the nurse. Other contraindications to heat therapy are:

- Acute inflammation
- Suspected appendicitis
- Dermatitis
- Deep vein thrombosis
- Peripheral vascular disease
- Open wound(s)
- Recent soft tissue injuries in which swelling or bleeding would be increased by heat
- Skin sensation impairment and/or paralysis
- Severe cognitive impairment
- Some physicians also recommend avoiding heat in children and pregnant women.

If a patient has any of these conditions, check with the RN before applying a heat application.

Apply direct heat cautiously (with close supervision) to patients:

- who are mentally confused, pediatric, and elderly
- with neurologic problems
- with impaired renal, cardiac, or respiratory function, arteriosclerosis or atherosclerosis

If you have any doubts about the patient's ability to tolerate the treatment, remain in the room for as long as necessary while the treatment is in place.

Dry Heat Treatments

Dry heat penetrates the tissue to a depth of about 1 centimeter. It does not affect deeper tissue because of the protective layer of subcutaneous fat and the blood vessels, which carry off and dissipate the heat. The use of heat in health care facilities is limited because of the safety risks associated with its use.

Hot Packs. Hot water bottles, reusable gel packs, and chemical hot packs are commonly used heat treatments. The normal treatment temperature for a hot water bottle is 105°F. The internal temperature of the water bottle should never exceed 110°F. The chemical hot pack is activated by striking it. Always strike it away from your face, as leakage of chemicals can occur. The chemical hot pack feels very warm when you first activate it. Use caution when applying it to patients who have circulatory or neurological problems. Cover both the water bottle and chemical pack with fabric. Test the temperature of the application on the inside of your forearm before applying it. The aquathermia pad is a safer, easier treatment that can be used in place of hot packs. Hot packs are contraindicated in:

- Paralysis or areas without sensation
- Acute edema or inflammation
- Infection
- Hemophilia
- Infants
- Cognitively impaired patients

Use hot packs with caution in very young and very old patients, and those with medical conditions such as:

- Impaired circulation
- Neurologic conditions
- Sensory impairment
- Cancer
- Rashes and open skin conditions

Procedure 96

Applying a Hot Water Bottle, Gel Pack, or Chemical Hot Pack

Supplies needed:
- Disposable exam gloves, if contact with blood or body fluids is anticipated
- Hot water bottle
- Hot tap water
- Pitcher
- Bath thermometer
- Chemical hot pack or gel pack, if used
- Protective cloth cover
- Tape or roller gauze, if needed
- Plastic bag for used supplies

1. Perform your beginning procedure actions.
2. Run tap water until it is hot. Fill a pitcher with water.
   OR
   If a gel pack is being used, warm it in hot water or a commercial warmer, according to type of product used and facility policies. Avoid the microwave, which may cause hot spots.
3. Check the water temperature. It should be 105°F (**Figure 12-1A**), or according to the RN's instructions. Adjust the temperature as needed.
4. Pour the hot water into the bottle, filling it approximately one-half to two-thirds full.
5. Expel air by squeezing the bottle gently until water reaches the neck (**Figure 12-1B** and **Figure 12-1C**).

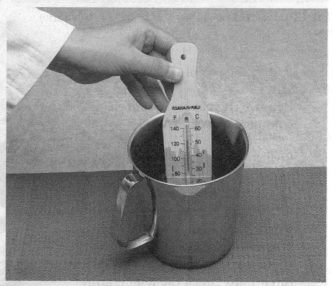

FIGURE 12-1(A) Use a thermometer to check the water temperature. The temperature should never exceed 105°F for adults, and 100°F for children and elderly persons.

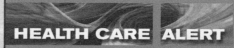

HEALTH CARE ALERT

A partially filled bottle is flexible and molds to the patient's body easily. The weight of a full bottle may cause pain to an injured area. A partially filled bottle with the air expelled stays warm longer. Extra air in the bottle cools the hot water.

(continues)

Procedure 96, *continued*

Applying a Hot Water Bottle, Gel Pack, or Chemical Hot Pack

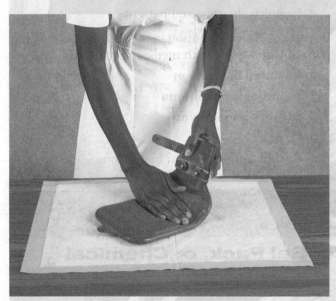

FIGURE 12-1(B) Flatten the bottle on the table to expel air.

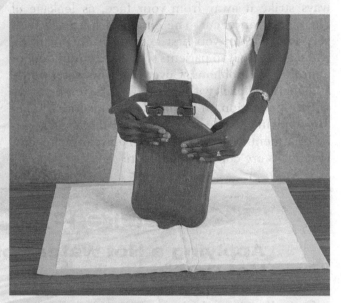

FIGURE 12-1(C) After filling, hold the bottle upright and squeeze gently until water reaches the neck to expel air. Dry the outside of the bag before placing the bag in a protective cover.

6. Fasten the top of the bottle.
   OR
   Remove the gel pack from the hot water or commercial warmer.
   OR
   Strike the chemical hot pack to activate it. Avoid striking the pack in front of your face, as the pack may break, spraying chemicals into your eyes and mucous membranes.
7. Cover the bag or activated pack with an absorbent cloth or cover.
8. Press the bag against the inside of your forearm to check the temperature.
9. Expose the area to be treated. Place the covered bag or pack on the area, and note the time.

10. Secure the device with tape or roller gauze, if necessary.
11. Following facility policy, periodically check the patient and the appearance of skin under the bag or pack.
12. Remove the source of heat after the designated length of time (usually 20 minutes).
13. Wash a reusable bag with soap and water, and hang to dry. Discard a chemical pack. Cleanse and care for the gel pack according to facility policies.
14. Perform your procedure completion actions.

Warmed Blankets. Sleep and rest are essential to enable the body to recover after illness or surgery. Patients will rest better if they are comfortable. A common complaint among hospitalized elderly patients is discomfort related to the cool environment. Many other factors, such as the hospital gown, lack of a blanket, incontinence, and some medical and nursing treatments, increase the sensation of coldness. The discomfort of feeling cold increases restlessness and muscle tension, aggravates pain, and decreases patient satisfaction with hospital care. Most hospitals have commercial warmers that are used to warm IV solutions and bath blankets. Although these are usually in the perioperative department, they may be available in other areas as well. A small body of evidence suggests that warmth promotes comfort, rest, and sleep, and reduces pain in elderly persons. Because of this, nurse researchers studied the effects of applying warmed blankets to comfort elderly patients (ages 65 to 98) who were cold, anxious, or uncomfortable. They measured the level of discomfort before and one hour after the application of a warm blanket. They found that the patients' ratings of discomfort were much less after receiving the warm blanket.[1]

Patients who could describe their discomfort said that they felt more comfortable. Nonverbal patients displayed fewer behavior problems and less body language suggesting discomfort. This small study proved that warmed blankets increase comfort and satisfaction of elderly patients in the cool hospital environment. Offering patients a warmed blanket is a simple nursing measure that the PCT can implement at any time. Helping to relieve pain and suffering is an important part of PCT care. Relieving discomfort is measured in improved quality of life. By using simple nursing measures such as a warmed blanket to increase patient comfort, you will be rewarded with improved patient satisfaction, quality of care, and quality of life.

Moist Heat Treatments

Moist heat penetrates deeper than dry heat. It is less drying to the skin, produces less perspiration, and is usually more comfortable for the patient. Moist heat also softens the skin, making it easier to eliminate crusts and exudates. Blood vessels dilate in response to the heat. This increases blood flow, which carries the heat away, so the effect is not long-lasting. However, moist heat is very effective for relieving muscle spasms.

[1]Robinson, S., & G. Benton. (2002). Warmed blankets: An intervention to promote comfort for elderly hospitalized patients. *Geriatric Nursing*, 23, 320–323.

Warm Soaks. Administering warm soaks (Figure 12-2) involves immersing part of the patient's body in water. The treatment should last no more than 20 minutes. The water temperature should not exceed 105° F, or as instructed by the RN.

SAFETY ALERT

Each state has laws governing the water temperature in patient care areas of the facility. These vary slightly from one state to the next, but in most, water temperature in patient care units and bathing areas should not exceed 120°F. The regulators sometimes fail, sending very hot water into the facility. However, water in bath and shower areas must be warm enough to bathe patients comfortably. Comfortable temperature for most people is 95°F to 105°F. Report water in bathing areas that does not warm up enough for comfortable bathing. Also report steaming water, or water that feels hot to the touch at any faucet in a patient care area. Use bath thermometers to check water temperatures before patient care whenever possible. If a thermometer is unavailable, check the temperature on the inside of your forearm or wrist.

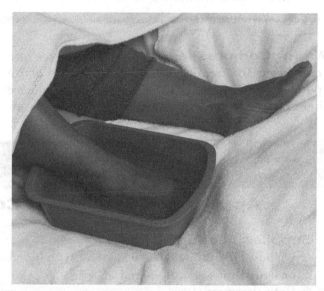

FIGURE 12-2 The patient is receiving warm soak therapy.

Procedure 97

Performing a Warm Soak

Supplies needed:
- Disposable exam gloves, if contact with blood or body fluids is anticipated
- Bath thermometer
- Washbasin

(continues)

Procedure **97**, *continued*

Performing a Warm Soak

▶ Pitcher
▶ Bath towels (2 or 3)
▶ Disposable underpads or large plastic sheet
▶ Bath blanket
▶ Plastic bag for used supplies

1. Perform your beginning procedure actions.
2. Take equipment to the bedside.
3. Cover the patient with a bath blanket.
4. Fanfold the bedding to the foot of the bed.
5. Expose the extremity to be soaked.
6. Raise the side rail on the far side of the bed, and assist the patient to move toward the rail. Position him or her for comfort.
7. Cover the bed with the underpads or plastic sheet and towel.
8. Fill the soak basin half-full with hot water at the sink. Check the temperature. It should not be more than 105°F.

9. Position the patient's extremity on the bed protector. Place the water basin on the bed protector. Assist the patient to place the limb in the basin. Cover with a towel to maintain temperature.
10. Check the water temperature every 5 minutes. Use the pitcher to warm the water, if needed. Remove the patient's limb before adding water to the basin.
11. Stop the procedure after the designated length of time (approximately 20 minutes).
12. Lift the patient's extremity out of the basin.
13. Slip the basin forward, or move it to the table.
14. Gently pat the patient's limb dry with the towel. If a foot soak was done, dry well between the toes.
15. Perform your procedure completion actions.

Warm Compresses. Warm compresses are soaks used for treating small areas. Warm gauze sponges or washcloths in hot water and squeeze them out. Fold the cloth and place it over the affected area. The compress cools quickly, so you must change it frequently. A hot water bottle or an aquathermia pad may be used to cover the application to keep it warm.

Procedure **98**

Applying Warm, Moist Compresses

Supplies needed:
▶ Disposable exam gloves, if contact with blood or body fluids is anticipated
▶ Bath thermometer
▶ Washbasin with prescribed solution at temperature ordered
▶ 4 × 4 gauze pads(unsterile, or according to RN's instructions) to use as compresses
▶ Water, sterile normal saline, or other prescribed solution
▶ Pitcher
▶ Pins or roller gauze
▶ Syringe

▶ Bath towels (2)
▶ Disposable underpads or large plastic sheet
▶ Bath blanket
▶ Plastic bag or covered hot water bottle, pack, or aquathermia pad, to maintain temperature
▶ Plastic bag for used supplies

NOTE: If you are applying compresses to an open postoperative area, use sterile technique, including sterile gloves, a sterile basin, sterile solution, and sterile 4 × 4 sponges. If a sterile thermometer is unavailable, pour some heated sterile solution into a clean container, check the temperature with a bath thermometer, then discard the test solution.

(continues)

Procedure 98, *continued*

Applying Warm, Moist Compresses

1. Perform your beginning procedure actions.
2. Take equipment to the bedside.
3. Cover the patient with a bath blanket.
4. Fanfold the bedding to the foot of the bed.
5. Expose the extremity to be treated.
6. Cover the bed with the underpads or plastic sheet and towel.
7. Apply gloves.
8. Check the temperature of the solution. It should not be more than 105°F, or as instructed by the RN. (For some treatments, the temperature may be as high as 110°F.) If using sterile solution, pour it into a small sterile bowl and heat the bowl in hot water, or heat a small bottle of solution in hot water.
9. Position the patient's extremity on the bed protector or towel (**Figure 12-3A**).
10. Moisten the compresses in the basin.

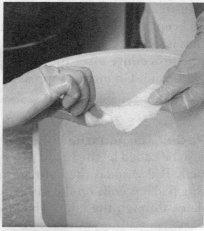

FIGURE 12-3(B) Dip the compress into the basin of hot water, then grasp the edges and twist to squeeze out excess liquid.

11. Squeeze out excess moisture (**Figure 12-3B**).
12. Apply compresses to the treatment area (**Figure 12-3C**).
13. Cover the compresses with a single layer cut from the plastic bag, or a properly covered hot pack or aquathermia pad, if ordered, to maintain temperature.
14. Secure the compress with a binder or roller gauze, if needed.
15. Following facility policy, periodically check the patient and the appearance of skin under the bag or pack. Maintain proper

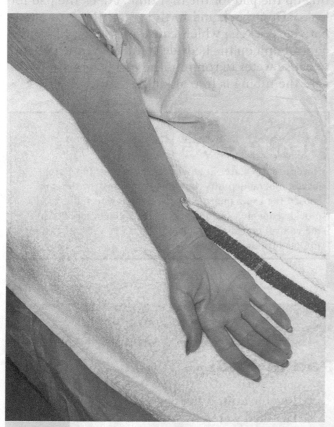

FIGURE 12-3(A) Protect the bed with a towel or underpad.

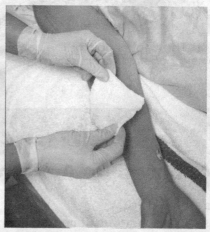

FIGURE 12-3(C) Open the compress and apply it to the treatment area.

(continues)

Procedure 98, *continued*

Applying Warm, Moist Compresses

temperature and moisture. A syringe may be used to keep compresses wet, if additional moisture is needed.

16. Stop the procedure after the designated length of time. Change compresses

as ordered, or at least once every 24 hours.

17. Discard used compresses in the plastic bag.
18. Gently pat the area dry with the towel.
19. Perform your procedure completion actions.

Heating Pads. The **aquathermia pad** (Figure 12-4) may also be called by the brand name, K-Pad, or Aquamatic K-Pad. *Aqua* is the Latin term for water. The plastic pad has coils on the inside. Distilled water circulates through the coils. The circulating water maintains a constant temperature. The pad is attached to a pump at the bedside. The temperature of the unit is preset between 95°F and 100°F. If you are responsible for setting the unit, you will adjust the temperature with a key. Remove the key before leaving so that the temperature cannot be changed. Like other heat applications, the plastic aquathermia pad should not contact the skin directly. Cover it with a pillowcase or flannel cover. Some facilities cover the pad with two pillowcases, providing extra protection against injury. When setting up the pad for the first time, check the pad for leaks. Tip it back and forth several times to eliminate air pockets, which cause hot spots. Place the control unit on the bedside stand above the patient, to cause water to run into the pad by gravity. Make sure the tubing is free of kinks.

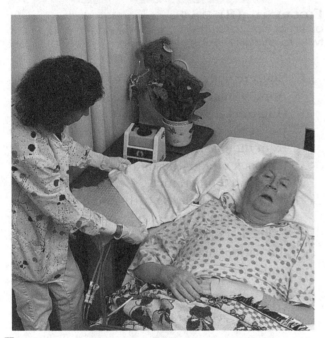

FIGURE 12-4 The control unit for the aquathermia pad maintains a constant temperature.

HEALTH CARE ALERT

Never use tap water in an aquathermia pad. Tap water leaves mineral deposits that damage or destroy the unit. Loosen the cap a quarter turn each time you fill it, to provide enough space for normal heat expansion. Placing the control unit slightly above the patient will assist water to flow into the coils.

Procedure 99

Applying an Aquathermia Pad (K-Pad)

Supplies needed:
- Disposable exam gloves, if contact with blood or body fluids is anticipated
- Aquathermia pad (K-Pad) and control unit
- Key for unit, if needed
- Distilled water
- Covering for pad

(continues)

Procedure 99, *continued*

Applying an Aquathermia Pad (K-Pad)

1. Perform your beginning procedure actions.
2. Check the cord and tubing for frayed or damaged insulation. Make sure the pad is free from cracks.
3. Place the control unit on the bedside stand.
4. Remove the lid of the control unit and check the level of distilled water. If low, fill the container two-thirds full or to the fill line using distilled water.
5. Screw the lid in place, then loosen it one-quarter turn.
6. If the temperature has not been set, check with the RN for the proper temperature to use. After setting the temperature, remove the key. Return the key to the designated area so it will not be lost.
7. Plug in the unit.
8. Cover the pad with the appropriate cover. Do not use pins to hold the cover in place.
9. Expose the area to be treated. Place the covered pad on the area, and note the time. Make sure the tubing does not hang over the edge of the bed. It should be coiled on the bed to promote the flow of liquid.
10. Following facility policy, periodically check the patient and the appearance of skin under the pad.
11. Remove the pad after the designated length of time (approximately 20 minutes).
12. Perform your procedure completion actions.

Moist Hot Packs. The **hydrocollator** is a rectangular tank containing very hot water. Hot packs usually contain a silicate gel in a cotton bag. The packs are placed between dividers in the tank. You may be responsible for applying the hot packs to patients' skin. They are commonly used on the back and neck. The packs (**Figure 12-5A**) are *very hot* to the touch. Always use tongs to remove them from the tank. Hold the tabs on the corners of the pack when removing a pack from the tank. Cover the pack with special, thick, layered terry cloth covers, or follow the directions in **Figure 12-5B** to cover it with folded towels. The thick cover maintains a barrier between the pack and the patient's skin. The packs are applied for 10 to 20 minutes, or as ordered. Before using hydrocollator hot packs, review the precautions for using heat applications in this chapter. Because the packs are extremely hot, they are contraindicated in many conditions, such as infancy, old age, and paralysis. They should be used with caution and close supervision for all patients.

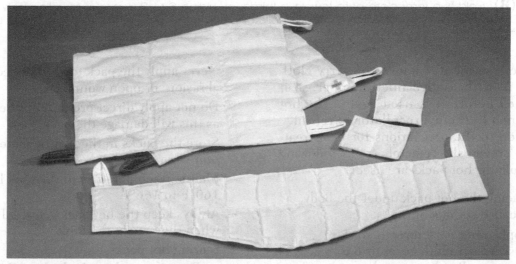

FIGURE 12-5(A) Select the hot pack that best conforms to the part of the body you are treating. (Courtesy of Briggs Corporation, Des Moines, IA; (800) 247-2343)

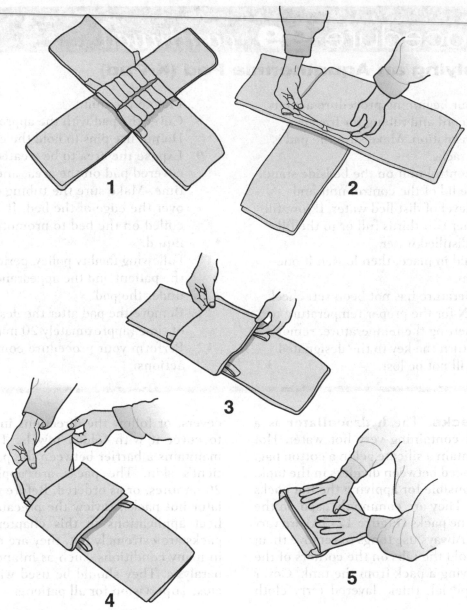

FIGURE 12-5(B) Fold two terry cloth bath towels in thirds, providing 6 to 8 layers of toweling between the hot pack and the patient's body. Position the hydrocollator pack in the center and fold the towels by following steps 2 through 5.

After the treatment, remove the terry cloth cover. Place it in the soiled linen hamper, so it can be washed before it is used again. The hot pack is returned to the hydrocollator to reheat.

In addition to the precautions for heat treatments listed previously, remember the following when hydrocollator hot packs are used:

- Avoid placing the hot pack under the body; this can cause serious burns.

- Never apply a hot pack directly to skin. Always use a terry cloth cover or 6 to 8 layers of dry terry toweling between the pack and the skin.

- Never apply the pack to an infected area, cut, abrasion, or open wound.

- Do not apply direct pressure to the hot pack, as this will damage the pack.

- Store the packs in the hydrocollator heating unit when not in use.

- Maintain temperature in the tank between 160°F to 166°F.

- Always keep the hot packs covered with water when they are in the tank.

- Storing hot packs
  - Return a pack to the hydrocollator immediately after use.

- Completely cover the pack with water and increase the temperature until the water temperature reaches 160°F.
- The pack must remain in the 160°F water for 20 minutes or longer before it can be used (or reused).
- Cleaning hot packs
  - Hand wash packs weekly, or according to facility policy, in a solution of 25 percent vinegar and 75 percent water. Rinse well. Disinfect with antimicrobial solution, according to facility policies. Never use a chlorine-based product.
- Cleaning the hydrocollator
  - Empty and disinfect the tank once a month, or according to facility policy.
  - Unplug the tank and remove the packs.
  - Carefully discard the hot liquid.
  - Allow the tank to cool before touching the inside surface.
  - When the tank is cool, scrub the inside with a facility-approved disinfectant or a solution of 25 percent vinegar and 75 percent water. (Some facilities pour 2 cups of calcium, lime, and rust remover into the tank, then fill with water until the heating element is covered. Let soak for 5 minutes and then drain. Rinse the tank well with clear water. Follow your facility policies and procedures.)
  - Disinfect the inside of the machine and racks with antimicrobial solution.
  - Remove the racks.
  - Rinse well to remove the chemicals.
  - Wipe the outside of the unit with disinfectant solution.
  - Replace the racks.

- After cleaning, refill the unit with fresh distilled water.
- Reheat the water to between 160°F and 166°F.
- Thoroughly wash all the hot packs.
- Return the clean packs to the tank.
- If a pack develops a bad smell, check the steam packs. Brown spots on them are most probably caused by contamination with a microbe or pathogen. This is caused by:
  - Water temperature below 160°F in the tank.
  - Packs left out too long in open air before being returned to the tank.
  - Packs not being cleaned regularly.
  - Hydrocollator tank not being cleaned and disinfected regularly.
- How to resolve:
  - Discard *all packs* that are in the unit. (The infection will spread to other packs.)
  - Clean the unit with a solution of 25 percent vinegar and 75 percent water, facility-approved disinfectant, or calcium, lime, and rust remover, according to facility policy. Rinse well.
  - Wipe the outside of the unit with disinfectant solution.
  - Clean and replace the racks.
  - After cleaning, refill the unit with fresh distilled water.
  - Reheat the water to between 160°F and 166°F.
  - Begin again with all new packs. Make sure the water temperature is at or above 160°F but at or below 166°F.

Procedure 100

Applying Moist Hot Packs (Hydrocollator Tank)

NOTE: In some states and facilities, PCTs are not permitted to perform this procedure. Your instructor will advise you if this is a PCT procedure in your state and facility. Perform this procedure only if you are permitted to do so by state law and facility policies.

Supplies needed:
- Disposable exam gloves, if contact with blood or body fluids is anticipated
- Bath towels
- Six-layer terry cloth cover for hot pack
- Disposable underpad
- Bath blanket
- Hydrocollator with hot packs heated to proper temperature
- Plastic bag for used supplies

(continues)

Procedure **100**, *continued*

Applying Moist Hot Packs (Hydrocollator Tank)

1. Perform your beginning procedure actions.
2. Prepare the hot pack in the clean utility room, therapy room, or designated area.
3. Unfold the terry cloth cover for the hot pack and place it flat on the counter.
4. Using the tongs, grasp the tabs on the corner of the hot pack and hold it over the hydrocollator tank.
5. Drip water off the pack into the tank.
6. Remove the pack, close the hydrocollator, and prepare the pack on a table.
7. Wrap the pack in the terry cloth cover and fasten the Velcro. The steam from the pack will penetrate the layers of toweling.
8. Wrap the pack in a towel to keep it warm. Promptly take it to the bedside.
9. Expose the part of the patient's body to be treated.
10. Cover the bed with the underpad, if needed.
11. Remove the outer towel and apply the covered hot pack to the affected area.
12. Check for patient comfort.
13. Adjust towel thickness by adding a bath towel if the patient complains that the pack is too hot.
14. Remain at the bedside. Check the skin under the pack after two to three minutes. Adjust towel thickness, if necessary.
15. Remove towel layers as the pack cools.
16. Stop the procedure after the designated length of time. A pack usually remains in place for 10 to 20 minutes.
17. After removing the pack, place it on the towel you used as an outer wrapper.
18. Assist the patient to reposition, as necessary.
19. Gather the pack and towel and return to the utility area.
20. Discard used linen in a plastic bag.
21. Return the pack to the hydrocollator.
22. Perform other necessary procedure completion actions.

HYDROTHERAPY

Hydrotherapy is water therapy. You may be asked to perform range-of-motion exercises on some patients in the whirlpool. The warm, circulating water relieves pain and muscle spasms, making movement easier. This type of water therapy is called **hydromassage,** because of the massaging effect of the agitating water. Hydrotherapy is contraindicated if the patient has unstable vital signs, fever, dehydration, or other fluid imbalances.

Whirlpool Therapy

Basins and small, portable whirlpools (**Figure 12-6A**) may be used for hydrotherapy and hydromassage on extremities. Portable whirlpool jets may be placed in regular bathtubs. Sometimes, you will immerse the patient's body in the regular whirlpool tub (**Figure 12-6B**) or Hubbard tank. Follow all safety precautions for the equipment you are using. Follow the RN's instructions for whirlpool temperature. **Figure 12-7** lists average therapeutic water temperature guidelines for the whirlpool bath.

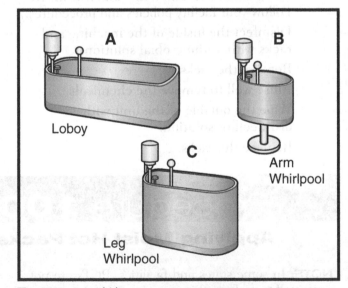

FIGURE 12-6(A) Select the whirlpool that best fits the part of the anatomy you are treating. (A) The "loboy" is similar to a Hubbard tank, but has lower sides. It is used to immerse the body when the lower limbs cannot hang down. (B) The arm whirlpool is used to treat the upper extremities, or areas below the knee. For small children, it may be used to immerse the entire body. (C) Leg whirlpools are used to treat the lower extremities.

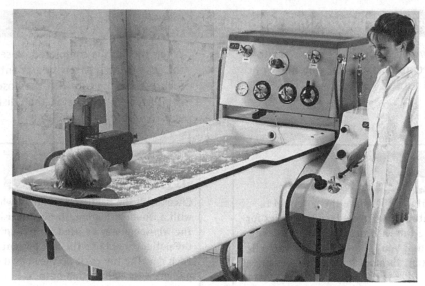

FIGURE 12-6(B) A whirlpool tub may be used for hydromassage or hydrotherapy. Fasten the safety belt and do not leave the room when the patient is in the tank.

Hot: 100°F to 110°F
Warm: 95°F to 105°F (this is the setting used for bathing and most treatments)
Tepid: 80°F to 93°F
Cool: 65°F to 80°F
Cold: 45°F to 60°F
• Never set the whirlpool for higher than 100°F without first checking with the RN.
• These guidelines may also be appropriate for other heat treatments; follow facility policies.

FIGURE 12-7 Average ordered water temperature for hydrotherapy treatments and procedures.

Guidelines for Giving a Whirlpool Bath

● Check with the RN before giving a whirlpool to a patient with an infection, recent surgical incision, or pressure ulcer.

● If the patient is combative or disoriented, check with the RN before giving the patient a whirlpool. The noise from the whirlpool may worsen the patient's agitation.

● Disinfect the whirlpool tub immediately before and after each use. Special techniques are necessary if the patient has an infection.

● Never leave a patient alone in the whirlpool tub, even for a minute.

● Always fasten the safety belt when moving a patient into or out of a whirlpool tub with a hydraulic lift seat. Keep the safety belt fastened throughout the procedure, even if the patient is alert.

● The patient may be frightened when using the hydraulic lift for the first time. Explain the procedure and reassure the patient.

● Drape the patient's genital area with a bath towel for modesty during the whirlpool bath.

● The water temperature in the whirlpool tub is usually set at 97°F to 100°F. This is a lower temperature than bath water because the temperature in the tub remains constant. The constant movement of warm water stimulates the patient's circulation.

● Use a low-suds or no-suds product designed specifically for whirlpool use.

● Never pour liquid soap or shampoo into the whirlpool tub. A tiny bit of liquid soap will result in an abundance of suds. If the patient accidentally creates a suds problem, rub a bar of soap against the walls of the tub to reduce the bubbles.

● The whirlpool activity provides a cleansing action. However, if you will be assisting the patient with bathing, apply the principles of standard precautions.

(continued)

Guidelines for Giving a Whirlpool Bath (Continued)

- Wrap the patient with a bath blanket for warmth and modesty immediately after removing him or her from the whirlpool tub.
- Limit hydrotherapy time to 20 to 30 minutes.

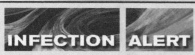

The jets in some whirlpool tubs have the potential to harbor dangerous pathogens. Follow facility policies for carefully cleaning the tub with the proper disinfectant solution. Make sure that you follow directions correctly and run the disinfectant through the tub for the correct length of time.

- When the bath is completed, raise the lift seat out of the soapy water. After the patient is dry, safe, and secure, rinse the tub with the hose, using comfortably warm water, then disinfect the tub according to facility policy.

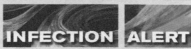

Check with the RN before giving a whirlpool to a patient with a wound infection, surgical incision, or pressure ulcer. The whirlpool may be used for patients with infections, but the patient should be the last patient to use the device each day. The tub must be specially disinfected after the patient with an infection bathes.

Hydrotherapy equipment has the potential to injure patients seriously if it malfunctions. Most tubs have a thermometer permanently mounted on the mechanism to check the water temperature. Occasionally, the internal thermometer fails, and the water comes out very hot. Use common sense; if the water is steaming, it is probably too hot. Use a second thermometer to double-check the water temperature. Test the water with your elbow before moving the patient into the tank. The maintenance department usually checks the equipment weekly. Report problems to your maintenance department or appropriate person in your facility.

Guidelines for Monitoring Hydrotherapy Equipment

- The temperature gauge should be within 2 degrees of the thermometer reading. Hot water in the tank should never exceed 105°F. Most tanks are set at 95°F to 97°F. Whirlpool bath temperature is slightly lower than for bathing in a tub or shower, because the whirlpool unit maintains a constant water temperature.
- The hydraulic lift is secured to the floor. Check the floor for hydraulic fluid or oil leaks; if present, do not use the lift until it has been repaired.
- The bolts holding the seat to the lift should not be corroded.

- The seat belt should lock securely. Belts must be present, working, and in good repair. Always lock the belt before lifting the patient to the tank. Keep the belt fastened throughout the procedure.
- Check the sides of fiberglass tanks for cracks.
- Spray hoses must be crack-free. Hot water leaks can cause burns.
- Follow facility policies and the manufacturer's instructions for the unit you are using. The operating instructions should be posted by the unit.

Disinfecting the Whirlpool. The whirlpool tub is drained after each use and cleaned with disinfectant solution. Follow the manufacturer's directions for the type of tub and disinfectant you are using. Suggested actions are to:

- Fill the tub with water and disinfectant.
- Turn on the whirlpool.

- Run the whirlpool action for 10 to 20 full minutes, or according to facility policy.
- Wipe areas that are not immersed in water with disinfectant solution. Let the full-strength solution sit on these areas while the whirlpool is running.
- Drain the tub while rinsing it well from top to bottom.

- Rinse the upper areas, working your way to the bottom of the tub.
- Rinse a second time from top to bottom.
- Dry the tub with a towel.

Disposing of Trash. Discard used protective equipment, soiled dressings, and cleaning cloths in a sealed plastic bag. Dispose of them according to facility policy.

Therapeutic Baths and Soaks

Therapeutic baths are usually given when patients have widespread skin problems. These baths involve the use of special products for bathing or soaking the skin, such as *colloidal oatmeal*. This oatmeal is very finely ground and pulverized. This product is used for many different skin conditions to relieve irritation, reduce itching, moisturize, soften, and protect the skin. When combined with the bath water, the tiny oatmeal molecules spread through the water, changing its consistency. The oatmeal granules do not sink to the bottom of the tub.

When bathing the patient, you may be instructed to use **tepid** (lukewarm) water instead of hot water. Tepid water should be between 80°F and 93°F. The patient may need a therapeutic bath up to three times a day, depending on the severity of the underlying condition. In addition to the bath, you may be instructed to assist the patient with using special lotions, soaps, and other topical products. When assisting with a therapeutic bath:

- Apply the principles of standard precautions.
- If an area of the patient's body is acutely inflamed, check with the RN before proceeding.
- Draw a tepid bath. Avoid hot water unless specifically instructed to use it. Hot water will further inflame the skin and absorb additional moisture rather than lubricating the skin.
- Add the required amount of colloidal oatmeal or other product to the tub as it is filling.
- Carefully assist the patient into the filled tub.
- The patient should soak for 10 to 20 minutes, or as listed on the care plan.
- Make sure that the patient does not get the treated bath water in the eyes.
- If the patient complains of feeling sticky after the bath, rinse with a few extra cups of tepid water from the faucet.

- The product may make the tub slippery. Instruct the patient to use the hand rail when rising from the tub, and provide assistance as needed.
- Pat (do not rub) the skin dry.
- Follow all facility policies and safety precautions that apply to bathing.

Colloidal oatmeal and other therapeutic bathing products bind to the skin. They act as a moisturizer because of their affinity for water. The products attract and hold water on the skin surface. Most products contain additional proteins to bind the moisturizers for long-lasting results. This improves the skin texture, making it feel softer and more elastic. Some products create a barrier that provides some protection from harmful substances. Therapeutic bath products help relieve redness and itching.

Tepid Sponge Bath

A tepid sponge bath is an older treatment that is sometimes used to reduce fever in adults and children. When performing the procedure for adults, you will give a variation of a bedbath. Children are usually given a tepid tub bath. You will monitor the patient's vital signs frequently. Obtain a rectal temperature, if possible. Avoid using the axillary method except as a last resort. A specific physician's order is needed for the tepid bath procedure. Follow the RN's instructions.

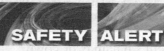

SAFETY ALERT

Some nurses recommend adding alcohol to a tepid sponge bath to further reduce body temperature. This is a dated practice, and alcohol should not be added without specific instruction from the RN. Alcohol evaporates from the skin more quickly than water, and cools the body faster. The recommended amount of alcohol to add varies from 20 percent to 40 percent. However, alcohol and rapid cooling can cause some patients to go into shock. Avoid the use of alcohol with infants, small children, pediatric or elderly patients. If alcohol is being used in the water, make sure it does not contact the mucous membranes of the eyes, nose, mouth, or genital area. Monitor the patient's rectal temperature and pulse closely during the procedure, and for at least 2 hours after the procedure if alcohol is used.

Procedure **101**

Giving a Tepid Sponge Bath to an Adult

Supplies needed:

▶ Disposable exam gloves, if contact with blood or body fluids is anticipated
▶ Bath towels (4 to 6)
▶ Washcloths (4 to 6)
▶ Washbasin with tepid water
▶ Alcohol, if ordered
▶ Bath thermometer
▶ Clinical thermometer to check the patient's temperature
▶ Bed linen and gown, as needed
▶ Disposable underpad, as needed
▶ Bath blanket
▶ Supplies to disinfect tub, as needed
▶ Plastic bag for used supplies

1. Perform your beginning procedure actions.
2. Take and record temperature and other vital signs to establish baseline values.
3. Place a bath blanket over the patient. Fanfold the top bedding to the foot of the bed.

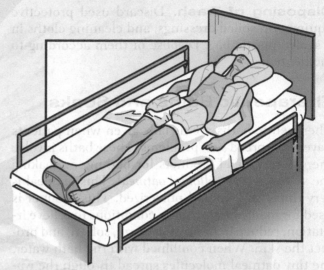

FIGURE 12-8A The head, groin, and axillae are the greatest areas of heat loss. Folding a cool washcloth and covering these areas will help reduce temperature.

HEALTH CARE ALERT

Using the bath blanket and towels to drape the patient is important during all bathing and personal care procedures, even if the room is completely private. Being exposed is uncomfortable for most people. Draping the patient properly provides a sense of dignity and protects the patient's modesty and self-esteem. Do not omit this important step for patients of any age.

4. Remove the patient's pajamas or gown.
5. Place a disposable underpad under the patient.
6. Obtain tepid water in the basin. Add alcohol only as instructed by the RN. Check the water temperature. Tepid water should be between 80°F and 93°F.
7. Place towels or washcloths in the solution.
8. Remove one moistened towel or washcloth and squeeze excess solution into the basin. Place the towel under the patient's arm. Repeat this step until you have a moist towel or washcloth in each axilla, one over the abdomen, and one on each side of the groin (Figure 12-8A). Fold a moist washcloth in thirds, and position it across the patient's forehead.

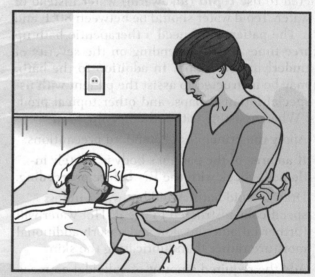

FIGURE 12-8B Expose only the part of the body on which you are working. Wash upward on the inner portion of the arm.

9. Replace towels or washcloths as they warm.
10. Expose only the part of the body on which you are working (Figure 12-8B). Keep the patient covered with towels and the bath blanket. Sponge the patient from the shoulder:
    • Across the upper chest.
    • Down the external portion of the exposed arm.
    • Upward on the inner portion of the arm. Repeat with the other arm.

(continues)

Procedure **101**, *continued*

Giving a Tepid Sponge Bath to an Adult

- Along the side of the body to the thigh. Sponge both sides of the body.
11. Sponge each leg.
12. Assist the patient to turn on his or her side, exposing the back.
13. Sponge the patient's back, backs of thighs, and legs.
14. Monitor the patient regularly throughout the procedure for chills, cyanosis, and increased pulse rate. Stop the bath and cover the patient with a blanket, if any of these signs is noted.
15. The bath should last 25 to 30 minutes. Take and record the TPR every 15 minutes

until it reaches 101°F, or the prescribed level.
16. Put the gown on the patient, remake the bed, and leave the patient dry and comfortable.
17. Because of the immediacy of this procedure, inform the RN of the current vital signs and other pertinent observations.
18. Take and record vital signs again 30 minutes following the bath, then every 30 minutes until the patient's temperature is stable.
19. Remove, clean, and store equipment. Discard the soiled linen.
20. Perform other necessary procedure completion actions.

Procedure **102**

Giving a Tepid Bath to a Child

Supplies needed:
- Disposable exam gloves, if contact with blood or body fluids is anticipated
- Bath towels
- Washcloths
- Paper or plastic cup
- Alcohol, if ordered
- Bath thermometer
- Clinical thermometer to check the patient's temperature
- Bath blanket
- Floor bath mat
- Rubber bath mat
- Supplies to disinfect tub, as needed
- Plastic bag for used supplies

1. Perform your beginning procedure actions.
2. Take supplies to the tub room. You may use a small, plastic tub for a child under the age of 3.
3. Clean the tub well with antibacterial cleaner.
4. Take and record the patient's temperature and other vital signs to establish baseline values.

5. Fill the tub with no more than 4 inches of tepid water. Add alcohol only as instructed by the RN. Check the water temperature. Tepid water should be between 80°F and 93°F.
6. Take the patient to the bathroom and assist him or her to undress and get into the tub.
7. Expose as much of the child's skin surface as possible to the water (you may use a cup to pour water over the child).
8. Sponge the patient from the shoulder:
   - Across the upper chest.
   - Down the external portion of the exposed arm.
   - Upward on the inner portion of the arm. Repeat with the other arm.
   - Down the torso to the waist. Sponge both sides of the body.
   - Down the back.
9. Monitor the patient regularly throughout the procedure for chills, cyanosis, and increased pulse rate. Stop the bath, remove the patient from the tub, dry, and cover the patient with a bath blanket, if adverse reactions are noted.

(continues)

Procedure 102, *continued*

Giving a Tepid Bath to a Child

10. The bath should last 25 to 30 minutes. Take and record the TPR every 15 minutes until it reaches 101°F, or the prescribed level. Use the rectal or tympanic method (Figure 12-9), if possible. Avoid using the axillary method except as a last resort.
11. Assist the patient from the tub and in drying.
12. Dress the patient in pajamas and return to bed.
13. Because of the immediacy of this procedure, inform the RN of the current vital signs and other pertinent observations.
14. Take and record vital signs again 30 minutes following the bath, then every 30 minutes until the patient's temperature is stable.
15. Remove, clean, and store equipment. Discard the soiled linen.

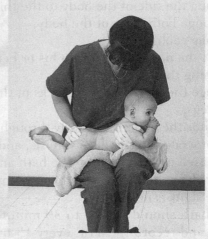

FIGURE 12-9 Take a rectal temperature every 15 minutes until it reaches 101°F, or the prescribed level.

16. Clean tub with antibacterial cleaner.
17. Perform other necessary procedure completion actions.

Sitz Bath

A sitz bath is usually done to relieve discomfort following childbirth, perineal surgery, or rectal surgery. Older hospitals may have permanent sitz bath tubs (Figure 12-10). In newer facilities, a portable (disposable) sitz bath kit is commonly used. It contains a plastic basin that fits over the toilet, and an irrigation bag with tubing and clamp.

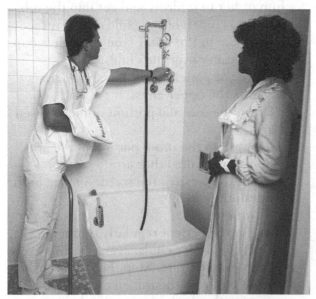

FIGURE 12-10 Many health care facilities have stationary sitz bath tubs.

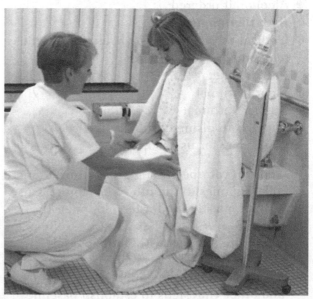

FIGURE 12-11 After the patient is seated, cover the lap (and shoulders, if desired) with a bath blanket.

The pelvic and perineal areas are immersed in warm water. Bathing this area enhances healing by reducing inflammation, stimulating circulation, and promoting wound healing. It is also very relaxing. The water temperature must be constant for maximum effect. Drape the patient's lower body with a bath blanket (**Figure 12-11**), and keep him or her warm throughout the procedure. Dress the patient promptly after the sitz bath to maintain body heat.

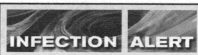

INFECTION ALERT

Infection occurs in about 6 percent of all postpartum patients. When assisting postpartum patients and patients who have had rectal surgery with toileting, have the patient stand up before flushing the toilet. This prevents spraying with contaminated water. Inform the RN promptly if a patient has an elevated temperature, chills, foul-smelling lochia, or other signs and symptoms of infection.

Procedure 103

Giving a Sitz Bath

Supplies needed:
- Disposable exam gloves
- Permanent sitz tub, portable sitz tub, or bathtub
- Bath towels (2 to 3)
- Bath blanket (2)
- Floor bath mat
- Rubber bath mat
- Bath thermometer
- Gown
- Footstool, if needed
- Overbed table
- Pitcher, if needed to refill irrigation bag
- IV standard (if needed, to hold irrigation bag)
- Dressings
- Supplies to disinfect tub, as needed
- Plastic bag for used supplies

1. Perform your beginning procedure actions.
2. Clean and disinfect the tub, if necessary.
3. Instruct the patient to void before beginning this procedure.
4. Remove dressings and/or peri pad, if used. If a dressing adheres to a wound, soak it off in the tub. Discard the used dressing in the plastic bag.
5. Fill the sitz tub (**Figure 12-12**) or bathtub one-third to one-half full, so that the water will cover the perineum, or will reach the patient's umbilicus if a permanent sitz tub is used. Use hot water, 105°F to 110°F, or as instructed by the RN. (The water will cool before the patient uses it; if the patient will be using it immediately, temperature should not exceed 105°F.)

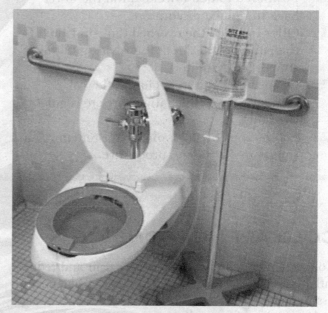

FIGURE 12-12 A portable sitz bath tub is placed under the base of the toilet after the seat is elevated.

6. Check the water temperature with a bath thermometer.
7. If you are using a disposable kit, fill the basin to the designated line.
8. Place the basin under the commode seat.
9. Close the plastic clamp on the irrigation tubing.
10. Fill the irrigation bag with 105°F to 110°F water. (The water will cool before use.)
11. Hang the solution bag from the towel bar, hook, or an IV standard.
12. Insert the irrigation tubing through the entry hole near the front of the plastic bowl.

(continues)

Procedure 103, *continued*

Giving a Sitz Bath

13. Pull the tubing inside the bowl.
14. Secure the tubing by snapping it into the channel in the center bottom of the bowl.
15. Make sure the small hole at the end of the tube faces up.
16. Assist the patient to sit on the seat. If the patient's legs do not reach the floor, support them on a footstool.
17. Cover the patient's shoulders and lap with a bath blanket.
18. Position a folded towel behind the lower back to reduce discomfort.
19. Offer to place the overbed table in front of the patient, if desired, to provide additional support and comfort.
20. Open the clamp to begin the flow of solution. Show the patient how to regulate the flow.
21. Follow your facility policies for remaining in the room during the procedure.

22. Frequently monitor the patient's color and condition. If he or she becomes dizzy or weak, check the pulse and blood pressure promptly. Use the call signal to get help. Return the patient to bed using a wheelchair.
23. Refill the irrigation bag when necessary.
24. After the prescribed time (usually 15 to 20 minutes), clamp the tubing.
25. Assist the patient to stand. Encourage him or her to use the hand rails. Monitor closely for dizziness, weakness, and feelings of faintness or nausea.
26. Assist the patient to dry, if necessary.
27. Apply a clean dressing or peri pad, if necessary.
28. Assist the patient to dress and return to his or her room.
29. Disinfect the sitz tub.
30. Store the disposable tub (these are often given to the patient upon discharge).
31. Perform your procedure completion actions.

COLD APPLICATIONS

Cold treatments are used to relieve pain and reduce inflammation. Cold slows and inhibits circulation and tissue metabolism, slows bleeding, reduces drainage and formation of pus, relieves congestion in blood vessels, slows bacterial activity, and reduces body temperature. The anti-inflammatory effect also helps relieve edema. Cold treatments are commonly used to treat strains, sprains, and bruises. Cold speeds the transition from the acute phase to the rehabilitation phase of injury treatment. It is a common treatment in the first 24 to 48 hours after a musculoskeletal injury.

Ice Packs, Collars, Gel, and Chemical Cold Packs

Ice packs, collars, gel and chemical cold packs (Figure 12-13) are the most common types of cold treatments. An ice pack is made by filling a hot water bottle or ice collar one-half full with crushed ice. Avoid sharp edges. After filling the container, lay it flat on the counter. Press to remove the excess air. Activate a chemical cold pack by striking it away

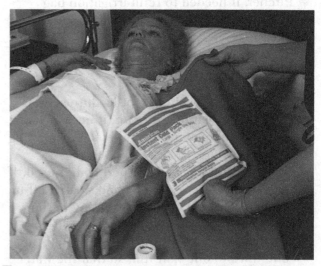

FIGURE 12-13 Cover the disposable cold pack before applying it to the patient.

from your face. Chemical packs are available in different sizes. The small packs do not stay cold for long, and may have to be replaced during the treatment. The larger packs stay cold for 20 to 30 minutes. Cover both types with fabric.

Paper or styrofoam cups of ice are sometimes used to massage an injured area. The person applying this treatment makes small, overlapping circles with the ice over the affected area for 20 minutes.

An examination glove filled with ice and secured with a rubber band is also sometimes used as an alternate ice application.

Procedure 104

Applying an Ice Bag, Ice Collar, Gel Pack, or Chemical Cold Pack

Supplies needed:
- Disposable exam gloves, if contact with blood or body fluids is anticipated
- Ice bag, collar, or gel, chemical cold pack
- Flannel cover for cold pack
- Paper towels
- Bath towel
- Spoon or small ice scoop
- Ice cubes or crushed ice
- Bath blanket
- Tape or roller gauze, if needed
- Plastic bag for used supplies

1. Perform your beginning procedure actions.
2. Fill the ice bag or collar with cold water to check for leaks. Empty the bag.
3. Use crushed ice, if possible. This is more comfortable for the patient, and the bag will be more flexible. If you will be using ice cubes, run them under water to remove sharp edges.
4. Fill the ice bag half full, using the scoop, a spoon, or paper cup (**Figure 12-14A**). Avoid contact between the scoop and the ice bag. Make sure the bag does not become too heavy. When finished, screw the top loosely in place.
5. Place the ice bag or collar on the paper towel on the counter. Loosen the top. Press on the bag to remove air (**Figure 12-14B**).
6. Tighten the top of the bag securely.
7. Wipe the ice bag with paper towels.
   OR
   Remove gel pack from freezer.
   OR
   Strike the chemical cold pack to activate it. Avoid striking the pack in front of your face, as the pack may break, spraying chemicals into your eyes and mucous membranes.

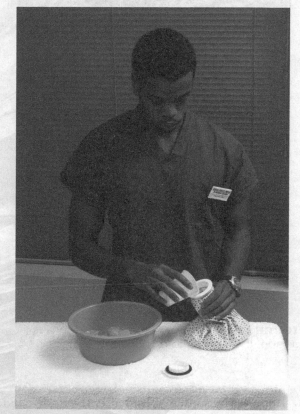

FIGURE 12-14(A) Fill the ice bag half full.

8. Cover the bag or activated pack with an absorbent cloth or flannel cover.
9. Press the bag against the inside of your forearm to check the temperature.
10. Expose the area to be treated. Place the covered bag or pack on the area, and note the time.
11. Secure the device with tape or roller gauze, if necessary. Wrap with a towel to maintain temperature (**Figure 12-15**).
12. Following facility policy, periodically check the patient and the appearance of skin under the bag or pack.

(continues)

Procedure 104, *continued*

Applying an Ice Bag, Ice Collar, Gel Pack, or Chemical Cold Pack

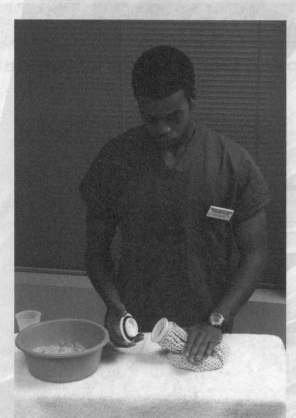

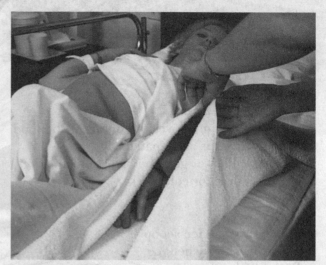

FIGURE 12-15 After positioning the cold pack, cover the application with a towel.

Cleanse and care for the gel pack according to facility policies.

15. Perform your procedure completion actions.

FIGURE 12-14(B) Place the ice bag on a flat surface, then press to remove the air.

13. Remove the source of cold after the designated length of time (usually 20 minutes).
14. Wash the reusable bag with soap and water, and hang it to dry. Discard a chemical pack.

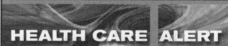

HEALTH CARE ALERT

Paper or styrofoam cups of ice are sometimes used to massage an injured area. The person applying this treatment makes small, overlapping circles with the ice for 20 minutes over the affected area. Ice massage may also be used to relieve pain or as a distraction during a painful procedure. An examination glove filled with ice and secured with a rubber band is also sometimes used as an alternate ice application.

Cold Compresses and Soaks

Like heat, cold compresses are soaks used for treating small areas. Place gauze sponges or washcloths in a basin of ice and water, then squeeze them out. Fold the cloth and place it over the affected area. The compress warms quickly, so you must change it frequently. An ice bag or chemical cold pack may be used to cover the application to keep it cool. Compresses are not used for more than 20 minutes.

Procedure **105**

Applying Cool, Moist Compresses

Supplies needed:

- Disposable exam gloves, if contact with blood or body fluids is anticipated
- Basin of ice chips
- Bath thermometer
- Washbasin with prescribed solution at temperature ordered
- 4 × 4 gauze pads (unsterile, or according to RN's instructions) to use as compresses
- Water, sterile normal saline, or other prescribed solution
- Pitcher
- Pins or roller gauze
- Syringe
- Bath towels (2)
- Disposable underpads or large plastic sheet
- Bath blanket
- Plastic bag, if needed to cover compress
- Ice bag, gel pack, or chemical cold pack with cover, to maintain temperature
- Plastic bag for used supplies

NOTE: If you are applying compresses to an open area, use sterile technique, including sterile solution, sterile gloves, a sterile basin, and sterile 4 x 4 sponges. If a sterile thermometer is unavailable, pour some sterile solution into a clean container, check the temperature with a bath thermometer, then discard the test solution.

1. Perform your beginning procedure actions.
2. Take equipment to the bedside.
3. Cover the patient with a bath blanket.
4. Fanfold the bedding to the foot of the bed.
5. Expose the extremity to be treated.
6. Cover the bed with the underpads or plastic sheet and towel.
7. Apply gloves.
8. Check the temperature of the solution. It should be approximately 65°F to 80°F, or as instructed by the RN. If using sterile solution, pour the solution into a small sterile bowl and pack the bowl in ice, or pack a small sterile solution bottle in ice.
9. Position the patient's extremity on the bed protector.
10. Moisten the compresses in the basin.
11. Squeeze out excess moisture.
12. Apply compresses to the treatment area.
13. Cover the compresses with a single layer cut from the plastic bag, or a properly covered cold pack or aquathermia pad, if ordered to maintain temperature.
14. Secure the compress with a binder, or roller gauze, if needed.
15. Following facility policy, periodically check the patient and the appearance of skin under the bag or pack. Maintain proper temperature and moisture. A syringe may be used to keep compresses wet, if additional moisture is needed.
16. Stop the procedure after the designated length of time. Change compresses as ordered.
17. Discard used compresses in the plastic bag.
18. Gently pat the area dry with the towel.
19. Perform your procedure completion actions.

Procedure **106**

Performing a Cool Soak

Supplies needed:

- Disposable exam gloves, if contact with blood or body fluids is anticipated
- Bath thermometer
- Washbasin
- Pitcher
- Ice cubes or crushed ice
- Bath towels (2 or 3)
- Disposable underpads or large plastic sheet

(continues)

Procedure **106**, *continued*

Performing a Cool Soak

▶ Bath blanket
▶ Plastic bag for used supplies

1. Perform your beginning procedure actions.
2. Take equipment to the bedside.
3. Cover the patient with a bath blanket.
4. Fanfold the bedding to the foot of the bed.
5. Expose the extremity to be soaked.
6. Raise the side rail on the far side of bed, and assist the patient to move toward the rail. Position him or her for comfort.
7. Cover the bed with the underpads or plastic sheet and towel.
8. Fill the soak basin half full with cool water at the sink. Check the temperature. It should be approximately 65°F to 80°F, or as instructed by the RN. Adjust the temperature by adding ice or room-temperature solution/water, as needed.

9. Position the patient's extremity on the bed protector. Place the water basin on the bed protector. Assist the patient to place the limb in the basin. Cover with a towel to maintain temperature.
10. Check the water temperature every 5 minutes. Use the pitcher or ice to cool the water, if needed. Remove the patient's limb before adding water to the basin.
11. Stop the procedure after the designated length of time (approximately 20 minutes).
12. Lift the patient's extremity out of the basin.
13. Slip the basin forward, or move it to the table.
14. Gently pat the limb dry with the towel. If a foot soak was done, dry well between the toes.
15. Perform your procedure completion actions.

WARM AND COOL EYE COMPRESSES

Many patients have dry, itchy eyes. This is especially problematic in elderly persons. The uncomfortable sensations may be caused by allergies, irritants, squinting, rubbing, or blinking the eyes. The eyes may appear red, with swollen eyelids. Scratching or rubbing the eyes increases the risk of infection. The patient may complain of:

- Burning
- Dryness
- Scratchy feeling
- Light sensitivity
- Difficulty moving the eyes
- Excess mucus production
- Severe pain
- Blurred vision
- Seeing halos

Observe the patient for:

- Drainage from eyes
- Redness of eyelid rims

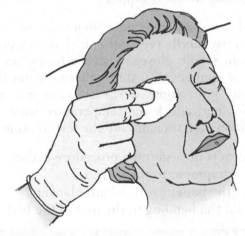

FIGURE 12-16 Instruct the patient to close his or her eyes. Apply one compress to the affected eye. Follow with a second compress.

- Scaly, flaky skin around the eyes
- Edema of the eyelids

Report your observations to the RN. You may be instructed to apply warm or cool soaks to the eyelids (**Figure 12-16**). Apply the principles of standard precautions when performing this procedure. For this procedure, using separate equipment for each eye is best. This will prevent an undiagnosed infection from spreading.

Procedure **107**

Applying Warm or Cool Eye Compresses

Supplies needed:
▶ Disposable exam gloves
▶ Towel
▶ Small bottle of sterile saline
▶ Small sterile basin
▶ Sterile gauze pads
▶ Ice, if cool compresses are ordered
▶ Plastic bag for used items

1. Perform your beginning procedure actions.
2. Position the patient for comfort. For warm compresses, assist the patient to a Fowler's or high Fowler's position, if possible. (This position helps reduce edema.) Cover the neck and shoulders with a bath towel.
3. Heat the bottle of sterile saline under hot running water, or place it in a second bowl of hot water. The solution should become comfortably warm, not hot. Check the temperature with a thermometer. It should be approximately 105°F.

NOTE: Never use a microwave to heat water for heat treatments.

If cool compresses are ordered, cool the bottle of saline by packing it in ice. Place some ice chips into the small, sterile basin. Pour the saline solution into the basin.

4. Pour the warm or cool solution into the small, sterile bowl.
5. Wash your hands, or use alcohol-based hand cleaner.
6. Apply disposable gloves.
7. Place the gauze pads into the bowl.

8. Remove a gauze pad from the bowl and squeeze out the excess solution.
9. Instruct the patient to close his or her eyes.
10. Apply one compress to the affected eye.
11. Remove a second gauze pad from the bowl and squeeze out the excess solution.
12. Apply the second compress on top of the first.
13. Repeat with the other eye, as directed.
14. If the patient complains that the compress is too hot or cold, remove it immediately.
15. Change the compresses every few minutes for the prescribed length of time. The treatment should not last longer than 15 to 20 minutes. Check the skin under the compress each time you change it.
16. You may be directed to cover the compress with an ice pack or warm pack. Make a small ice pack by placing ice chips in a sandwich bag or disposable glove. Squeeze the air out of the bag and tie the end. Keep the pack size small. Cover the compress with the pack, as directed. Remove it immediately if the patient complains of pain.
17. After 15 to 20 minutes, or as directed, remove the compresses. Discard them in the plastic bag.
18. Use the remaining clean gauze pads to dry the eye. Pat gently from the inner corner to the outer corner. Use each gauze pad once, then discard it in the plastic bag.
19. Perform your procedure completion actions.

HYPOTHERMIA

Human survival depends on each person's ability to maintain a stable body temperature between 97°F and 100°F. Normally, your nervous system controls your body responses to heat and cold, and regulates temperature automatically to keep the body at optimum operating temperature. When heat loss exceeds heat production, the nervous system will trigger certain involuntary responses, such as shivering, to restore the balance. If the cold stress is great, and the person's system is overwhelmed, body temperature decreases. **Hypothermia** is a lowering of **core body temperature** to 95°F or below. Core body temperature is the temperature of the body center, or core. This is the normal body operating temperature. The core temperature value reflects the temperature in deep structures of the body such as the liver. The severity of hypothermia is determined by the degree to which core temperature is lowered:

- Mild hypothermia—93°F to 95°F
- Moderate hypothermia—86°F to 93°F
- Severe hypothermia—less than 86°F

Untreated, the patient's condition will progress, and dehydration, liver failure, and kidney failure develop. In the early stages, the pulse, respirations, and blood pressure may rise. If the temperature drops below 90°F, these vital signs decrease significantly. If the temperature drops to 86°F, most people become comatose. If the temperature continues to drop to 82°F or below, serious ventricular dysrhythmias will occur.

Hypothermia may be classified as primary or secondary. **Primary hypothermia** occurs as a result of overwhelming cold stress (Figure 12-17). The greatest area of heat loss is from the head, so if the head is wet or exposed to temperature extremes, internal body temperature will decrease rapidly. **Secondary hypothermia** is part of other clinical conditions. These conditions are usually acute and severe, such as shock and sepsis. The highest mortality rates occur in infants and elderly persons. Many chronic medical conditions, such as post polio syndrome, diabetes, malnutrition, infection, thyroid disease, spinal cord injuries, and stroke, further impair temperature-regulating ability. Males are at higher risk than females. Nonwhite

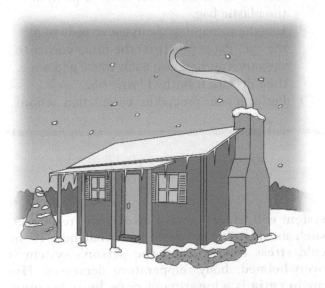

FIGURE 12-17 Primary hypothermia occurs as a result of overwhelming cold stress, which commonly occurs during exposure to a cold environment.

persons may have a higher risk. The mortality increases if symptoms are present. Unfortunately, the signs and symptoms are very nonspecific, and may be caused by many other conditions. Hypothermia may be very difficult to identify in infants and young children, cognitively impaired patients, and patients with communication barriers.

Accurate diagnosis of hypothermia is done by measuring the *core* body temperature. The thermometers used in health care facilities typically measure 94°F to 105°F. Some have a narrower range. To measure core body temperature accurately, a rectal thermometer that measures from 77°F to 104°F must be used. Some facilities use a tympanic thermometer, but this is not as desirable because variations in user technique may yield inaccurate values. In situations of possible hypothermia, the temperature measurement must be accurate.

Treatment for Primary and Secondary Hypothermia

Keep patients with hypothermia NPO, unless instructed to give a warm beverage by the RN. (This treatment may be used for patients with mild hypothermia who are alert and able to swallow.) Cover these patients' heads. Avoid rubbing the skin. Handle the patient gently and as little as possible. Patients with moderate and severe hypothermia will be treated in the intensive care unit. Special, gradual rewarming techniques are needed. Improper rewarming can cause fatal dysrhythmias. For mild to moderate decrease in body temperature, the hypothermia-hyperthermia blanket may also be used.

Perioperative Hypothermia

During the perioperative period, many factors interfere with the patient's normal temperature-regulating mechanisms. Normally, we shiver when we are cold. The blood vessels constrict. **Perioperative hypothermia** develops in the operating room. Anesthesia and some sedatives disrupt the internal ability to regulate temperature. The drugs promote heat loss by reducing the shivering response and preventing blood vessel constriction. Underlying factors such as age, presence of chronic disease, and body size also affect temperature regulation.

The operating room is a very cool environment. Open body cavities and administration of blood and IV fluids further contribute to temperature loss. In the first 30 minutes after being given general anesthesia, body temperature usually decreases. The

American Association of Nurse Anesthetists (AANA) recommends continuous temperature monitoring on pediatric patients receiving general anesthesia and, when indicated, on all other patients. Some experts recommend checking the temperature at 15- to 30-minute intervals while the patient is in the operating room.

The body cannot return the temperature to normal until the concentration of anesthetic in the brain decreases and the normal temperature-regulating responses are triggered and can take over. Pain further decreases the effectiveness of these responses. Because of these factors, return to normal temperature may take 2 to 5 hours, depending on the degree of hypothermia and the age of the patient. Perioperative outcomes are better if the patient does not become hypothermic.

To maintain patient temperature during and after surgery, the hyperthermia-hypothermia blanket is commonly used. The circulating water is known to be a very effective warming mechanism. The blankets may be used under or over the patient, but are most effective when positioned over the patient's body.

HEAT-RELATED ILLNESS

Like hypothermia, the very young and very old are at high risk for complications of heat-related illness. Abnormally high body temperature is called **hyperpyrexia** or **hyperthermia.** When environmental temperature exceeds body temperature or the humidity is high, the body retains heat, increasing core temperature. The normal mechanisms that cause you to feel thirsty or to drink fluids are reduced. Aging and many chronic diseases further reduce the effectiveness of sweating to cool the body.

Heat Exhaustion

Heat exhaustion is also called *heat prostration*. It develops as a result of overexposure to heat. This prolonged exposure stimulates and increases perspiration, which eliminates fluid and salt from the body, upsetting the electrolyte balance. When this occurs, heat exhaustion develops.

Caring for a Patient with Heat Exhaustion. Keeping the patient in a cool environment, giving IV fluids, and increasing fluid intake (if the patient can swallow) are usually enough to reverse heat exhaustion. Vital signs must be frequently monitored. A tepid sponge bath or other

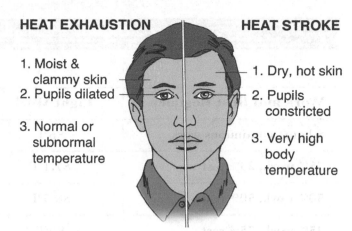

HEAT EXHAUSTION

1. Moist & clammy skin
2. Pupils dilated
3. Normal or subnormal temperature

HEAT STROKE

1. Dry, hot skin
2. Pupils constricted
3. Very high body temperature

FIGURE 12-18 Comparison of heat exhaustion and heat stroke

bath may be used to reduce the patient's temperature, or the hypothermia-hyperthermia blanket may be used.

Heat Stroke

Heat stroke is also called *sunstroke*. This is a very serious condition suggesting a profound disruption of the internal mechanisms that control heat in the body. It is caused by extended exposure to heat, especially when there is little air movement. **Figure 12-18** compares heat exhaustion with heat stroke. Table 12-2 lists American Conference of Government Industrial Hygienists (ACGIH) recommendations for work and rest in high temperatures.

Nursing Care for Heat Stroke. Heat stroke is a medical emergency. In the early stages, the patient will be treated in the emergency department and transferred to the intensive care unit. Monitor the patient's airway, breathing, and circulation. Keep him or her NPO. You will assist the RN in cooling the patient's body as rapidly as possible by immersing the patient in tepid or cool water (if awake and alert), or sponging with tepid water. The hypothermia-hyperthermia blanket may also be used.

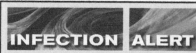

INFECTION ALERT

Always read the instructions before using a hyperthermia-hypothermia blanket. Some units are manually operated. This means that the blanket will maintain the preset temperature regardless of the patient's temperature. You will have to adjust the temperature setting manually. Make sure you are familiar with the directions for the unit you are using.

Table 12-2 Criteria for High Heat and Physical Labor

Work and Rest Regimen	Permissible Limits		
	Light Work	Moderate Work	Heavy Work
8 hours continuous work	86°F	80.1°F	77°F
75% work, 25% rest	87.1°F	82.4°F	78.6°F
50% work, 50% rest	88.5°F	84.9°F	82.2°F
25% work, 75% rest	90°F	88°F	86°F

Adapted from: American Conference of Governmental Industrial Hygienists. (2001). 2001 TLVs and BEIs: Threshold limit values for chemical substances and physical agents and biological exposure indices (pp. 171–172). Cincinnati, OH.

THE HYPOTHERMIA-HYPERTHERMIA BLANKET

The **hypothermia-hyperthermia blanket** (Figure 12-19) is a full-size aquathermia pad, similar to a K-Pad. It is used to raise, lower, or maintain the patient's temperature. It is commonly used to lower the body temperature in patients with fever. It may be used to maintain body temperature during sur-

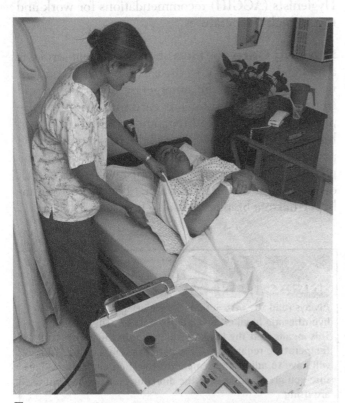

FIGURE 12-19 Hypothermia-hyperthermia blanket

gery, or when the patient is in shock. Sometimes it is used to manage severe pain or bleeding.

The blanket is operated either manually or automatically. For manual operation, the unit is set to a predetermined temperature, which is ordered by the physician. The blanket maintains this temperature, regardless of changes in the patient's temperature. When the unit is set for automatic operation, it monitors the patient's temperature through a rectal, skin, or esophageal probe. The probe is secured with tape to prevent injury. The blanket temperature changes according to the patient's temperature. The goal is to maintain the patient's body temperature. An alarm will sound for abnormal temperature variations.

Before using the blanket, check it for cracks, tears, or leaks. Do not use it if there are cracks or an electrical malfunction.

Using the Hypothermia-Hyperthermia Blanket

The patient should wear a hospital gown when the blanket is used. Use a gown with tie closures. Snaps, pins, or other metal may cause injury to the skin. Before beginning the procedure, check and record the patient's baseline vital signs as a basis for comparison.

One or two aquathermia blankets may be used. The RN may instruct you to place one under the patient and cover him or her with the other. Each blanket must be covered with a disposable cover, sheet, or bath blanket to absorb perspiration and prevent complications. Avoid using pins to cover the blanket. These can puncture the unit or injure the patient's skin by causing hot or cold spots. Use tape or Velcro fasteners, if necessary, to cover the unit.

The blanket should be set up and preheated or precooled before it is applied to the patient. Connect the blanket to the control unit by plugging in the tubing. Set the blanket for automatic or manual operation, then set the desired body temperature or blanket temperature. The RN will instruct you what temperature values to use. Turn the device on, then add distilled water to the reservoir. Position the controls at the foot of the bed. After the device has reached the designated tempera-

ture, apply it to the patient. If the patient will be lying on a blanket, place a pillow or folded bath blanket under the head.

The patient's head should not contact the blanket. A combination of the heat or cold and the surface of the blanket promotes skin breakdown on the back of the head. Apply lanolin or another designated produce to the skin in exposed areas that contact the blanket directly. You may wrap the patient's hands and feet to prevent chilling, if desired.

Procedure 108

Applying the Hypothermia-Hyperthermia Blanket

Supplies needed:
- Disposable exam gloves
- Hypothermia-hyperthermia blanket
- Blanket cover
- Sterile distilled water
- Skin or rectal probe
- Tape
- Thermometer
- Blood pressure cuff
- Stethoscope
- Bath blankets, 2
- Gowns, 2
- Towel
- Covers for the patient's hands and feet, if desired
- Plastic bag for used supplies

1. Perform your beginning procedure actions.
2. Take the patient's vital signs and record them.
3. Cover the patient with a bath blanket for modesty.
4. Turn the patient on the side. Fold the blanket in half lengthwise, then fold it

again, as you would the bottom sheet in the occupied bedmaking procedure. Slide the blanket halfway across the bed, on top of the sheet. Align the top edge of the blanket with the patient's neck.

5. Turn the patient on the opposite side, then unfold the blanket.
6. Fold a bath blanket under the patient's head, or use the pillow, as instructed by the RN.
7. Apply lanolin to exposed areas of the patient's skin.
8. If the blanket is set for automatic operation, apply gloves and insert the rectal probe. Tape the probe in place.
9. Remove gloves and discard according to facility policy.
10. Cover the patient with a sheet or a second blanket, as directed by the RN. Pull the bath blanket out without exposing the patient.
11. Wrap the patient's hands and feet to prevent chilling, if desired.
12. Perform your procedure completion actions.

Caring for the Patient Using a Hypothermia-Hyperthermia Blanket

Monitor the patient's vital signs every 5 minutes until the temperature reaches the designated value. After that, take vital signs every 15 minutes, or as directed by the RN. The blanket's texture increases

the risk of skin breakdown. Reposition the patient every 30 to 60 minutes to prevent skin breakdown. Change the gown and top sheet as often as necessary if the patient is actively perspiring. If the patient has a catheter, the RN may direct you to monitor the intake and output hourly. Report changes listed in the Observe & Report box to the RN immediately.

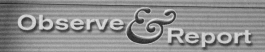

Observe & Report

Hypothermia–Hyperthermia

Changes in skin color
Cyanosis of the lips or nail beds
Sudden changes in temperature
Marked changes in pulse, respirations, or blood pressure
Respiratory distress
Pain
Changes in sensation
Edema
Shivering and chills
Urinary output below 50 mL/hour

Discontinuing the Blanket

The RN will inform you when to discontinue use of the blanket. Follow manufacturer's directions for the type of blanket you are using. Turn the unit off. Some types must remain plugged in for 30 to 60 minutes to dry condensation inside the unit. Dry the patient's skin and assist him or her into a dry gown. Position the patient in a comfortable position. Remove the aquathermia blanket from the bed after the designated time. Continue checking vital signs and intake and output every 30 minutes for the first 2 hours, then hourly or as directed by the RN.

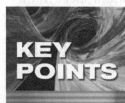

KEY POINTS

▶ Heat and cold treatments are commonly used to treat musculoskeletal conditions.

▶ Cold treatments are often applied immediately after an injury.

▶ Moist applications penetrate deeper than dry applications.

▶ A localized application delivers heat or cold to a specific area.

▶ Localized heat and cold applications that contact the skin must always be covered.

▶ A generalized application delivers heat or cold to the entire body.

▶ Infants and elderly patients are very sensitive to heat and cold.

▶ Heat should not be used if bleeding or edema is present.

▶ Sleep and rest are essential to enable the body to recover after illness or surgery. Patients rest better if they are comfortable.

▶ A small body of evidence suggests that warmed blankets promote sleep and help reduce pain in elderly persons.

▶ Distilled water circulates through the coils of the aquathermia pad. The circulating water maintains a constant temperature. This pad is used in place of a dry heating pad.

▶ The hydrocollator is a rectangular tank containing very hot water. It is used to heat hot packs containing silicate gel in a cotton bag.

▶ Hot packs must always be covered with special, thick, layered terry cloth covers when they are used to treat a patient.

▶ Hydrotherapy is water therapy.

▶ Never pour liquid soap or shampoo into a whirlpool tub. A tiny bit of liquid soap will result in an abundance of suds. If suds are a problem, rub a bar of soap against the walls of the tub to reduce the bubbles.

▶ Therapeutic baths are usually given when patients have widespread skin problems.

▶ Therapeutic baths involve the use of special products for bathing or soaking the skin, such as colloidal oatmeal.

(continues)

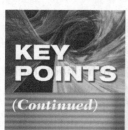

KEY POINTS

(Continued)

▶ Tepid baths are an older treatment that may be ordered to reduce temperature.

▶ A sitz bath is usually done to relieve discomfort following childbirth, perineal surgery, or rectal surgery.

▶ Warm and cool compresses are commonly ordered to treat dry, itchy eyes.

▶ Hypothermia is a lowering of core body temperature to 95°F or below.

▶ Primary hypothermia occurs as a result of overwhelming cold stress.

▶ The greatest area of heat loss is from the head, so if the head is wet or exposed to temperature extremes, internal body temperature will decrease rapidly.

▶ Secondary hypothermia is part of other clinical conditions, such as sepsis.

▶ Perioperative hypothermia is hypothermia that develops in the operating room as a result of anesthesia and some other drugs, open body cavities, and administration of cold fluids.

▶ Abnormally high body temperature is called hyperpyrexia or hyperthermia.

▶ Heat exhaustion develops as a result of overexposure to heat.

▶ Heat stroke suggests a profound disruption of the internal mechanisms that control heat in the body. It is caused by extended exposure to heat, especially when there is little air movement.

▶ The hyperthermia-hypothermia blanket is used to raise, lower, or maintain the patient's temperature.

▶ Never use pins or gowns that have snaps with the hyperthermia-hypothermia blanket.

▶ When using the hyperthermia-hypothermia blanket, monitor the patient's vital signs every 5 minutes until the temperature reaches the designated value. After that, take vital signs every 5 minutes, or as directed by the RN.

▶ Reposition a patient who is using a hyperthermia-hypothermia blanket every 30 to 60 minutes to prevent skin breakdown.

▶ When using the hyperthermia-hypothermia blanket, report to the RN:

   ▶ Changes in skin color

   ▶ Cyanosis of the lips or nail beds

   ▶ Sudden changes in temperature

   ▶ Marked changes in pulse, respiration, or blood pressure

   ▶ Respiratory distress

   ▶ Pain

   ▶ Changes in sensation

   ▶ Edema

   ▶ Shivering and chills

   ▶ Urinary output below 50 mL/hour

CLINICAL APPLICATIONS

1. You are assigned to apply a hot water bottle to Mr. Ng, a 59-year-old alert patient. He speaks very little English. You check the water temperature of the application and find that it is 105°F. You apply the flannel cover and immediately apply it to the treatment area. When you apply the bottle, Mr. Ng quickly removes it and says, "Hot, hot." What action will you take?

2. Dr. McGhie is an 87-year-old mentally confused resident from the local long-term care facility. His body language suggests that he is having pain. He moans when he is being moved. It is 3:00 A.M., and the patient has not slept since you began your shift at 10:00 P.M. The nurse gave the patient some Tylenol and asked you to "make him comfortable" so he could go to sleep. How can you help this patient?

3. Mrs. Yeary had an order for an aquathermia pad to her low back. Five minutes after applying the pad, you return to her room and find that you forgot to remove the key from the unit. The temperature has been increased to 120°F. The patient denies changing the setting, but you are certain it was set to 100°F when you left the room. What action will you take?

4. You give Ms. Romcevich a whirlpool bath. When you lift the seat out of the water, the resident begins to shiver and complains of "freezing." You drape a bath towel across her shoulders, but she continues to complain. What action will you take?

5. You are caring for Mrs. Blumenfeld, a 73-year-old mentally confused resident from a nursing facility. She was admitted with a diagnosis of severe urinary tract infection. She is on an antibiotic, but the culture and sensitivity report has not come back from the lab yet. When you take the routine 8:00 A.M. vital signs using a tympanic thermometer, the patient's temperature is 94°F. The patient is lethargic. What action will you take?

6. Mr. Long develops a postoperative infection, with a fever of 104°F. The nurse instructs you to apply the hypothermia blanket. After 60 minutes, Mr. Long's temperature drops from 104°F to 99°F, and he begins shivering. What action will you take?

CHAPTER REVIEW

Multiple-Choice Questions

Select the one best answer.

1. When applying a heat or cold application:
   a. gloves are not necessary.
   b. wear a gown and gloves.
   c. apply the principles of standard precautions.
   d. apply the principles of transmission-based precautions.

2. Following an injury, heat should not be used for:
   a. 2 hours.
   b. 24 hours.
   c. 36 hours.
   d. 48 hours.

3. Heat and cold applications are usually not left in place longer than:
   a. 20 minutes.
   b. 40 minutes.
   c. 1 hour.
   d. 2 hours.

4. Cold therapy should not be used for patients with:
   a. congestive heart failure.
   b. peripheral vascular disease.
   c. orthopedic surgery.
   d. sprains with edema.

5. Heat therapy should not be used for patients with:
   a. intravenous infiltration.
   b. low back pain.
   c. arthritis.
   d. paralysis.

6. The aquathermia blanket:
   a. should not contact the patient's skin directly.
   b. should be pinned to the sheet to maintain position.
   c. is turned on after the patient is covered with the unit.
   d. should be wrapped around the patient's body.

7. When applying heat and cold treatments, the nursing assistant should:
   a. always remain in the room for the duration of the treatment.
   b. check the temperature of the solution with his or her elbow.
   c. monitor the skin under the application every 30 minutes.
   d. remove jewelry, buttons, or zippers that may conduct heat or cold.

8. When caring for a patient using an aquathermia blanket, the nursing assistant should:
   a. regulate blanket temperature at least every 15 minutes.
   b. give the patient plenty of iced liquids to drink to reduce fever.
   c. monitor the patient for cyanosis or changes in vital signs.
   d. turn the patient at least every 2 hours.

9. The term *cryotherapy* refers to:
   a. heat therapy.
   b. cold therapy.
   c. moist therapy.
   d. water therapy.

10. Before using a heat or cold application, you should know all of the following *except:*
   a. all the patient's medical diagnoses.
   b. the area of the patient's body to be treated.
   c. the length of time the application is to remain in place.
   d. proper temperature of the application.

11. Heat may be used to:
   a. reduce wound drainage.
   b. reduce edema.
   c. relieve muscle spasms.
   d. constrict blood vessels.

12. Which of these is an example of a dry heat treatment?
   a. aquathermia pad
   b. hot water bottle
   c. hydrocollator pack
   d. warm compress

13. Strike the chemical cold pack by:
   a. breaking it in front of your body.
   b. hitting it with a hammer.
   c. striking it away from your face.
   d. stepping on it.

14. Moist heat:
   a. is not as effective as dry heat.
   b. should not be used to treat muscle spasms.
   c. is used to relieve edema.
   d. penetrates much deeper than dry heat.

15. Fill the aquathermia pad with:
   a. hot water.
   b. distilled water.
   c. sterile saline.
   d. ice water.

16. The cover slips off the aquathermia pad. Fasten it with:
   a. pins.
   b. staples.
   c. glue.
   d. tape.

17. The water temperature in the hydrocollator should be between:
   a. 160°F and 166°F.
   b. 180°F and 196°F.
   c. 95°F and 115°F.
   d. 120°F and 126°F.

18. Store the hot packs for the hydrocollator:
   a. in the freezer.
   b. hanging to dry.
   c. submerged in water in the unit.
   d. soaking in a chlorine solution.

19. Brown spots on the hydrocollator packs suggest that:
   a. the packs are getting old.
   b. the packs have been burned.
   c. the packs are contaminated with a pathogen.
   d. chemicals from the tank have stained them.

20. The whirlpool bath should be set at:
   a. 120°F to 130°F.
   b. 110°F to 115°F.
   c. 100°F to 109°F.
   d. 97°F to 100°F.

21. A tepid sponge bath is used to:
   a. treat skin conditions.
   b. reduce fever.
   c. relieve muscle spasms.
   d. relieve pain.

22. A sitz bath is applied to the:
   a. perineum.
   b. shoulder.
   c. arm.
   d. leg.

23. Hypothermia is body temperature:
   a. above 100°F.
   b. below 100°F.
   c. below 95°F.
   d. above 90°F.

24. The greatest area of heat loss is from the:
   a. chest.
   b. groin.
   c. torso.
   d. head.

25. Secondary hypothermia is commonly caused by:
   a. prolonged heat exposure.
   b. shock and sepsis.
   c. diabetes and heart failure.
   d. prolonged cold exposure.

26. Patients with severe hypothermia should be:
   a. rewarmed gradually.
   b. immersed in warm water.
   c. wrapped in blankets.
   d. rewarmed rapidly.

27. Perioperative hypothermia:
    a. results from environmental temperature below 60°F.
    b. usually develops before surgery.
    c. occurs primarily as a result of anesthetics.
    d. develops as a result of blood vessel constriction.

28. Abnormally high body temperature is:
    a. hypothermia.
    b. cryotherapy.
    c. diathermy.
    d. hyperpyrexia.

29. Fill the hyperthermia-hypothermia control unit with:
    a. alcohol.
    b. sterile distilled water.
    c. sterile normal saline.
    d. tap water.

30. When a patient begins using the hyperthermia-hypothermia blanket, check the vital signs every:
    a. 5 minutes until the patient's temperature reaches the designated value.
    b. 15 minutes until the patient's temperature reaches the designated value.
    c. 30 minutes until the patient's temperature reaches the designated value.
    d. 60 minutes until the patient's temperature reaches the designated value.

E X P L O R I N G   T H E   W E B

AORN Malignant Hyperthermia Guideline	http://www.aorn.org
Aquatic Therapy	http://www.advancefornurses.com (See past articles 2/11/02)
Complications and Treatment of Mild Hypothermia	http://www.or.org
Environmental Patient Standards	http://www.equip.ac.uk
Guide to Hypothermia & Hyperthermia	http://www.outdoored.com
Heat and Cold Applications	http://www.imperial.edu
Heat and Cold Therapy	http://www.genufix.com
Heat in Motion: Evaluating and Managing Temperature	http://www.findarticles.com
Hot and Cold Therapies	http://www.spineuniverse.com
Malignant Hyperthermia: Perianesthesia Recognition, Treatment, and Care	http://www.aspan.org
Managing Pain with Heat and Cold	http://www.arthritis.org
Managing Pain with Heat and Cold	http://www.orthop.washington.edu
Post Acute Pools	http://www.advancefornurses.com (See past articles 9/9/02)
Principles of Heat and Cold: Clinical Application	http://jan.ucc.nau.edu
Recommended Practices for Safe Care Through Identification of Potential Hazards in the Surgical Environment	http://www.findarticles.com
Temperature Troubles	http://healthgate.partners.org
Thermal Emergencies	http://www.cpem.org
Use of Heat and Cold in Pain	http://www.kasenterprises.com
Using Heat and Cold	http://www.silvercross.org
Water World	http://www.advancefornurses.com (See past articles 10/7/02)

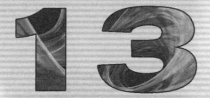

CHAPTER 13

Caring for Patients with Special Needs

OBJECTIVES:

After reading this chapter, you should be able to:

- Spell and define key terms.
- State the guidelines for working with interpreters.
- Define domestic violence and list the signs and symptoms of relationship violence.
- List the causes, signs, and symptoms of delirium.
- Identify the various types of seizures and the signs and symptoms of each.
- List seizure precautions and describe how to care for a patient who is having a seizure.
- Differentiate paraplegia from tetraplegia (quadriplegia), and flaccid paralysis from spastic paralysis.
- State the causes, signs, and symptoms of autonomic dysreflexia.
- Describe the nursing care given, observations made, and precautions taken when caring for patients who are receiving chemotherapy, radiation therapy, or immunotherapy.
- Identify some members of the rehabilitation team and describe the services provided by each.
- List the principles of rehabilitation and restoration.
- List four types of pain and describe the characteristics of each.
- List observations of patients' pain that should be reported to the RN.
- Describe the PCT care of patients who use transcutaneous electrical nerve stimulation, epidural catheters, or implanted medication pumps.

SPECIAL-NEEDS PATIENTS

The disorders described in this chapter are relevant to PCT practice, but are subjects that may not be committed to memory. Some information is difficult to find in other sources. However, the subjects in this chapter are not related to each other. The chapters of this book are logically organized, with similar subject matter grouped together. This format enables you to find the information for which

you are accountable quickly. This chapter is different from the others, in that it draws skills from other chapters, but covers content areas that are not related to each other. Nevertheless, everything is important. Determining which subject is the most important would be impossible. Committing this information to memory or using it as a reference for patient care will enhance the care you provide to special-needs patients who do not fit into the categories listed elsewhere in this book.

WORKING WITH INTERPRETERS

Some people have special communication needs because of aging changes, injury, or illness. Most experienced PCTs have learned and practiced communication skills in class, and have become proficient in communicating with patients who have communication disorders. Occasionally, you will care for a patient who does not speak your language, and communication may be limited. Gestures and body language are not universal, either. For example, in the United States, we move the head up and down to mean *yes*. We shake the head from side to side to signify *no*. In India, these gestures mean just the opposite: Shaking the head from side to side means *yes*, and moving it up and down means *no*. Because of differences in culture and language, there may be times when you need the assistance of a communication professional.

Suggestions for Working with Interpreters

An **interpreter** is a communication professional who mediates between speakers of different languages. Interpretation is an activity that consists of establishing, either simultaneously or consecutively, oral or gestural communication between two or more speakers who do not speak the same language. Some interpreters speak. Others use sign language (Figure 13-1) to establish communication between a hearing person and a nonhearing person. A qualified interpreter is very familiar with the language, cultural values, beliefs, gestures, body language, and verbal and nonverbal expressions that are used in the languages he or she is interpreting. Clearly, this is a great responsibility.

In health care, the terminology and technical information are complex. Health care interpreters receive special education to facilitate accurate communication. The facility is required to furnish

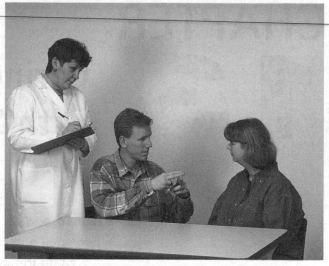

FIGURE 13-1 Learning to be a medical sign language interpreter takes special skill.

interpreters in certain situations, according to federal law. State laws may be more stringent regarding requirements for furnishing interpreters for patients. There are times, however, when using an interpreter will be essential, such as in obtaining consent for a procedure.

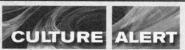

CULTURE ALERT

Personal space is a comfortable distance in which to communicate with others. In the United States, comfortable personal space is 18 to 36 inches. Eye contact is acceptable and expected. Lack of eye contact may be viewed as lack of self-esteem or untruthfulness. We also accept handshakes as a normal greeting. A limp handshake is often interpreted as discomfort or a lack of self-esteem. In other countries, personal space may be very close. Touching may be considered offensive. Eye contact is frequently avoided, as a sign of respect. Shaking hands may not be acceptable for women. Men are dominant in many cultures. Show respect for the patient's culture. If you are unsure about something, ask. Asking is not offensive. It shows that you sincerely care about meeting your patients' needs.

Guidelines for Working with Interpreters in the Health Care Facility

- Use a medical interpreter, whenever possible. Persons who are unfamiliar with medical terms and procedures may not be able to interpret them correctly.

- Avoid using the patient's minor children or grandchildren as interpreters. This may upset the child or family social order. The child's language skills

and social experience may not be well developed in either language, causing inaccurate translation. Some medical subject matter may frighten children.

- Consider the ethnic group, age, and sex of the interpreter. Members of some ethnic groups may prefer an interpreter of the same sex, especially if

(continued)

Guidelines for Working with Interpreters in the Health Care Facility (Continued)

the subject matter is sensitive or embarrassing. Older patients may prefer a more mature interpreter.

- Avoid asking another patient to interpret for you.
- Avoid using nonqualified support staff as interpreters, except in an emergency.
- Medical interpreters are communication professionals, not caregivers, companions, or babysitters. Do not ask a medical interpreter to monitor a patient, provide direct care, or keep a patient company.
- Document the use of an interpreter. List the interpreter's name and the language spoken.
- Give the interpreter an overview of the situation before meeting with the patient.
- If the interpreter is signing, provide written materials to review in advance. The interpreter will be unable to look at the written materials and interpret simultaneously.
- Greet the patient and make eye contact. If you are unsure about how to approach the patient, ask the interpreter for appropriate greeting tips. He or she may also advise you about essential cultural aspects of care.
- Ask the patient's permission for the interpreter to be present. Introduce the interpreter. Allow the interpreter to greet the patient and explain his or her role. Inform the RN and document when the patient refuses an interpreter.
- Make sure that you pronounce the patient's name correctly. Ask the patient how he or she prefers to be addressed.
- Make sure patients understand that the interpreter is not in charge, and is not present on the unit at all times. The purpose of the interpreter is to facilitate communication.
- Allow enough time for conversations, questions, and explanations. Everything must be said twice, so communication may take a long time.
- When speaking, look at the patient, not the interpreter.
- If the patient needs a sign language interpreter, let the interpreter arrange the seating so the patient can see both the interpreter and the persons speaking.
- For accurate interpretation, the sign language interpreter listens to the message for concepts and ideas, not just words.
- Monitor the patient's body language. Ask the interpreter for help with understanding the meaning of nonverbal communications, if necessary.

- Ask the interpreter for cultural clarification, if needed.
- Ask the interpreter to inform you if it seems that the patient is expressing a culture-related idea or concept that you may not understand.
- Speak slowly and clearly. Avoid raising your voice.
- Keep information as simple as possible. Do not expect the interpreter to remember long explanations. Speak one sentence, then pause for the interpreter to translate. For accurate translation, avoid providing too much information at once. It may take the interpreter longer to say something than it took you to say it in English.
- Avoid slang and medical terminology. Use simple, straightforward language.
- The interpreter may ask open-ended questions to clarify a patient's responses.
- Avoid interrupting the patient and interpreter.
- Allow adequate time for the patient to ask questions or have information clarified.
- Confirm your understanding and/or agreement with the patient.
- Ask the interpreter to clarify terms with you, as needed. If necessary, ask the interpreter to have the patient repeat his or her understanding of the communication.
- It is not necessary to say "tell her," or "ask him," or "find out if she." The interpreter will communicate the message in the first person, such as saying, "I plan to be there" rather than, "He says he plans to be there."
- Interpreters will not omit, delete, or add meaning to any of the interpretation. Ask the interpreter to tell you if he or she does not understand your message, then clarify as needed.
- Learning a few basic signs (**Figure 13-2**) or words in the patient's native language is a pleasant gesture that will be appreciated by the patient. For example, learn how to say hello and goodbye, and to ask how the patient feels. If the patient has a recurrent problem, such as pain or nausea, learn how to ask about the problem in the patient's language. You do not have to learn to speak in sentences. For example, the word "douleur" is French for pain. You do not have to ask, "Are you having pain?" (translated into French, this is, "Avez-vous mal?") Simply ask the patient, "Douleur?" The inflection in your voice will indicate that you are asking a question.

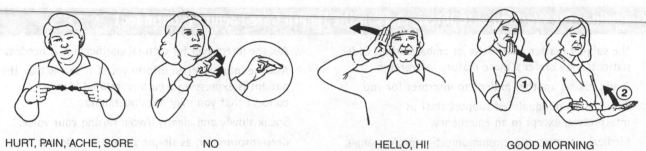

HURT, PAIN, ACHE, SORE   NO   HELLO, HI!   GOOD MORNING

FIGURE 13-2 Basic signs.

DOMESTIC VIOLENCE

Domestic violence is a newly emerging health care problem. The behaviors are perpetrated by a family member or another party who is or was involved in an intimate relationship with the victim. Relationship violence occurs in all ages, races, and socioeconomic groups. Although females are most commonly abused, males may also be abused by women. Abuse can occur in both heterosexual and homosexual relationships, and among other couples who are married or unmarried. Violence sometimes occurs in teen dating relationships.

The American Nurses Association (ANA) supports the education of health care providers in recognizing signs of domestic violence, and learning the skills necessary for prevention of domestic violence. ANA believes there is a critical need for attention to and increased awareness of the problems of domestic violence particularly against women. Calling attention to the problem will reduce the physical and psychological injuries associated with this crime. Repeated episodes of domestic violence potentiate or **exacerbate** chronic health problems. A problem that is exacerbated is escalated, magnified, aggravated, intensified, or worsened by certain factors, such as abuse.

Health promotion is the process of enabling people to increase control over and improve their health. Many factors influence health. Among these are environment, lifestyle, and behavior choices. The abuse of women by their partners must be viewed in context of the social and economic context of their lives.

Domestic violence against women is a pattern of forced behaviors that may include repeated battering and injury, psychological abuse, sexual assault, and progressive social isolation, deprivation, and intimidation (**Figure 13-3**). It can occur in both heterosexual and same-sex couples. The abuser has not lost control. He or she is using violence (verbal, nonverbal, or physical) as a deliberate means of controlling another person. In addition to other methods of violence listed here, the abuser may leave the victim in a dangerous place, or deprive her of medical care.

LEGAL ALERT

Most states have laws prohibiting abuse of children and elderly adults. These laws often require mandatory reporting of suspected patient abuse to police and state agencies. The penalties for abuse can be severe, and may include imprisonment. Stress commonly triggers the abuse. Learn and practice methods of reducing personal stress for optimal mental, emotional, and physical health. Recognize signs of stress in yourself and others, such as:

- Difficulty sleeping
- Irritability
- Feelings of sadness
- Anxiety
- Guilt
- Indecisiveness
- Loss of appetite
- Loss of interest in sexual activity
- Isolation
- Loss of interest in work
- Hopelessness
- Drug or alcohol misuse
- Inability to concentrate

Follow your state reporting laws. Usually, you are responsible only for reporting suspected abuse to the RN. He or she will assess the patient and investigate.

Battered woman syndrome is a pattern of signs and symptoms, such as fearfulness, hopelessness, and helplessness, which are commonly seen in women who have experienced physical and emotional abuse over a long period of time. Women with this condition often become depressed and cannot take action to escape the abuse. Most individuals with this condition have low self-esteem, and believe that the abuse is their fault. They will usually refuse to press charges against the abuser. The woman typically refuses offers of help, and may become aggressive toward those who offer assistance. It is similar to posttraumatic stress disorder, and is seen in people threatened with death or serious injury in extremely stressful situations, such as war. More than half the

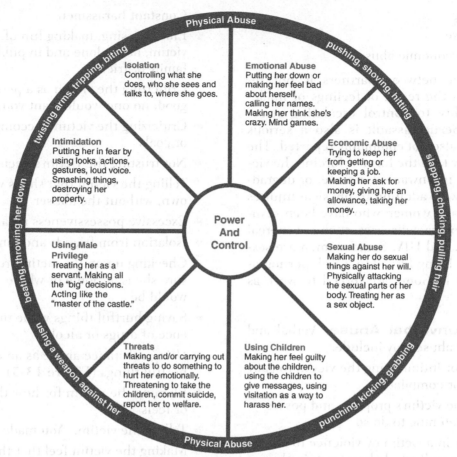

FIGURE 13-3 Domestic violence is a pattern of forced behavior that may include repeated battering and injury, psychological abuse, sexual assault, and progressive social isolation, deprivation, and intimidation. The behaviors are perpetrated by a family member or person who is or was involved in an intimate relationship with the victim. (Courtesy of Minnesota Program Development, Inc. Domestic Abuse Intervention Project, Duluth, MN)

women involved in violent relationships live in households with children under the age of 12. Violence against women is present in all racial, ethnic, and socioeconomic groups. It is more prevalent against women in lower socioeconomic groups, but educated women in higher-income homes are not exempt. Many women in lower socioeconomic status also become victims of poverty and abuse. The victim may be unable to hold a job because of the abuse. The rates of violence against minorities exceed those against Caucasian women.

Scope of the Problem

The key elements of domestic abuse are intimidation, humiliation of the victim, and physical injury. Ninety-five percent of serious assaults in relationships are committed by men battering women. Abuse is a leading cause of injury, and homicide is a major cause of death to women. However, the ex-

act numbers of victims are not known. An estimated 1.5 to 3.9 million women are physically abused by spouses or significant others every year. *Physical violence* is deliberate behavior intended to harm another person. It includes pinching, biting, burning, hitting, slapping, kicking, punching, pushing, using objects as weapons, choking, breaking bones, holding, restraining, confining, or causing injury or death by use of a gun, knife, or other weapon. Physical violence is both an assault and a crime. Injuries include contusions, concussions, lacerations, fractures, and gunshot wounds. Domestic violence can also occur in the form of:

- Verbal abuse
- Mental abuse
- Sexual abuse
- Neglect
- Stalking (at home, work, on the telephone or in person)

- Cyberstalking
- Spiritual abuse
- Financial or economic abuse

Most violence between partners is not reported. It is often the result of feelings of inadequacy and inability to control escalating stress (**Figure 13-4**). Sexual assault is also a serious problem, but it is also not commonly reported. The sexual assault may take the form of forcing the victim to participate in unwanted, unsafe, or degrading sexual activity. In addition to physical injuries and emotional scars, women who have been sexually abused may contract diseases, such as venereal disease, hepatitis, and HIV. Some women are sexually exploited by being forced to watch pornography, then imitate it. Some are forced to work as prostitutes.

Verbal and Nonverbal Abuse. Verbal and mental/emotional abuse may include:

- Threatening or intimidating the victim to gain cooperation or compliance
- Destroying the victim's property and possessions, or threatening to do so
- Instilling fear in a victim by violence to an object, such as a wall or a beloved pet, in the presence of the victim
- Yelling or screaming
- Name-calling

- Constant harassment
- Embarrassing, making fun of, or mocking the victim, both alone and in public, or in front of family or friends
- Criticizing the victim as a person (fat, ugly, no good, no one would want you)
- Criticizing the victim's accomplishments or goals
- Not trusting the victim's decision making
- Telling the victim that she is worthless on her own, without the abuser
- Excessive possessiveness regarding the victim
- Isolation from friends and family
- Checking up on the victim frequently to make sure she is at home or where she said she would be
- Saying hurtful things while under the influence of drugs or alcohol
- Using substance abuse as an excuse for saying hurtful things (**Figure 13-5**)
- Blaming the victim for how the abuser acts or feels
- Telling the victim, "You made me do it"
- Making the victim feel that there is no way out of the relationship

Results of Domestic Violence

Domestic violence and abuse contribute to depression, alcohol and substance abuse, and chronic pain. It is estimated that a violent event occurs in one of every eight relationships annually. Abuse also occurs in dating and cohabiting relationships. Estimates are that one-sixth to one-fourth of all

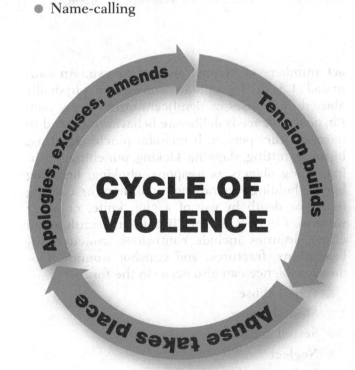

FIGURE 13-4 Stress escalates until abuse occurs.

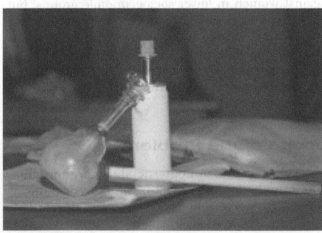

FIGURE 13-5 Crack and other drugs perpetuate domestic violence. (Photo courtesy of UPI/Corbis)

dating relationships are affected by violence. Physical abuse often begins during pregnancy: 25 to 30 percent of pregnant women report abuse before or during pregnancy. Women who are involved in abusive relationships are most likely to deliver a low-birth-weight infant.

Health care professionals are often reluctant to look for or identify incidents of domestic violence with their patients. The reasons for this discomfort vary. Stated reasons for overlooking the problem include personal experience; social norms; the structure and philosophy of medicine; lack of education, skills, and knowledge; short staffing and other priorities; and the structure of the health care system. Some health care workers do not view domestic violence as a health issue. The statistics and magnitude of the problem are not widely known or agreed upon. Some will not ask about abuse because they do not know how to respond. Some may avoid the problem because addressing it with patients may force them to deal with the reality of violence in their own lives.

Failure to identify and recognize signs and symptoms contributes to the overall domestic violence problem. Domestic violence and abuse are very uncomfortable subjects to discuss. Avoiding the subject is much easier. Victims of domestic violence usually feel helpless, hopeless, and very lonely. Overcoming the discomfort surrounding this subject makes an enormous difference by making the abused person feel hopeful, that she is not alone, and that she has options. Women in violent relationships will usually not complain about or admit to being abused, even if the caregiver recognizes the signs. They need compassionate, considerate, skillful care, as well as assistance in finding resources. The RN and social worker will work with the patient to develop a plan of care to keep the victim safe and find a long-term solution to break the cycle of violence.

Signs and Symptoms of Domestic Abuse

Identification of the signs and symptoms of domestic violence and abuse may begin by observing the behavior of both the abuser and the person being abused. The abuser may:

- Appear overly controlling or coercive
- Attempt to answer all questions for the abused partner
- Isolate the abused partner from others as much as possible
- Refuse to let the abused partner out of his or her sight
- Act very jealous of those who pay attention to her, especially other men

When both partners are observed together in the same interaction, the abused woman may:

- Appear quiet and passive
- Show signs of depression, such as crying
- Show signs of low self-esteem, such as poor eye contact
- Appear embarrassed, ashamed, or frightened
- Act inappropriately nonchalant
- Display frightened, timid behavior
- Be very ambivalent

Signs and symptoms of domestic violence are listed in Table 13-1.

Table 13-1 Signs and Symptoms of Domestic Violence	
Behavioral signs and symptoms	• Frequent visits to the physician's office or emergency department • Frequent hospital shopping, or uses emergency department instead of primary physician • Children acting out • Unusual behavior in children • Interpersonal difficulties in family • Often delays seeking medical attention for injuries, misses appointments, does not see a health care provider • Sees health care providers frequently, but has no physical examination findings to account for her symptoms • Substance abuse, including alcohol, prescription drugs, and illicit drugs (This occurs as a result of the relationship; it is not a cause of the violence.)

(continues)

Table 13-1 Signs and Symptoms of Domestic Violence (Continued)

Psychological signs and symptoms	• Anxiety • Depression • Chronic fatigue • Suicidal tendencies or attempts • Lack of trust in others • Feelings of abandonment • Anger • Sensitivity to rejection • Inability to concentrate

Physical signs and symptoms	The signs and symptoms may resemble injuries from other causes. The patient may have a plausible excuse for the injuries. However, the types and locations of injuries should increase suspicion of domestic violence.
	
	• Bruises in various stages of healing
	• Ruptured eardrum
	• Loose or broken teeth
	• Injury to the rectal or genital area
	• Scrapes, bruises, contusions on the head
	• Scrapes, bruises, cuts, or fractures to the face; scrapes and bruises to the neck
	• Cuts or bruises to the abdomen
	• Cuts or bruises to the arms
	
	The distribution of injuries often follows certain patterns:
	
	• Centrally located injuries are common
	• Injuries occur in a "bathing suit" pattern, in areas that are covered by clothing and cannot be seen, such as the breasts, torso, back, buttocks, and genitals
	• The head and neck account for approximately half of all abusive injuries
	
	Characteristic types of injuries:
	
	• Cigarette burns
	• Bite marks
	• Rope burns
	• Bruises
	• Welts with a recognizable outline, such as a belt or belt buckle
	• Puncture wounds
	• Scars in genital or rectal area
	• Injuries involving both sides of the body, usually the arms and legs
	• Defensive injuries to parts of the body used to fend off an attack; the injuries are not consistent with the explanation given. The type or severity of the injury does not fit with the history provided, or the cause of injury would not produce the signs and symptoms:
	
	  • The small-finger side of the forearm (used to block blows to the head and chest)
	  • Palms of hands (used to block blows to the head and chest)
	  • Bottoms of the feet (used to kick away an assailant)
	  • Back, legs, buttocks, and back of the head (when the victim is on the floor)
	
	<div align="right">*(continues)*</div>

Table 13-1 Signs and Symptoms of Domestic Violence (Continued)	
Noninjury physical signs and symptoms	Women experiencing ongoing abuse and stress in their lives may develop medical complaints as a direct or indirect result. Some abused women are noncompliant in their management of chronic diseases. Some typical medical complaints are: • Headache • Neck pain • Chest pain • Insomnia • Abdominal pain • Panic attacks • Heart palpitations • Choking sensations • Appetite disturbances • Numbness and tingling • Painful sexual intercourse • Vaginitis • Pelvic pain • Urinary tract infection

ANA Recommendations

The American Nurses Association supports:

- Education of health care providers in the detection, prevention, or initial intervention in situations of violence against women.
- Routine screening of all women for signs of abuse.
- Maintenance of strict confidentiality if abuse is identified.
- The provision of culturally sensitive care and problem solving within a framework of choice and safety planning.
- Education of all women about the cycle of violence, potential for homicide, and community resources for prevention and care.
- Development and evaluation of nursing models for evaluation, intervention, and treatment for abused women, their children, and perpetrators of violence.

PCT Responsibilities

As a PCT, you are not responsible for questioning a patient about domestic violence. You are not responsible for counseling or treating the patient. Your responsibility is to be aware of the domestic violence problem, and monitor patients for signs and symptoms. You are closer to the patients than most other workers. If you recognize signs of domestic violence, report them to the RN. The RN depends on the accuracy of your observations. Take confidence in the knowledge that you have made a difference in the life of your patient.

Health care facility staff must work as an interdisciplinary team to benefit the patients. The expression "It takes a village to raise a child" has an analogy in health care. In this situation, it takes the expertise of an entire interdisciplinary team of professionals and paraprofessionals to care for each patient. For effective care, lines of communication must be open and precise. Documentation must be concise and accurate. Team members must communicate with each other regularly. Team members use the nursing process in the care of patients, and this process is very effective in helping victims of domestic violence find a solution to their problems.

By helping to identify victims of domestic violence, you are supporting your patients. You help break the cycle of aggression. You help the patient feel human, knowing that someone cares. You help make a horrible experience more bearable. In short, you fulfilled the highest calling. You worked as a member of the nursing team to provide care and service to someone who most probably felt hopeless. You identified a need that will help prevent future pain and suffering, and that is the true essence of nursing.

DELIRIUM

You will care for many elderly patients in the hospital. Some of these patients will appear to have cognitive impairment or mental confusion. This is not a normal aging change, and is often caused by reversible conditions. **Delirium** is an acute confusional state caused by reversible medical problems. It is common in the elderly, particularly those over the age of 75. However, it can occur in patients of any age, because of medical problems. Delirium is a nonspecific symptom of acute illness and dehydration in the elderly. It may also occur when elderly adults are given anesthesia or some other medications. Sensory losses, including uncorrected vision or hearing, may cause the patient to be unable to interpret the environment correctly and thus appear confused. Changes in patient routines and the environment, as well as complications of many different medical conditions, can cause delirium.

Figure 13-6 lists common causes of delirium. These conditions can occur simultaneously, and can worsen other problems in patients who have dementia. Because so many factors contribute to

- Unfamiliar environment: relocation to a new room or new facility
- Vascular insufficiency
- Central nervous system infection
- Trauma
- Tumors or masses, malignancies
- Chemotherapy
- Seizures
- Migraine
- Decreased cardiac output, reduced blood flow, interrupted blood flow
- Urinary retention
- Urinary tract infection
- Pressure ulcers
- Hypotension
- Inadequate oxygenation
- Pneumonia or other lung infection
- Systemic infections, acute and chronic
- Metabolic disorders
- Anemias
- Decreased renal function
- Endocrine system disorders
- Nutritional deficiencies, malnutrition
- Emotional stress

- Pain
- Surgery, anesthesia
- Alteration in temperature regulation (hyperthermia, hypothermia)
- Dehydration, fluid and electrolyte imbalances
- Depression
- Anxiety
- Grief over loss of family member or close friend
- Fatigue
- Sensory/perceptual deficiencies
- Sensory deprivation/isolation, confinement to a restricted area
- Sensory overload
- Immobility, bedrest
- Exposure to toxic substances
- Restraints
- Medication reactions
- Use of invasive equipment such as nasogastric tube or catheter
- Lack of prosthetic devices, including glasses, hearing aid, dentures
- Lack of items that complete body image, such as canes, purses, walkers
- Loss of family contact
- Loss of control over body processes

FIGURE 13-6 Common causes of delirium.

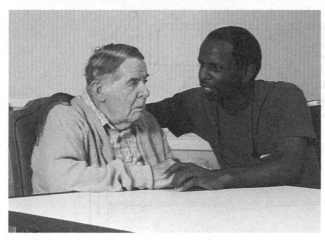

FIGURE 13-7 Delirium is a reversible mental confusion. The patient has a decreased environmental awareness and poor safety judgment, making him a high risk for injury.

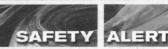

SAFETY ALERT

Patients with delirium have very poor safety judgment and are at high risk for falls and other injuries. Monitor these patients frequently. Avoid use of restraints whenever possible. Consider alternatives, such as distraction, before applying restraints. If restraints are necessary, the RN should make the decision regarding the type of restraint to use in keeping with physician orders. Remove and reapply the restraint every 2 hours. Offer comfort measures, including food, fluids, and toileting, as appropriate. Provide distraction and calm touch, if appropriate.

delirium, it is often misunderstood, and may be confused with dementia. Delirium is a very serious condition. Unrecognized and untreated, the mortality rate is high, particularly in patients with chronic disease, mental problems, or dementia. This is unfortunate, because delirium can be reversed if promptly identified and treated.

Signs and Symptoms of Delirium

Delirium develops rapidly. Usually, the onset is within a few hours or days. Delirium may not be recognized until the patient is critically ill. Staff believe that the patient became ill suddenly because of the rapid onset of mental changes, but a closer look often reveals subtle changes in the patient's physical or mental condition over several days before the onset of delirium. *Any change in a patient's mental status is significant.*

Patients with acute delirium develop disorientation, behavioral changes, and decreased awareness of the environment (**Figure 13-7**). Other common signs and symptoms are:

- Reduced or fluctuating levels of consciousness
- Misinterpretation of the environment, misunderstanding or misinterpretation of conversations
- Hallucinations
- Illusions
- Delusions
- Insomnia and disturbance of sleep-wake cycle
- Change in motor activity
- Mental confusion and memory impairment

PCT Responsibilities

Early identification and careful observation are essential to preventing more serious problems. As a PCT, you will work more closely with patients than most other caregivers. This places you in an ideal position to notice subtle changes in mental status and other signs of dehydration, infection, or physical illness that may lead to delirium. You will become familiar with the patient's usual or normal condition. If something differs from the patient's usual condition, do not overlook it. Monitor changes in patients carefully, and report them to the RN promptly. Keep changes in patient routines and environment minimal. Monitor for and promptly report signs and symptoms of physical illness to the RN.

CARING FOR PATIENTS WITH SEIZURE DISORDERS

In the mid-1800s, Hughlings Jackson described a seizure as "an abnormal electrical discharge of the brain." Today, this description continues to characterize our understanding of this condition. A **seizure** or convulsion (**Figure 13-8**) is a sudden, spontaneous episode of excessive and scrambled electrical activity caused by interference with impulses in the brain. Seizures are transient alterations in awareness that disrupt the patient's ability to control physical processes. They can interfere with the mental and behavioral processes of the individual. They may also cause changes in awareness, body movements, sensations, and/or emotions. Seizures are seen in epilepsy and some other diseases. Injuries, medication, fever, and infection can also cause seizures. Some appear mild, whereas others appear severe. They can be characterized by jerking and shaking of the body, or other abnormal sensations or problems, depending on the type of seizure. The most common types of seizures are related to epilepsy. These are described in Table 13-2.

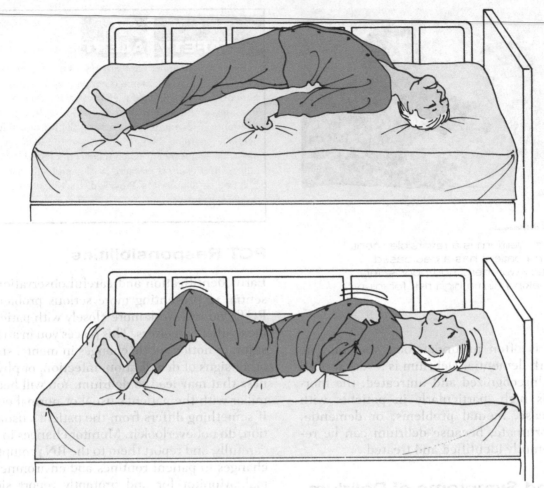

FIGURE 13-8 Generalized tonic-clonic seizures involve the entire body. Side rails should be padded for patients with seizure disorder. The side rails are down in this picture for clarity.

Table 13-2 Seizures		
Type of Seizure	**Signs of Seizure Activity**	**Comment**
Generalized tonic-clonic seizure (grand mal seizure)	May be preceded by an aura. Loss of consciousness, convulsive activity, characterized by rigid stiffening of muscles and jerking movement of the arms and legs. Saliva runs from the mouth. Patient's color may change because of lack of oxygen, incontinence of bowel and bladder.	Usually lasts three to four minutes. The patient may be very tired after the seizure and may have a headache. The patient may be mentally confused, have slurred speech, and be very weak. The patient will not remember the seizure. *(continues)*

Table 13-2 Seizures (Continued)

Type of Seizure	Signs of Seizure Activity	Comment
Absence seizure (petit mal seizure)	Staring, blinking, or stopping what the patient is doing. The patient may stare blankly. One muscle group may twitch or jerk. The seizure begins without warning, and consists of a period of unconsciousness, in which the patient blinks rapidly, stares blankly, breathes rapidly, or makes chewing movements. The seizure lasts 2 to 10 seconds, then ends abruptly. The patient usually resumes normal activity immediately. Because these seizures are mild, they may go unnoticed. Children with absence seizures may have learning problems if the seizures are not identified and treated.	Petit mal seizures usually last less than a minute, but may occur many times a day.
Simple-partial (Jacksonian)	Involves only part of the brain. Can be a sensation or feeling with no abnormal muscle activity. If muscle spasms occur, they begin with spasms of the face, hands, or feet. Starts at one extremity, such as an arm or leg, and progressively moves upward on that side of the body.	May spread to other areas in the brain, resulting in a grand mal seizure
Complex-partial (psychomotor)	Abnormal acts, irrational behavior, or loss of judgment due to a temporary change in consciousness. Automatic behavior, such as typing or eating, may continue normally. The patient may uncontrollably smack the lips, wander aimlessly, or uncontrollably twitch part of the body.	Usually lasts only a few seconds. The patient usually does not remember the seizure.
Myoclonic	Consists of one or more myoclonic jerks. The patient remains conscious but cannot control the muscle movement.	The patient is aware that an extremity is jerking but is unable to stop it. The patient remains conscious throughout and can remember the seizure activity.
Status epilepticus	Multiple seizures occurring simultaneously with no break between seizures. When this seizure begins, the patient cries out, then falls to the floor. The muscles stiffen (tonic phase), then the extremities begin to jerk and twitch (clonic phase). The patient may lose bladder control. Consciousness returns slowly. After this seizure, the patient may feel tired, or be confused and disoriented. This may last from a few minutes to several hours or days. The patient may fall asleep, or gradually become less confused until full consciousness returns.	Status epilepticus may be precipitated by sudden withdrawal of antiseizure medications, fever, and infection. This type of seizure is dangerous and can lead to decreased mental function, neurological impairment, and death.

A seizure is a serious medical emergency. The goal of seizure care is to prevent injury. Some patients have a sensation called an **aura** immediately before a seizure. An aura is a sensation, vision, smell, taste, or light that signals the onset of a seizure.

Some people have service dogs that warn them of an impending seizure so they can take safety precautions before the seizure begins. Dogs' sense of smell is much more sensitive than that of humans. It is believed that the dog smells a chemical reaction that signals the onset of a seizure. All states have access laws regarding service animals, but these vary widely. In this situation, the federal laws supersede state laws, and hospitals are required to permit patients to keep their service animals, with stipulations. The Association of Professionals in Infection Control has guidelines for hospitals to follow. Your facility will have policies regarding the use of service animals while patients are hospitalized.

Status epilepticus is a seizure that lasts for a long time, or repeats without recovery. It is a life-threatening condition. Death may result if the patient is not treated immediately. Status epilepticus can be convulsive (tonic-clonic) or nonconvulsive (absence). A person in nonconvulsive status epilepticus may become confused or appear dazed. The highest incidence of status epilepticus occurs during the first year of life and after the age of 60. In elderly adults, most cases are related to cerebrovascular accidents.

Seizure Precautions

Safety is a primary concern for patients diagnosed with seizure disorder and those who are at risk for seizures because of other medical conditions, such as stroke and head injury. The care plan or critical pathway will list individualized precautions to take. **Seizure precautions** are individualized measures that keep the patient safe during an unexpected seizure. Some seizure precautions are:

- Follow facility policies for remaining in the room while the patient is in the tub or shower. The patient on seizure precautions should not be left alone in the tub. A shower is preferred, but the door should not be locked. Encourage the patient to sit on a shower stool or chair. Fasten the safety strap.

- Make sure the patient has a call signal in reach at all times.

- Apply side rail pads (Figure 13-9) to the bed. If commercial pads are not available, use 6

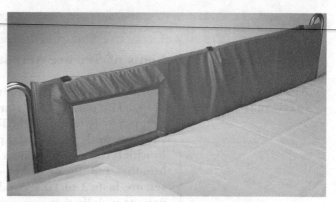

FIGURE 13-9 When a patient is on seizure precautions, apply commercial side rail pads or wrap the side rails with bath blankets. (Courtesy of Skil-Care Corporation, Yonkers, NY, (800) 431-2972).

bath blankets to pad the bed. Wrap each rail with two bath blankets. Tape the blankets in place with adhesive tape. Fold a bath blanket to pad the headboard and footboard, then tape it in place.

- When the patient is in bed, keep the side rails up and the bed in low position. A mat may be placed on the floor as an extra precaution, or a low bed without side rails may be used as an alternative (Figure 13-10). If a mat is used on the floor, pick it up when the patient is out of bed so it is not a fall hazard.

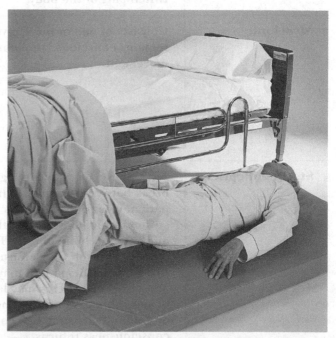

FIGURE 13-10 A floor mat may used as an extra precaution, or a low bed without side rails may be used as an alternative. If a mat is used on the floor, pick it up when the patient is out of bed so it is not a fall hazard. (Courtesy of Skil-Care Corporation, Yonkers, NY, (800) 431-2972).

- Keep an oral airway readily available at the bedside.
- Keep a suction machine at the bedside, or readily available.
- Oxygen equipment should be readily available.
- Avoid taking oral temperatures. Take tympanic (preferred), rectal, or axillary temperatures.
- If the patient has prolonged or frequent seizures, you may be instructed to insert a heparin lock for emergency venous access.
- Always protect the head if the patient has a seizure. If he or she is on the floor, move furniture or place padding in front of hard or sharp objects, as necessary.

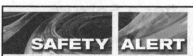

SAFETY ALERT

You may have heard an old wives' tale that describes how patients swallow their tongues when having a seizure. Years ago, caregivers placed a spoon in the seizure patient's mouth, which often resulted in broken teeth and other injuries to both the patient and the nurse. Never try to force the mouth open or place your hands or any other object in the patient's mouth during a seizure. The jaw clenches and becomes rigid, and you may be bitten. Never try to forcibly restrain the patient during a seizure. This could cause serious injury to the patient. If he or she is in a chair, try to get the patient to the floor. If he or she is on the floor, move hard or sharp objects away from the head, or place a pillow between the head and the furnishings. Monitor the patient's activities and the times of each, as well as the time the seizure began and ended. This information will help the physician identify the seizure cause and type.

Procedure 109

Caring for the Patient Who Is Having a Seizure

1. Stay with the patient and call for help.
2. Use standard precautions if contact with blood or moist body fluids (except sweat) is likely.
3. If the patient is in bed, remove the pillow and raise the side rails.
4. If the patient is not in bed, gently lower the patient to the floor, protecting the head.
5. Turn the patient on the side. If this is not possible, turn the head to the side. This allows secretions to drain from the patient's mouth.
6. Move any hard objects, or pad objects that may injure the patient with pillows, blankets, or other available items, such as chair cushions.
7. Loosen tight and restrictive clothing.
8. Provide privacy by asking onlookers to leave, closing the door to the patient's room, and pulling the privacy curtain.
9. Avoid restraining the patient in any way.
10. Do not try to place any object in the patient's mouth. Doing this could break teeth and cause injury to the patient and yourself.
11. Check the patient's vital signs as requested by the RN. You may be instructed to check vital signs frequently until the patient is stable.
12. Assist the RN as directed. The patient may need suction, oxygen, or medication to stop the seizure.
13. When the seizure stops, orient the patient to where he or she is and what happened. Assist the patient to bed. The patient will be very tired. Allow him or her to sleep.
14. Leave the patient in a position of comfort and safety. Leave the call signal and needed personal items within reach.
15. Remove gloves, if worn, and dispose of them according to facility policy.
16. Wash your hands, or use alcohol-based hand cleaner.
17. Report to the RN:
    - Any change in the patient before the seizure, such as an aura, confusion, or change in behavior.
    - Loss of control of bowel or bladder, eyes rolling upward, rapid blinking, biting tongue.
    - Time the seizure started and stopped.
    - A description of the way the seizure looked, including the body parts involved.
    - Condition of the patient after the seizure.
    - Vital signs.

Nursing Care after a Seizure

When the seizure stops, tell the patient where he or she is and what happened. Assist him or her to bed. Make the patient comfortable and allow him or her to sleep. Put the side rails up, unless instructed otherwise by the RN. The patient may be drowsy, confused, and require periodic reorientation. Some health workers incorrectly call this condition *postictal*. However, **postictal** is not a sign or symptom. It is the period of time immediately after a seizure. During the postictal period, the patient is often drowsy or sleepy. Leave him or her in a position of comfort and safety with the call signal and needed personal items within reach. Other care includes:

- Providing incontinent care, if necessary
- Checking the vital signs as instructed; you may take vital signs frequently until the patient is stable
- Monitoring the patient closely for return of seizure activity
- Administering oxygen or suctioning, as directed

Report to the RN:

- Any change in the patient before the seizure, such as an aura, confusion, or change in behavior
- A description of the way the seizure looked, including the body parts involved
- Loss of bowel or bladder control, eyes rolling upward, rapid blinking, biting tongue
- The time the seizure started and stopped, if known
- Condition of the patient after the seizure
- Vital signs

SPINAL CORD INJURIES

Some patients are admitted to the facility because of injuries or other conditions of the spinal cord that result in **paralysis.** This is loss of movement and impairment of various parts of the body (**Figure 13-11**). In spinal cord injury, paralysis develops immediately below the level of injury. Paralysis affects sensation and voluntary movement below the level of injury (**Figure 13-12**). These patients are at great risk for developing pressure sores and other skin injuries. Because sensation is impaired, they will not feel the pain that serves as a warning sign when the skin begins to break down. Pressure ulcers commonly progress to Stage IV, and patients

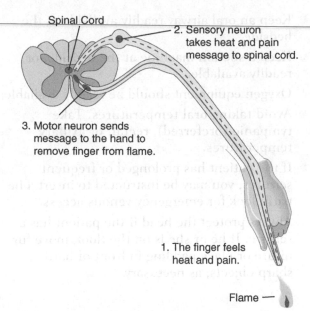

Spinal Cord

2. Sensory neuron takes heat and pain message to spinal cord.

3. Motor neuron sends message to the hand to remove finger from flame.

1. The finger feels heat and pain.

Flame —

FIGURE 13-11 A reflex arc.

often develop sepsis and other serious complications. Pressure ulcers are always easier to prevent than treat. Take preventive skin care very seriously in patients with paralysis.

The most common cause of paralysis is trauma. Conditions such as tumors, infection, cerebral palsy, **congenital disorders** (conditions present at birth), and neurological diseases can also cause paralysis. **Paraplegia** is paralysis of the lower half of the body, including both legs. Bowel and bladder control are also lost. **Tetraplegia** is paralysis affecting the arms and legs. **Quadriplegia** is an older term for this condition. **Flaccid paralysis** involves loss of muscle tone and absence of tendon reflexes. Some patients have **spastic paralysis.** These patients have no voluntary movement. The extremities move in an involuntary pattern, similar to muscle spasms. The patient is aware of the movements, but cannot stop them. The type of paralysis is determined by the level of injury. Patients with upper motor injuries are more likely to exhibit spastic paralysis.

Loss of Independence

Most dictionaries define the term *independent* as self-reliant or self-supporting. In reality, it is much more than this. People who are independent move about and complete activities of daily living (ADLs) at will, without assistance. In some ways, independence is a state of mind. It is freedom to do what we want, when we want, within the constraints of per-

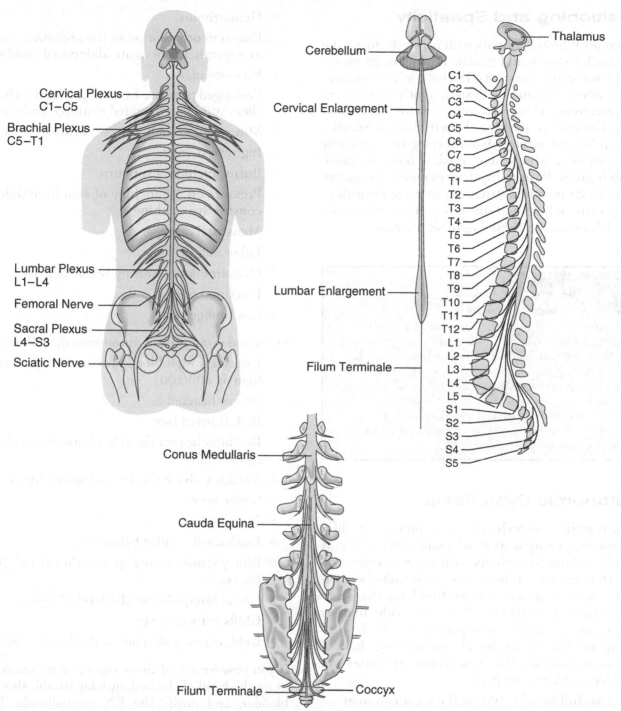

Cervical Plexus
C1–C5

Brachial Plexus
C5–T1

Lumbar Plexus
L1–L4

Femoral Nerve

Sacral Plexus
L4–S3

Sciatic Nerve

Cerebellum

Cervical Enlargement

Lumbar Enlargement

Filum Terminale

Thalamus

C1
C2
C3
C4
C5
C6
C7
C8
T1
T2
T3
T4
T5
T6
T7
T8
T9
T10
T11
T12
L1
L2
L3
L4
L5
S1
S2
S3
S4
S5

Conus Medullaris

Cauda Equina

Filum Terminale

Coccyx

FIGURE 13-12 The spinal cord and nerves

sonal ethics and the law. Independence is a tangible thing that most people take for granted. We do not realize how greatly we value it until we lose it. Loss of independence is an enormous loss. People who were suddenly paralyzed lost their independence in seconds. Imagine the shock of living normally one minute, then developing an injury or medical condition that renders you completely unable to care for yourself. Imagine the loss of your income. Imagine

the inability to earn a living, then having to wait for months for government assistance to be approved. Imagine the shame of having to ask for it in the first place! People with paralysis have experienced devastating losses. Because of this, some seem to have an attitude or behavior problem. Be honest and sincere with the patient. Allow him or her to direct the care that you give. This gives the patient a measure of control, and improves self-esteem.

Positioning and Spasticity

When positioning patients with paralysis, move the extremities slowly and gently. Rapid, rough movements will cause spasticity. If a patient's extremities move into a position of flexion, gently move them into extension. If the extremities move into a position of extension, position them in flexion. Spasticity can be very strong. Avoid forcing the extremity into position, which may break a bone or cause other injuries. Positioning devices may be necessary to maintain position. Attention to proper positioning is extremely important to prevent contractures and deformities in these high-risk patients.

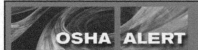

OSHA ALERT

Patients with spinal cord injury can provide limited to no assistance with positioning, moving, and transfers. Elevate the bed to the high position when giving care (make sure the rail is up on the opposite side of the bed). To prevent injury to your back, never move a patient who has a spinal cord injury by yourself. Make sure that another assistant is available to help you. Using lift sheets, mechanical lifts, and other adjunctive devices make moving the patient easier for both the patient and the PCT.

Autonomic Dysreflexia

Autonomic dysreflexia is a potentially life-threatening complication of spinal cord injury. It usually occurs in patients with injuries above the mid-thoracic area. It indicates uncontrolled sympathetic nervous system activity. Problems that seem minor can trigger this condition. As a rule, injuries that would normally cause pain below the level of the spinal damage set this life-threatening chain of events in motion. The most common causes are bladder problems, such as:

- Overfull bladder (this is the most common cause)
- Irritation of the bladder wall
- Urinary retention
- Urinary infection
- Blocked catheter
- Noncompliance with intermittent catheterization schedule

Other potential causes of autonomic dysreflexia are:

- Overfilled urinary drainage bag or leg bag
- Constipation or fecal impaction
- Hemorrhoids
- Infection or irritation in the abdomen, such as appendicitis or acute abdominal conditions
- Pressure ulcers
- Prolonged pressure by an object in the chair, shoe, sitting on wrinkled clothing, and the like.
- Minor injury, such as a cut, bruise, or abrasion
- Ingrown toenails
- Burns, including sunburn
- Pressure on or pinching of skin from tight or constrictive clothing
- Menstrual cramps
- Labor and delivery
- Overstimulation during sexual activity
- Fractured bones
- Gas (indigestion)

Signs and symptoms of autonomic dysreflexia are:

- Extremely high blood pressure (may be as high as 200/100)
- Severe headache
- Red, flushed face
- Red blotches on the skin above the level of spinal injury
- Sweating above the level of spinal injury
- Stuffy nose
- Nausea
- Bradycardia (pulse below 60)
- Blurry vision, seeing spots, other visual disturbances
- Goose bumps below the level of injury
- Chills without fever
- Cold, clammy skin below the level of injury

If you observe any of these signs and symptoms, elevate the head of the bed, quickly troubleshoot the bladder, and notify the RN immediately. Treatment for this condition involves rapidly identifying the offending stimulus and removing it. If you believe something has triggered the condition, inform the nurse.

PCTs who work with patients with spinal cord injury must be able to recognize autonomic dysreflexia quickly and take appropriate nursing action. Become familiar with your patients' average blood pressures. People with spinal cord injury often have normal or low blood pressure. An increase in blood pressure of 20 mm Hg suggests the onset of symptoms. Undetected, the blood pressure will continue to rise to dangerously high levels. The outcome of this condition is largely determined by how quickly personnel identify it.

DIFFICULT PATIENT ALERT

Autonomic dysreflexia is most common in people with spinal cord injuries above the sixth thoracic vertebra. Although the description sounds casual, this is a true medical emergency. Any irritation can trigger this condition, but the most common cause is a full bladder. Other common problems are a full rectum or something pinching the skin. Any irritant can cause it. The irritation triggers a reflex reaction that causes the blood pressure to increase markedly. The pulse also increases and may become irregular. Because the nerves in the spinal cord are damaged, they cannot correct or control the situation. The only way to remedy the problem is to quickly identify the cause and return the blood pressure to normal. Although the patient may recognize the symptoms, he or she does not know what is causing the blood pressure elevation. People with spinal cord injury may describe autonomic dysreflexia with the phrase "going hyper."

PCT Care for the Patient with Autonomic Dysreflexia

Immediate interventions for autonomic dysreflexia are to:

- Position the patient in a high Fowler's (sitting) position or elevate the head of the bed 90 degrees, or as tolerated; lower the patient's legs.
- Remove tight and constricting clothing, shoes, and appliances.
- Check with the RN regarding removal of appliances such as ace wraps, binders, or antiembolism hosiery.
- Monitor blood pressure every 2 to 3 minutes.
- Avoid movements or activities that would cause the patient to bear down as if having a bowel movement. Bearing down has the potential to worsen the syndrome.
- Be calm and reassuring. This condition can be very frightening for the patient.

Problems related to the catheter are among the most common causes of this condition, so your first priority is to check the catheter and drainage bag for problems. The RN may instruct you to change the catheter. If no catheter is in place, you may be instructed to insert one. PCT actions include:

- Checking the catheter for potential problems.
- Making sure tubing is positioned correctly and that urine is not refluxing into the bladder.
- Removing kinks or obstructions in tubing, if found.
- Emptying the leg bag or urinary drainage bag.
- Irrigating the catheter. Insert a small volume (15 mL) of room-temperature solution at one time. A cold solution may worsen the condition.

If the catheter is not draining, or the urine contains a large amount of sediment, you will be instructed to replace the catheter immediately. If the patient has an intermittent catheterization schedule, you will be instructed to do a straight catheterization immediately to ensure that the bladder is empty. When inserting a catheter for a patient with this condition, empty the bladder *slowly*. Rapid drainage may worsen the condition by causing bladder spasms. The RN may instruct you to use a special anesthetic lubricant during catheterization procedures.

Problems related to the bowel are the second most likely cause of autonomic dysreflexia. The RN may instruct you to check for a fecal impaction. If found, remove it carefully. The nurse may first insert an anesthetic lubricating jelly into the rectum to numb the mucous membranes. This will take effect in about 2 to 5 minutes. The RN may instruct you to use additional jelly instead of the lubricant normally used for this procedure.

Skin-related problems are the third most likely cause of autonomic dysreflexia. Undress and reposition the patient and carefully check the entire body for pressure ulcers and other problems, such as ingrown toenails.

Once the offending stimulus has been identified and treated, monitor the patient for rebound hypotension. This condition is most likely to occur if the blood pressure was lowered by giving medications. (Medications are not usually necessary if the noxious causative stimulus is identified and eliminated.) Continue to check the blood pressure every 5 minutes after the episode has resolved. You must check the blood pressure frequently for the remainder of the shift, as instructed by the RN. Monitoring frequency will vary from every 5 minutes to every 30 minutes, depending on the patient's baseline condition and response to treatment.

Patients who have experienced autonomic dysreflexia are always at risk for a recurrence. Prevention is the preferred treatment goal, so the care plan will be modified to emphasize preventive care.

CARING FOR PATIENTS WHO ARE RECEIVING CHEMOTHERAPY

Chemotherapy uses medications or drugs to destroy cancer. Unfortunately, healthy cells may also be destroyed. The goals of chemotherapy vary, depending on the type of cancer, stage, and situation. Goals might be to:

- Completely eliminate the cancer
- Control and slow the growth of cancer to prolong the patient's life
- Reduce the size of the cancer to eliminate pain and improve quality of life

COMMUNICATION ALERT

A cancer diagnosis evokes strong feelings and emotions in patients and their families. These may be difficult to understand and cope with. Patients or families may lash out in anger at you or their loved ones. They are not angry with you. They are angry with their circumstances. Avoid responding with anger. Keep your temper even, and do not take comments personally. Saying, "I see you are upset," or validating their feelings is the best way to respond. Providing compassionate care, listening, and giving sincere, solid emotional support will help patients and family members cope during this difficult time.

Chemotherapy is given by many different routes. Some patients can take oral medications. Others must receive the drugs in the muscles, veins, or other organs and body cavities. If the drugs are given intravenously, a central intravenous catheter is usually inserted to avoid repeated needlesticks and reduce the risk of vein irritation and collapse. Chemotherapy drugs are very potent and can irritate the skin, eyes, and mucous membranes of caregivers. Because of this, special measures are used to handle the drugs. Never eat, drink, or chew gum in an area where chemotherapy is being prepared. If you accidentally contact a chemotherapy drug with your hands or mucous membranes, flush the contacted area well with water and seek medical attention. These drugs and the containers they are dispensed in require special handling and disposal.

Side Effects of Chemotherapy

Chemotherapy targets rapidly regenerating cells, such as cancer cells. The drugs cannot differentiate cancer cells from normal cells, so other cells that regenerate rapidly may also be affected. Other cells in the body that are commonly affected are:

- Blood cells, such as red blood cells, white blood cells, and platelets
- Hair and nail cells
- Gastrointestinal cells

DIFFICULT PATIENT ALERT

Hair is important to everyone's self-esteem and appearance. Some diseases and medications cause hair loss. Some cause changes to the volume and texture of hair. Some medications cause hair to become dry and brittle. Patients who have problems with their hair may become anxious or angry, because the appearance of the hair affects their self-esteem. If the patient is experiencing problems with the hair, treat it gently. Use products such as baby shampoo and conditioner. Use tepid water. Pat the hair dry. Do not rub it with a towel. Use a wide-toothed comb to style the hair gently. Avoid braids and rubber bands, which may worsen hair loss or breakage. Assist the patient to wear a scarf or turban, if desired.

Side effects of cancer drugs can range from mild to life-threatening. Patients who are receiving these drugs need special monitoring. Sometimes the dose and scheduling must be changed to reduce side effects. Common side effects are:

- Alopecia, or hair loss. This commonly starts within two weeks after chemotherapy begins. It may take up to five or six months to regrow the hair.
- Nausea and vomiting, depending on the drugs used. Sometimes it occurs immediately, but may be delayed until several days after the drug is given.
- Anorexia, or loss of appetite. This is sometimes caused because the drugs cause changes in the taste buds. In other patients, loss of appetite is due to nausea.
- Anemia, a deficiency of the red blood cells. This is caused by changes in the body due to the chemotherapy drugs. Sometimes special medications are given to reverse the anemia.
- Fatigue; patients often become very tired. Anemia and reduced red blood cells are the most likely cause.
- Low white blood cell count, which increases the risk of infection. This usually begins within a week of beginning therapy and may

last a long time. Precautions are taken to prevent exposure to infection.

- A reduction in the number of platelets in the blood, which increases the risk of bleeding. Precautions must be taken to prevent injury.
- Destruction of the mucous membranes of the mouth. This causes burning, pain, redness, and breakdown inside the mouth.

Many other side effects are caused by chemotherapy drugs. The RN will advise you what to watch for in each patient.

Disposal of Body Fluids and Wastes

Patients who are receiving chemotherapy may excrete the drugs in their waste and body fluids. Discard gloves and other protective apparel, if worn, in a leakproof container. Follow facility policies for discarding this equipment in biohazardous waste or other contaminated area. Because the drugs are excreted in body waste, linens that have contacted blood, body fluids, or excretions require special handling. Wear gloves when handling linen, and always apply the principles of standard precautions. Soiled items should be bagged in specially marked bags before they are sent to the laundry.

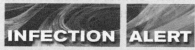
INFECTION ALERT

Patients with leukemia (cancer of the blood) are at high risk of infection. You may have learned that these patients have many white blood cells, which would normally help protect the patient from infection. Patients with leukemia do have many white cells, but the cells are immature and do not offer protection from infection. Conscientiously apply the principles of standard precautions in all patient care. Notify the RN promptly of signs or symptoms of infection.

Observations and PCT Care

Observe chemotherapy patients for side effects of the drugs and report them to the RN promptly. Monitor the patient for bruising, and abnormal skin lesions. Inform the RN promptly if fever is present. Encourage fluids of the patient's choice, as tolerated. Provide nursing comfort measures, such as good mouth care and daily bathing. Routinely take precautions to prevent injuries and infection. For example, you may be instructed to remind the patient to cough and deep breathe to keep the lungs clear. You may be asked to take vital signs every 2 to

4 hours. Rectal temperatures should not be taken in some patients. Check with the RN before taking a rectal temperature. Report a fever over 101°F or chilling to the RN immediately. Other signs of infection to report are:

- Swelling, redness, or irritation inside the mouth
- Rectal pain or tenderness
- Change in bowel or bladder habits
- Pain or burning on urination
- Redness, swelling, open area, or pain on the skin
- Cough or shortness of breath
- Decreased level of consciousness
- Decreased urine output
- Warm, flushed, dry skin
- Hypotension (below 100/60, or as instructed)

Because of the risk of bleeding, patients may have to take special precautions, such as blowing the nose gently, or using an electric razor. A very soft toothbrush will probably be necessary. Special mouthwash products may be ordered. The care plan and the RN will provide special directions.

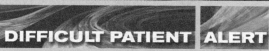
DIFFICULT PATIENT ALERT

Monitor the chemotherapy patient for bruising and abnormal skin lesions. Inform the RN promptly if fever is present. Encourage fluids of the patient's choice, as tolerated.

Promoting good nutrition and hydration is very important. You may be asked to serve the patient six small meals a day. High-protein drinks may also be ordered. Encourage fluids, and record intake and output, including emesis. Alternate periods of rest with periods of activity to reduce fatigue. Plan your care to allow frequent rest periods. Inform the RN if the patient:

- Has nausea or vomiting
- Is not eating or drinking
- Complains of changes in the taste buds affecting the ability or desire to eat
- Complains of constipation or diarrhea
- Has white patches or unusual areas inside the mouth (**Figure 13-13**)
- Complains of signs of a vaginal infection
- Develops bruising or bleeding (**Figure 13-14**)

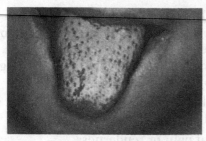

FIGURE 13-13 Monitor for and report white patches in the mouth to the RN. (Courtesy of Daniel J. Barbaro, MD, Fort Worth, Texas)

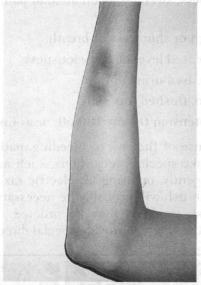

FIGURE 13-14 Bruises are a sign of internal bleeding. Report them promptly.

DIFFICULT PATIENT ALERT

Liquid nutritional supplements are very filling, which is why they are usually served between meals and not with meals. Most patients prefer them cold. If the beverage is warm, the patient may not accept it. Because some of these products are milk-based, serving them warm can also be an infection control hazard. When serving supplements and nourishments, make sure the patient is able to consume the beverage independently. Do not set it on the table and walk out. Pour the beverage into a cup, if preferred by the patient. Pour it over ice, as desired by the patient, if it is warm. Provide a straw. If the patient cannot consume the product independently, assist him or her. Document the percentage consumed on the proper form. Record the amount if the patient is on intake and output. Inform the RN if the patient expresses a preference or dislike for a certain product or flavor.

Because the chemotherapy drugs are so toxic, you must observe the patient closely when he or she is receiving them. Inform the RN promptly if:

- There are signs of intravenous infiltration, such as redness, swelling, or pain at the needle insertion site
- The patient's mental status changes
- The patient's vital signs change

Assisting the Patient with Body Image

Cancer surgery and chemotherapy may change body appearance. This is often very upsetting to the patient. Hair loss may be especially traumatic, particularly in females. The eyebrows and eyelashes may also fall out. Be calm and reassuring. The hair will grow back, although the color or texture may be different. Assist the patient to wear a turban, scarf, or wig, if desired.

CARING FOR THE PATIENT WHO IS RECEIVING RADIATION THERAPY

Radiation therapy involves the use of high-energy, ionizing beams directed to the site of the cancer (Figure 13-15). The objective is to destroy the cancerous tissue without damaging healthy tissue. Several different types of radiation therapy may be used. Common side effects of radiation that should be reported to the RN are:

- Fatigue
- Nausea, vomiting
- Diarrhea
- Skin redness, irritation, peeling

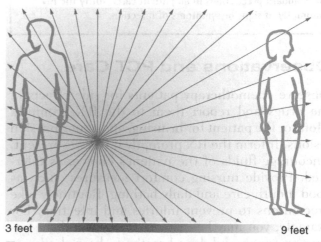

3 feet   9 feet

FIGURE 13-15 Radiation therapy is a treatment for certain types of cancers.

- Change in taste
- Irritation of mucous membranes
- Cough
- Shortness of breath

Special Care

The patient may have markings on the skin at the site where radiation is delivered. Do not wash these off. The radiation may be very irritating to the patient's skin. Check the skin daily for problems and report them to the RN, if found. Special skin care may be listed on the care plan. You may be instructed to:

- Wash the patient with lukewarm water and mild soap; in some situations no soap is used
- Avoid rubbing or creating friction on the skin
- Avoid shaving areas near the treatment field
- Avoid using tape on the patient's skin near the treatment field
- Avoid using lotions and cosmetics near the treatment field
- Avoid tight-fitting garments; dress the patient in loose, comfortable clothing

Brachytherapy

Brachytherapy is another form of radiation therapy in which tiny radioactive seeds or pellets are implanted directly inside the body. This treatment is very successful and preferred over traditional radiation therapy for some patients, because it has fewer side effects. Brachytherapy may be used to treat conditions such as prostate, lung, cervical, and endometrial cancer. The dosage varies with the area being treated and type of cancer. Treatment may last from several hours to several days. The brachytherapy seeds used to treat prostate cancer may be left in place permanently. Brachytherapy may be used in combination with traditional radiation therapy.

Care of the Patient Who Is Receiving Radiation Therapy and Brachytherapy

Sources of radiation are sometimes implanted inside the patient's body. If this is the case, you will be instructed as to special precautions to follow to reduce your risk of radiation exposure. The patient will be in a private room. Usually, the hospital has designated rooms that are used only for radiation therapy patients. The patient may be on bedrest to prevent dislodgment of the radioactive device(s). To prevent radiation exposure, visitors will be restricted with regard to how close they may get to the patient and how long they may stay in the room. Pregnant women and children below the age of 18 are not permitted to enter the room. Prostate cancer may be treated with permanent implantation of radioactive seeds. The patient will be instructed to stay away from pregnant women and children for a designated period of time, such as six months.

You will be assigned a personal monitoring badge, called a **dosimeter.** This is a small instrument that measures the radiation dose to which each individual is exposed when working with the patient. Always wear the badge between your waist and collar when you enter the room. Never borrow someone else's badge. Use only the badge that was issued to you. Do not take the badge home. When off duty, store it according to facility policy, away from sources of radiation.

DIFFICULT PATIENT ALERT

The patient should have a lead-lined container and long-handled forceps in a corner of the room. The radiation safety personnel will mark a "safe line" on the floor with masking tape approximately 6 feet from the bed. The line is a warning to visitors to minimize their radiation exposure. If desired, place a portable lead shield in the back of the room to use when providing care. If the patient has an implant in the neck or mouth, an emergency tracheotomy tray will be placed in the room.

Guidelines for Working with Radiation Therapy and Brachytherapy Patients

- If you think you may be pregnant, do not enter the room. Inform the RN.
- Plan and organize your time before entering the patient's room. Provide necessary care, but try to minimize time spent with the patient.
- You may be required to apply gloves and shoe covers when entering the patient's room. Remove them before leaving.
- Wear a mask if the patient has a tracheostomy or signs of a respiratory infection.

(continued)

Guidelines for Working with Radiation Therapy and Brachytherapy Patients (Continued)

- Work behind mobile shields whenever possible.

- Work no closer to the patient than necessary. Stay at least three feet away from the patient unless direct care is being given.

- Think about what you are doing. Conscientiously apply the principles of standard precautions for all patient care.

- A separate sink may be designated for handwashing. If so, use only this sink.

- The care plan, critical pathway, or radiation isolation sign will list where to find special safety precautions, including the maximum length of time to remain in the room. The radiation isolation sign is not an infection control sign. After the radioactive material has been given to the patient, he or she will be restricted under "Radiation Precautions." The sign bearing a radiation symbol (Figure 13-16) will be affixed to the door to the room. This sign has a black or magenta tri-blade on a white or yellow background, with the words "Caution: Radioactive Material." No one should enter the room without consulting medical, nursing, or radiation safety staff. Become familiar with the patient's individual precautions, and follow them carefully.

- Monitor the length of time visitors stay in the room. Make sure they do not stay beyond the specified time.

- The location of chairs and other furniture in the room will be specified to be a certain distance away from the patient. Do not move the furniture. Instruct visitors not to move the chairs closer to the patient.

- Explain the purpose of the mobile safety shield, and ask visitors to remain behind it.

- Do not allow pregnant women or children under the age of 18 into the radiation isolation room to visit.

- Follow facility policies for cleaning the room, and serving and removing meal trays. In many facilities, personnel from the dietary and housekeeping departments are not permitted to enter the room.

- Do not remove items from the room without permission from the radiation safety personnel.

- If a radiation source has become dislodged from the patient, avoid touching it. Ask visitors to leave the room. Try to move the source to a corner by using a tool, such as a yardstick. Inform the RN or radiation safety personnel.

- Find out if special precautions are necessary for handling soiled linens, tissues, or dressings.

- Strain all urine of patients who have brachytherapy seeds near the bladder. Some seeds may be lost through urination. Follow facility policies for straining urine in a catheter bag. In some facilities, careful visual inspection of the catheter bag is sufficient. If a seed is found, do not attempt to remove it. Inform the RN or radiation safety personnel.

- Place a small radioactive-labeled container in the patient's bathroom. Do not remove it. The container will be used to dispose of the dislodged seeds, if any.

- Follow the RN's instructions if you are directed to obtain a urine specimen after brachytherapy seeds have been implanted.

- Patients receiving certain types of therapy will require special urine collection. Bottles and special collection shields will be provided. Teach the patient to be responsible for urine collection, if possible. The urine collection bottles will be removed by radiation safety personnel.

- Notify the radiation safety personnel if there is a large spill of urine.

- Contaminated items must be incinerated if possible. A separate container will be used to discard these items, such as tissues, gauze sponges, shoe covers, and gloves.

- Use a separate, designated laundry bag for items that have been contaminated with body fluids, such as vomitus, incontinence, wound drainage, or profuse perspiration.

When the patient is discharged, you should:

- Discard disposable utensils, such as bedpans, urinals, and basins, with the radioactive waste.

- You will use the same permanent equipment items for the patient from admission until discharge. Wash them well with soap and running water. Radiation safety personnel must check the items before they are returned to floor stock.

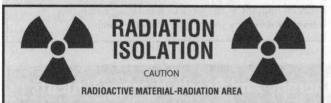

FIGURE 13-16 The radiation precautions sign has a black or magenta tri-blade on a white or yellow background, with the words "Caution: Radioactive Material." No one should enter the room without first consulting medical, nursing, or radiation safety staff.

(continued)

Guidelines for Working with Radiation Therapy and Brachytherapy Patients (Continued)

- Wear utility gloves when washing potentially contaminated equipment. When you have finished, wash the gloves with soap and water, then dry them before removing them. (This is the only exception to the rule that states you should never wash your gloved hands. It is a radiation precaution, not an infection control problem.)

- After the patient is discharged, the room will require special cleaning. Follow the radiation safety department's instructions. The room must not be used again until after it has been cleared by the radiation safety department.

CARING FOR THE PATIENT WHO IS RECEIVING IMMUNOTHERAPY

Immunotherapy is a treatment in which various biologic agents are given to alter the patient's immune response, to eliminate cancer. The vital signs must be regularly and closely monitored when these agents are given. Side effects of therapy usually cease within a week after beginning treatment. Care of the patient receiving immunotherapy involves:

- Monitoring vital signs every 2 to 4 hours, or as instructed
- Monitoring capillary refill
- Advising the patient to remain in bed if the systolic blood pressure is below 100, or according to the RN's instructions
- Weighing the patient daily and informing the RN of weight gain

Notify the RN promptly if the patient:

- Has fever or chills
- Has a pulse over 100, or respirations over 24
- Becomes cyanotic
- Is short of breath
- Is restless and/or apprehensive
- Has diarrhea, nausea, or vomiting
- Complains of itching

THE REHABILITATION SERVICES TEAM

As a PCT, you will be exposed to, work with, and assist many different types of therapists and individuals who are members of the rehabilitation team. Members of this team are listed in Table 13-3. This chart is not all-inclusive. Many other workers provide therapy and rehabilitation services, such as psychologists, dance therapists, and art thera-

pists. The positions listed here are the most common for rehabilitation workers in the health care facility.

Many hospitals are also beginning to offer CAM services. **Complementary** and **alternative medicine (CAM)** is a group of diverse systems, practices, and products that are not presently considered part of conventional medicine. This is an area of much research and scientific study. Because of this, practices listed as CAM change continually. New practices and techniques are always emerging. Some CAM practices have been proven unsafe or ineffective and are no longer used. Others have proven safe and effective and have moved into mainstream health care. Hospitals that offer alternative and complementary services will have additional types of therapists, such as those who provide acupuncture. **Acupuncture** (Figure 13-17) is a popular CAM therapy. It is an ancient practice dating back thousands of years that is used to treat

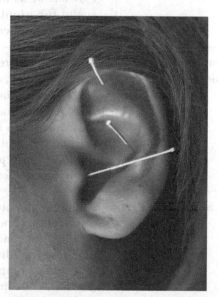

FIGURE 13-17 Acupuncture is used to treat many different conditions by correcting energy imbalances throughout the body. The needles are usually left in place from 5 to 20 minutes.

many acute and chronic conditions. Tiny, thin needles are placed in various parts of the body to correct imbalances in energy. It is safe and painless when done by a qualified practitioner.

The **rehabilitation team** emphasizes the uniqueness, value, and worth of all patients. The team includes workers from many professions, depending on the patient's individual needs. It is composed of licensed therapists, licensed and certified therapy assistants, restorative nurses, and restorative nursing assistants. The rehabilitation team begins to work with a patient early in the illness. This team evaluates and treats patients; designs rehabilitation and restorative programs; teaches the patient, facility staff, and family members; and serves as consultant when needed. You may be familiar with some rehabilitation (rehab) skills, such as range of motion, from your nursing assistant class. Your instructor will teach you procedures you will use if you will be expected to assist members of the rehabilitation team.

Table 13-3 Rehabilitation Team Members	
Type of Therapist	**Description of Licensure and Responsibilities**
Audiologist	A person with a degree, license, and certification in audiology (science of hearing) who measures hearing, identifies hearing loss, and participates in rehabilitation of hearing impairment. A certified audiologist will use the letters CCC-A or FAAA after his or her name.
Massage therapist	Massage therapists complete an intensive educational program. In the United States, the requirements vary from one state to the next. Most programs require more than 500 hours of education. Upon program completion, the therapist must pass written and skills examinations to be licensed by the state. Massage improves the function of the body's connective tissues and muscles by kneading and manipulation. It is believed to stimulate the immune system to fight disease.
Music therapist	An allied health service that uses principles similar to those underlying occupational therapy and physical therapy. The music therapist has a baccalaureate degree in music therapy. Although music therapy is an enjoyable activity, it is not done strictly for fun and games. Music therapy consists of using music to address physical, psychological, cognitive, and/or social functioning. Music therapy is relaxing and pleasurable to most people and is used successfully in the care of patients of all ages and disabilities.
Occupational therapist (OT)	A highly educated, licensed individual who evaluates and treats patients for self-care, work, and ADLs. OTs assess functioning in activities of everyday living that are essential for independent living, including dressing, bathing, grooming, meal preparation, writing, and driving. He or she modifies tasks and the environment to help the patient become independent. Occupational therapists are knowledgeable about using activity, exercise, splints, and positioning. The therapist helps prepare for the patient's discharge home, and makes arrangements for home modifications and adaptive devices, if necessary.
Physical therapist (PT)	A highly educated, licensed individual who prevents physical disability; uses physical methods to evaluate and treat pain, disease, and injury. He or she specializes in muscle development and motor coordination. Responsible for teaching mobility, ambulation, and transfers. The physical therapist evaluates and treats components of movement, including: muscle strength, muscle tone, posture, coordination, endurance, and general mobility. He or she develops and establishes an individualized treatment program to help the patient achieve functional independence.

(continues)

Table 13-3 Rehabilitation Team Members (Continued)

Type of Therapist	Description of Licensure and Responsibilities
Respiratory care practitioner (RCP) (also called respiratory therapist [RT])	Respiratory therapists have completed either a two-year associate's degree or a four-year baccalaureate degree. The RCP is a licensed professional who specializes in the care of patients with disorders of the cardiopulmonary system, respirations, and sleep disorders that affect the patient's breathing. The RCP will be highly involved in the care of patients with cardiac and respiratory problems and the specialized equipment used for treatment. Works with patients who have problems with oxygenation, and performs breathing treatments.
Social worker (LSW)	A licensed individual who works with normal and disturbed patients; he or she talks with patients and their families about emotional, social, or physical needs, and finds them support services. Within the hospital, the social worker counsels and assists in the emotional, social, environmental, and financial needs of the patient and family. He or she works as a liaison with other professionals, coordinates patient discharge from the hospital, and oversees contact with other services or organizations to ensure that the patient receives needed services in the community. The social worker helps facilitate the patient's reentry into family and community life.
Speech language pathologist (SLP) (may also be called speech therapist [ST])	A highly qualified, licensed professional who evaluates patients and plans, and directs care for patients who have problems with chewing, swallowing, speech, comprehension, communication, or memory loss. He or she evaluates the patient, develops a plan of care, and oversees the special techniques and skills used in helping patients who have communication and swallowing disorders.
Therapeutic recreation specialist (TRS)	Promotes the development of functional independence and helps patients develop and maintain an appropriate leisure lifestyle in consideration of their mental, physical, emotional, and/or social limitations. Some activities are designed to provide exercise. Others are developed to provide positive self-esteem. Activities reduce social isolation by providing opportunities for patients to socialize with others.

Rehabilitation versus Restorative Nursing Care

Rehabilitation and restorative care are based on a belief in the dignity and worth of each patient. Being dependent on others negatively affects self-esteem. Members of the rehabilitation team work to restore the patient to the highest level of independence possible (Figure 13-18). Each patient is a unique individual. Both services are designed to assist patients to attain and maintain the highest level of function possible. The maximum level is viewed in the context of the patient's individual needs. Restorative nursing care is given by nursing staff. Rehabilitation is skilled care given by licensed therapy staff and their assistants.

A patient's physical condition affects self-esteem and quality of life. Restorative nursing care is given 24 hours a day, 7 days a week. It is simply good, goal-oriented, hands-on nursing care that can be given in any setting. To be successful, all staff must be aware of the restorative program. Each time a restorative service is needed, the care given is in keeping with the restorative goals and approaches established by the interdisciplinary team. Keys to success of the restorative nursing program are:

- Consistency
- Continuity of care
- Good communication
- Use of the care plan or critical pathway

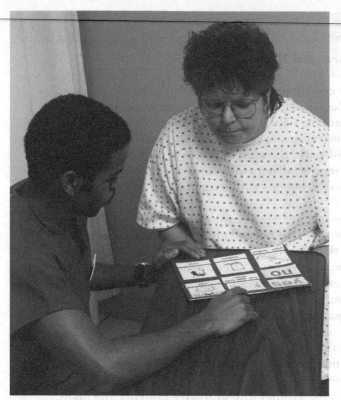

FIGURE 13-18 The PCT is using communication cards to communicate with an aphasic patient.

Consistency and continuity of care mean that all staff care for the patient in the same manner.

In contrast, rehabilitation is provided by licensed therapists. The goal of care is the same as restorative care. However, the skill level of the caregiver is higher. The care is more complex and specialized. Some facilities use the terms *rehabilitation* and *restoration* interchangeably. However, rehabilitation is really a higher level of care. It is always provided by licensed personnel. The terms *restoration, restorative care,* and *restorative nursing care* are interchangeable.

Rehabilitation is a program designed by a therapist to help patients regain lost skills or teach new skills. Therapists teach patients, families, and staff members techniques for reinforcing and maintaining what the patient has learned. Restorative nursing does not compete with skilled rehabilitation. Instead, it complements it. When you follow the restorative care plan, you reinforce what the therapists are teaching, and the patient masters the skill more quickly. The restorative approach provides continuity of care. This is because many nursing staff members are working on the same goals. They are using the same approaches to the patient's problems. The patient benefits from the continuity and consistency. Most progress quickly when restorative care is given.

Principles of Rehabilitation and Restoration

The principles of rehabilitation and restoration are the same, and apply to all patients. They are:

- Begin treatment early (**Figure 13-19**). Starting restorative care early in the disease or admission will improve the outcome.

- Activity strengthens and inactivity weakens. Keep the patient as active as possible, considering his or her medical condition. Encourage patients to be as independent as possible. For example, giving passive range-of-motion exercises prevents deformities and complications. However, active range-of-motion exercises done by the patient will prevent deformities *and strengthen muscles.*

- Prevent further disability. Follow the care plan to prevent injury and deformity. Practice safety.

- Stress the patient's ability and not the disability. Emphasizing what the patient can do gives the patient confidence and provides hope. Instead of saying, "You cannot use your right arm," say, "You can use your left arm."

- Treat the whole person. You have learned that you cannot isolate the medical problem from the rest of the person. Consider all of the patient's strengths and needs. Use and build on the strengths to overcome the needs. Communicate strengths, so others can use them to help the patient as well.

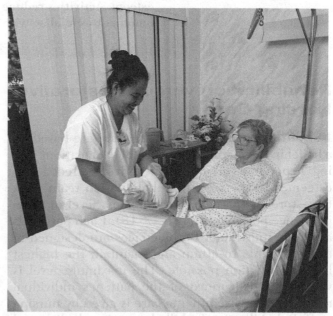

FIGURE 13-19 Patients who have had an amputation benefit from early treatment.

The care plan or critical pathway will guide you in the approaches to use. If you discover something that works for the patient, inform the RN. He or she will add it to the care plan so that all staff are aware of it. Good communication is also an important part of restorative nursing care.

THE PAIN PROBLEM

Many facilities have made a commitment to ensuring pain relief. These facilities consider pain to be the "fifth vital sign." Pain is regularly and frequently evaluated. Pain is a major preventable public health problem that slows recovery in individuals with acute illness, and increases health care costs. Relieving pain has always been an important nursing responsibility. Nursing staff must identify patients who are having pain, and those who are at risk for pain, then take the appropriate action(s) to ensure that all patients are made as comfortable as possible.

Evaluating Pain

Pain affects well-being and quality of life. Patients have the right to timely pain assessment and management. Many factors affect patients' reactions to pain. The reactions may be different from one moment to the next, and one patient to the next. Four types of pain are listed in Table 13-4. Monitor the patients' body language for signs of pain (Figure 13-20). Regularly ask patients if they are in pain. Some will not volunteer this information if not asked directly. Some patients will moan or grimace during transfers or movement. Confused patients may cry or yell out. This may be interpreted as confusion instead of pain.

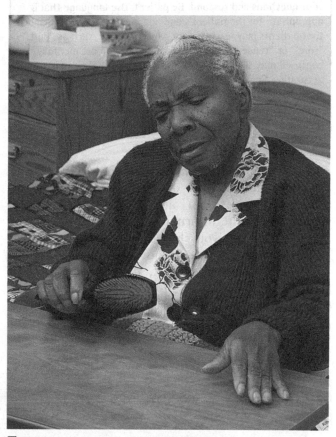

FIGURE 13-20 Monitor the patient's facial expression and body language for signs of pain.

Table 13-4 Types of Pain	
Type of Pain	**Description**
Acute pain	Occurs suddenly and without warning. Acute pain is usually the result of tissue damage, caused by conditions such as injury or surgery. Typically, acute pain decreases over time, as healing takes place.
Persistent pain	Persistent pain that lasts longer than six months. (Another, older term for this type of pain is *chronic pain*.) It may be intermittent or constant. Persistent pain may be caused by multiple medical conditions.
Phantom pain	Phantom pain occurs as a result of an amputation. The patient has had a body part, such as a leg, removed, but complains of pain in the toes of the missing limb. The pain is real, not imaginary.
Radiating pain	Radiating pain moves from the site of origin to other areas. For example, when a patient is having a heart attack, the pain may radiate from the chest to the jaw or arm.

COMMUNICATION ALERT

When asking patients about pain, make sure the patient can see and hear you. Allow enough time for the patient to process your questions and respond. Be patient. Use language that is appropriate for the patient's age and mental status. Remember that patients may use different words for pain, such as "hurt," "sore," or "tender." Children and patients who are mentally confused may surprise you. Some can describe their pain accurately. Some will admit to having pain only if you ask them directly, so do not omit this important step. Always ask patients who are crying, those whose body language suggests pain, and those whose behavior suggests pain.

A nursing assessment of pain involves many different factors. Your observations contribute to the RN's assessment and patients' well-being. Other important information you may see, hear, and observe that you should report to the RN are listed in the Observe & Report box.

Always remember that, despite outward appearances, *the patient's self-report of pain is the most accurate indicator of the existence and intensity of pain,* and should be respected and believed. Avoid making assumptions about a patient's pain.

Constipation

Constipation is a common side effect of pain medication, particularly narcotic medications. Many side effects go away over time, but constipation is an ongoing problem. Monitor the patient's bowel activity carefully and document it on the flow sheet. If the patient uses the bathroom without assistance, do not be embarrassed to ask whether he or she has had a bowel movement each day. Problems can become very serious if not carefully monitored. Encourage patients to eat fiber foods on trays, drink liquids, and be as active as possible in keeping with the plan of care. Report patient complaints or signs of constipation to the nurse. Inform the RN if the patient has not had a BM in three days.

PAIN MANAGEMENT PROCEDURES

Patients may be admitted to the hospital for pain management. Intermittent and continuous medication infusion may be used to manage pain after major surgery, or when the patient has cancer

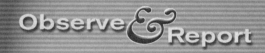

Pain Observations

- Change in vital signs
- Change in body language, facial expressions, or behavior
- Verbal expressions of pain, such as crying or moaning
- Change in skin color
- Location of pain (specific site of pain on the body)
- Radiation, if any (movement of pain to other areas)
- Time of onset (when the pain began)
- Duration (how long the pain lasts)
- Frequency (how often it occurs)
- Pain quality (nature and type of pain)
- Pain intensity (strength and description of pain, in the patient's own words)
- Aggravating and alleviating factors (things that improve or worsen the pain)
- Character (properties, features, characteristics)
- Variation or patterns of pain (changes in pain or cycles of pain)

- Pain management history, if any (things the patient tells you about past history of pain and things that make it better or worse)
- Present pain management regimen, if any, and its effectiveness (things the patient does to relieve pain, including response to comfort measures and medications)
- Effect of pain on activities of daily living, sleep, appetite, relationships, emotions, concentration, and so on
- Direct observation of abnormalities at the site of the pain
- Other observations, such as facial expressions, body language, movements, nausea or vomiting
- Side effects of analgesic (pain-relieving) medications, if applicable
- Response to pain medications and other forms of treatment, if applicable

or another chronic, painful condition. Pain management may be provided by a combination of methods:

- Oral medications
- Injectable medications
- Intravenous medications
- Implanted medication pumps
- Other implanted devices
- Transcutaneous electrical nerve stimulation (TENS)

Other approaches, such as massage, physical therapy, and alternative treatments such as acupuncture, may also be provided in combination with nursing comfort measures. Patients receive regular pain medications, and the medication regimen is adjusted until the patient receives the maximum benefit. Patients are more willing to participate in their care plans when they are not having pain, and are usually more satisfied with their care.

Pain Management with an Epidural Catheter

Continuous medication infusion may be used to manage pain after major thoracic, abdominal, and orthopedic surgery. This therapy works by blocking transmission of pain at the spinal cord. Patients receiving **continuous epidural analgesia** receive stable, consistent doses of pain medication rather than experiencing the peaks and valleys associated with most other pain control methods.

An epidural catheter is implanted under the patient's skin. It is inserted into the epidural space near the spinal cord (**Figure 13-21**). Medication is administered either intermittently or continuously through the catheter into the epidural space. Narcotic pain-relieving medications and local anesthetics are usually given together, but either drug can be given individually. The patient may have leg numbness and weakness for the first 24 hours after the catheter is inserted. Limited mobility in areas not affected by the medication and decreased

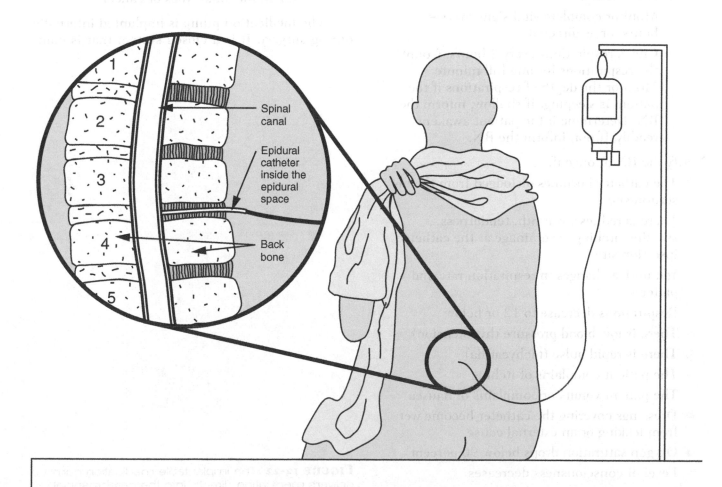

FIGURE 13-21 The epidural catheter is used for intermittent or constant pain medication.

blood pressure when rising from bed are also common reactions.

Patient Care. Instruct the patient to call for assistance in getting out of bed. Other routine PCT procedures are:

- Elevate the head of the bed 30° or 40°.
- Monitor the vital signs frequently. For the first 24 hours:
  - Check blood pressure and pulse at least every hour for the first 2 hours after the catheter is inserted, then every 2 hours for 24 hours.
  - Monitor temperature every 4 hours.
  - Check respirations *every hour*. Count the respirations for one full minute. Monitor the depth of respirations if the patient is sleeping. If shallow, inform the RN. Determine if the patient awakens readily. If not, inform the RN.
- After 24 hours,
  - Monitor complete vital signs every 4 hours, or as directed.
  - Check respirations every 2 hours. Count the respirations for one full minute. Monitor the depth of respirations if the patient is sleeping. If shallow, inform the RN. Determine if the patient awakens readily. If not, inform the RN.

Notify the RN at once if:

- The catheter becomes dislodged from the insertion site
- There is redness, warmth, tenderness, swelling, itching, or drainage at the catheter insertion site
- You notice changes in respiration rate and pattern
- Respirations decrease to 12 or below
- There is low blood pressure (hypotension)
- There is rapid pulse (tachycardia)
- The patient complains of itching
- The patient vomits or complains of nausea
- Dressings covering the catheter become wet from leaking or an external cause
- Oxygen saturation drops below 90 percent
- Level of consciousness decreases
- There is urinary retention (the patient complains of a need to urinate, but cannot)

- Hives appear
- The patient complains of inability to move the legs
- The patient complains of severe low back pain
- The patient complains of change in sensation or motor function

Implantable Medication Pumps

Implantable medication pumps are sometimes used for long-term medication delivery, in both adults and children. The pumps are surgically placed under the abdominal skin. A tiny catheter is threaded under the skin from the pump to the spine (Figure 13-22). Medications are infused directly into the cerebrospinal fluid. This type of therapy has become common for patients with:

- Chronic, severe pain
- Severe spasticity (sudden, frequent, involuntary muscle contractions that impair function)
- Treatment for some types of cancer

The medication pump is implanted internally during surgery. It is a closed system that is com-

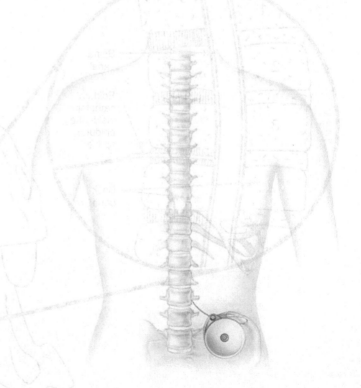

FIGURE 13-22 The implantable medication pump delivers medication directly into the cerebrospinal fluid. (Courtesy of Medtronic, Minneapolis, MN; (800) 505-5000)

pletely under the skin, with no external parts. The patient will have two surgical sites: one on the abdomen and a smaller one near the spine. A physician or specially educated RN will use a programming computer (**Figure 13-23**) to adjust the medication dose gradually until the desired response is achieved.

The patient may remain on bedrest for 2 to 20 hours after surgery, depending on physician preference and patient response. An abdominal binder (Chapter 5) may be used after surgery. The RN may instruct you to apply a cool application or ice pack (Chapter 12) to the site where the catheter tunnels under the skin. Some physicians permit patients to resume normal activity immediately, if they are able. If you are assisting the patient with transfers, *avoid using the transfer belt until the surgical insertion site is well healed.* This restriction usually lasts for several months after surgery, according to the physician's order and facility policy. In some facilities, a wide transfer belt is always used (even after the insertion site has healed) for these patients to prevent pressure on the pump or surgical site.

Patients with newly implanted medication pumps may have a complicated medication regimen in which they slowly withdraw from oral medications and depend increasingly on medications administered through the pump. Notify the RN if the patient:

- Has decreased responsiveness
- Has respirations of 12 or below
- Has a temperature of more then 100°F orally
- Complains of headache
- Experiences fluid leakage
- Develops a collection of blood or fluid under the skin at the insertion site
- Has redness, warmth, tenderness, swelling, itching, or drainage at the surgical sites
- Complains of a feeling of tightness over the pump site
- Is unable to move the legs
- Has sudden loss of bowel or bladder control

Monitor the patient for changes in neurological status, breakthrough pain, and dehiscence in the postoperative period. **Dehiscence** is splitting or gaping open of the suture line. The greatest risk is infection. Although it may occur in anyone, patients who are in poor health, those with poor nutrition, and those who are small in stature are at greatest risk of postoperative infections. With an implanted pump, this can be quite serious, because the location of the catheter provides a direct passageway to the brain. Because of this, careful monitoring and observation are necessary. Meningitis and other brain infections may develop, but these complications are rare. Change the dressings as ordered. Always use sterile technique for this procedure.

The implanted medication pump in the patient's abdomen will sound an alarm if the flow of medication is interrupted, or the chamber is low or empty. The alarm will sound every 15 minutes until it is turned off by computer. You will not be able to silence the sound. Medication disruption is a potentially serious condition. The patient could experience drug withdrawal and other complications, including high fever, seizures, and death, if the drug is suddenly withdrawn.

Precautions. The patient should not engage in activities involving altitude, pressure, or temperature changes. This includes exposure to a very hot environment or hot water. These changes can cause the pump to alter the amount of medication dispensed, which creates the potential for underdose or overdose.

Most pumps are not compatible with MRIs. Temporary disruption of therapy may occur with

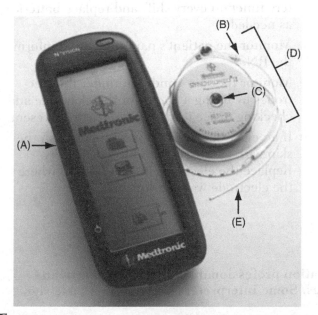

FIGURE 13-23 A computer sets the dosage and time for medication infusion. The dosage can be varied or constant throughout the day. The computer shows how much medication is left in the pump, and when it has to be filled. An alarm will sound if the pump volume is low. Parts of the computer include the: (A) programming computer; (B) plastic connector; (C) Medication refill port; (D) implantable pump and (E) spinal catheter. (Courtesy of Medtronic, Minneapolis, MN; (800) 505-5000)

MRI exposure. Check with the RN before sending the patient for an MRI. A CT scan should not interfere with pump activity. If the MRI is essential, the physician must make provisions to check the pump with the programming computer and ensure that it is working properly immediately after the procedure. The MRI may turn the pump off completely, so it must be checked promptly to prevent medication withdrawal and other complications.

The patient may complain of pain if tight pants (such as jeans) or an elastic waistband is positioned directly over the pump. A tight waistband also has the potential to obstruct or break the spinal catheter or its connector. Position the waist of the pants above or below the pump. Let the patient's comfort guide you. If the pants are uncomfortable in relation to the pump, readjust them.

If a patient with a pump dies, the funeral home must be informed about the implanted medication pump. If cremation is planned, the pump must be removed. The patient will have a pump identification card. This should be given to the funeral home. If the card is not available, supply the pump manufacturer's contact information. The manufacturer will provide information regarding pump removal, and furnish a mailer so that the funeral home can return the pump to the manufacturer.

Transcutaneous Electrical Nerve Stimulation

Transcutaneous electrical nerve stimulation (TENS) is a nondrug method of managing pain. Mild, harmless electrical current stimulates nerve fibers to block transmission of pain to the brain. Electrodes are taped to the patient's skin. The location of the electrodes is determined by the area of pain. The electrodes are attached to wires in a con-

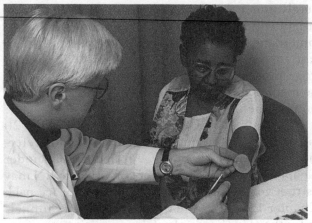

FIGURE 13-24 A TENS unit is used to relieve pain.

trol box (Figure 13-24). The RN (or the patient) will adjust the intensity of stimulation on the control box.

PCT responsibilities in caring for a patient with a TENS unit are:

- Check the unit each shift to make sure that the lead wires are connected to the electrodes and stimulator.
- A light on the TENS unit blinks when the device is functioning properly. Check the battery function every shift and replace batteries as needed.
- Monitor the patient's pain relief, and inform the RN.
- Monitor the skin condition under the electrodes by lifting a corner of the electrode and checking to see if irritation or rash is present.
- If an electrode becomes detached, wash the skin with gentle soap and water. Pat dry. Replace the electrode in proximity to where the electrode was previously.

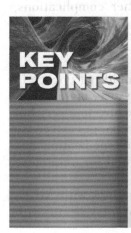

KEY POINTS

▶ An interpreter is a communication professional who mediates between speakers of different languages. Some interpreters speak. Others use sign language to communicate.

▶ A qualified interpreter is very familiar with the language, cultural values, beliefs, gestures, body language, and verbal and nonverbal expressions used in the languages he or she is interpreting.

▶ Domestic violence against women is a pattern of forced behaviors that may include repeated battering and injury, psychological abuse, sexual assault, progressive social isolation, deprivation, and intimidation.

▶ Domestic violence is a deliberate means of controlling another person.

(continues)

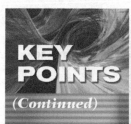

KEY POINTS
(Continued)

▶ The key elements of domestic abuse are intimidation, humiliation of the victim, and physical injury.

▶ Helping to identify signs of domestic violence is a way of supporting the patient. The PCT is responsible for monitoring patients for signs and symptoms of domestic violence. If recognized, report signs of domestic violence to the RN, who depends on the accuracy of the PCT's observations.

▶ Delirium is an acute confusional state caused by reversible medical problems. It is common in the elderly.

▶ Any change in a patient's mental status is significant.

▶ A seizure is a sudden, spontaneous episode of excessive and scrambled electrical activity caused by interference with impulses in the brain. Seizures disrupt the patient's ability to control physical processes, interfere with mental and behavioral processes, and cause changes in awareness, body movements, sensations, and/or emotions.

▶ An aura is a sensation, smell, taste, or bright light that precedes the onset of a seizure.

▶ Status epilepticus is a serious medical emergency that may result in death. It is a seizure that lasts for a long time, or repeats without recovery.

▶ Seizure precautions are individualized measures that keep the patient safe during an unexpected seizure.

▶ Paralysis is loss of movement and impairment of various parts of the body. It develops immediately below the level of spinal cord injury, and affects sensation and voluntary movement.

▶ Paraplegia is paralysis of the lower half of the body, including both legs. Bowel and bladder control are also lost.

▶ Tetraplegia (quadriplegia) is paralysis affecting the arms and legs.

▶ Flaccid paralysis involves loss of muscle tone and absence of tendon reflexes.

▶ Spastic paralysis is a condition in which there is no voluntary movement. The extremities move in an involuntary pattern, similar to intense muscle spasms. The patient is aware of the movements, but cannot stop them.

▶ Autonomic dysreflexia is a potentially life-threatening complication of spinal cord injury that commonly develops in patients with injuries above the mid-thoracic area.

▶ Problems that seem minor can trigger autonomic dysreflexia. As a rule, injuries that would normally cause pain below the level of spinal cord damage will trigger this condition. Bladder problems are the most common cause.

▶ Chemotherapy is the use of medications or drugs to destroy cancer. It cannot differentiate cancer cells from other cells, so healthy cells may also be destroyed.

▶ Radiation therapy involves the use of high-energy, ionizing beams at the site of a cancer to destroy the cancerous tissue without damaging healthy tissue.

▶ Brachytherapy is a form of radiation therapy in which tiny radioactive seeds or pellets are implanted directly inside the body.

(continues)

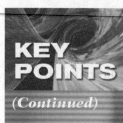

▶ A radiation isolation sign is not an infection control sign. It lists where to find special safety precautions, including the maximum length of time to remain in the radiation therapy patient's room.

▶ Women who are pregnant and children under the age of 18 must not enter a room where radiation therapy is being given.

▶ Provide necessary care, but try to minimize time spent with the radiation therapy patient.

▶ Immunotherapy is a cancer treatment that involves the use of biologic agents to alter the patient's immune response and eliminate cancer.

▶ The rehabilitation team includes workers from many professions, depending on the patient's individual needs. Team members include licensed therapists, licensed and certified therapy assistants, restorative nurses, and restorative nursing assistants.

▶ The rehabilitation team begins to work with patients early in the illness. They will evaluate and treat patients; design rehabilitation and restorative programs; teach the patient, facility staff, and family members; and serve as consultants when needed.

▶ Rehabilitation and restorative nursing care are based on a belief in the dignity and worth of each patient.

▶ Being dependent on others negatively affects self-esteem.

▶ Members of the rehabilitation team work to restore the patient to the highest level of independence possible.

▶ Restorative nursing care is good, hands-on nursing care that is given 24 hours a day, in any setting.

▶ Keys to success of the restorative nursing program are consistency, continuity of care, good communication, and using the care plan or critical pathway.

▶ Pain is considered the fifth vital sign. It is a major preventable public health problem that slows recovery and increases health care costs.

▶ Identifying patients who are having pain, and those who are at risk for pain, then taking the appropriate action(s) to make patients comfortable are important nursing responsibilities.

▶ Constipation is a common side effect of pain medication, particularly narcotic medications. Other side effects go away over time, but constipation is an ongoing problem. Monitoring and documenting the patient's bowel activity are important PCT responsibilities.

▶ Implantable medication pumps are surgically placed under the abdominal skin, and are used for long-term medication delivery.

▶ Avoid using a transfer belt on a patient who has an implantable medication pump until the surgical insertion site is well healed.

▶ Continuous epidural analgesia is the intermittent or continuous infusion of pain medication through a catheter into the epidural space.

▶ Transcutaneous electrical nerve stimulation is a nondrug method of managing pain by directing mild, harmless electrical current into nerve fibers to block transmission of pain to the brain.

CLINICAL APPLICATIONS

1. Mr. Hoover is a 76-year-old confused patient. He ambulates in his room and is normally pleasant and talkative, although he does not always make sense. He recognizes you as his primary caregiver. Mr. Hoover uses the urinal for elimination. When you enter his room to give AM care, you find him sleeping in the chair, which is unusual. His skin is hot to the touch, and he is lethargic. He is much more confused than usual. You notice his urinal on the floor next to his chair. The urine in the urinal is reddish and has mucus threads in it. What should you do? What do his signs and symptoms suggest?

2. Mrs. Bugee is a 26-year-old mother of a 3-year-old daughter who was admitted to your unit for complications of a new pregnancy. She tells you that the sonogram shows she is having a boy, whom they have decided to name after her husband. Mrs. Bugee is on bedrest. Last night she did not eat her main dish. When you asked if she wanted a substitute, her husband said, "She doesn't like the food. She wants a hamburger, but she is getting so fat that it won't hurt her to skip a meal." The patient said nothing, and you forgot about it. Today, you noticed bruises in various stages of healing on both the patient's arms. She said, "I ran into a door at home in the dark." Her husband visits again, and you hear him criticizing the patient. He says, "You had better not lose my namesake or else." The patient is crying quietly. When her husband leaves, you ask if she needs anything. She apologized for crying and says, "I just feel so ashamed that I am such a bother, and just don't know where to turn." What do you think the problem is? How can you help this patient? What action will you take?

3. An interpreter has been assisting you in communicating with Mrs. Shams, a 73-year-old resident of Pakistan who became ill while visiting her daughter in your city. The patient wears a long nightgown when in bed and pulls the covers up to her neck if a male staff member enters the room. The patient does not speak English, and no interpreter is available right now. You are assigned to walk her in the hallway to the shower room. How will you explain the procedures to the patient? What are the cultural considerations of walking this patient to the shower room?

4. Mrs. Kowalek is a nursing home resident who was admitted to your unit with a diagnosis of transient ischemic attack. Her daughter tells you that the patient previously spoke English, but stopped after she had her first stroke several years ago. The patient is crying and trying to speak with you in her native language. You do not understand what she is trying to say. She keeps saying something that sounds like, "Mosca wudja." No interpreter is available. However, you know another patient who speaks this patient's language. That patient has Stage I Alzheimer's disease, but can communicate and responds appropriately to your questions when you care for him. Someone tells you that there may be a bilingual worker who speaks Polish in the housekeeping department. What action will you take?

5. Mr. Farago is a quadriplegic who has been admitted to your unit. He has an indwelling catheter and is out of bed much of the day. The care plan states that he should return to bed for an hour after each meal, but he refuses to lie down. He says it is "too much trouble," and he prefers to be up. He operates an electric wheelchair with one finger, and has limited use of his arm. He has been up in the chair all day when you take his 4:00 p.m. vital signs. They are 99.2°F (PO)-96-18-254/168. The patient's face is flushed. Upon questioning, he says, "I feel OK," and wants to stay up until after supper. What action will you take? What do you think is causing his signs and symptoms?

6. Mrs. Carswell is an obese patient who was admitted to your unit after surgery to implant a medication pump in her abdomen to treat persistent pain. She has post polio syndrome and needs help with transfers. She cannot ambulate. The patient is up in the chair and asks you to help her with toileting. You realize that you cannot transfer the patient by yourself. How will you assist this patient?

Multiple-Choice Questions

Select the one best answer.

1. Delirium is:
   a. a sign of mental illness.
   b. caused by reversible medical problems.
   c. a sign of cognitive impairment.
   d. caused by autonomic dysreflexia.

2. Signs and symptoms of delirium are:
   a. abdominal pain and nausea.
   b. mental confusion and memory impairment.
   c. pain, pallor, and paralysis.
   d. headache and sore throat.

3. The RN informs you that Mr. Gianassi's condition is exacerbated by certain inhalants, including cigarette smoke. This means that the inhalants will cause the medical problem to:
   a. improve.
   b. worsen.
   c. stabilize.
   d. become unstable.

4. The key elements of domestic abuse include all of the following *except*:
   a. intimidation.
   b. humiliation.
   c. alcoholism.
   d. physical injury.

5. The abusive domestic partner will often:
   a. isolate the victim from others.
   b. seek medical care for the injured partner.
   c. leave the room when the RN assesses the patient.
   d. care for the patient himself.

6. The interpreter is responsible for:
   a. assisting with all complex patient care.
   b. staying with a patient when he or she is lonely.
   c. teaching the staff how to speak the patient's language.
   d. facilitating communication between the patient and others.

7. An interpreter is:
   a. a low-level worker.
   b. a communications professional.
   c. at the facility 24 hours a day.
   d. always a U.S. citizen.

8. A patient tells you that she sometimes smells roses before having a seizure. This is most probably a/an:
   a. aura.
   b. hallucination.
   c. delusion.
   d. catastrophic reaction.

9. A seizure is a/an:
   a. insignificant event.
   b. incident.
   c. serious medical emergency.
   d. accident.

10. Staring, blinking, or stopping what the patient is doing are signs of:
    a. a tonic-clonic seizure.
    b. an absence seizure.
    c. a myoclonic seizure.
    d. status epilepticus.

11. Seizure precautions are:
    a. methods of preventing a seizure.
    b. highly technical nursing skills.
    c. emergency measures to use during a seizure.
    d. methods of keeping a seizure patient safe.

12. A patient with paraplegia has:
    a. paralysis of the legs.
    b. paralysis of the legs and arms.
    c. bowel and bladder control.
    d. problems controlling secretions.

13. A patient with tetraplegia has:
    a. paralysis of the legs.
    b. paralysis of the legs and arms.
    c. bowel and bladder control.
    d. problems controlling secretions.

14. Spastic paralysis is a/an:
    a. voluntary movement.
    b. lower motor neuron disorder.
    c. involuntary movement.
    d. indication that muscle tone has returned.

15. The most common causes of autonomic dysreflexia are related to:
    a. bladder problems.
    b. unstable temperature.
    c. systemic infection.
    d. constipation.

16. Chemotherapy involves the use of:
    a. radiation to destroy cancer.
    b. biologic agents to change the immune system.
    c. tiny radioactive seeds and pellets.
    d. medications to destroy cancer.

17. Common side effects of chemotherapy include:
    a. unstable blood pressure and seizures.
    b. alopecia and loss of appetite.
    c. blood clots from increased platelets.
    d. flatus and constipation.

18. Radiation therapy markings on the patient's skin should be:
    a. left alone.
    b. removed with alcohol.
    c. scrubbed off each day with soap.
    d. treated with lotion every shift.

19. Patients who are receiving chemotherapy and radiation therapy:
    a. may not have visitors who are under the age of 18.
    b. must wear a mask when out of their rooms.
    c. may excrete drugs or radiation in their urine.
    d. are usually placed in strict airborne precautions.

20. A dosimeter is commonly used to measure the:
    a. dosage of drugs given to the patient.
    b. PCT's exposure to radiation.
    c. patient's maximum dose of brachytherapy.
    d. distance from the radiation source to your body.

21. A patient who is in radiation isolation:
    a. has an infectious disease.
    b. is receiving chemotherapy.
    c. has radioactive devices in his or her room.
    d. should not have visitors who are under the age of 18.

22. Brachytherapy involves:
    a. implanting radioactive seeds inside the body.
    b. placing thin needles in various parts of the body.
    c. treating a patient for bradycardia with drugs.
    d. complementary and alternative treatments.

23. Rehabilitation and restorative nursing care are:
    a. highly skilled services that are given only by licensed personnel.
    b. used only for patients with stroke, trauma-related injuries, and physical disorders.
    c. duplicative services that compete with each other.
    d. given to assist patients to attain and maintain their highest level of function.

24. The principles of rehabilitation and restorative nursing include:
    a. doing as much as possible for patients who have physical limitations.
    b. stressing the patient's ability and not the disability.
    c. making sure the patient rests at least 23 hours a day.
    d focusing only on the patients' diagnoses and medical conditions.

25. All of the following are true about pain *except:*
    a. Pain is a major preventable public health problem.
    b. Pain is the responsibility of licensed personnel.
    c. Pain slows recovery in individuals with acute illness.
    d. Pain increases health care costs.

26. Phantom pain:
    a. is the result of an amputation.
    b. is imaginary pain.
    c. is similar to an aura.
    d. moves away from the site of origin.

27. Persistent pain:
    a. results from an acute injury.
    b. is caused by an amputation.
    c. moves about the body.
    d. lasts more than six months.

28. The most accurate indicator of the presence and intensity of pain is/are:
    a. based on a nursing assessment.
    b. abnormal vital signs.
    c. the patient's self-report.
    d. abnormal body language.

29. When providing postoperative care for the patient with a newly implanted epidural catheter, you should:
    a. elevate the head of the bed 30° to 40°.
    b. monitor the respirations every 4 hours.
    c. check the temperature every hour.
    d. encourage the patient to resume normal activity.

30. When caring for a patient who uses a TENS unit, you should:
    a. rotate the electrodes every shift.
    b. remove the adhesive by scrubbing with alcohol.
    c. lift a corner of the electrode to check the skin.
    d. check the power light to make sure it is not blinking.

EXPLORING THE WEB

About.com	http://nursing.about.com
Accucare Pain Medicine	http://www.accucarepainmedicine.com
Acute Delirium	http://www.neuroland.com
Advance for Nursing	http://www.advancefornurses.com
Ambulation Program for Restorative Nursing	http://www.mpcrf.org
American Academy of Pain Medicine	http://www.painmed.org
American Association of Neuroscience Nurses	http://www.aann.org
American Cancer Society	http://www.cancer.org
American Epilepsy Society	http://www.aesnet.org
American Occupational Therapy Organization	http://www.aota.org
American Physical Therapy Association	http://www.apta.org
Association of Rehabilitation Nurses	http://www.rehabnurse.org
Autonomic Dysreflexia	http://www.noah-health.org
Autonomic Dysreflexia	http://www.spinalcord.org
Autonomic Dysreflexia (Hyperreflexia)	http://calder.med.miami.edu
Autonomic Dysreflexia Resources	http://www.spinalcord.uab.edu
Breast Cancer Awareness Crusade	http://www.avoncompany.com
Canadian Breast Cancer Network	http://www.cbcn.ca
Cancer Clinical Services Quality Assurance Project	http://qap.sdsu.edu
Cancer Immunity	http://www.nlm.nih.gov
Cancer News	http://www.cancernews.com
Cancer Risk Assessment	http://users.rcn.com
CancerEducation.com	http://www.cancereducation.com
CancerFacts.com	http://www.cancerfacts.com
CancerPage.com	http://www.cancerpage.com
CancerSource.com	http://www.cancersource.com
CancerTrack	http://www.cancertrack.com
CancerWeb	http://cancerweb.ncl.ac.uk
City of Hope Mayday Pain Resource Center	http://www.cityofhope.org
Combined Health Information Database	http://chid.nih.gov
Cultural Profiles Project	http://cwr.utoronto.ca
Delirium	http://www.clevelandclinicmeded.com
Delirium	http://www.mentalhealth.com
Diagnostic Medical Exposures: Advice on Exposure to Ionizing Radiation During Pregnancy	http://www.hpa.org.uk

Documenting Domestic Violence: How Health Care Providers Can Help Victims	http://www.ncjrs.org
Domestic Violence Policies and Procedures	http://www.4nursingmanagers.com
Domestic Violence: The Challenge for Nursing	http://www.nursingworld.org
Electronic Journal of Oncology	http://elecjoncol.org
Epilepsy Action	http://www.epilepsy.org.uk
Epilepsy Foundation	http://www.epilepsyfoundation.org
EthnoMed	http://ethnomed.org
Everything Spinal	http://www.everythingspinal.com
The Fifth Vital Sign	http://www.advancefornurses.com (See past articles 2/4/02)
Gait Belt Procedure	http://www.texashste.com
General Comfort Questionnaire	http://www.uakron.edu
The Implications of Service Animals in Health Care Settings (APIC State-of-the-Art Report)	http://www.apic.org
Information on the Intrathecal Baclofen Program for Spasticity	http://www.drbarolat.com
Intelihealth Pain Scales	http://www.intelihealth.com
International Cancer Alliance	http://www.icare.org
Jabboury Foundation for Cancer Research	http://www.jabboury.org
JNCI Cancer Spectrum	http://jncicancerspectrum.oupjournals.org
The Management of Acute, Chronic and Cancer Pain	http://www.asahq.org
Management of Chronic Pain in Older Persons (American Geriatrics Society)	http://www.americangeriatrics.org
Medline Plus	http://www.nlm.nih.gov
Medtronic Pain Therapies	http://www.medtronic.com
Medtronic SynchroMed II Programmable Infusion System	http://www.medtronic.com
Merck Manual—Delirium	http://www.merck.com
Movement Disorder Virtual University	http://www.mdvu.org
National Cancer Institute	http://www.cancer.gov
National Foundation for Cancer Research	http://www.researchforacure.com
OncoLink	http://www.oncolink.com
Oncology Nursing	http://www.jcjc.cc.ms.us
Oncology Nursing Society	http://ons.org
Oncology Tools	http://www.fda.gov
Oregon Health & Science University Hematology and Medical Oncology Division	http://www.ohsu.edu
Pain in Children and Adults	http://www.nursing.uiowa.edu
Pain Management: TENS and Electrothermal Therapy	http://my.webmd.com

Pain.com	http://www.pain.com
Physical Therapist Online	http://physicaltherapist.com
Physical Therapy Clinical Toolbox	http://physicaltherapy.about.com
Rehabilitation Nursing—What? Why? How?	http://www.rcna.org.au
Restorative Nursing PowerPoint Presentation	http://www.michigan.gov
RobertsReview	http://www.robertsreview.com
Screening for Delirium, Dementia, and Depression in Older Adults	http://www.rnao.org
Spasticity	http://www.mdvu.org
Spasticity: Take Charge of Your Options	http://www.medtronic.com
Spinal Cord Injuries	http://www.spinalcordinjuries.net
Spinal Cord Injury Complications: Autonomic Dysreflexia	http://lifecenter.rehabchicago.org
Spinal Cord Injury Information Network	http://www.spinalcord.uab.edu
Spinal Cord Injury Nursing Care	http://www.muw.edu
Spinal Cord Injury: Treatment Advances and Rehabilitation	http://www.onlinece.net
Transcultural and Multicultural Health Care	http://www.iun.edu
Transcutaneous Electrical Nerve Stimulation (TENS)	http://www.spineuniverse.com
Trauma Nursing: Intimate Partner Violence	http://www.rnweb.com
University of Maryland Shock Trauma Manual (spinal cord injuries)	http://safetycenter.umm.edu
Violence Against Women Document Library	http://www.vaw.umn.edu
What Is "Autonomic Dysreflexia"?	http://www.northeastrehab.com

CHAPTER
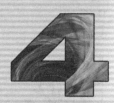

Respiratory Procedures

OBJECTIVES:

After reading this chapter, you should be able to:

- Spell and define key terms.
- Identify the effects of carbon dioxide buildup in the body.
- List six conditions that cause the patient to be at high risk of poor oxygenation.
- State the purpose of checking capillary refill.
- Describe how the pulse oximeter works.
- State the purpose of oxygen therapy.
- List the components of an oxygen delivery system, and describe the purpose of each.
- Describe the care of patients who are receiving oxygen therapy.
- List safety precautions for oxygen administration.
- List the indications and contraindications for oropharyngeal and nasopharyngeal airways.
- State the purpose of suctioning.
- State the purpose of a small-volume nebulizer treatment.
- State the purpose of CPAP and BiPAP therapy.
- State the purpose of postural drainage and describe the positions used.

- Nose
- Pharynx (throat)
- Larynx (voicebox)
- Trachea (windpipe)
- Bronchi
- Lungs

COMMUNICATION ALERT

Oxygen is a basic need at the lowest level of Maslow's hierarchy of needs. Needs at the lower levels must be fulfilled before needs at the higher levels become important. The patient who is having trouble breathing cannot focus on much else. Keep conversation short and succinct. Give the patient verbal and nonverbal reassurance. Find alternate means of communicating, such as furnishing pen and paper, if necessary.

STRUCTURE AND FUNCTION OF THE RESPIRATORY SYSTEM

The respiratory system (Figure 14-1) extends from the nose to the alveoli (tiny air sacs in the lungs). The organs of the respiratory system are the:

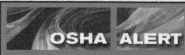

OSHA ALERT

We all know that respiratory infections are spread by the airborne and droplet methods of transmission. Handwashing is an often overlooked means of preventing the spread of respiratory infection. Secretions containing pathogens make their way to the environment. You pick up these pathogens on your hands. Good handwashing is the best method for preventing infection, including respiratory infection.

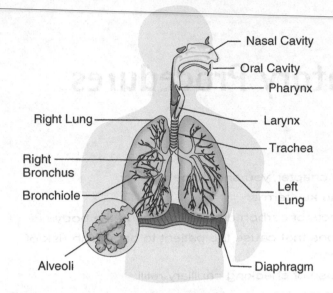

FIGURE 14-1 The respiratory system.

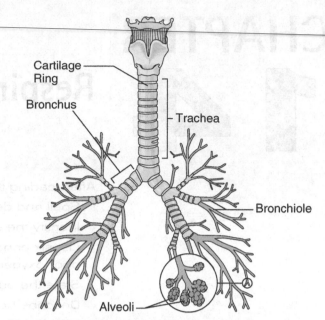

FIGURE 14-2 The lower respiratory tract.

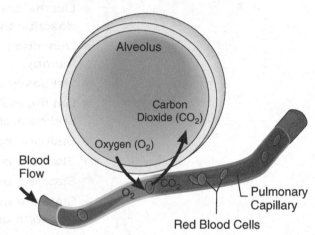

FIGURE 14-3 Oxygen and carbon dioxide are exchanged in the alveoli.

The sinuses, diaphragm, and intercostal muscles between the ribs are auxiliary structures.

Air is warmed, moistened, and filtered by the hairs in the nose as it passes through the nasal cavities, which are separated by a septum. The air passes through the pharynx, which is a passageway for both air and food, into the larynx and trachea. It then moves into the bronchi to join the upper respiratory tract to the lungs. Within the lungs, the bronchi branch into smaller and smaller divisions called *bronchioles*. The *alveoli* are tiny air sacs that extend from the bronchioles. It is at this level that exchange of gases occurs (**Figure 14-2**).

The alveoli, bronchioles, and the important pulmonary blood vessels form the lungs. The way in which oxygen and carbon dioxide are exchanged between the alveoli and capillaries is shown in **Figure 14-3**. As you can see, there is a close connection between the respiratory and circulatory systems.

The purpose of the respiratory system is to take in oxygen (O_2) to meet cellular needs and to remove **carbon dioxide (CO_2)**. Each cell in the body must have a constant supply of oxygen. Oxygen is delivered throughout the body by means of the bloodstream. Oxygen is necessary to sustain life, because it is used to produce the energy needed for cellular activity (**Figure 14-4**).

Carbon dioxide is a gaseous, metabolic waste product produced by the cells. The human body eliminates three main waste products. You have already learned about urinary and bowel elimination. The third waste product is carbon dioxide, which is produced by every cell in the body. This waste product is transported in venous blood. When it reaches the lungs, it is exhaled into the atmosphere. When the body does not eliminate carbon dioxide, this gas creates chemical reactions that cause an acid buildup. The buildup of acid will become life-threatening unless it is promptly identified and corrected. Death will result if levels of acid and carbon dioxide become too high. Signs and symptoms that suggest problems with oxygenation are listed in the Observe & Report box.

Nutrients + Oxygen = (yields) energy + water + CO_2

FIGURE 14-4 Oxygen produces energy for cellular activity.

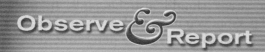

Observe & Report

Monitoring for Breathing Adequacy

- The patient can talk, respirations are between 12 and 20, and there is no apparent distress.
- The respiratory rhythm is regular.
- The patient's color is normal, with no cyanosis or gray coloration.
- The patient's chest should expand equally with each inspiration.
- Listen for breath sounds; place your ear next to the patient's nose and mouth, if necessary. The sounds should be quiet, without gurgling, wheezing, gasping, or other abnormal sounds.
- Feel for breath movement on your cheek and ear.
- Pulse oximeter reading should be at or above 95 percent.
- Capillary refill should be 2 to 3 seconds or less.

Signs and Symptoms of Inadequate Breathing and Decreased Oxygenation to Report to the Nurse Immediately

- Movement in the chest is absent, minimal, or irregular.
- Breathing movement appears to be in the abdomen, not the lungs.
- Air movement cannot be detected by listening and feeling for breath sounds on your cheek and ear.
- Respiratory rate is irregular, slow, or rapid.
- Respirations are gasping, very deep, or shallow.
- Respirations appear labored.
- Respirations are noisy.
- The patient is short of breath, or is having difficulty breathing.
- The patient is having Cheyne-Stokes respirations.
- The patient's skin, lips, tongue, earlobes, mucous membranes, lining or roof of mouth, or nail beds are dusky, pale, blue or gray.
- The patient has cool, clammy skin.
- The patient is unable to speak at all, or cannot speak in sentences because he or she is short of breath.
- Nasal flaring is present during inspiration.
- The muscles below the ribs and/or above the clavicles retract inward during respiration.
- Vomiting occurs while the patient has an oxygen mask, CPAP, or BiPAP mask in place.
- The patient has tachycardia.
- There are changes in the patient's mental status, including decreased responsiveness, drowsiness, **lethargy** (abnormal sleepiness for no apparent reason), restlessness, anxiety, disorientation, increasing confusion.
- The patient is wheezing.
- The patient is coughing (dry or moist/productive)
- The patient is having retractions (the chest appears to sink in just below the neck, and/or under the breastbone or rib cage with each inhalation in an effort to take more air into the lungs).

Nursing care is directed toward making breathing easier and preventing transmission of infection.

CARING FOR PATIENTS WHO HAVE RESPIRATORY CONDITIONS

You will care for many patients who have problems related to the respiratory system. Some conditions are caused by diseases within the lungs. Others are complications of other conditions. Nevertheless,

attention to the patient's oxygenation is a very important responsibility.

Patients Who Are at Risk of Poor Oxygenation

Certain patients have a known high risk of developing **hypoxemia.** This is a condition in which there is insufficient oxygen in the blood. It can occur in anyone, and is not a disease. Many of the patients who are at high risk for developing hypoxemia are not in the intensive care unit, where monitoring of oxygenation is routine. They are on medical and surgical units, in the long-term care facility, and in other patient care areas. Patients who are immobile and those on bedrest have an increased risk of hypoxemia. When hypoxemia develops, immobility is a barrier to positive outcomes. Other high-risk conditions are:

- Cardiac disease
- Pulmonary disease
- Postoperative status, for up to a week after surgery
- Sleep apnea
- Decreased level of consciousness
- Neuromuscular diseases
- Morbid obesity
- Kyphoscoliosis (curvature of the spine)

CAPILLARY REFILL

Checking **capillary refill** is a quick, easy, painless test to evaluate how well oxygen is getting to body tissues. Capillary refill is an indication of the patient's peripheral circulation and shows how well the tissues are being nourished with oxygen. In a light-skinned person, the skin should be pink, indicating an adequate supply of oxygen. The nail beds, mucous membranes, and lips are also an indication of how well the patient is using oxygen. The color

of these areas should also be pink. In a dark-skinned person, you must look at the nail beds, mucous membranes, and lips to determine how well the person is using oxygen, because you cannot evaluate the skin. If the skin, nail beds, mucous membranes, or lips are cyanotic, this indicates a problem with oxygen delivery. This may be due to a lack of oxygen in the blood or poor circulation.

The capillary refill test will help you determine the patient's circulation. Delayed capillary refill indicates a problem. Perform a capillary check on all four extremities, or according to facility policy. Although capillary refill varies with age, it should return to normal within 2 to 3 seconds in all patients. The color should be restored to the nail bed in the length of time it takes you to say the words *capillary refill*.

Nail Polish

Several of the procedures in this chapter involve using and evaluating the patient's fingernail beds. The color of the fingernails is a good indication of how much oxygen is in the blood. Nail polish will interfere with your ability to evaluate the patient. Follow your facility policy for removing nail polish. Some facilities remove polish from one finger only. Some facilities remove all nail polish. If a female patient has acrylic or sculpted nails, remove the polish with a non-acetone polish remover. Some facilities completely remove one acrylic nail. Know and follow your facility policy.

Procedure **110**

Checking Capillary Refill

1. Perform your beginning procedure actions.
2. Inspect the nails, noting the color.
3. Press on a nail for a few seconds, until the skin underneath blanches or turns white.

4. Release the nail and evaluate the time it takes for the skin to return to the normal color. If oxygenation is normal, this will occur within 2 to 3 seconds.
5. Perform your procedure completion actions.

You can check capillary refill whenever you are taking vital signs or caring for the patient. If the capillary refill time is more than 3 seconds, inform the RN of your findings.

THE PULSE OXIMETER

Pulse oximetry is another simple, painless test to determine how well oxygen is being carried in the body. Some health care professionals call pulse oximetry

the "fifth vital sign." The **pulse oximeter** (Figure 14-5) is an instrument that measures the level of saturation of the patient's hemoglobin with oxygen. *Hemoglobin* is the part of blood that carries oxygen to the cells to nourish them. The pulse oximeter measures how full the hemoglobin molecules are with oxygen. The measurement is usually done continuously, but can be intermittent. Having this data readily available enables the RN to treat the patient quickly. Pulse oximetry often detects critical changes in the

DIFFICULT PATIENT ALERT

In 2004, researchers at Massachusetts General Hospital published a paper entitled, "The Effect of Chronic or Intermittent Hypoxia on Cognition in Childhood: A Review of the Literature," in Pediatrics. The researchers concluded that mild oxygen desaturation of the blood, once thought to be of limited harm, contributes to long-term impaired mental function and behavioral disorders, such as attention deficit/hyperactivity disorder (ADHD), in children. This is an area of ongoing research and study. Many additional studies and clinical resources are listed in the Masimo web site in the "Exploring the Web" section at the end of this chapter.

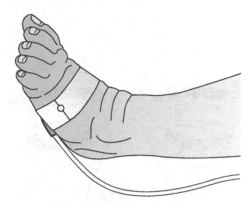

FIGURE 14-6(A) Adhesive neonatal sensor.

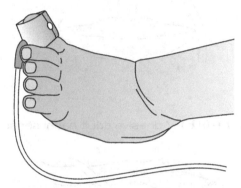

FIGURE 14-6(B) Adhesive infant sensor.

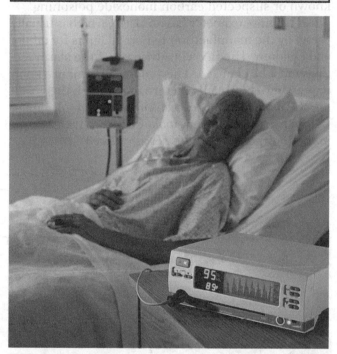

FIGURE 14-5 The pulse oximeter shows the oxygen saturation of the patient's blood as a percentage on the display. (Courtesy of Ohmeda, Louisville, CO)

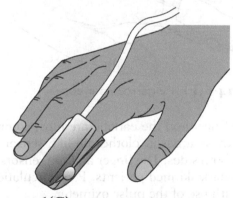

FIGURE 14-6(C) Adhesive pediatric sensor.

patient's oxygen levels before the skin color changes. This makes it a valuable tool that provides details about changes in the patient's condition immediately, as soon as they occur. The patient's outcome is usually better when early treatment is provided.

Before applying the pulse oximeter, check the patient's oxygen, if being used. Make sure the oxygen liter flow is set as ordered by the physician. Document the liter flow.

How the Pulse Oximeter Works

The pulse oximeter sensor is attached to the patient's skin. Several different sensors are available. These can be placed on the finger, toe, earlobe, foot, forehead, or bridge of the nose (Figure 14-6A–F). The

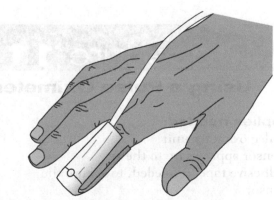

FIGURE 14-6(D) Adhesive adult sensor.

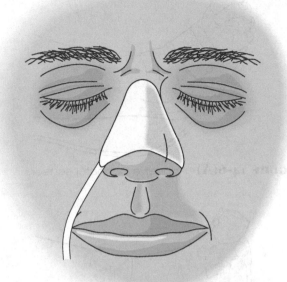

FIGURE 14-6(E) Adhesive adult nasal sensor.

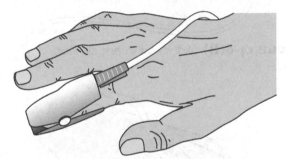

FIGURE 14-6(F) Finger-clip sensor.

tip of the finger and the earlobe are most commonly used. In these areas, a clothespin-like sensor is attached to both sides. The finger and toe sensors work best with dark-skinned patients. Poor circulation interferes with use of the pulse oximeter.

The unit has two light-emitting diodes (LEDs). One is red, the other is infrared. The sensor contains a photodetector that measures the light as it passes through the tissue (**Figure 14-7**). This measures the amount of oxygen in the patient's arterial blood. The pulse oximeter converts this into a percentage, which reads out on a digital display. The physician will order what he or she wants the minimum oxygen saturation to be. The RN will give you this information. A measurement of 95 percent to 100 percent is considered normal. Readings below 90 percent suggest complications. When the reading reaches 85 percent, there may not be enough oxygen for the tissues. Values below 70 percent are life-threatening. The pulse oximeter is not used in patients with known or suspected carbon monoxide poisoning.

The pulse oximeter has an alarm, which is usually preset by the manufacturer to normal limits for adults and children. The RN will advise you if the alarm settings must be changed. This is done by turning a knob or pressing a button. If you turn the unit off, then back on, the oximeter will reset itself to the default limits. Before leaving the room, make sure that the alarm is in the "on" position, and is set as ordered.

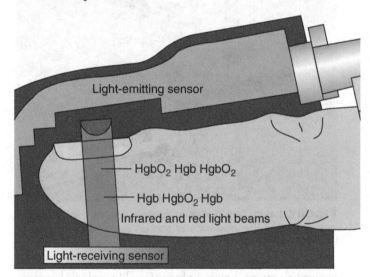

FIGURE 14-7 As the light passes through the tissue, a photodetector measures the amount of oxygen in the patient's arterial blood.

Procedure 111

Using a Pulse Oximeter

Supplies needed:
- Pulse oximeter unit
- Sensor appropriate to the site
- Adhesive tape, if needed, to secure the sensor

1. Perform your beginning procedure actions.
2. Select and apply the sensor. If the sensor has position markings, align them opposite each other to ensure an accurate reading.

(continues)

Procedure 111, *continued*

Using a Pulse Oximeter

Fasten the sensor securely, or the reading will not be accurate. Make sure the sensor is not wrapped so tightly with tape that it restricts blood flow.

3. Attach the sensor to the patient cable on the oximeter.
4. Turn the unit on. You will hear a beep with each pulse beat. Adjust the volume as desired. Some units also have light bars that indicate the strength of the pulse. Note the percentage of oxygen saturation. Inform the RN, or document according to facility policy.
5. Note the patient's pulse rate, if the unit provides this reading. Compare with the patient's actual pulse to make sure the unit is picking up each beat. Inform the RN, or document according to facility policy.
6. Monitor the patient's respirations and general appearance. Inform the RN, or document according to facility policy. If the patient's general condition changes at any time, notify the RN.
7. Perform your procedure completion actions.

Monitoring the Patient

You must monitor the patient regularly when the pulse oximeter is being used. Reporting to the RN is part of your procedure completion actions. In this case, make sure to report the patient's initial pulse oximeter reading and vital signs. This is important information on which the nurse will act. He or she will further assess the patient and provide care for abnormal values. The RN must know the initial values as a basis for comparison.

If the patient's vital signs or appearance change significantly from your baseline values, notify the RN. Also inform the RN immediately if the patient's pulse oximetry value is less than the level ordered by the physician. Monitor the patient's oxygen, if used, each time you are in the room. Make sure it is set at the liter flow ordered by the physician.

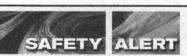

SAFETY ALERT

Always monitor the patient and not the equipment. For example, the pulse oximeter alarm sounds and the oxygen saturation value reads 63 percent. You know this suggests that the patient is in distress. However, the patient is visiting with his family, smiling and talking. His color is good, nail beds and mucous membranes are pink, and the capillary refill time is less than 2 seconds. You are having an equipment problem, not a patient problem. If you cannot identify and correct the problem, ask the RN or respiratory professional to help. Advise the RN of your findings and evaluation of the patient.

Rotate the position of the finger sensor every 4 hours. A spring-clip sensor should be moved every 2 hours. Rotating the location of the sensor reduces the risk of skin breakdown and complications related to pressure. If adhesive tape is used to secure the sensor, monitor for signs and symptoms of a reaction to the tape. If a rash, itching, or other signs of tape allergy occur, move the sensor to a different location. Apply a spring-clamp sensor, or attach it with hypoallergenic tape.

OXYGEN THERAPY

Oxygen is necessary for life. Humans take in oxygen from the air during breathing. Some diseases and conditions prevent enough oxygen from feeding the body's tissues, so supplemental oxygen is administered. Some patients have normal oxygen levels, but are given oxygen because their medical condition puts them at risk for hypoxemia. Oxygen is a prescription item, and a physician's order is necessary to administer it to a patient. The physician will order additional oxygen to be given through an oxygen delivery system. He or she will specify how much oxygen to use and the method of oxygen delivery. Depending on your facility policy, oxygen may also be given at the RN's discretion, according to protocol or clinical practice guidelines. You should not start, stop, or change the flow rate of oxygen unless you are trained in the procedure, are permitted to do it in your facility, and have an order to make the change.

The PCT's responsibilities for oxygen administration are determined by facility policy. In many facilities a respiratory care practitioner (RCP) administers oxygen therapy. Nursing personnel monitor patients who use oxygen and notify the RCP as needed. He or she will see the patient one or more times each shift. Although an RCP may be responsible for the patient's oxygen needs, you must still have a working knowledge of oxygen administration. You must also know where oxygen cylinders are stored, how to assemble them, and how to transport them safely, as the RN may send you for the portable oxygen supply in an emergency.

Oxygen Delivery Systems

Oxygen is usually piped in through the wall in hospitals. The flow meter is plugged into an adapter in the wall (**Figure 14-8**). Oxygen is delivered when the flow meter is turned on. Some units have more than one adapter. Oxygen is color-coded with a green label in the United States. Read carefully when initiating oxygen through a piped-in system. Make sure you are using the correct adapter and plug. Never modify the equipment to make it fit together. If you cannot assemble the components of the system, request help from the RN or RCP. Portable cylinders (**Figure 14-9**) are used for transporting patients from one area to another, and may be used in emergencies in hallways or other areas without a piped-in source.

Most long-term care facilities use oxygen cylinders or concentrators (**Figure 14-10**). The oxygen concentrator converts room air to oxygen and delivers it to the patient. Oxygen also comes in a liquid canister (**Figure 14-11**). The canister

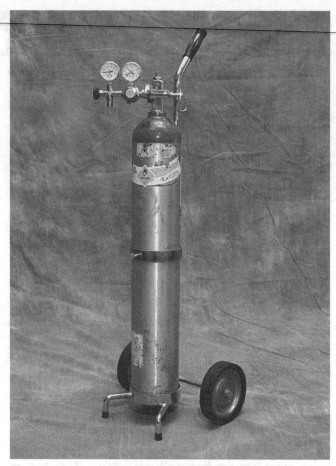

FIGURE 14-9 Portable emergency oxygen tank.

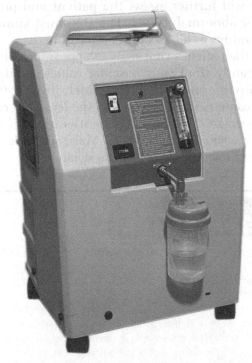

FIGURE 14-10 Oxygen concentrators convert room air into oxygen. They are typically used in long-term care facilities and home care settings. A concentrator is ineffective for liter flows over 5.

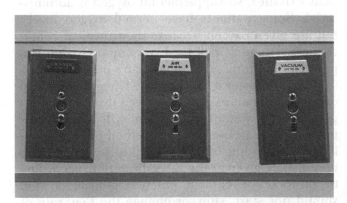

FIGURE 14-8 Typical fittings for piped-in oxygen and other gases. The fitting on the left is for oxygen, the center outlet is used for air, and the fitting on the right is used for a vacuum system.

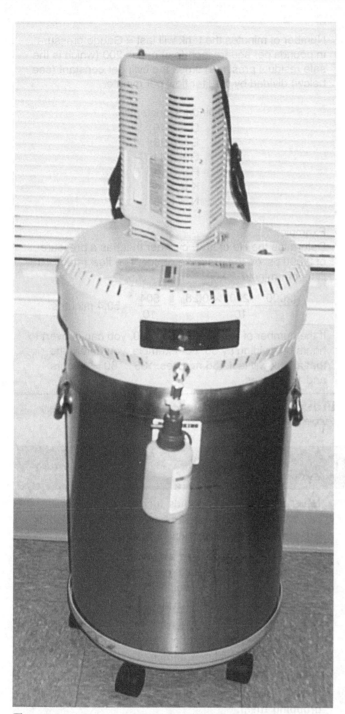

FIGURE 14-11 A liquid oxygen canister. The portable tank on top is detachable.

delivers a higher concentration of oxygen than a concentrator, and is portable and convenient. It does not require electricity to operate. The canister is quiet compared with a concentrator, which has an electric motor and makes a humming noise. Liquid and cylinder oxygen are more expensive than a concentrator.

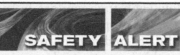

SAFETY ALERT

In 2001, the FDA sent a warning to all U.S. health care facilities regarding the risks in connecting a gas other than oxygen into the oxygen system. (See the FDA Public Health Advisory in the "Exploring the Web" section at the end of this chapter.) The most significant problems occurred when:

• The person connecting the vessel to the oxygen system did not understand that connection incompatibility is a built-in safeguard
• The person making the connection did not examine the label to ensure that the product was medical oxygen before connecting it to the oxygen supply system

The FDA memo lists recommendations to prevent mixups of medical gases. Because of this memo, several states changed their laws to reduce the risk of injury.

Flow Meters

Oxygen flow is regulated by a flow meter (**Figure 14-12**) that shows how many liters of oxygen are being delivered to the patient each minute. Flow meters come in several different sizes and shapes, but work the same way. However, the various size cylinders use different gauges. If you are setting up a cylinder, make sure you have gauges that fit. The flow of oxygen is increased by turning the knob on the flow meter clockwise, and decreased by turning it counterclockwise. Always read the label on the flow meter before applying it, to ensure that it is intended for use on oxygen tanks. Do not depend on color-coding in this case. Colors are not always consistent with flow meters, as they are for oxygen.

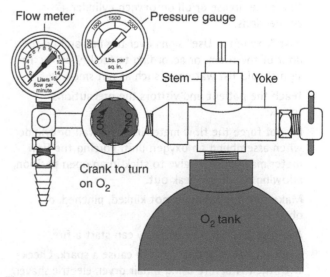

FIGURE 14-12 The flow meter shows the amount of oxygen being delivered. The pressure gauge shows how much oxygen remains in the tank.

~~Check the liter flow each time you are in the~~ room to be sure it is set at the proper rate. If you notice a difference from the ordered rate, correct it, if permitted. If not, report this important information to the RN. Oxygen is a prescription product, similar to prescription drugs. Because of this, you may not be allowed to adjust the flow rate.

Pressure Gauge

The pressure gauge is connected to the flow meter on an oxygen cylinder. This gauge shows how much oxygen is in the cylinder. Oxygen is measured in pounds. Follow your facility policy for checking the gauge. Notify the appropriate person before the cylinder is empty. Many facilities consider cylinders empty when the pressure reaches 500 pounds, and change them when this pressure is reached. You may have to estimate how long a cylinder will last. This varies with the cylinder size and the number of liters per minute of oxygen use. The formula for calculating the duration of oxygen cylinder use is listed in **Figure 14-13**. See the following guidelines for using oxygen safely.

Number of minutes the tank will last = Gauge pressure in pounds per square inch (psi) minus 200 (which is the safe residual pressure) times the cylinder constant (see below) divided by the liter flow per minute.

Cylinder Constants
D = 0.16
E = 0.28
G = 2.41
H = 3.14
K = 3.14
N = 1.56

Example:
Determine the life of an E cylinder that has a pressure of 2,000 psi on the pressure gauge. The flow rate is 10 liters per minute.

$$\frac{(2000 - 200) \times 0.28}{10} = \frac{504}{10} = 50.4 \text{ minutes}$$

If the number of minutes exceeds 60, you can convert to hours by dividing by 60. For example, you determine that a tank will last 135 minutes. 135 ÷ 60 = 2 hours and 15 minutes.

FIGURE 14-13 Formula for determining oxygen remaining in a tank.

Guidelines for Oxygen Safety

- Before initiating oxygen therapy, check the patient's room to make sure it is safe for oxygen delivery.
- When using cylinder oxygen, identify the contents of the cylinder. Oxygen cylinders are always green in the United States. Read the label listing the contents as a double-check.
- Never use grease or oil on oxygen cylinder connections.
- Post "Oxygen in Use" signs over the bed and on the door of the room, or according to facility policy. The sign should list warnings, such as not smoking.
- Teach the patient and visitors the precautions to take.
- Do not force the flow meter into the wall or cylinder when assembling an oxygen unit. Forcing the flow meter may cause a valve to stick in an open position, allowing oxygen to leak out.
- Make sure the tubing is not kinked, pinched, or obstructed.
- Avoid sparks. Static electricity can start a fire.
- Some electrical appliances can cause a spark. Check with the RN before using a hair dryer, electric shaver, fan, radio, or television.

- Never use flammable liquids such as nail polish remover or adhesive tape remover. Flammable liquids are combustible and will burn readily.
- Avoid using alcohol-based aftershave, cologne, perfume, or other products on patients who are using oxygen.
- Cylinder oxygen should be secured in a base or chained to a carrier or the wall. Avoid dropping the tank. Cylinders can explode if the tank is dropped and the cylinder valve is damaged.
- Transport oxygen cylinders carefully. They should be chained to a carrier during transport. Avoid dropping them.
- Smoking is not allowed in the room when oxygen is in use.
- Cover the patient with a cotton blanket. Avoid using wool and synthetic blankets and clothing.
- Some facilities remove the call signal and replace it with a bell that is used manually. The call signal may cause a spark.
- Patients receiving oxygen receive frequent oral and nasal care because the oxygen dries the mucous membranes. Avoid using petroleum jelly or other

(continued)

Guidelines for Oxygen Safety (Continued)

petroleum products as lubricants. Consult the RN for a water-soluble lubricant.

- Respond to equipment alarms, including oxygen equipment, immediately. Take corrective action or notify the appropriate person.

- If oxygen equipment makes an unusual noise, take corrective action or notify the appropriate person. If you suspect that a cylinder or wall outlet is leaking, remove the patient from the room and close the door.

- Learn how to turn off oxygen in case of a fire emergency. Piped-in oxygen may be turned off at a zone valve in the hallway. Cylinders, canisters, and concentrators must be turned off at the unit.

- Learn facility policies for emergency transport and evacuation of patients who need continuous oxygen.

- Follow infection control precautions when caring for patients who use oxygen, such as keeping the cannula covered when not in use. Keep the oxygen cannula and tubing off the floor.

- Learn facility policies for using liquid oxygen. When liquid oxygen is used, high concentrations of oxygen build up quickly. Some materials are very flammable when saturated with oxygen. Follow all safety precautions for preventing sparks and fires.

- Liquid oxygen should be filled and used a minimum of 5 feet away from electrical appliances such as electric wheelchairs, television sets, radio and stereo equipment, air conditioners, fans, electric razors, and hair dryers.

- Liquid oxygen is nontoxic, but will cause severe burns upon direct contact. Avoid opening, touching, or spilling the container. If your skin or clothing contacts the liquid oxygen, flush the area immediately with a large amount of water. Never seal the cap or vent port on the liquid oxygen. Doing so will increase pressure within the system, creating a potentially dangerous situation. If a bottle falls or tips, evacuate yourself and the patient from the room and close the door. Follow facility policies for getting assistance in this type of emergency.

- Do not transfer oxygen from one container to another in patients' rooms. Such transfers must be done only in designated areas that meet certain fire and ventilation standards. These rooms must be separated from areas in which patients are housed.

- Do not fill liquid oxygen bottles unless you are qualified to perform this procedure, and are wearing the correct protective equipment. PPE for handling cryogens includes a full face shield *over safety glasses,* loose-fitting thermal insulated or leather gloves, a long-sleeved shirt, and pants without cuffs. Gloves must be loose-fitting so they can be removed quickly if cryogenic liquid is spilled on them. Insulated gloves are not made for use in cryogenic liquid. They will provide only short-term protection from accidental contact. In an emergency, self-contained breathing apparatus (SCBA) may be required. In addition, safety shoes are recommended for people involved in the handling of containers. Depending on the application, additional protective apparel may be advisable. As you can see, this job is best left to maintenance or safety personnel.

Procedure 112

Preparing Wall-Outlet Oxygen

Supplies needed:
- Flow meter
- Sterile humidifier bottle, if used
- Oxygen precautions sign(s)
- Triangular adapter, if necessary (this is commonly called a Christmas tree because of its shape and color)

1. Perform your beginning procedure actions.
2. Select the correct flow meter. Oxygen is color-coded green in the United States and air is coded black. You cannot put the flow meter in the wrong outlet because the connectors are different sizes.
3. Attach the male adapter in the flow meter to the female adapter in the oxygen plate in the wall by pushing it in securely. You may need to push hard.
4. Hold the flow meter in your hand as you gradually release the pressure. If the flow

(continues)

Procedure **112**, *continued*

Preparing Wall-Outlet Oxygen

meter is not securely in place, it may pop out, causing injury.

5. Gently pull on the flow meter to make sure it will not fall off the wall.

6. Attach the sterile humidifier bottle (Procedure 114), if used.

7. If the humidifier is not used, you must screw the triangular adapter to the bottom

of the flow meter. Connect the tubing to the point of the triangle.

8. Post the oxygen precautions sign(s) according to facility policy.

9. Perform your procedure completion actions.

Procedure **113**

Preparing the Oxygen Cylinder

Supplies needed:
- Oxygen cylinder
- Wrench, depending on type of flow meter used
- Handle or wrench for opening cylinder valve
- Flow meter to fit cylinder
- Sterile humidifier bottle, if used
- Sterile distilled water for humidifier

- Tubing and delivery device
- Oxygen precautions sign(s)

1. Perform your beginning procedure actions. Refer to **Figure 14-14** as you review this procedure.

2. Obtain the cylinder. Check the color and read the label to identify the contents.

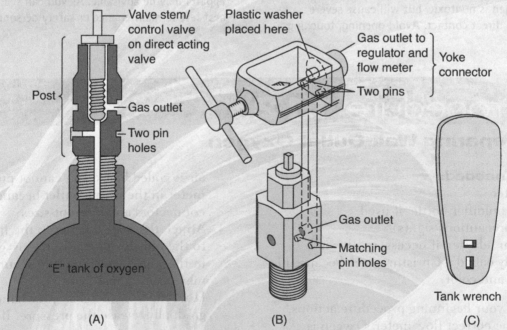

FIGURE 14-14 Directions for preparing an "E" tank of oxygen.

(continues)

Procedure **113**, *continued*

Preparing the Oxygen Cylinder

3. Transport the cylinder to the designated area. Chain the cylinder to a wheeled dolly, if necessary.
4. Position the cylinder upright on the dolly, upright in a base, or chained to the wall.
5. Stand to the side. Do not stand directly over the cylinder. Remove the metal or plastic cap, or wrapper protecting the outlet.
6. Attach the handle to the cylinder. Crack the main valve for one second. Close the valve.
7. Position the cylinder valve gasket on the regulator port.
8. Check the regulator. Turn the knob to make sure the regulator port is closed.
9. Align the two holes in the outlet with the two pins in the regulator, or thread the nut onto the male adapter on the outlet. Tighten the t-screw for the pin yolk, or use a wrench to tighten the threaded outlet. Note: For small, cylinder-type regulators, a Teflon "O" ring must be in place, or the connection will leak.
10. Turn the cylinder on and check the pressure gauge. Make sure the cylinder is full. Listen for air leaks. If a leak is present, turn the cylinder off, remove the regulator, and reapply.
11. Attach the humidifier filled with sterile distilled water, tubing, and delivery device, if ordered.
12. Post the oxygen precautions sign(s) according to facility policy.
13. Perform your procedure completion actions.

Humidifiers

In some facilities, a **humidifier** (Figure 14-15) is attached to the oxygen administration equipment if the patient's liter flow exceeds 5 liters. Use of oxygen humidifiers is a controversial subject. Humidification is not necessary for liter flows below 5.

The humidifier is a water bottle that moistens the oxygen for comfort and prevents drying of the mucous membranes in the nose, mouth, and lungs. The bottle screws into a male adapter on the flow meter. Oxygen passes through the water in the humidifier, picking up moisture, before it reaches the patient. The delivery device plugs into a male adapter on the side of the humidifier. You may be responsible for checking or changing the humidifier. Avoid tap water. Sterile distilled water is always used in the humidifier. Inhalation of tap water is associated with an increased incidence of Legionnaire's disease. The water level in the humidifier should always be at or above the "minimum fill" line on the bottle.

When the oxygen delivery system is functioning correctly, the water in the humidifier will bubble. Oxygen will not exit the tubing into the mask or cannula if the tubing is kinked or obstructed. If this occurs, pressure builds up in the unit and discharges through a pressure relief valve. When setting up a humidifier, check this valve by turning the oxygen on and pinching the connecting tubing.

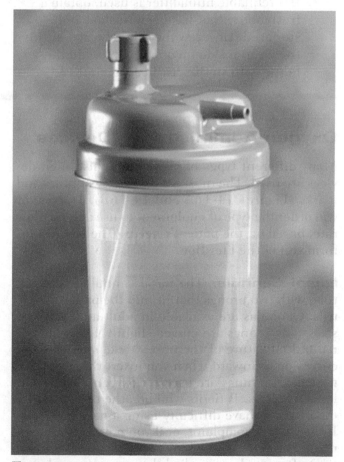

FIGURE 14-15 A humidifier. (Courtesy of Hudson RCI, Temecula, CA, USA)

Types of Humidifiers. Two types of humidifiers are used. The *prefilled* type of humidifier is commonly used in acute care hospitals. This unit is usually changed once a week, when it is empty, or according to the manufacturer's directions. Discard the bottle after replacing it with a new one. Your facility may require you to attach a sticker to the bottle listing the date and time it was changed, and your initials.

Refillable humidifiers are washed with soap and water or 2 percent alkaline gluteraldehyde solution every 24 hours. They are rinsed well, then sterilized.

Refill the sterile bottle with sterile distilled water. Never add water to a partially filled humidifier. A sticker is also attached to this bottle showing the date and time it was changed.

Procedure 114

Attaching the Humidifier to the Oxygen Flow Meter or Regulator

Supplies needed:
▶ Sterile disposable or refillable humidifier bottle
▶ Sterile distilled water for refillable humidifier

1. Perform your procedure completion actions.
2. Open the package for the humidifier and remove the bottle.
3. If a refillable humidifier is used, obtain a fresh bottle that has been washed and sterilized. Unscrew the lid and place it with the clean inside up on the table. Fill the bottle with sterile distilled water, then

replace the lid. Do not touch the inside of the bottle or lid with your fingers.
4. Connect the female adapter in the top of the humidifier bottle to the male adapter on the flow meter. Tighten the nut securely.
5. Connect the tubing on the cannula or mask to the male adapter on the side of the humidifier bottle.
6. Turn on the flow of oxygen. Pinch the connecting tubing to ensure that the safety valve pops off.
7. Perform your procedure completion actions.

Oxygen Administration Devices

Many different types of oxygen administration devices are used. The most common are cannulas and masks (**Figures 14-16A and 14-16B**). The doctor will order the type of equipment to use and the flow rate, based on the patient's needs. The RN will inform you of the liter flow.

Nasal Cannula. The nasal cannula is a small tube with two prongs that fit into the patient's nostrils. Cannulas are available in adult and pediatric sizes. The prongs are curved slightly, following the natural curvature of the nose. Make sure that the curves point inward when you insert them into the nostrils. Cannulas are used for oxygen delivered at low liter flows. Patients who breathe through their mouths may have difficulty using a nasal cannula. If the patient complains, or if you notice a problem, notify the RN. Asking him or her to assess the patient after you have applied the oxygen cannula is a good idea.

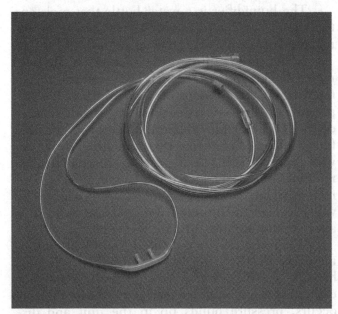

FIGURE 14-16(A) An oxygen cannula with extension tubing.

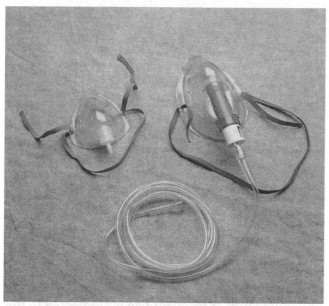

FIGURE 14-16(B) Oxygen masks without tubing and with tubing.

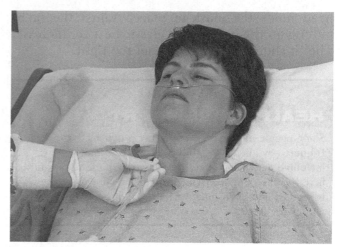

FIGURE 14-17 Slip the bead up and adjust for a comfortable fit.

HEALTH CARE ALERT

When caring for patients who have COPD, pace activities. Help them to conserve energy as much as possible. Minimize activities involving raising the arms over the head. Avoid exposing patients to aerosol sprays.

Two types of straps are used to hold the cannula in place. The single elastic strap is positioned at the back of the patient's head. Adjust the tension on the elastic at the sides of the cannula to make it tighter or looser. Another type of cannula has thin plastic tubes that are slipped over the ears. A bead under the chin is raised or lowered to adjust the fit (Figure 14-17). This type of adjustment is similar to that on a child's cowboy hat.

Procedure 115

Administering Oxygen through a Nasal Cannula

Supplies needed:
▶ Oxygen cannula

1. Perform your beginning procedure actions.
2. Connect the end of the cannula tubing to the male adapter on the humidifier or flow meter by pushing it securely in place.
3. Turn the oxygen on to the designated flow rate by adjusting the knob on the flow meter.
4. Place your hand in front of the nasal prongs to feel the flow of oxygen.
5. Position the cannula in the patient's nostrils. Tighten the adjustment on the strap so it is secure, but not too tight.
6. Perform your procedure completion actions.

Simple Mask. The oxygen mask fits over the patient's nose, mouth, and chin. A small tube connects the mask to the oxygen source. Masks are available in adult and pediatric sizes. A special mask fits over a tracheostomy. Using an oxygen mask is necessary when high liter flows of oxygen are or-

dered. Masks may also be used for mouth-breathers (individuals who breathe through their mouths). A mask should not be used with liter flows under 5 because it may cause rebreathing of the patient's exhaled carbon dioxide, and have a smothering effect. An elastic strap that slips over the back of the head holds the mask in place. Adjust the fit by pulling on the ends of the elastic next to the mask. The fit should be snug, but not too tight.

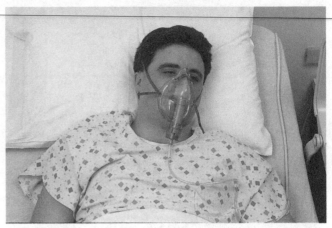

FIGURE 14-19 The air entrainment (Venturi) mask.

has one-way plastic flaps on the sides. The patient's exhalations escape through these flaps, but outside air cannot enter. A reservoir bag is connected to the bottom of the mask. The combination of bag and mask increases the amount of oxygen delivered to the patient. The bag should be inflated at all times. Make sure it does not collapse more than halfway during inspiration.

Air Entrainment Mask. The **air entrainment mask** (Figure 14-19) is also called a **Venturi mask, venti mask,** and **high airflow with oxygen enrichment (HAFOE) mask.** This is similar to a simple mask, but it has a large plastic tube at the bottom. The mask mixes oxygen with room air to obtain the percentage of oxygen ordered by the physician. The settings on the mask are changed according to the physician's order. When this mask is used, make sure the patient does not inadvertently change the setting.

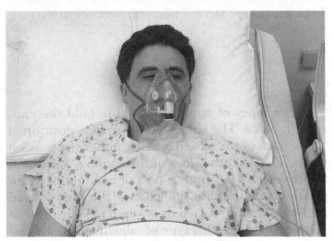

FIGURE 14-18 The nonrebreathing mask is commonly used for hypoxemic patients.

Nonrebreathing Mask. The nonrebreathing mask (Figure 14-18) is a modification of the simple oxygen mask. This mask is used for patients with severe hypoxemia. The nonrebreathing mask

Procedure **116**

Administering Oxygen through a Mask

Supplies needed:
▶ Oxygen mask

1. Perform your beginning procedure actions.
2. Connect the end of the mask tubing to the male adapter on the humidifier or flow meter by pushing it securely into place.
3. Turn the oxygen on to the designated flow rate by adjusting the knob on the flow meter.
4. Place your hand in front of the inlet and feel for the flow of oxygen.
5. Position the mask over the patient's nose, mouth, and chin. Mold the metal band at the top of the mask to the patient's nose.
6. Slip the elastic strap behind the patient's head.
7. Tighten the adjustment on the elastic strap so that the mask is secure, but not too tight.
8. Perform your procedure completion actions.

Caring for a Patient Who Is Receiving Oxygen Therapy

Elevate the head of the bed when the patient is receiving oxygen. This will make it easier to breathe. A patient who is using an oxygen mask cannot eat while wearing the mask. The physician may order a nasal cannula at mealtime. Follow the instructions on the care plan or critical pathway for patient care measures.

Being unable to breathe is very frightening. Patients who are receiving oxygen may need reassurance and emotional support. Check on the patient frequently and spend as much time in the room as possible. Difficulty in breathing makes it hard to talk. The patient may be unable to hold a normal conversation. Just being with the patient without talking is very reassuring.

You will care for patients who are using different devices for the administration of oxygen. Carefully check the skin under the device. Make sure that it does not become red or irritated from the elastic that holds it in place. Report any skin problems to the RN. Because oxygen is drying, patients who are receiving oxygen may need extra liquids to drink. They also need frequent care of the mouth and nose. Sometimes patients feel warm and will perspire heavily. Extra bathing and linen changes may be necessary. You may need to adjust the temperature in the room and help the patient change into a hospital gown. Cover him or her with a sheet. The care plan or critical pathway will provide information on patient preferences and needs.

Safety Measures for Oxygen Use

You must know general safety measures for oxygen use. Keep sources of ignition out of the room, including matches and lighters, cigarettes, and some electrical appliances. Extra oxygen in the air may cause

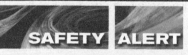

Oxygen is a prescription item, like a medication. Using oxygen is safe if you follow facility policies and safety guidelines. Never change the fittings from one type of oxygen bottle to another. Make sure you use the correct adapter and plug for the unit. Make sure the oxygen cylinder is secure in a base or chained to a wall or carrier in an upright position. If a cylinder is accidentally knocked over, it has the potential to turn into a missile, causing great damage. If you think that an oxygen tank or liquid oxygen canister is leaking, remove the patient from the room and close the door. Report the problem to the proper person. Never attempt to carry or move an oxygen cylinder or canister if it is leaking.

objects to burn much faster than they normally would. By itself, oxygen is not explosive or flammable. However, the patient's gown and linens on the bed absorb extra oxygen from the air, so they will burn readily.

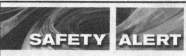

Bed linens can absorb oxygen. Any time oxygen is in use, avoid sparks. Static electricity can start a fire.

Discontinuing Use of an Oxygen Cylinder

Your facility will have policies and procedures for cleaning and storing oxygen cylinders after they have been used. A portable emergency cylinder or transport cylinder is often returned to the storage area for reuse. Before storing an oxygen cylinder, you must turn the oxygen off. When this is done, a certain amount of oxygen remains in the gauges. Bleeding the cylinder ensures that no oxygen remains in the gauges. Bleed the gauge by turning the oxygen supply from the cylinder to the flow meter off by turning the valve on top. Next, turn the flow meter on. Although the cylinder is turned off, the flow meter will rise momentarily, then the liter flow will drop to zero. This ensures that all free oxygen is removed from the gauges.

Use of Oxygen in an Emergency

There are several differences between routine oxygen use and use of oxygen in an emergency. In an emergency, high concentrations of oxygen are necessary. A concentrator will not deliver an adequate amount of oxygen for emergencies. Cylinders, liquid oxygen, or oxygen piped in through the wall are used. Concentrators cannot deliver liter flows over 5. Most facilities use small, portable cylinders for emergency purposes. Oxygen may be delivered dry. Do not take the time to search for a humidifier. In an emergency, the patient requires high liter flows of oxygen immediately. Use a nonrebreather mask if possible.

OROPHARYNGEAL AIRWAY

An **oropharyngeal airway** (Figure 14-20), or oral airway, is a curved plastic or rubber device that is inserted into the mouth to the posterior pharynx. It is used to keep the airway open in unconscious patients. Conscious patients cannot tolerate this device. Inserting this airway into a conscious or semiconscious patient will induce vomiting. If the patient is awake enough to spit the airway out, he or she does not need it.

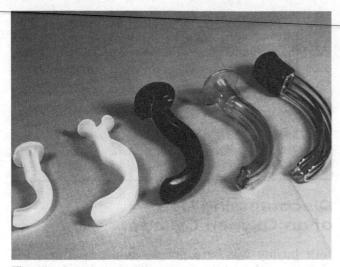

FIGURE 14-20 Various types and sizes of oral airways.

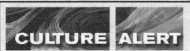

Many individuals have tongue piercings, and may wear tongue studs or other ornaments to make a fashion statement. Many risks accompany this procedure. Inform the RN promptly if a patient with a tongue piercing has pain, bleeding, increased flow of saliva, swelling, or signs of infection in the mouth. Swelling of the tongue can become severe, closing off the airway. To prevent patient injury, tongue piercings and ornaments will probably have to be removed when an oral airway is inserted. Check with the RN.

The most common cause of airway obstruction is the tongue. The oral airway prevents the tongue from falling to the back of the throat, obstructing the airway. The airway has a flange at the end, which fits between the patient's lips. The curve of the airway holds the tongue forward. It is not the airway of choice for patients who have recently had oral surgery, or those with loose teeth.

Oral airways come in several sizes. Using the correct size is important; a wrong-size airway will worsen the obstruction or cause other complications. Check the airway size by positioning the flat flange end at the corner of the patient's mouth, with the curved part down. The tip of the airway should reach the earlobe on the same side (Figure 14-21). If the airway is too long or short, select another size. Never use an airway without checking the size.

In many situations, the airway must be inserted quickly. Use caution, however, to avoid tooth and tissue damage. To insert an oral airway, position the patient supine with the neck extended, if this is not contraindicated. Apply gloves and other personal protective equipment as needed to maintain the principles of standard precautions. If the patient coughs, gags, chokes, or moves a hand to the face during airway insertion, stop the procedure. The patient is too responsive to use this type of airway.

After inserting the airway, position the patient on his or her side. Make sure the patient's tongue and lips are not positioned between the airway and the teeth.

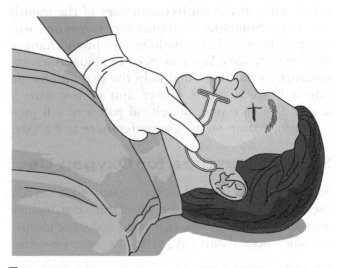

FIGURE 14-21 Measure the airway and select the correct size.

Procedure 117

Inserting the Oropharyngeal Airway

Supplies needed:
- Disposable exam gloves
- Oral airways of various sizes
- Tongue blade (optional)

1. Perform your beginning procedure actions.
2. If the patient's mouth is not open, use a tongue blade or cross the thumb and forefinger of one gloved hand. Position your

(continues)

Procedure **117**, *continued*

Inserting the Oropharyngeal Airway

fingers in the corner of the mouth, on the upper and lower teeth. Spread your fingers apart to open the mouth.

3. Select the airway size and position it with the tip pointing sideways, toward the cheek.

4. Insert the airway into the mouth, sliding it along the tongue past the tissue in the back of the throat until you meet resistance. Check the tongue to make sure it is not against the back of the throat. An alternate method is to press the tongue down and forward with the tongue blade. Insert the airway with the tip pointing downward. This method is preferred in infants and children.

5. Gently rotate the airway 90 degrees, until the tip is pointing down (Figure 14-22).

6. Check the tongue to make sure it is not against the back of the throat. The flange of the airway should be between the patient's lips.

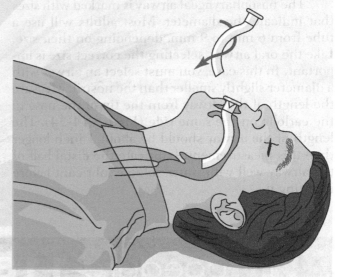

FIGURE 14-22 Rotate the airway. When it is properly inserted, the flange will rest on the patient's lips.

7. Check the patient's respirations to ensure that they are adequate.

8. Perform your procedure completion actions.

After you have inserted the airway, check the patient often. Make sure the airway remains in the correct position. Avoid taping the airway in position. The patient's behavior is a clue to guide you on airway removal. The patient may gag or cough as he or she becomes more alert. The patient may reach up and remove the airway. Do not try to replace it if the patient removes it or spits it out. Check the patient's respirations immediately after the airway is removed to ensure that they are adequate. If you have concerns about the patient's ability to maintain his or her own airway, discuss them with the RN.

NASOPHARYNGEAL AIRWAY

A **nasopharyngeal airway** (Figure 14-23) is a curved, soft rubber device that is inserted through one nostril. It extends from the nostril to the posterior pharynx area, keeping the tongue off the back of the throat. This airway may be used in responsive patients. It is the airway of choice for patients who have recently had oral surgery, who have loose teeth

or trauma of the mouth, and who need frequent nasal suctioning. You may hear others call this airway a "nasal trumpet." The nasopharyngeal airway should not be used for patients who are receiving anticoagulant (blood thinning) medications, or for patients who have nasal deformity, bleeding disorders, or sepsis.

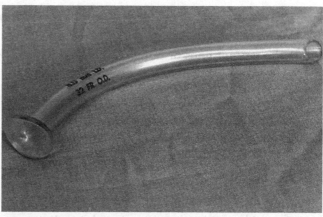

FIGURE 14-23 The nasopharyngeal airway may safely be used for conscious patients.

To insert the airway, position the patient in the supine position with the head extended, unless contraindicated. Apply gloves and other personal protective equipment as needed to observe the principles of standard precautions.

The nasopharyngeal airway is marked with sizes that indicate the diameter. Most adults will use a tube from 6 mm to 9 mm, depending on their size. Like the oral airway, selecting the correct size is important. In this case, you must select an airway with a diameter slightly smaller than the nostril. Measure the length of the airway from the tip of the nose to the earlobe on the same side (Figure 14-24). The length of the airway should be about 1 inch longer than this measurement. Lubricate the distal half of the airway well with water-soluble lubricant before inserting it.

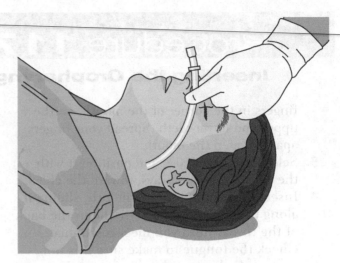

FIGURE 14-24 Measure the nasal airway from the tip of the nose to the earlobe. It should be approximately one inch longer than this distance.

Procedure 118

Inserting the Nasopharyngeal Airway

Supplies needed:
▶ Disposable exam gloves
▶ Water-soluble lubricant
▶ Nasopharyngeal airways, assortment of sizes
▶ Tongue blade

1. Perform your beginning procedure actions.
2. Select the correct size airway: slightly smaller than the diameter of the nostril, and approximately 1 inch longer than the distance from the tip of the nose to the earlobe.
3. Lubricate the distal half of the airway with water-soluble lubricant.

4. With your nondominant index finger, push up on the tip of the patient's nose.
5. Hold the airway in your dominant hand. Insert it into the nostril and gently thread the tube until the flange is at the tip of the nose. Avoid forcing the airway. If you meet resistance, remove the airway and notify the RN.
6. After the airway is inserted, depress the tongue with a tongue blade. Look for the airway behind the soft tissue at the back of the throat. Next, close the patient's mouth. Place your finger in front of the airway to feel for air movement.
7. Perform your procedure completion actions.

If the patient gags or coughs after you have inserted the airway, it may be too long. Remove the airway and insert a shorter one. Most facilities remove the airway every shift, perform nasal care, and check for irritation in the nose. The airway is cleaned before it is reinserted. Follow your facility policies.

SUCTION

Suction is used to remove fluid, food, and secretions from the patient's nose, mouth, and airway, reducing the risk of aspiration. This keeps the air-

way clear in patients who are unable to cough effectively to maintain it on their own. There is usually no fixed interval for suctioning. It is done as often as necessary to remove secretions.

A flexible, plastic suction catheter (Figure 14-25A) or rigid plastic suction, called a **Yankauer catheter** (Figure 14-25B), or tonsil tip, are used for suctioning. The flexible catheter is inserted into the mouth or nose to remove secretions. The Yankauer is used only for oral suctioning (Figure 14-25C). Apply the principles of standard precautions when caring for the patient and handling suc-

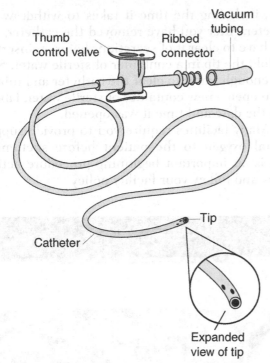

FIGURE 14-25(A) Flexible suction catheter with thumb control valve.

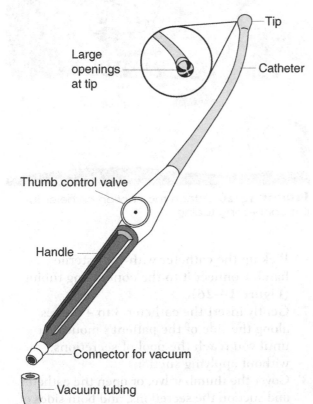

FIGURE 14-25(B) Yankauer suction catheter.

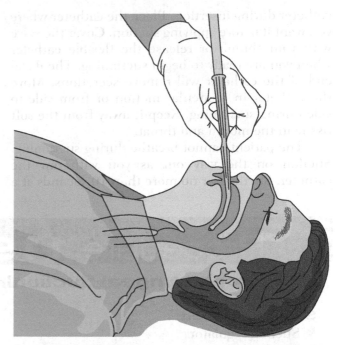

FIGURE 14-25(C) The Yankauer catheter should never be placed farther back than the base of the tongue.

tion equipment. Wear a mask and face protection if this is your facility policy, or if there is a risk that the patient will cough in your face. In many facilities, oropharyngeal suctioning is a sterile procedure

because the catheter may inadvertently slip into the patient's trachea. Follow your facility policies.

Some suction regulators have an adjustable pressure setting. The pressure may be set between 80 and 120 mm Hg. The RN or respiratory care practitioner will set the pressure or advise you what setting to use. Before beginning, block the end of the suction connecting tubing or pinch the tubing to check the pressure. If it is below 80 or above 120, check with the RN or RCP before continuing.

For safety, measure the plastic suction catheter from the corner of the patient's mouth to the earlobe on the same side. Do not insert the catheter more than this distance. Insert the catheter gently. When using a tonsil tip, measuring is not necessary. You should never lose sight of the tip of the rigid suction catheter. Leave the airway in place. Do not remove it for suctioning. Whenever possible, position the patient in the high Fowler's position. If this is not possible, the semi-Fowler's position can be used, or the patient can be positioned on his or her side. Instruct the patient to cough and deep breathe several times before you begin suctioning, if possible. This helps loosen secretions and may reduce the amount of suctioning necessary.

Depending on the type of catheter used, you will have to start and stop the suction. Most suction catheters have a thumb control valve. Leave the valve open, or bend or pinch the flexible suction catheter during insertion. Place the catheter where you want it before applying suction. Cover the valve with your thumb or release the flexible catheter when you are ready to begin suctioning. The distal end of the catheter will remove secretions. Move the catheter in a circular motion or from side to side during suctioning. Keep it away from the soft tissue in the mouth and throat.

The patient cannot breathe during suctioning. Suction on the way out as you withdraw the catheter. Suction for no more than 10 seconds at a time, including the time it takes to withdraw the catheter. After you have removed the catheter, you may have to clear it of secretions before reinserting it. Hold the tip in a container of sterile water. Suction enough water to clear the catheter and tubing. If you open a new container of sterile water, label it with the date and time it was opened.

Many facilities require you to provide supplemental oxygen to the patient before suctioning. This is an important beginning procedure action. Know and follow your facility policy.

Procedure 119

Oropharyngeal Suctioning

Supplies needed:
- Suction regulator
- Sterile gloves
- Other personal protective equipment as needed or according to facility policy
- Yankauer suction catheter, or sterile #12 or #14 French suction catheter for an adult
- Sterile water or normal saline
- Small sterile basin
- Plastic bag for used supplies

1. Perform your beginning procedure actions.
2. Open the sterile water. Pour some into the sterile basin.
3. Attach the connecting tubing to the suction regulator, if this has not been done. Turn the suction on. Place your finger over the distal end of the connecting tubing to check the suction while the tube is blocked.
4. Open the suction catheter. Attach the connecting tubing to the proximal suction catheter. Maintain sterility by exposing only the connecting end of the catheter. Keep the distal (patient) end covered inside the wrapper.
5. Apply sterile gloves. Consider your dominant hand sterile and your nondominant hand unsterile. Use your nondominant hand to pick up objects and to open the catheter package so you can remove it with your sterile hand. You can use your nondominant hand to open and close the thumb valve while your dominant hand controls the position of the catheter.

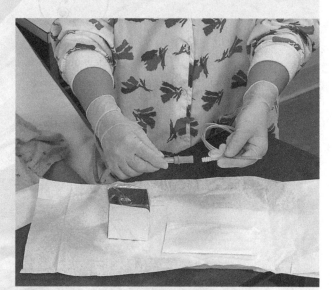

FIGURE 14-26 Attach the suction catheter to the connecting tubing.

6. Pick up the catheter with your sterile hand. Connect it to the connecting tubing (Figure 14-26).
7. Gently insert the catheter 3 to 4 inches along the side of the patient's mouth, or until you reach the pool of secretions, without applying suction.
8. Cover the thumb valve, or open the catheter and suction the secretions, and both sides of the mouth in a continuous rotating motion.
9. Suction for no longer than 10 seconds, including the time it takes you to withdraw the catheter.

(continues)

Procedure **119**, *continued*

Oropharyngeal Suctioning

10. Allow the patient to breathe normally before reinserting the catheter. If you will be reinserting the catheter, wrap it around your dominant hand, leaving the distal end free, to avoid contamination.

11. If secretions are thick, insert the tip of the catheter into the sterile water, suctioning water into the catheter and connecting tubing to clear it.

12. Repeat the suctioning until gurgling or bubbling stops and the patient's respirations are silent.

13. Perform your procedure completion actions.

Nasopharyngeal Suctioning

Nasopharyngeal suctioning is an uncomfortable procedure. To minimize discomfort, alternate suctioning between nostrils. If the patient has a nasopharyngeal airway, suction through the airway. This minimizes discomfort and trauma to the sensitive nasal tissue. Exercise great care when performing this procedure. Do not advance the catheter too far. If the patient's heart rate increases or decreases during suctioning, discontinue the procedure immediately and notify the RN. Stay with the patient and use the call signal. A nerve in the airway may be stimulated by the suction catheter. This nerve will cause changes in the heart rate, which could cause serious problems. Because of this high risk, some facilities do not permit PCTs to perform this procedure. Some facilities permit the PCT to perform the procedure only if a nasopharyngeal airway is in place. Know and follow your facility policies.

Many facilities require you to provide supplemental oxygen to the patient before nasopharyngeal suctioning. This is an important beginning procedure action. Know and follow your facility policy.

Procedure **120**

Nasopharyngeal Suctioning

Supplies needed:
- Suction regulator
- Sterile gloves
- Other personal protective equipment as needed or according to facility policy
- Sterile #12 or #14 French suction catheter for an adult
- Sterile water or normal saline
- Small sterile basin
- Water-soluble lubricant
- Plastic bag for used supplies

1. Perform your beginning procedure actions.
2. Open the sterile water and sterile basin. Pour some water into the sterile basin.
3. Attach the connecting tubing to the suction regulator, if this has not been done. Turn the suction on. Place your finger over the distal end, then remove it to check the suction.
4. Open the suction catheter. Attach the connecting tubing to the proximal suction catheter. Maintain sterility by exposing only the connecting end to the catheter. Keep the distal (patient) end covered inside the wrapper.
5. Apply sterile gloves. Consider your dominant hand sterile and your nondominant hand unsterile. Use your nondominant hand to pick up objects and to open the catheter package so you can remove it with your sterile hand. Use your nondominant hand to open and close the

(continues)

Procedure **120**, *continued*

Nasopharyngeal Suctioning

thumb valve while your dominant hand controls the position of the catheter.

6. With your nondominant hand, apply a small amount of water-soluble lubricant on the sterile area.

7. Pick up the catheter with your sterile hand. Lubricate the tip with the water-soluble lubricant.

8. With your nondominant index finger, push up on the tip of the patient's nose. *If a nasopharyngeal airway is in place, omit this step.*

9. Gently insert the catheter into the nostril. If the patient has a nasopharyngeal airway in place, insert the catheter through the lumen of the airway. Thread it carefully, 5 to 6 inches, until you reach the pool of secretions, or the patient begins to cough. Do not force the catheter. Withdraw if you meet resistance. Do not apply suction during catheter insertion.

10. Cover the thumb valve, or open the catheter and suction the secretions, in a continuous rotating motion.

11. Suction for no longer than 10 seconds, including the time it takes you to withdraw the catheter.

12. Allow the patient to breathe normally before reinserting the catheter. If you will be reinserting the catheter, wrap it around your dominant hand, leaving the distal end free, to avoid contamination.

13. If secretions are thick, insert the tip of the catheter into the sterile water, suctioning water into the catheter and connecting tubing to clear it.

14. Repeat the suctioning until gurgling or bubbling stops and the patient's respirations are silent.

15. Perform your procedure completion actions.

Complications of Suctioning

Allow the patient to rest after suctioning, while you continue observing him or her. Patients may become anxious, short of breath, cyanotic, or have other respiratory complications as a result of suctioning. The risk of complications related to nasopharyngeal suctioning is great. Perform this procedure exactly as you were taught. If the patient has signs or symptoms of distress during the procedure, stop suctioning. If he or she begins to vomit, turn the patient on the side. Use the suction to clear the airway, if necessary. Stay with the patient and use the call signal to notify the RN. Check the patient's pulse, respirations, and color before leaving the room. If you notice abnormalities, call the RN immediately. Do not leave the patient alone.

Discarding Suction Equipment

Suction catheters are sterile. This means that they are used once, then discarded. Some facilities have policies permitting you to reuse a catheter in certain circumstances. The Yankauer is commonly reused several times before being discarded. Know and follow your facility policy. If your facility reuses suction catheters, you must find out how to store the used catheter after each use. In many facilities, the catheter is rinsed well by suctioning sterile water, then stored by covering it with its original package or a plastic bag. The suction catheter should never be left uncovered, on a table, or on the suction machine.

Because the suction catheter has come into contact with body secretions, it contains biohazardous material. Follow your facility policies for discarding it in the proper container.

SMALL-VOLUME NEBULIZER TREATMENT

You may be assigned to give small-volume nebulizer treatments to patients. A **nebulizer** (Figure 14-27) is an inhalation dispenser that converts liquid medicine into a mist that can be inhaled by the patient. A nebulizer may be large, small, ultrasonic, or placed inside ventilator tubing. It may be

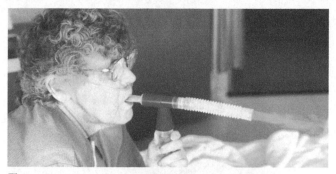

FIGURE 14-27 The handheld, small-volume nebulizer.

powered by oxygen or compressed air. Typically, drugs are ordered to open obstructed airways for patients with COPD, asthma, and allergies. The nebulizer helps loosen and lubricate secretions so the patient can cough them up. The RN or RCP will evaluate the patient's lung sounds before the treatment is given. After a nebulizer treatment, encourage the patient to cough. Have tissues and an emesis basin available in case the patient needs them. The RN or RCP will reassess the patient for improvement after medication delivery.

Procedure 121

Administering a Small-Volume Nebulizer Treatment

Supplies needed:
- Thermometer
- Blood pressure cuff
- Stethoscope
- Pressurized gas source
- Flow meter
- Oxygen tubing
- Nebulizer cup
- Mouthpiece or mask
- Normal saline solution or sterile distilled water
- Prescribed medication
- Syringe
- Tissues
- Emesis basin
- Plastic bag for used supplies

1. Perform your beginning procedure actions.
2. Position the patient in a high Fowler's or orthopneic position to promote lung expansion and distribute the medication. Instruct the patient to take slow, even breaths during the treatment.
3. Take the patient's vital signs to establish a baseline.
4. Draw up the prescribed medication.
5. Inject the medication into the nebulizer cup.
6. Add the prescribed amount of saline solution or water to the cup.
7. Attach the mouthpiece, mask, or other delivery device.

8. Attach the flow meter to the gas source.
9. Fasten the nebulizer to the flow meter.
10. Adjust the flow to at least 10 L/minute (or as specified by the RN).
11. Check the outflow port to ensure that steam is coming out.
12. Instruct the patient to put the mouthpiece in his or her mouth and inhale the steam.
13. Remain with the patient, if instructed, during the treatment.
14. Upon treatment completion, recheck vital signs.
15. Encourage the patient to breathe deeply, cough, and expectorate, or suction if necessary. Offer the tissues and emesis basin, if necessary.
16. Clean or change the nebulizer cup and tubing according to facility policy.
17. Perform your procedure completion actions.

DIFFICULT PATIENT ALERT

Monitor pediatric patients for signs of fluid overload and overhydration. Weight gain within several days of beginning therapy is a cardinal sign. Report abnormalities to the RN. If oxygen is being given while the patient uses the nebulizer, monitor the mist when the patient inhales. If it disappears, the gas flow will have to be increased. Inform the RN or RCP.

NONINVASIVE MECHANICAL VENTILATION

Some patients need respiratory support, but do not require an artificial airway. These patients do not have continuous oxygenation problems, can manage their secretions, and do not have an airway obstruction. For example, some obese patients require support because the chest is so heavy that expanding the lungs fully is very difficult. Patients with sleep apnea require ventilatory assistance while they sleep.

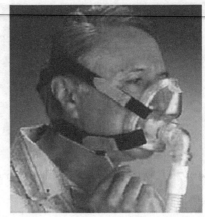

FIGURE 14-28 The CPAP mask applies pressure to keep the airway open while the patient sleeps, preventing sleep apnea.

Continuous Positive Airway Pressure

Some patients stop breathing periodically while they sleep. This condition is called **sleep apnea.** It is commonly caused by a blockage or obstruction in the airway created when the patient falls asleep and the muscles relax. Patients with sleep apnea may stop breathing hundreds of times a night, and they snore loudly when they start to breathe again. This interrupts their sleep, although they are unaware of it, so they are often very tired during the day. A common treatment is use of a device that delivers pressure to the airway while the patient sleeps, keeping the airway open.

The CPAP (pronounced *see-pap*) device holds the airway open. CPAP means **continuous positive airway pressure** (Figure 14-28). CPAP maintains constant airway pressure, which makes breathing easier. The CPAP maintains positive pressure in the chest throughout the respiratory cycle. The result is that the increased pressure opens partially or fully closed alveoli, providing more surface area for gas exchange. The additional surface area results in increased oxygenation. CPAP therapy also helps prevent premature airway closure, which traps air in the chest, interfering with normal breathing and gas exchange.

To use the CPAP, you will place a mask on the patient's face, then secure it with a head strap. Large-diameter corrugated tubing connects the mask to a device (sometimes called a blower) that creates low levels of pressure. Because there is always pressure in the system, the mask must fit tightly against the face. The amount of pressure ranges from approximately 2 cm H_2O to 20 cm H_2O. The level is ordered by the physician. The device is initially set up by a respiratory care practitioner, who works with the patient to identify the mask that will be most effective and comfortable. The RCP will probably set the pressure to the ordered value by making an adjustment on the device.

Many patients will put on their own masks at bedtime. Remind them to wash and dry the face thoroughly before putting the mask on so that less skin oil will get on the mask. You should help monitor the patient while he or she is connected to a CPAP machine. Check to make sure the mask is comfortable. Air leaks around the top will direct air into the patient's eyes, which is very irritating. If this happens, adjust the mask to reduce the leak. If the mask is too tight, the patient may feel pain or may develop redness or skin breakdown on or near the nose.

If the patient complains of excessive dryness in the nasal passages, the RCP may add a humidifier to the CPAP system. The physician may order saline spray or nose drops to reduce the irritation. Always avoid the use of petrolatum products with respiratory devices. These products increase flammability, and some will erode the plastic. If a patient swallows a lot of air, belches frequently, and/or feels pressure in the abdomen, elevate the head of the bed to see if this reduces air swallowing.

Wash the mask in soap and water each morning, after the patient takes it off. Wash it with soap and water, or according to facility policy. Store it in a clean plastic bag until use at bedtime.

Bilevel Positive Airway Pressure

Bilevel positive airway pressure (BiPAP) is similar to CPAP. In fact, some health care workers confuse the two devices, or think they are the same. CPAP maintains pressure only during the inspiratory phase of the respiration cycle. BiPAP maintains positive airway pressure during both inspiration and expiration. The device is set to regulate the flow according to the patient's needs. The system changes if patient needs and other factors (such as air leaks) create the need for a change in pressure.

The BiPAP device cycles between inspiratory and expiratory pressure at a specific time or in response to the patient's respiratory effort. The BiPAP senses when the patient is making an effort to inhale, and delivers a higher pressure on inhalation while maintaining lower pressure during exhalation. By doing this, the BiPAP reduces the effort of breathing. It keeps the airway open by reducing the need for high alveolar opening pressure. BiPAP is usually administered through a nasal mask, and the patient exhales through the mouth. You will see this device being used in patient care, but in most facilities the RCP is responsible for setting and applying the BiPAP device. He or she will check the patient several times each shift, and will inform the RN if adjustments are made to the BiPAP. Respond to equipment alarms quickly and notify the RN promptly of changes in the patient's condition.

Complications of CPAP and BiPAP

Patients using CPAP and BiPAP must be alert, have a patent airway, and be able to manage secretions. Patients who are edentulous (missing all teeth) and those who have full beards may have problems with air leaks, making ventilation difficult or impossible. Complications are:

- Nasal bridge ulceration
- Nasal congestion
- Eye irritation
- Gastric distention
- Aspiration

Inform the RN if signs or symptoms of these problems are present.

POSTURAL DRAINAGE

Postural drainage is a technique in which gravity is used to help drain and remove secretions from the lungs. Current respiratory care standards recommend using this technique only for patients who have cystic fibrosis or certain types of pneumonia. However, some physicians order the treatment for other respiratory conditions. The procedure is contraindicated if the patient has cancer in the area being treated, osteoporosis, unstable vital signs, or cyanosis. This procedure should be performed by a licensed health care professional. In most facilities, this is a respiratory care practitioner. You will assist with positioning, monitoring, and comfort measures.

The respiratory care practitioner will listen to the lungs before and after the procedure. He or she will administer medications, if necessary. The RCP determines if the patient can safely be repositioned. You will be instructed on the position to use (**Figure 14-29**). Positioning the patient exactly as ordered is very important. Some positions involve placing the head and chest lower than the legs. Change the position immediately if the patient shows signs of respiratory distress. The patient remains in each position for 5 to 10 minutes. Use foam, pillows, or props to position the patient during the procedure.

Bring the suction to the room before you begin positioning the patient and before beginning the procedure. If the patient cannot cough, the respiratory care practitioner will suction to remove secretions. Apply the principles of standard precautions when assisting.

The physician may order **percussion** during postural drainage (**Figure 14-30**). The patient's back is usually covered with a towel. The respiratory care practitioner cups his or her hands and claps against the patient's chest wall to loosen secretions. Dress the patient in a gown or pajamas. Make sure the patient is covered with clothing or a thin layer of cloth. Move buttons, snaps, and zippers away from the areas of percussion. You will be given specific instructions for positioning the patient. The licensed person will perform the procedure.

DIFFICULT PATIENT ALERT

Postural drainage is not painful. Some patients describe it as relaxing. Others fall asleep. The position of your hand creates a clapping sound, making it appear that you are hitting the patient much harder than you really are. This activity may give the impression that percussion hurts. This treatment is effective and useful. Do not avoid it for fear of hurting the patient.

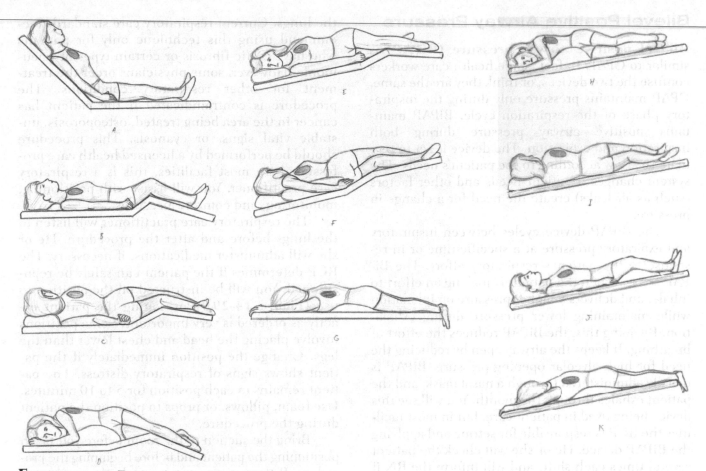

FIGURE 14-29 Postural drainage positions.

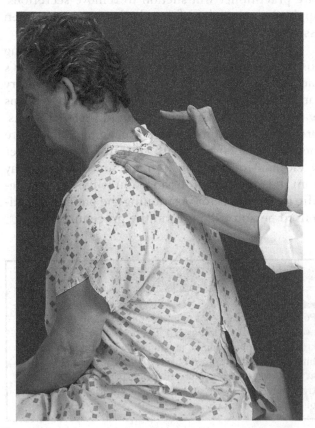

FIGURE 14-30 Chest percussion.

Monitor the patient closely after the procedure. He or she will cough up secretions. Do not leave the room until you are certain the patient is stable. Notify the RN or respiratory care practitioner immediately if the patient shows signs of respiratory distress, the vital signs are unstable, the patient is cyanotic, or the patient shows signs of cardiopulmonary distress. Stay in the room and call for help by using the call signal. Report complaints of pain or exhaustion after the treatment. Provide tissues, an emesis basin, and mouthwash, and assist the patient to use them as needed. Make the patient as comfortable as possible.

DIFFICULT PATIENT ALERT

The positioning and procedure for postural drainage are very time-consuming, and increase patient dependence. Some patients, such as those with cystic fibrosis, require postural drainage several times each day. These patients may bring a portable high-frequency chest compression vest with them to the hospital. This device uses an inflatable vest with hoses connected to a high-frequency pulse generator. The generator pumps air into the vest, vibrating the chest. This method is believed to be more effective than conventional percussion, and the patient can use the device independently.

Procedure 122

Assisting with Postural Drainage

Supplies needed:
- Disposable exam gloves
- Emesis basin
- Tissues
- Mouthwash
- Cup
- Straw
- Pillows
- Props
- Plastic bag for used supplies

1. Perform your beginning procedure actions.
2. Position and support the patient as directed, using foam wedges or pillows.

3. Provide an emesis basin, tissues, and bag in which to discard secretions.
4. Remain in the room with the patient during and after the procedure. Monitor for signs and symptoms of respiratory distress. Monitor vital signs as directed. Provide comfort measures as necessary.
5. Offer the patient mouthwash to rinse the mouth.
6. Perform your procedure completion actions.

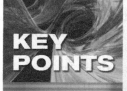

KEY POINTS

▶ Every cell in the body produces carbon dioxide. When CO_2 is not eliminated, it causes an acid buildup. Death will result if levels of acid and carbon dioxide become too high in the body.

▶ Hypoxemia is a condition in which there is insufficient oxygen in the blood.

▶ Patients at high risk of hypoxemia include those with cardiac or pulmonary disease, postoperative patients for up to a week after surgery, and those with sleep apnea, decreased level of consciousness, or neuromuscular diseases.

▶ Remove nail polish to check the patient's capillary refill and pulse oximeter readings.

▶ Capillary refill is an indication of the patient's peripheral circulation and shows how well the tissues are being nourished with oxygen.

▶ Capillary refill should return to normal in 2 to 3 seconds.

▶ The pulse oximeter measures the level of saturation of the patient's hemoglobin with oxygen.

▶ A pulse oximeter measurement of 95 percent to 100 percent is considered normal. Readings below 90 percent suggest complications. When the reading reaches 85 percent, there may not be enough oxygen for the tissues. Values below 70 percent are life-threatening.

▶ The pulse oximeter is not used in patients with known or suspected carbon monoxide poisoning.

▶ Oxygen is necessary for life. Some diseases and conditions cause the patient to be unable to take in enough oxygen, so supplemental oxygen is administered.

▶ The most common method of oxygen delivery in the hospital is through piped-in wall outlets. Oxygen is also administered through portable cylinders. Long-term care facilities commonly use oxygen concentrators, cylinders, and liquid oxygen.

(continues)

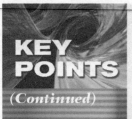

▶ Oxygen flow is regulated by a flow meter that shows how many liters of oxygen are being delivered to the patient each minute.

▶ The pressure gauge shows how much oxygen is in the cylinder.

▶ In some facilities, a humidifier is attached to the oxygen administration equipment if the patient's liter flow exceeds 5 liters; humidification is not necessary with liter flows below 5.

▶ Avoid using tap water in oxygen humidifiers; it is associated with an increased risk of Legionnaire's disease. Fill humidifiers with sterile distilled water.

▶ Nasal cannulas are used for oxygen delivered at low liter flows.

▶ An oxygen mask is used for liter flows over 5.

▶ A nonrebreathing mask is used for patients who are severely hypoxemic.

▶ Avoid matches, lighters, and other sources of ignition when oxygen is in use; follow all safety measures for oxygen administration.

▶ In an emergency, the patient requires high liter flows of oxygen, delivered through a nonrebreathing mask.

▶ An oropharyngeal airway, or oral airway, is a curved plastic or rubber device that is inserted into the mouth to the posterior pharynx. It is used to keep the airway open in unconscious patients.

▶ The most common cause of airway obstruction is the tongue.

▶ A nasopharyngeal airway may be used in responsive patients. It is the airway of choice for patients who have recent oral surgery, loose teeth, or trauma of the mouth, and those who need frequent nasal suctioning.

▶ The suction machine is used to remove fluid, food, and secretions from the patient's nose, mouth, and airway, reducing the risk of aspiration.

▶ Suction for no more than 10 seconds at a time, including the time it takes to withdraw the catheter.

▶ Notify the RN immediately if the patient shows signs and symptoms of complications of suctioning; stay in the room and use the call signal to get help.

▶ A nebulizer is an inhalation dispenser that converts liquid medicine into a mist that is inhaled by the patient. It helps loosen and lubricate secretions so the patient can cough them up.

▶ Patients with sleep apnea snore loudly and may stop breathing hundreds of times a night. This condition is usually caused by a blockage or obstruction in the airway that occurs when the patient falls asleep and the muscles relax. Sleep is interrupted and the patient may be very tired during the day.

▶ The continuous positive airway pressure device holds the airway open. It maintains positive pressure in the chest throughout the respiratory cycle, providing more surface area for gas exchange. CPAP therapy also helps prevent premature airway closure.

▶ Bilevel positive airway pressure maintains positive airway pressure during inspiration and expiration. It regulates pressure to meet the patient's needs by sensing when the patient is trying to breathe. BiPAP makes breathing easier and keeps the airway open.

▶ Postural drainage is a technique in which gravity is used to help drain and remove secretions from the lungs. It is used for patients who have cystic fibrosis or certain types of pneumonia. Monitor the patient closely for complications following the procedure.

CLINICAL APPLICATIONS

1. Mrs. Jackson is an African American patient who had a hysterectomy this morning. You are checking Mrs. Jackson's vital signs an hour after she returned to the unit from surgery. Her pulse is 120, respirations 22, and blood pressure 98/60. You decide to check her capillary refill, and discover it takes 5 seconds for her nail beds to return to normal color. Are these findings normal for a patient who has just returned from surgery? What actions will you take, if any?

2. Mr. Pagano is very diaphoretic. He has a pulse oximeter applied, but the tape keeps coming off because of his profuse sweating. What can the PCT do?

3. Mr. Pagano's pulse oximeter reading was 95 percent when you applied the sensor. You en-ter his room and discover that the reading is now 89 percent. The sensor is securely in place and has not slipped. Is this change significant? Why or why not? What action will you take?

4. During report, you write down that Mrs. Chang has a physician's order for oxygen at 12 liters per minute through a nonrebreathing mask. When you enter the patient's room shortly after your shift begins, you notice that she is using a simple mask. The patient is tolerating the mask well and does not appear to be in acute distress. Is any nursing action necessary? Why or why not? What action will you take?

5. Mr. Hateem has a nasopharyngeal airway. He tells you that his nose is very sore, but thinks this is probably normal because of the size of the airway. What action will you take?

CHAPTER REVIEW

Multiple-Choice Questions

Select the one best answer.

1. Patients at risk for hypoxemia include those with:
   a. ulcers.
   b. Parkinson's disease.
   c. congestive heart failure.
   d. urinary tract infection.

2. Capillary refill should return to normal color in:
   a. 1 second.
   b. 2 to 3 seconds.
   c. 4 to 6 seconds.
   d. 8 to 10 seconds.

3. The component of the blood that carries oxygen to cells to nourish them is:
   a. hemoglobin.
   b. leukocytes.
   c. hematocrit.
   d. white blood cells.

4. Pulse oximetry:
   a. measures the total amount of hemoglobin in the blood.
   b. determines the percentage of capillary refill.
   c. is a complicated invasive test.
   d. measures the amount of oxygen in the blood.

5. A pulse oximeter reading of 84 percent:
   a. is normal in geriatric patients.
   b. is normal for patients with cardiac disease.

   c. suggests that the patient will become short of breath.
   d. indicates that there may not be enough oxygen in the tissues.

6. The device used to determine the rate of oxygen administration is the:
   a. flow meter.
   b. pressure gauge.
   c. humidifier.
   d. inlet valve.

7. An oxygen cylinder is always:
   a. blue.
   b. yellow.
   c. red.
   d. green.

8. When caring for a patient who is receiving oxygen therapy:
   a. always apply a cannula at mealtime.
   b. elevate the head of the bed.
   c. keep the room temperature very warm.
   d. apply a wool blanket for warmth, as oxygen has a chilling effect.

9. An oropharyngeal airway is contraindicated in a patient who is:
   a. recovering from anesthesia.
   b. positioned in the lateral position.
   c. receiving anticoagulants.
   d. conscious.

10. Suction the patient for no more than:
    a. 3 to 5 seconds.
    b. 10 seconds.
    c. 15 seconds.
    d. 30 seconds.

11. When caring for a patient who is receiving oxygen therapy, always:
    a. inform the RN if the capillary refill is 2 seconds.
    b. inform the RN if the pulse oximeter value is 95 percent.
    c. check the mucous membranes for normal blue-gray color.
    d. monitor the patient, not the equipment.

12. You are missing a part for an oxygen setup, which is needed quickly. You should:
    a. ask for help from the RN or RCP.
    b. modify a part from the nitrous oxide setup.
    c. tape the parts so they fit together.
    d. go to another unit to find the part.

13. A nebulizer:
    a. is set to ventilate the patient's lungs.
    b. keeps the airway open.
    c. converts liquid medicine into a mist for inhalation.
    d. is a common treatment for patients who have sleep apnea.

14. The CPAP device:
    a. administers negative pressure.
    b. maintains positive pressure.
    c. administers inhalation medication.
    d. provides intermittent airway pressure.

15. The BiPAP device:
    a. maintains positive pressure during inhalation and exhalation.
    b. maintains negative pressure during inhalation and exhalation.
    c. maintains positive pressure during inhalation only.
    d. maintains positive pressure during exhalation only.

EXPLORING THE WEB

Alternative Airways: CPAP, BiPAP	http://www.acutedoc.com
American Association for Respiratory Care	http://www.aarc.org
American Lung Association	http://www.lungusa.org
American Sleep Apnea Association	http://www.sleepapnea.org
American Society for Asthma, Allergy, and Immunology	http://allergy.mcg.edu
Breathin' Easy	http://www.breathineasy.com
Breathing Disorders	http://www.breathingdisorders.com
Campaign for Tobacco-Free Kids	http://www.tobaccofreekids.org
Canadian Society for Respiratory Therapy	http://www.csrt.com
Emphysema Foundation for Our Right to Survive	http://www.emphysema.net
FDA Public Health Advisory	http://www.fda.gov
Global Initiative for Chronic Obstructive Lung Disease	http://www.goldcopd.com
Masimo Company (pulse oximetry)	http://www.masimo.com
Mask CPAP/BiPAP Procedure	http://www.umdnj.edu
Merck Manual of Geriatrics: Respiratory Failure	http://www.merck.com
National Association for Medical Direction of Respiratory Care	http://www.namdrc.org
Nebulizer Small Volume	http://www.nebulizersite.com
Noninvasive Positive Pressure Ventilation to Treat Respiratory Failure	http://www.annals.org

Patient Orientation Handbook—CPAP or BiPAP	http://www.norco-library.com
Patient Orientation Handbook—Oxygen Equipment	http://www.norco-library.com
Pulmonary Education and Research Foundation	http://www.perf2ndwind.org
Pulmonary Nebulizers	http://www.nebulizerinfo.com
The Pulmonary Paper	http://www.perf2ndwind.org
PulmonaryChannel.com	http://www.pulmonarychannel.com
Pulse Oximetry	http://www.utmb.edu
Respiratory Infection Tracker	http://www.rtialert.com
Respiratory Therapy Society of Ontario	http://www.rtso.org
Society of Thoracic Surgeons	http://www.sts.org
Special Patient Care Procedures—Care of Respiratory Therapy Equipment (Walter Reed Army Hospital)	http://www.wramc.amedd.army.mil

CHAPTER

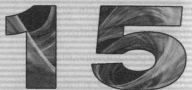

15

Advanced Respiratory Procedures

OBJECTIVES:

After reading this chapter, you should be able to:

- Spell and define key terms.
- State the purpose of endotracheal intubation and describe how to assist with this procedure.
- Describe the care of a patient who has an endotracheal tube.
- State the purpose of a tracheotomy.
- Describe the parts of the tracheostomy apparatus.
- Demonstrate the care of a patient who has a tracheostomy.
- Compare and contrast a laryngectomy and tracheostomy.
- State the purpose of chest tubes, and list PCT responsibilities in the care of patients with chest tubes.
- Differentiate a pneumothorax, hemothorax, tension pneumothorax, and pleural effusion.
- Describe PCT care for a patient who uses a ventilator.

ENDOTRACHEAL INTUBATION

Endotracheal intubation is a measure that provides complete control over the airway. It is commonly called *intubation*. An **endotracheal tube (ET tube)** is passed through the mouth, or less commonly the nose, into the patient's lungs (Figure 15-1). Endotracheal tubes are available in many sizes, ranging from pediatric to adult. Most adults use sizes 6.0 through 9.0. The patient is ventilated and suctioned through the tube. Patients are routinely intubated for many surgical procedures. Intubation is also commonly performed in some

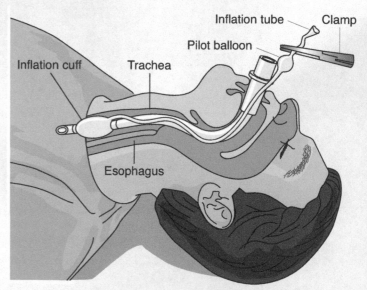

FIGURE 15-1 A properly placed endotracheal tube.

emergencies, including code situations. Intubating the patient has many advantages over other methods of controlling the airway. Some of these are listed in **Table 15-1**. Risks of endotracheal intubation are listed in **Table 15-2**.

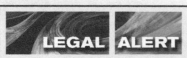

LEGAL ALERT

In some states and facilities, PCTs are not permitted to perform the procedures in this chapter. Your instructor will explain your responsibilities in your state and facility. Perform these procedures only if you are permitted to do so by state law and facility policies. Doing only tasks that you have been instructed to do, and doing things in the way that you were taught, protects patients from injury. Working in this way also protects you from injury, legal exposure, and liability.

Table 15-1 Advantages of Endotracheal Intubation

- Provides a means of delivering 100 percent oxygen directly to the lungs

- Provides a method for delivering positive pressure ventilation in a code or other emergency in which the patient requires ventilation assistance

- Protects the airway in patients who are at risk for aspiration

- Maintains a patent airway in patients who develop an airway obstruction, despite the presence of an oral or nasal airway

- Maintains a patent airway in patients with burns, inhalation injuries, or ingestion of caustic substances that cause swelling in the throat or lower airway

- Provides a pathway through which the health care professional can suction the lungs

- Does not cause **gastric distention** (a condition in which the stomach fills with air) during artificial ventilation

Table 15-2 Risks and Complications of Endotracheal Intubation

- Intubation of the esophagus, in which the tube is passed into the esophagus instead of the lungs; this condition is critical because the lungs will not be oxygenated

- Inadvertently passing the endotracheal tube into the right mainstem bronchus, so that only one lung is ventilated

- Injury to the teeth, lips, mouth, and structures in the throat

- Aspiration

- Apnea, reflex breath holding, reduced oxygen delivery

- Laryngeal edema

- Oral or nasal erosion; similar to a pressure ulcer

- Oral or nasal necrosis; similar to that seen with a pressure ulcer

- Bleeding

- Hypoxemia; low oxygenation of blood

- Bradycardia; slow pulse

The endotracheal tube is inserted by a qualified health professional who is certified in advanced cardiac life support (ACLS). As a PCT, you may assist with the insertion procedure or care for patients who have been intubated.

Direct Laryngoscopy

The **laryngoscope** is the instrument used to perform the intubation procedure. It consists of two parts: a handle containing batteries, and a blade. The

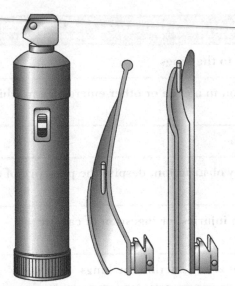

FIGURE 15-2 The laryngoscope handle and blades.

blade has a tiny light bulb to permit the health care professional to visualize the structures in the throat when the tube is inserted. Two different blades are available (**Figure 15-2**). The blades are available in pediatric and adult sizes. A straight blade or curved blade can be used, depending on the health care professional's preference. The straight blade is used to lift the epiglottis (**Figure 15-3**), exposing the vocal cords. The endotracheal tube is passed between the vocal cords, then into the lungs. The curved blade is

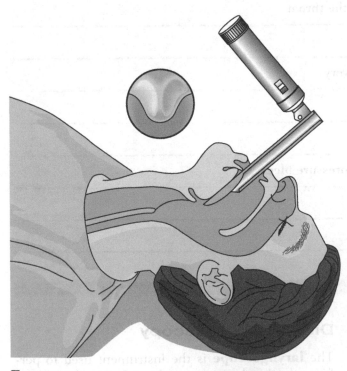

FIGURE 15-3 Visualization of the epiglottis.

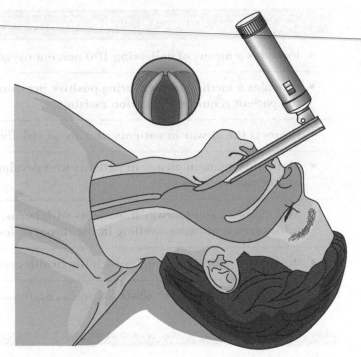

FIGURE 15-4 Visualization of the vocal cords.

designed so the health care professional can slip the tube between the base of the tongue and the epiglottis. Visualization of the larynx (**Figure 15-4**), vocal cords, and structures in the back of the throat with a laryngoscope is called *direct laryngoscopy.*

The laryngoscope is usually kept in the crash cart. Extra batteries are usually stored with the instrument. Check the light before each use, and when checking the crash cart, or according to facility policy. The light should be white, bright, and steady. If it is dull, yellow, or flickers, replace the batteries. A yellow or flickering light distorts the ability to see the structures in the back of the throat. The batteries can also become loose, causing the light to fail. Gently check the bulb to ensure that it is in the socket tightly. Make sure an extra bulb and batteries for the handle are available in case the bulb burns out or the batteries fail.

Assisting with Endotracheal Intubation

A physician, RN, or RCP will perform the intubation procedure. The patient must be well oxygenated before the endotracheal tube is inserted. This is performed by mouth-to-mask or bag-valve-mask resuscitation. After setting up for the procedure, you may be asked to provide oxygenation, allowing the health care professional time to check and prepare the equipment for intubation. The patient is completely without oxygen while the intubation is being performed, so the endotracheal tube must be inserted rapidly.

Your role and responsibility for assisting with this procedure will vary with facility policies. You may set up equipment and position the patient. He or she should be supine, with no pillow under the head. The shoulders may be propped on a towel, if necessary. Position the patient's head in the **sniffing position** (Figure 15-5) for the procedure. The position is so named because the patient appears to be sniffing a flower or other object. The neck is flexed and the head extended. The equipment used is pictured in **Figure 15-6.**

During the intubation procedure, you may be instructed to apply pressure on the lower neck. This closes the esophagus, reducing the risk of gastric distention, a condition in which the stomach fills with air. The air occupies a great deal of space, making it difficult for the lungs to expand. Several other serious complications are associated with gastric distention. You will be given very specific instructions for assisting with this procedure. Listen carefully and follow the directions of the licensed health care professional.

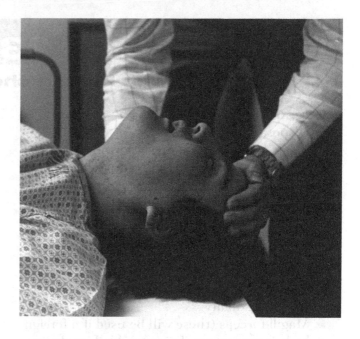

FIGURE 15-5 The sniffing position.

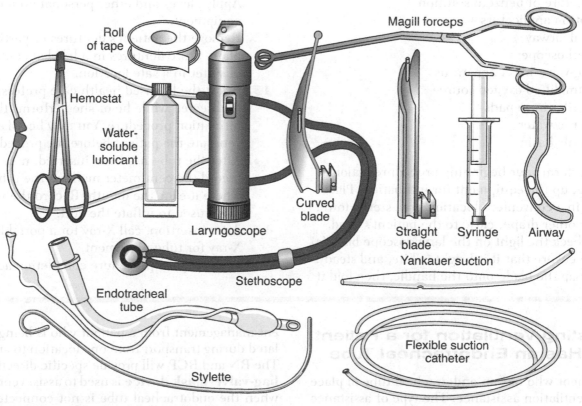

FIGURE 15-6 Primary intubation equipment.

Roll of tape

Magill forceps

Hemostat

Water-soluble lubricant

Laryngoscope

Curved blade

Straight blade

Syringe

Airway

Yankauer suction

Stethoscope

Endotracheal tube

Stylette

Flexible suction catheter

Procedure 123

Assisting with Endotracheal Intubation

Supplies needed:
- Disposable exam gloves
- Mask, face shield, or other personal protective equipment depending on the patient situation and facility policy
- Sterile towel or drape
- Laryngoscope handle and blades
- Endotracheal tubes, assorted sizes; ask the licensed professional to select the proper size tube
- **Stylette,** a wire inserted through the tube to reduce flexibility
- Magill forceps (these will be used if a foreign body is present, or if nasotracheal intubation is necessary)
- 10-mL syringe
- Kelly clamp or other hemostat
- Water-soluble lubricant
- Suction, set up with flexible catheter
- Tape, 1- and 2-inch sizes, or endotracheal tube holder
- Tincture of benzoin solution
- Cotton applicators
- Oral airway
- Stethoscope
- Bag-valve-mask apparatus
- Humidified oxygen source
- Sterile gauze pads
- Sterile water
- Sterile basin

1. Perform your beginning procedure actions.
2. Set up the equipment for intubation. Place it in a convenient location on a sterile towel or other drape, close to the patient's head.
3. Check the light on the laryngoscope blade(s) to ensure that it is bright, white, and steady. Snap the blade onto the handle, then fold it up and down. When pulled up, the light should go on. Folding it down turns the light off.
4. Open the sterile package containing the endotracheal tube. Leave the tube within the package, removing only the inflation port for the cuff. The tube must remain sterile.
5. Pull the plunger back on the syringe. Attach it to the inflation port on the endotracheal tube. Slowly inject air into the inflation port to check the cuff for leaks. Pull back on the plunger to deflate the cuff.
6. Lubricate the entire stylette, and place it on the table next to the endotracheal tube.
7. Tear the tape and place it over the edge of the table, or in another convenient location.
8. Squeeze water-soluble lubricant onto a sterile gauze pad.
9. Prepare the humidified oxygen.
10. Set up the suction.
11. Apply gloves and other personal protective equipment.
12. Remove the patient's dentures or partial plate. Store dentures in a labeled container of water in a safe location.
13. Assist the licensed health care professional as directed while he or she performs the intubation procedure. You may be asked to ventilate the patient before the procedure.
14. After the tube has been inserted, note and record the centimeter mark on the tube where it exits the mouth. Record the volume of air used to inflate the cuff.
15. After insertion, call X-ray for a portable X-ray for tube placement.
16. Perform your procedure completion actions.

Assisting Ventilation for a Patient Who Has an Endotracheal Tube

The patient who has an endotracheal tube in place needs ventilation assistance. The type of assistance necessary is determined by the patient's needs. For example, a patient in cardiac arrest will need different management from a patient who is being ventilated during transport from one location to another. The RN and RCP will provide specific directions. A **bag-valve-mask device** is used to assist ventilation when the endotracheal tube is not connected to a mechanical ventilator. The mask is removed and the bag is connected directly to the endotracheal tube.

Procedure 124

Ventilating an Endotracheal Tube Using a Bag-Valve Device

Supplies needed:
- Disposable exam gloves
- Eye protection and face mask
- Bag-valve-mask device
- Oxygen source with nipple adapter for connecting tubing
- Oxygen connecting tubing

1. Perform your beginning procedure actions.
2. Connect the bag-valve-mask device to the connecting tubing. Attach the connecting tubing to the oxygen flow meter.
3. Turn the flow meter on to 15 liters per minute, or as instructed.
4. If the bag-valve mask is assembled, remove the mask by twisting and pulling slightly.
5. Connect the bag valve to the endotracheal tube.
6. Squeeze the bag with sufficient force to cause the patient's chest to rise. Release the bag. Repeat at a rate of once every 3 to 5 seconds, or as directed. The rate may vary depending on the purpose of the procedure.
7. Upon completion, disconnect the bag-valve device and reconnect the endotracheal tube to the ventilator, or as instructed.
8. Perform your procedure completion actions.

Caring for the Patient Who Has an Endotracheal Tube

Patients who are intubated need a great deal of care, comfort measures, and reassurance. Because of the position of the tube, the patient will be unable to speak. Patients who are intubated are ventilated mechanically. This often involves using a ventilator, a positive pressure device that forces air into the patient's lungs. The RCP and RN will care for the ventilator and will suction through the endotracheal tube, if needed. The patient may be restrained to prevent him or her from removing the endotracheal tube. A patient who is restrained will need total nursing care, including turning and repositioning, and restraint care and observation. The care plan or critical pathway will provide instructions. The RN will guide you if you have questions. In general, care for a patient who is intubated involves:

- Monitoring the patient frequently and anticipating his or her needs.
- Keeping the head of the bed elevated in the semi-Fowler's or Fowler's position, as directed.
- Keeping the patient's head turned to the side if an oral or nasal airway is used; turning the head helps prevent aspiration.
- Suctioning oral secretions. Avoid suctioning the endotracheal tube. If the patient is using a mechanical ventilator, a licensed professional will suction the tube.
- Inserting an oropharyngeal or nasopharyngeal airway and removing the airway once each shift for cleaning.
- Providing oral and nasal care as directed.
- Keeping the lips and mucous membranes moist.
- Repositioning the patient every 2 hours, or more often, if indicated.
- Monitoring restraints, if used, and releasing restraints according to facility policy.
- Monitoring the bony prominences for signs of redness, irritation, or breakdown.
- Monitoring the tube insertion site for signs of redness, irritation, or breakdown.
- Monitoring vital signs and capillary refill, and reporting abnormalities to the RN immediately.
- Monitoring for signs of respiratory distress, and reporting to the RN immediately.
- Reassuring the patient and family.
- Developing a means for communicating with the patient, such as using a magic slate, or by writing.

PATIENTS WHO BREATHE THROUGH THE NECK

A **tracheotomy** is a surgical procedure to create an opening into the neck through which to breathe. The procedure is performed for airway obstruction, which may have many causes. The opening into the airway is called a **tracheostomy** (Figure 15-7). The external opening on the skin surface is the stoma. Eventually, the stoma will heal and remain permanently open. An indwelling tube is inserted through the stoma to maintain patency. This tube is the **cannula.** An outer and inner cannula are used. Several types of outer cannulae are available. The most common has an inflatable cuff. The cuffed cannula is used to prevent aspiration. It seals or reduces the air flow to the nose and throat, so virtually all ventilation is done through the tracheostomy. The outer cannula has a flat plate, with a flange on each side that is fastened to twill tape or a Velcro fastener that encircles the patient's neck. The tape helps hold the device securely in place. The inner cannula has an adapter on the distal end that can be attached to a bag-valve mask. The parts of the tracheostomy apparatus are pictured in **Figure 15-8.**

Cancer of the larynx may require removal of the larynx (voicebox), resulting in a loss of voice. A **laryngectomy** is the surgical removal of the larynx. During this procedure, the airway is separated from the mouth, nose, and esophagus. When the larynx is removed, there is no longer a connection between the upper and lower airways (Figure 15-9). A person who has had this surgery may be called a **laryngectomee.** The patient breathes through an artificial opening in the neck and trachea.

A patient with a laryngectomy breathes through a permanent stoma in the neck. A laryngectomy stoma is a special kind of opening in the neck. Though it may look like a regular tracheostomy, it is very different. If you are caring for a patient with a stoma, you must know whether it is a tracheostomy stoma or a laryngectomy stoma. If the patient has a

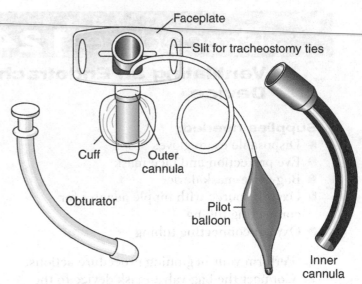

FIGURE 15-8 Parts of the tracheostomy.

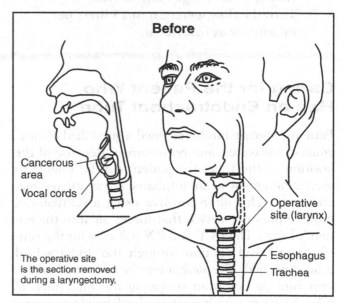

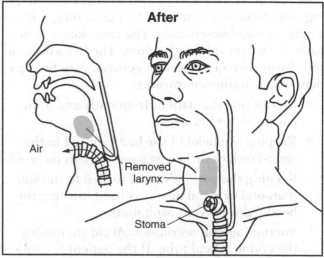

FIGURE 15-9 The anatomy of the face and neck before and after laryngectomy surgery.

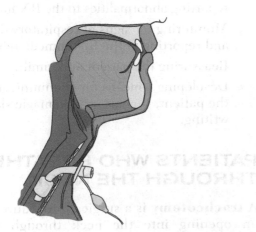

FIGURE 15-7 A tracheostomy with the cuff inflated.

tracheostomy, the passageway from the mouth and nose through the trachea remains intact. Patients can still smell odors, blow their noses, and suck on a straw. If a patient has a laryngectomy, the larynx has been completely removed. The upper airway is no longer connected to the trachea. The patient will be unable to talk, smell, blow his or her nose, whistle, gargle, or suck on a straw. He or she retains the ability to swallow, although initially a tube feeding may be used to promote healing and prevent irritation of the esophagus.

Loss of voice is very traumatic. Just think how frustrated you would feel if you could no longer use your voice to express your thoughts, feelings, wants, and needs to others. During the immediate postoperative period, writing is the major form of communication. A "magic slate" is often used. Later, a speech language pathologist will work with the patient to teach him or her to use electronic speech or esophageal speech.

In most people, the structures in the nose and mouth capture microbes and other foreign particles, preventing them from entering the airway. In addition, the body moistens and warms air before it enters the lungs. Inhaling cold, dry air is very uncomfortable, as well as irritating to the lungs. Because the tracheostomy bypasses the normal breathing structures, the patient's body cannot use its normal protective mechanisms to warm, moisten, or filter the air. Thus, care is designed to replace these body functions. Warm, humidified oxygen is often administered to patients with a tracheostomy.

The stoma now provides a direct passageway into the lungs. The risk of aspirating a foreign particle is greatly increased. Avoid getting water, powder, lint, dust, or other objects near the stoma. Likewise, the opening in the neck provides an open pathway for bacteria to enter and cause serious infection. Using faultless sterile technique and precise medical asepsis and practicing frequent handwashing are also very important.

Patient Care for Neck Breathers

Patients may expel secretions through the stoma in the neck. The patient has no control over this. If he or she is expelling secretions, in addition to gloves, you should wear a gown, mask, and eye protection during patient care.

The stoma in the neck is the patient's primary airway. If the tube becomes blocked, dislodged, disconnected, or otherwise disrupted, the patient's airway will be severely compromised. Be especially careful when turning and bathing the patient. Encourage deep breathing and coughing every 2 hours. Monitor the patient's skin color closely. Watch for cyanosis, changes in the color of the nail beds or mucous membranes, or respiratory distress. Monitor for restlessness, dyspnea, anxiety, increased heart rate, lethargy, or disorientation. These are signs of ineffective airway clearance and poor gas exchange. Review the Observe & Report box in Chapter 14 to make sure you are familiar with important observations for patients who have respiratory disorders.

Ventilating a Patient Who Has a Tracheostomy

Some patients with a tracheostomy breathe room air. Some use humidified oxygen delivered through a special tracheostomy mask (Figure 15-10). Others are dependent on a ventilator to maintain respirations. If the ventilator is disconnected, a bag-valve mask, with the mask removed, is used to ventilate the patient. A bag valve is also used for emergency ventilation.

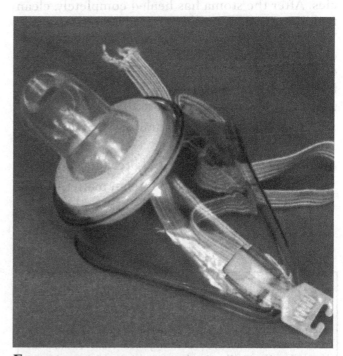

FIGURE 15-10 An adult tracheostomy oxygen mask.

Procedure 125

Ventilating a Tracheostomy Using a Bag-Valve Device

Supplies needed:
- Disposable exam gloves
- Eye protection and face mask
- Bag-valve-mask device
- Oxygen source with nipple adapter for connecting tubing
- Oxygen connecting tubing

1. Perform your beginning procedure actions.
2. Connect the bag-valve-mask device to the connecting tubing. Attach the connecting tubing to the oxygen flow meter.
3. Turn the flow meter on to 15 liters per minute, or as instructed.

4. If the bag-valve mask is assembled, remove the mask by twisting and pulling slightly.
5. Connect the bag valve to the adapter on the inner cannula.
6. Squeeze the bag with sufficient force to cause the patient's chest to rise. Release the bag. Repeat at a rate of once every 3 to 5 seconds, or as directed. The rate may vary depending on the purpose of the procedure.
7. Upon completion, disconnect the bag-valve device and reconnect the cannula to the ventilator, or as instructed.
8. Perform your procedure completion actions.

Tracheostomy Care

Caring for a new tracheostomy is a sterile procedure. This procedure is performed only by RNs in most facilities. Know and follow your facility policies. After the stoma has healed completely, clean technique may be used by the patient in the home. You may be permitted to care for healed tracheostomies. In health care facilities, tracheostomy care is done under sterile conditions because of the increased risk of infection. The goals of tracheostomy care are to:

- Keep the stoma and cannulae clean and free from obstruction
- Prevent skin irritation and breakdown
- Prevent water and solid foreign matter from entering the lungs
- Prevent infection

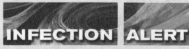

INFECTION ALERT

The nasal hairs and tonsils filter pathogens and other substances from the air, preventing them from reaching the lungs. A patient with a tracheostomy does not have this advantage. The stoma provides a direct, unfiltered passageway to the lungs for irritating foreign substances and pathogens. Practice good infection control techniques when caring for a patient who has a stoma.

The PCT should perform these procedures only on patients who have established (healed) tracheostomies. Avoid disconnecting patients from mechanical ventilation devices to perform the procedures. Perform these skills only on patients who are not ventilator-dependent.

Caring for a patient who has a tracheostomy is easiest if you have an assistant, because of the need to open extra sterile supplies. The assistant can ventilate the patient with the bag-valve device. Always ventilate according to the patient's natural breathing rhythm. Do not ventilate against the patient's breathing, as this will increase pressure within the airway. This has the potential to cause serious complications.

Suctioning a tracheostomy stimulates coughing, so wearing face and eye protection is necessary. A gown is optional, but preferred. When the patient coughs, secretions are expelled through the cannula. The patient cannot control the cough or direction in which the secretions will travel.

Like oropharyngeal and nasopharyngeal suctioning, pressures in the suction machine should not be below 80 or above 120. If the suction pressure is not within this range, notify the RN or RCP before proceeding. Suctioning the tracheostomy may increase the patient's anxiety, because it is uncomfortable. He or she cannot breathe during suctioning. Be calm and reassuring. Always explain what you are doing, and state why the procedure is important. Stop immediately and signal for the RN if the patient's color changes, or if he or she begins coughing uncontrollably or becomes short of breath. After suctioning, check the patient's vital signs. Report your observations to the RN. Special observations to report are listed in the Observe & Report box.

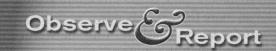

Observe & Report

Tracheostomy Suctioning

Patient's reaction to and tolerance of the procedure
Change in vital signs
Changes in the patient's color
Changes in the pulse oximeter or cardiac monitor
Color and character of secretions; they should be thin, white, or translucent; secretions are slightly sticky. Report:
  – thick secretions
  – yellow, green, brown, or red sputum
  – red streaks in sputum

Set up the supplies on a sterile field on the overbed table before beginning. Position the patient in the semi-Fowler's position. Drape a towel or sterile towel across the patient's chest, according to facility policy. A sterile towel or drape is best because it enlarges the sterile area you have to work in.

Follow the RN's instructions for tracheostomy care. You may be instructed to suction the patient's mouth after suctioning the trachea. Follow the guidelines in Procedure 119 for oropharyngeal suctioning.

DIFFICULT PATIENT ALERT

Suction catheters are measured in millimeters. When suctioning a tracheostomy or endotracheal tube, the outer diameter of the suction catheter should be no greater than one-half the inner diameter of the airway. Suction catheter sizes are measured in French, similar to catheters. To determine the correct size, double the size of the artificial airway (which is also measured in mm). For example, a patient with an 8–mm endotracheal tube may be suctioned safely with a size 16 French catheter.

Procedure 126

Suctioning a Tracheostomy

Supplies needed:
▶ Sterile gloves
▶ Eye protection
▶ Surgical mask
▶ Gown
▶ Sterile towel, according to facility policy
▶ Sterile drape to set up sterile field
▶ Sterile suction catheter
▶ Sterile normal saline
▶ Sterile basin
▶ Sterile, lint-free sponges
▶ Alcohol sponge
▶ Bag-valve-mask device
▶ Plastic bag for used supplies

1. Perform your beginning procedure actions.
2. Prepare the sterile field, if you have not done so previously. Pour sterile normal saline into the sterile basin.
3. If the bag-valve-mask device is assembled, remove the mask by twisting and pulling slightly.

4. Connect the bag valve to the tracheostomy and firmly ventilate the patient 4 or 5 times. Synchronize your ventilations with the patient's respirations. Avoid squeezing the bag while the patient is exhaling.
5. Apply sterile gloves.
6. Drape the sterile towel across the patient's upper chest.
7. Attach the suction catheter to the connecting tubing. The hand that touches the connecting tubing is no longer sterile.
8. Turn the suction on with the nonsterile hand.
9. Holding the catheter with your sterile hand, insert the tip into the saline. Suction a small amount of saline through the catheter to lubricate the inside. Secretions will flow through the catheter more readily if the inside is lubricated first.
10. Gently insert the suction catheter into the inner cannula (**Figure 15-11**) until you

(continues)

Procedure **126**, *continued*

Suctioning a Tracheostomy

meet resistance (approximately 6 inches), then withdraw 2 to 3 cm (1½ inches). If the patient begins to cough, do not insert the catheter further. Withdraw the catheter 2 to 3 cm. If the patient coughs violently, wait a few seconds before proceeding.

11. Cover the thumb port and apply suction for no more than 10 seconds. While suctioning, rotate the catheter gently. Rotation is important

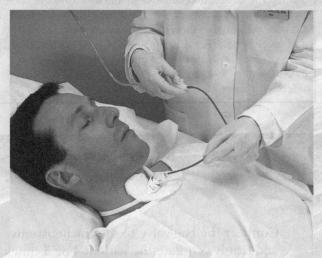

FIGURE 15-11 Insert the suction catheter into the inner cannula.

to prevent the suction from removing tissue. Continue suctioning as you pull the catheter out. Remember, the entire procedure should take no more than 10 seconds.

12. Insert the suction catheter into the sterile saline and flush the tubing.

13. Connect the bag-valve device and give the patient 4 or 5 breaths. Ask another PCT to do this, if possible, to avoid contaminating your gloves.

14. Allow the patient to rest a few minutes before repeating the suctioning. During this time, observe the patient's response and skin color, and color and character of the secretions, to report to the RN upon procedure completion.

15. Repeat steps 7 through 11 until the airway is clear of secretions. Do not suction more than 2 to 4 times, or according to facility policy.

16. Upon conclusion, connect the bag-valve device and give the patient 4 or 5 additional breaths.

17. Wipe the connection of the bag-valve device well with alcohol. Cover the connection with a sterile gauze sponge or sterile glove.

18. Discard used supplies in the plastic bag.

19. Perform your procedure completion actions.

Procedure **127**

Giving Tracheostomy/Stoma Care Using a Nondisposable Inner Cannula

Supplies needed:

- Sterile gloves, 3 pair
- Towel or sterile towel, according to facility policy
- Sterile normal saline
- Hydrogen peroxide
- Sterile suction catheter and suctioning supplies

- Sterile tracheostomy care kit OR
  - Sterile drape to set up sterile field
  - Sterile tracheostomy brush
  - Two small sterile basins
  - Sterile applicators
  - Sterile, lint-free gauze pads
  - Sterile tracheostomy dressing
- Plastic bag for used supplies

(continues)

Procedure **127**, *continued*

Giving Tracheostomy/Stoma Care Using a Nondisposable Inner Cannula

1. Perform your beginning procedure actions.
2. Open the plastic trash bag. Place it at the foot of the bed or other location where you can reach it without crossing over the sterile field.
3. Set up the sterile field and open sterile supplies, if this was not done previously. Pour a mixture of equal parts of normal saline and hydrogen peroxide into a basin. Pour plain normal saline into the second basin.
4. Apply sterile gloves and suction the tracheostomy (Procedure 126), using sterile technique.
5. Remove your gloves. Discard the gloves and suction catheter in the plastic bag.
6. Wash your hands.
7. Apply new sterile gloves.
8. Moisten a sterile sponge in sterile normal saline, then squeeze out excess water. Wipe the area under the flanges and twill tapes on the sides. Begin near the stoma, working your way outward. Use moist cotton applicators, if necessary, to clean around the stoma and under the flanges (**Figure 15-12**). Keep water out of the stoma, cleaning only the outside. Use each sponge or applicator only once. Discard used sponges and applicators in the plastic bag.

9. Moisten a second sponge or applicator and repeat. Use each sponge only once, working from the clean, inner area outward.
10. Pat the area dry with a sterile gauze sponge or applicator.
11. Remove your gloves and discard them in the plastic bag.
12. Wash your hands.
13. Apply new sterile gloves.
14. With your nondominant hand, discard the tracheostomy dressing, if not done previously. Discard it in the plastic bag.
15. With your nondominant hand, carefully hold the flange to the outer cannula. Turn the inner cannula counterclockwise to unlock it.
16. Remove the inner cannula by pulling it out, then down. Place the cannula in the basin with the hydrogen peroxide mixture.
17. With your dominant hand, insert the small brush into the inner cannula to scrub secretions on the inside, using the hydrogen peroxide mixture (**Figure 15-13**).
18. Place the inner cannula into the basin of normal saline for 10 seconds, and agitate it to rinse it thoroughly.

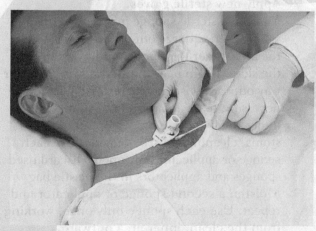

FIGURE 15-12 Use an applicator or gauze pad to clean under the faceplate.

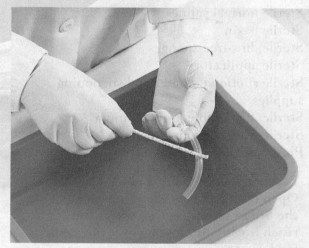

FIGURE 15-13 Clean the inner cannula with hydrogen peroxide to remove secretions.

(continues)

Procedure **127**, *continued*

Giving Tracheostomy/Stoma Care Using a Nondisposable Inner Cannula

19. Check the cannula to ensure that it is clean, then tap it on the inner edge of the basin to remove excess water.
20. Reinsert the inner cannula. Turn the adapter on the distal end clockwise to lock it in place, then check to make sure it is secure.
21. Apply a clean tracheostomy dressing and ties (Figure 15-14).
22. Perform your procedure completion actions.

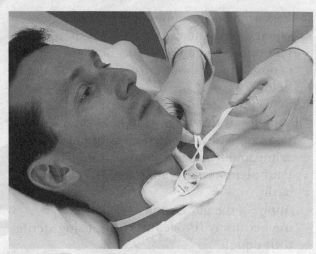

FIGURE 15-14 Change the twill tape ties.

Procedure **128**

Giving Tracheostomy/Stoma Care Using a Disposable Inner Cannula

Supplies needed:
- Sterile gloves, 2 pair
- Towel or sterile towel, according to facility policy
- Sterile normal saline
- Sterile basin
- Sterile, lint-free sponges
- Sterile applicators
- Sterile suction catheter and suctioning supplies
- Sterile, disposable inner cannula
- Sterile tracheostomy dressing
- Plastic bag for used supplies

1. Perform your beginning procedure actions.
2. Open the trash bag. Place it at the foot of the bed or other location where you can reach it without crossing over the sterile field.
3. Set up the sterile field and open sterile supplies, if this was not done previously.

4. Apply sterile gloves, and suction the tracheostomy (Procedure 126), using sterile technique.
5. Remove your gloves. Discard the gloves and catheter in the plastic bag.
6. Wash your hands.
7. Apply new sterile gloves.
8. Moisten a sterile sponge in sterile normal saline, then squeeze out excess water. Wipe the area under the flanges and twill tapes on the sides. Begin near the stoma, working your way outward. Use moist cotton applicators, if necessary, to clean around the stoma and under the flanges. Keep water out of the stoma, cleaning only the outside. Use each sponge or applicator only once. Discard used sponges and applicators in the plastic bag.
9. Moisten a second sponge or applicator and repeat. Use each sponge only once, working from the clean, inner area outward.

(continues)

Procedure **128**, *continued*

Giving Tracheostomy/Stoma Care Using a Disposable Inner Cannula

10. Pat the area dry with a sterile gauze sponge or applicator.
11. Remove your gloves and discard them in the plastic bag.
12. Wash your hands.
13. Apply new sterile gloves.
14. With your nondominant hand, carefully hold the outer flange to support it. Turn the inner cannula counterclockwise to unlock it.
15. Lift the inner cannula free from the outer cannula by pulling it out, then down.
16. Check the inner cannula for the presence of secretions.

17. Discard the cannula in the plastic bag.
18. Pick up the new, sterile inner cannula, touching only the locking adapter on the end.
19. Insert the inner cannula into the outer cannula.
20. Turn the adapter on the distal end of the cannula clockwise to lock it in place. Check the connection to make sure it is secure.
21. Apply a clean tracheostomy dressing and ties.
22. Perform your procedure completion actions.

Tracheostomy Dressing and Ties

The tracheostomy dressing is used to absorb perspiration and secretions, preventing skin irritation. It is a lint-free, composite 4 × 4 sponge. The dressing is split in the center so it can be positioned around the outer cannula. When the dressing is inserted, the split faces up, toward the patient's face. Regular gauze sponges should not be cut because lint and threads in the gauze may accidentally enter the stoma. If a split dressing is not available, a sterile gauze sponge may be folded and inserted surrounding the cannula (**Figure 15-15**). Foreign particles that enter the stoma or cannula will be inhaled into the lungs.

In most facilities, a Velcro band is used to secure the outer cannula. However, twill ties are also often used. The procedure here describes twill ties, but the method for inserting Velcro is similar.

The tracheostomy ties are inserted into a hole in the flange on either side of the neck. The ties are made of twill tape, which does not fray or unravel. Gauze roller bandage should not be used because it will unravel, increasing the risk of aspiration of threads and particles. The tape is inserted through the flange, then drawn securely around the neck. It is tied in two double knots at the side. The old ties are not removed until the new ties are in place. Avoid tying in the back of the neck, as pressure from the knot may cause skin breakdown. The tape is tied tightly enough to hold the cannula securely. The flat

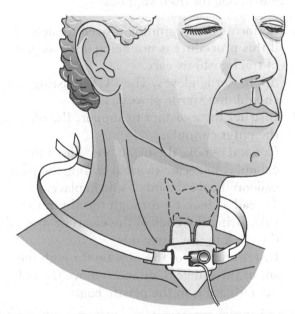

FIGURE 15-15 A 4 × 4 gauze sponge can be folded if a split tracheostomy dressing is not available.

plate to the outer cannula should be flat against the patient's neck. You should be able to place one or two fingers between the tape and the neck. The ties should hold the tracheostomy firmly in place so it cannot be coughed out, but should not be too tight.

When changing the ties, ask another PCT to hold the outer cannula in place. If the patient begins to cough after the old tie is cut, the plate and outer cannula may be expelled. The stoma may close quickly, so this has the potential to become a serious emergency. If a tracheostomy becomes dislodged during any care, stay with the patient and call for the RN or RCP immediately. A second, smaller tracheostomy set is kept at the bedside at all times. A smaller set is used to accommodate immediate closing of the stoma. A cannula of the original size may not fit.

The dressing and ties are usually replaced during tracheostomy care. However, they should be replaced any time they become moist with secretions or perspiration. Wear face protection and a surgical mask when performing this procedure, because manipulating the cannulae may cause the patient to cough.

Procedure 129

Applying a Tracheostomy Dressing and Ties

Supplies needed:
- Sterile gloves, 2 pair
- Sterile tracheostomy dressing
- Sterile twill tape tie, approximately 24 to 30 inches long
- Face mask or goggles
- Surgical mask
- Gown
- Plastic bag for used supplies

1. Perform your beginning procedure actions, if this procedure is not being done as part of tracheostomy care.
2. Apply sterile gloves. The PCT assisting you should don sterile gloves as well.
3. Instruct the assistant to support the plate on the outer cannula.
4. Cut and remove the tie on one side of the cannula. Take care to avoid cutting the pilot balloon. Leave the other side in place.
5. Thread a clean tie through the slit in the side. Bring the ends of the clean tie around the neck to the other side.
6. Insert one end of the new tie through the slit in the flange. Cut and remove the old tie. Discard it in the plastic bag.

7. Pull the ends of the tie so that the tape is snug, but not tight. One or two fingers should fit between the ties and the neck.
8. Tie the ties in a double knot on the side of the neck. To do this, cross the right tie over the left tie, then under. Next, slip the left tie over the right tie, then cross under. Pull tightly.
9. Tie a second double knot on top of the first. The next time the ties are changed, tie the knot on the opposite side of the neck.
10. Trim the ends of the tie with scissors.
11. Instruct your assistant to release pressure on the flange.
12. Inspect the sterile tracheostomy dressing for lint and gauze. If noted, replace the dressings.
13. Separate the sides of the split tracheostomy dressing slightly. Slide the dressing up from the bottom of the outer cannula so the open ends face the patient's head.
14. Perform your procedure completion actions.

NOTE: This is a two-person procedure. If you are performing the procedure alone, **do not** remove the old ties until the new ties are securely in place.

CHEST TUBES

Chest tubes (Figure 15-16) are sterile plastic tubes that are inserted through the skin of the chest, between the ribs, and into the spaces between the pleural membrane that covers the lung and the pleural membrane that lines the chest wall. They are used after surgery to drain any bloody fluid from the chest. These tubes also al-

low air to escape if there is a leak of air at the suture line after lung surgery.

Chest tubes are used to treat **pneumothorax**. This is free air in the chest cavity outside the lung. The free air presses against the lung, so that the lung cannot expand properly. **Hemothorax** is a similar condition, in which there is blood in the chest cavity. Spontaneous lung collapses are rare. This condition usually occurs as a result of trauma,

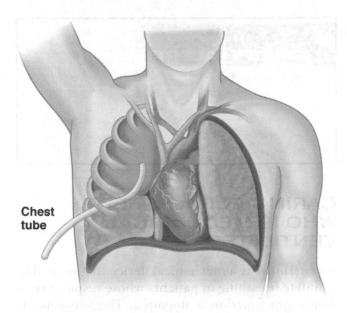

Chest
tube

FIGURE 15-16 Chest tubes are sterile plastic tubes that are inserted through the skin of the chest, between the ribs, and into the space between the pleural membrane that covers the lung and the pleural membrane that lines the chest wall.

such as the injury that occurs in an automobile accident. A fractured rib may also cause an air leak from the lung.

A small pneumothorax without underlying disease may resolve on its own. A larger pneumothorax usually requires chest-tube placement to evacuate the air and allow the lungs to re-expand. You are most likely to see patients with chest tubes for three reasons:

- To reinflate a lung affected by pneumothorax or hemothorax.
- To correct an air leak that is slow to heal after lung surgery.
- To drain fluid that collects around the lungs in patients who have cancer. (This fluid is called a **pleural effusion.**)

The chest tube is attached to a drain of some sort (Figure 15-17). The nurse will manage the system.

Caring for a Patient Who Has a Chest Tube

PCT monitoring and care for a patient who has a chest tube includes:

- Making sure that the bottle is always lower than the patient's heart

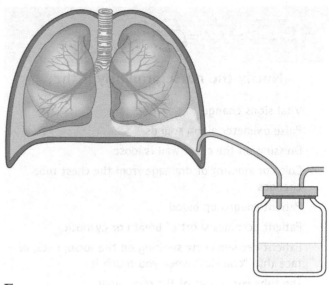

FIGURE 15-17 Chest tubes are always attached to a drainage bottle, which must be kept lower than the insertion site.

- Making sure that nothing pulls on the tube
- Making sure that the chest tube is taped to the chest distal to the insertion site
- Making sure the junction of the chest tube and the drainage tube is taped to prevent accidental separation
- Positioning the drainage system upright and below the level of the heart at all times
- Repositioning the patient every 2 hours, or as instructed
- Making sure that the chest tube is never twisted, kinked, or obstructed
- Coiling the tubing that connects the chest tube to the drain on the bed, similar to the way you would position tubing for a Foley catheter
- Checking with the RN before disconnecting a drain that is connected to a vacuum regulator
- Keeping the patient mobile; getting the patient up in a chair regularly
- Making sure that the patient always has oxygen and suction sets at the bedside
- Making sure that a tray of emergency equipment is kept in the room; never remove these items
- Informing the RN if the patient develops any of the signs and symptoms listed in the Observe & Report box

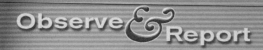

Notify the nurse promptly if the:

- Vital signs change
- Pulse oximeter alarm sounds
- Dressing on the chest wall is loose
- Color or amount of drainage from the chest tube changes
- Patient coughs up blood
- Patient becomes short of breath or cyanotic
- Patient develops new swelling on the torso, neck, or face that "crackles" when you touch it
- The tube comes out of the chest wall

Emergency Care for a Patient Who Has a Chest Tube

The most common nursing complications of chest tube use are accidental tube dislodgement or removal, and breakage of the drainage bottle. If either of these situations occurs, you must observe the patient for signs of **tension pneumothorax,** a very serious condition in which the air cannot escape, leading to a steady buildup of pressure. Signs and symptoms of tension pneumothorax are:

- Chest pain
- Hypotension
- Distended neck veins
- Tracheal shift to one side
- Hypoxemia
- Rapid, weak pulse
- Dyspnea
- Rapid respirations
- Diaphoresis

If the chest tube comes out, promptly cover the site with 4 × 4 gauze pads or petroleum gauze pads from the emergency supply kit. Tape them in place. If a glass drainage bottle accidentally breaks, a plastic drainage bottle cracks, or a tube disconnects, clamp the chest tube as close to the insertion site as possible by using the rubber-tipped clamp in the emergency tray. Stay with the patient and use the call signal to get help. Monitor the vital signs every 10 minutes, or as instructed.

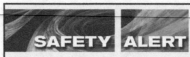

SAFETY ALERT

In many hospitals, the Kelly or other clamp is sealed in a sterile package or covered in plastic. The package is taped next to or over the head of the bed to keep it from being misplaced, and is visible to all if needed in an emergency. (This procedure may also be used for the clamps used to manage broken central intravenous catheters.)

CARING FOR A PATIENT WHO IS MECHANICALLY VENTILATED

A **ventilator** is a mechanical device that is used to facilitate breathing in patients whose respiratory or diaphragm function is impaired. The ventilator is connected to an endotracheal tube or the tracheostomy. Ventilators are used primarily in intensive care and subacute care units. Patients who are using ventilators usually have serious medical problems, and may be very unstable. Most of the skilled services will be provided by the RN or RCP. You will assist with ADLs and routine nursing care, as directed by the RN. The risk of infection is a great concern for patients who are mechanically ventilated. Use good handwashing (or alcohol-based hand cleaner) and be conscientious in using standard precautions and aseptic technique. Your job description and facility policy and procedure manuals will list your specific responsibilities in the care of patients who are mechanically ventilated. Generally, the following are PCT responsibilities in the care of mechanically ventilated patients:

- Make sure that the alarm is on at all times. It should never be turned off. Respond to alarms immediately. Remember, if an alarm sounds, check the patient first, not the machine.
- Provide frequent oral and nasal care. Monitor the mucous membranes for signs of pressure, irritation, and breakdown from the breathing apparatus.
- Observe for changes in respiratory rate and depth, shortness of breath, and use of accessory muscles in breathing.
- When monitoring the vital signs of patients who are using mechanical ventilation, count spontaneous respirations as well as ventilator-delivered breaths.
- Check for tube displacement or misplacement each time you are in the room. The endotra-

cheal tube is usually marked at the lips, teeth, or nares, so you can see if the tube has moved.

- Make sure that the endotracheal tube is taped securely.
- Visually inspect the chest. If it does not appear symmetrical upon breathing, inform the RN.
- Monitor the patient regularly for complaints of pain, and report them to the RN.
- Elevate the head of the bed 60 to 90 degrees, or as directed.
- Remember that elevation of the head of the bed increases the risk of skin breakdown. Reposition the patient every 2 hours or more often. Provide preventive skin care with lotion. Apply a therapeutic mattress, if ordered.
- Elevate the heels off the surface of the bed to prevent pressure ulcers. Heel protectors relieve friction and shearing. They do not prevent pressure.
- Suction, if permitted, using sterile technique.
- Condensation in the ventilator tubing will cause resistance to air flow and increase the risk of aspiration. Condensate must be drained into a collection trap, or the patient must be disconnected from the ventilator long enough to empty the tubing. Inform the RN if condensation forms. Do not attempt to perform this procedure unless you have been taught to do so, and are permitted to disassemble the ventilator parts. Never empty condensation in the ventilation tubing backward into the humidifier or in a way that causes you to get sprayed in the face with contaminated fluid.
- Use disposable saline irrigation units to rinse in-line suction.
- Make sure adequate sterile supplies are quickly available in the room.
- Monitor the patient for constipation.
- Provide active and passive range of motion, according to the plan of care. Use positioning aids as necessary to reduce the risk of contractures.
- Monitor the patient's tolerance to the ventilator by checking pulse oximetry, vital signs, cardiac monitor, anxiety, ability to sleep, and mental status. Suction as needed and if permitted.

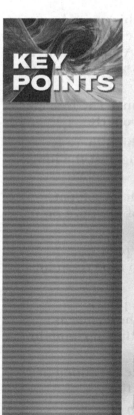

KEY POINTS

▶ Endotracheal intubation is a measure that provides complete control over the airway.

▶ An endotracheal tube is passed through the mouth, or less commonly the nose, into the patient's lungs.

▶ A laryngoscope is the instrument used for intubation.

▶ The light on the laryngoscope blade should be white, bright, and steady.

▶ Visualization of the larynx, vocal cords, and structures in the back of the throat with a laryngoscope is called direct laryngoscopy.

▶ The patient must be well oxygenated before the endotracheal tube is inserted.

▶ The patient's head should be placed in the sniffing position for endotracheal tube insertion.

▶ When ventilating a patient with an endotracheal tube or tracheostomy using a bag-valve device, connect the oxygen to the bag; set the flow to 15 liters per minute.

▶ Patients who are intubated need a great deal of care, comfort measures, and reassurance.

▶ A tracheotomy is a surgical procedure to create an opening into the neck through which to breathe.

▶ A tracheotomy is performed for airway obstruction related to many causes.

(continues)

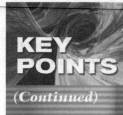

KEY POINTS
(Continued)

▶ The opening into the airway created during a tracheotomy is called a tracheostomy.

▶ The external opening on the skin surface created during the tracheotomy is the stoma.

▶ The cannula is an indwelling tube inserted through the stoma to maintain airway patency.

▶ Several types of outer cannulae are used for a tracheostomy, but the most common is held in place by an inflatable cuff.

▶ Tracheostomy care is a sterile procedure.

▶ When ventilating a patient who has an endotracheal tube or tracheostomy, squeeze the bag once every 3 to 5 seconds, or as directed.

▶ The goals of tracheostomy care are to keep the area clean and free from obstruction, to prevent skin irritation and breakdown, and to prevent infection.

▶ To remove the inner cannula, turn the adapter at the end counterclockwise. Pull the cannula out, then down.

▶ The tracheostomy provides a direct route to the lungs; avoid getting powder, lint, moisture, or other substances in the cannula.

▶ The tracheostomy dressing is split in the center. It is made of lint-free composite material. The open end of the dressing faces the patient's head.

▶ The ties that hold the outer tracheostomy cannula in place are knotted at the side to avoid pressure on the back of the neck.

▶ A laryngectomy is surgical removal of the larynx. During this procedure, the airway is always separated from the mouth, nose, and esophagus. The patient breathes through a permanent stoma in the neck. A patient with a laryngectomy cannot speak, smell, blow his or her nose, whistle, gargle, or suck on a straw. He or she retains the ability to swallow.

▶ Pneumothorax is free air in the chest cavity outside the lung. The free air presses against the lung so that the lung cannot expand properly.

▶ Hemothorax is a condition similar to pneumothorax, in which there is blood in the chest cavity. The collection of blood presses against the lung, so that the lung cannot expand properly.

▶ Tension pneumothorax is a very serious condition in which air cannot escape from the chest cavity, leading to a steady buildup of pressure on the lung.

▶ If a chest tube comes out, cover the site with 4 × 4 gauze pads or petroleum gauze pads from the emergency supply kit, then tape them in place.

▶ If a glass chest tube drainage bottle accidentally breaks, a plastic drainage bottle cracks, or a tube disconnects, clamp the chest tube as close to the insertion site as possible by using the rubber-tipped clamp in the emergency tray.

▶ A ventilator is a mechanical device that is used to facilitate breathing in patients who have impaired respiratory or diaphragm function.

▶ Patients who are mechanically ventilated are at a very high risk of infection.

CLINICAL APPLICATIONS

1. Mrs. Papadakis experienced a cardiac arrest. She was intubated in the emergency department. She awakens when you are caring for her in the special care unit. She cannot speak because of the tube. Her eyes are wide and she looks afraid. She reaches up with her right hand as if to pull the tube. What action will you take?

2. Mrs. Papadakis is unstable. A bed becomes available in the intensive care unit and the RN informs you that the patient will be transferred there. The ventilator cannot be used while the patient is being moved. The RN instructs you to ventilate Mrs. Papadakis once every 3 to 5 seconds during the transfer. How will you move this patient? How will you perform the ventilations? How many assistants do you think will be necessary to transfer the patient safely?

3. You enter Mr. Jennison's room. He is coughing forcefully, expelling secretions out of his tracheostomy. His color is dusky. What action will you take?

4. The RN arrives in Mr. Jennison's room and directs the activity. The patient stabilizes quickly. After the emergency is over, you notice that the patient's gown is wet from secretions. The ties and dressing on the tracheostomy are also wet and soiled. What actions will you take? State the PPE you will wear while you are providing this care.

5. Later in the shift, you are performing tracheostomy care for Mr. Jennison. You insert the suction catheter and Mr. Jennison begins to cough uncontrollably. What action will you take?

CHAPTER REVIEW

Multiple-Choice Questions

Select the one best answer.

1. You are assisting the RCP with endotracheal intubation. You are setting up for the procedure, and check the light on the laryngoscope blade. To perform the procedure correctly, the light should be:
   a. yellow.
   b. white.
   c. flickering.
   d. dim.

2. The RCP is ready to begin the intubation procedure. You will position the patient's head:
   a. to the right side.
   b. as far back as it will go.
   c. as far forward as it will go.
   d. in the sniffing position.

3. During intubation, you may be asked to apply pressure to the lower neck. You know that this is done to:
   a. keep air from entering the esophagus.
   b. prevent air from entering the lungs.
   c. maintain the airway, making intubation easier.
   d. enlarge the trachea.

4. When using the bag-valve device to ventilate a patient who has an endotracheal tube, squeeze the bag to inflate the lungs once every:
   a. second.
   b. 2–4 seconds.
   c. 3–5 seconds.
   b. 10 seconds.

5. When caring for a patient with an endotracheal tube, position him or her in the:
   a. supine position.
   b. semi-Fowler's position.
   c. lateral position.
   d. sniffing position.

6. A surgical procedure to create a hole in the neck through which to breathe is a:
   a. laryngectomy.
   b. laryngotomy.
   c. tracheostomy.
   d. tracheotomy.

7. The hole in the skin surface through which the outer and inner cannulae are inserted is the:
   a. stoma.
   b. tracheotomy.
   c. ostomy.
   d. appliance.

8. When oxygen is administered to a patient who has a tracheostomy:
   a. a nasal cannula is used.
   b. a Venturi mask is used.
   c. the oxygen is humidified.
   d. the oxygen is dry.

9. When using a bag-valve-mask apparatus to ventilate a patient who has a tracheostomy, connect supplemental oxygen set to:
    a. 2 liters per minute.
    b. 6 liters per minute.
    c. 10 liters per minute.
    d. 15 liters per minute.

10. To replace the ties on the outer cannula of a patient's tracheostomy, use:
    a. roller gauze.
    b. twill tape.
    c. sterile string.
    d. elastic bandage.

11. A person who has had the voicebox surgically removed may be called a:
    a. tracheostomy.
    b. laryngectomy.
    c. stoma.
    d. laryngectomee.

12. A patient who has had a laryngectomy:
    a. can blow his or her nose.
    b. cannot suck on a straw.
    c. can smell unpleasant odors.
    d. cannot swallow.

13. Signs of ineffective airway clearance and poor gas exchange include:
    a. restlessness, anxiety, increased heart rate, lethargy.
    b. hypertension, chest pain, bradycardia, anxiety.
    c. elevated temperature, tachycardia, hypertension, chest pain.
    d. lethargy, hypertension, bradycardia, disorientation.

14. Pneumothorax and hemothorax are treated with a:
    a. laryngectomy.
    b. chest tube.
    c. tracheostomy.
    d. ventilator.

15. The drainage bottle for the chest tube should be:
    a. on the table next to the bed.
    b. above the level of the patient's heart.
    c. below the level of the patient's heart.
    d. 16 to 24 inches above the bed.

16. Supplies used for providing tracheostomy care for the ventilator-dependent patient should be:
    a. sterile.
    b. clean.
    c. sanitized.
    d. disinfected.

17. When the alarm on a ventilator sounds, you should:
    a. call the RN.
    b. check the ventilator.
    c. check the patient.
    d. promptly find the RCP.

18. If a glass chest tube bottle accidentally breaks, you should:
    a. use the rubber-tipped clamp to clamp the chest tube.
    b. quickly find another container to use for drainage.
    c. pad the chest tube insertion site with 4 × 4 and tape.
    d. use the rubber-tipped clamp to clamp the drainage tube.

19. When caring for a patient who uses a ventilator, you should:
    a. keep the head of the bed elevated 15 degrees.
    b. position the patient in the semiprone position.
    c. empty condensation in the tubing into the humidifier.
    d. give mouth care and monitor mucous membranes.

20. Signs and symptoms of tension pneumothorax include:
    a. mental orientation.
    b. hypoxemia.
    c. hypertension.
    d. elevated temperature.

EXPLORING THE WEB

Aaron's Tracheostomy Page	http://tracheostomy.com
Action-Plan for Airway Problems	http://medi-smart.com
Adult Ventilation Management	http://www.corexcel.com
Chest Tubes and Drainage Systems	http://www.nursewise.com
Different Chest Tubes Present Different Clinical Challenges	http://www.atriummed.com
Laryngectomy Basics	http://www.larynxlink.com

Laryngectomy Life	http://www.laryngectomylife.com
Management of Chest Tubes	http://www.hsc.usf.edu
Nurse Bob's MICU Survival Guide	http://rnbob.tripod.com
Nursing Policy: Oral Care for Intubated, Trached, and Intensive Care Patients	http://www.scmcweb.com
Nursing Strategies to Prevent Ventilator-Associated Pneumonia	http://www.aacn.org
Passy-Muir Tracheostomy and Ventilator Speaking Valves	http://www.passy-muir.com
Post-Acute Care of the Ventilator-Dependent Patient	http://www.careplanners.net
Postoperative Care of Patients with an Endotracheal Tube	http://www.perspectivesinnursing.org
Pulmonary Concepts in Critical Care Airway Management	http://rnbob.tripod.com
Rotherham Clinical Policies and Procedures	http://www.rotherhampct.nhs.uk
Total Laryngectomy	http://www.mdanderson.org
Tracheostomy	http://medicine.creighton.edu
Tracheostomy Care	http://www.headandneckcancer.org
Tracheostomy Care	http://www.healthsquare.com
Tracheostomy: Easing the Transition from Hospital to Home	http://www.perspectivesinnursing.org
Tracheostomy: Postoperative Recovery	http://www.perspectivesinnursing.org
Tracheostomy Primer on Critical Care for Patients and Their Families	http://www.thoracic.org
Understanding Chest Drainage	http://www.nursingceu.com
Voice Rehabilitation after Laryngectomy	http://www.utmb.edu
What Is a Tracheostomy?	http://www.tracheostomy.com
Working with Chest Tubes	http://tegrity.cscc.edu/tegrity

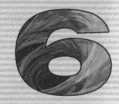

CHAPTER 16

Cardiac Care Skills

OBJECTIVES:

After reading this chapter, you should be able to:

- Spell and define key terms.
- State the purpose of the cardiac monitor and electrocardiograph.
- Describe the pathway that an electrical impulse takes as it travels through the heart.
- Describe the heart action corresponding to each wave on the electrocardiograph paper and cardiac monitor.
- Identify common dysrhythmias.
- Describe how to take the apical pulse, apical-radial pulse, and femoral pulse.
- Identify the locations for taking the posterior tibial and dorsalis pedis pulses.
- Demonstrate how to use a Doppler instrument to hear body sounds.
- Explain why hypertension is a silent killer.
- List the blood pressure values for normal blood pressure, prehypertension, Stage I hypertension, and Stage II hypertension.
- State the indications and guidelines for electronic blood pressure monitoring.
- Describe the care of a patient following an angiogram or arteriogram.
- Describe the care of a patient following cardiac catheterization.

ELECTRICAL CONDUCTION OF THE HEART

Cardiovascular disorders are the leading cause of death in the United States. The cardiac monitor and **electrocardiograph (ECG or EKG)** are important diagnostic equipment used in health care facilities. These devices measure electrical activity within the heart and display the information on a screen. This information helps guide health care professionals in diagnosis and treatment of the patient. As a PCT, you will assist by performing ECGs, applying the cardiac monitor to patients, and recognizing the rhythm displayed. Report abnormalities to the RN immediately.

The heart is a very strong muscle. It has four chambers, two atria, and two ventricles (**Figure 16-1**). The heart has very sensitive tissue that can conduct electrical impulses. This electrical activity causes the heart to beat. In a healthy heart, electrical activity begins in the right atrium. The electrical impulse moves through the conduction pathway in the AV node, through a series of fibers, to the ventricles, which contract. This contraction causes the heartbeat. The cycle repeats itself hundreds of times each day. The **cardiac cycle** consists of two phases, **contraction** and **relaxation.** During contraction, the heart beats, pumping blood to the body. During the relaxation phase, the heart rests and recovers. Understanding the normal conduction of the heart

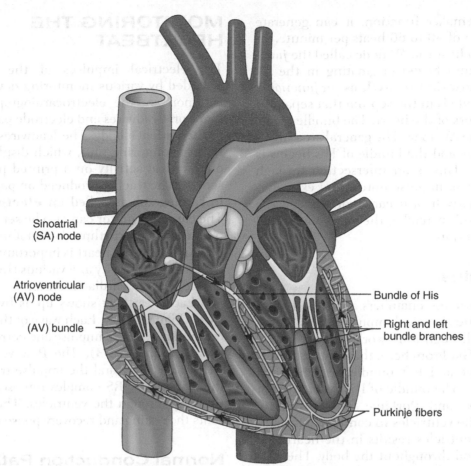

Sinoatrial
(SA) node

Atrioventricular
(AV) node

(AV) bundle

Bundle of His

Right and left
bundle branches

Purkinje fibers

FIGURE 16-1 The conduction system of the heart.

is very important to understanding how to interpret a cardiac rhythm.

The Pacemaker

The electrical activity that results in a heartbeat begins in the pacemaker. Any tissue in the heart can function as the pacemaker, if necessary. However, the normal pacemaker is in the right atrium, and is called the **sinoatrial node (SA node).** Although any tissue in the heart can function as the pacemaker, the SA node fires most rapidly, 60 to 100 times each minute. When the SA node fires, the cells of the atria contract simultaneously.

Because the SA node fires so rapidly, other tissue within the heart does not need to fire to begin the cardiac impulse. However, if the number of impulses generated by the SA node falls below 50 beats per minute, other tissues within the heart may send impulses to pace the heartbeat. The number of pacemaker impulses that can be fired from each area of the heart is listed in **Table 16-1.**

After the SA node fires, the electrical impulse moves downward through a network of **junctional**

Table 16-1 Pacemaker Rates	
SA node	60–100 beats per minute
AV node (AV junction)	40–60 beats per minute
Ventricles	20–40 beats per minute

fibers. The fibers are long, thin conduction cells. They help move the electrical impulse downward, on its way to the ventricles.

The Atrioventricular Node

The **atrioventricular node (AV node)** is located on the bottom of the atrium, just above the ventricles. If the heart is functioning normally, the AV node conducts the electrical impulse downward, into the ventricles. However, if the AV node must assume the pacemaker function, it can generate impulses at a rate of 40 to 60 beats per minute.

You may also hear the AV node called the *junction.* Rhythms (and beats) originating in the AV node are called **junctional rhythms** (or *junctional beats*). The AV node is in the septum that separates the lower chambers of the heart. The bundle of His descends from the AV node. The general area where the AV node stops and the bundle of His begins is the AV junction. This is an intersection through which the electrical impulse enters and exits. Because of this, many health care workers call the area the "junction," instead of the more proper "AV node" or "AV junction."

The Ventricles

The **ventricles** are the chambers at the bottom of the heart. After the electrical impulse leaves the AV node, it travels through a network of fibers called the **bundle of His.** From here, the impulse travels through the right and left bundle branches and **Purkinje fibers.** The bundle of His, left and right bundle branches, and Purkinje fibers work together, causing the ventricles to contract. The contraction of the ventricles results in the heartbeat, which forces blood throughout the body. The ventricles can also function as the pacemaker if the SA node and AV node fail. However, they generate a very slow impulse, at 20 to 40 beats per minute.

The ventricles rest momentarily after they contract; then the SA node fires and begins the cycle again. The working phase of the heart is called **systole.** The resting phase is called **diastole.** You are familiar with these terms from learning about blood pressure. The systolic pressure is the pressure in the arteries when the heart is working, whereas the diastolic pressure is the resting pressure.

MONITORING THE HEARTBEAT

The electrical impulses of the heart can be recorded by various monitoring devices. The most common are the electrocardiograph and cardiac monitor. Leadwires and electrode pads are attached to the patient's body. The leadwires are connected to the monitoring unit, which displays the pattern of electrical activity on a printed paper or display screen. The tracing produced on paper by the electrocardiograph is called an **electrocardiogram.** The cardiac monitor can also be set to print a paper tracing of the rhythm. Understanding the basic conduction of the heart is important to interpreting the electrical activity and various rhythms displayed on the ECG or cardiac monitor.

Each heartbeat shows up as five waves on the ECG (**Figure 16-2**). Each wave of the heartbeat represents an electrical impulse and corresponding heart action (**Figure 16-3**). The P wave represents the pacemaker firing and the impulse traveling through the atria. The QRS complex represents the impulse traveling through the ventricles. The T wave represents the resting and recovery phase of the heart.

Normal Conduction Pathway

The normal conduction pathway begins in the SA node, with the P wave. The QRS complex begins in the AV node.

ECG Paper

Understanding the significance of the blocks on the ECG paper (**Figure 16-4**) is important to understanding the various waves on the ECG. The ECG paper consists of many small and large blocks.

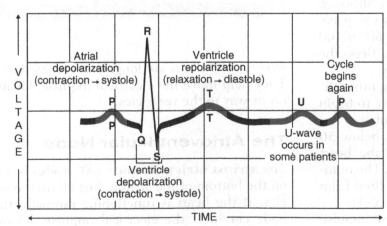

Q wave is a negative deflection or wave.

R wave is a positive deflection or wave.

S wave is a negative wave.

T wave is a positive wave and represents ventricular repolarization.

U wave (occasionally seen in some patients) is a positive deflection and associated with repolarization.

FIGURE 16-2 The conduction of the heart on a normal ECG.

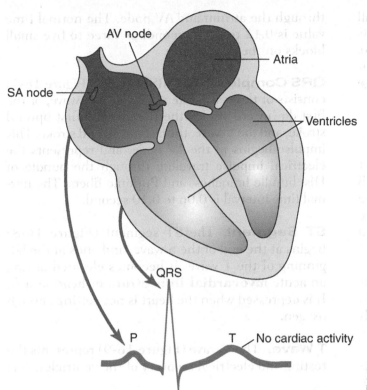

FIGURE 16-3 Waves representing an electrical impulse being transmitted through the heart.

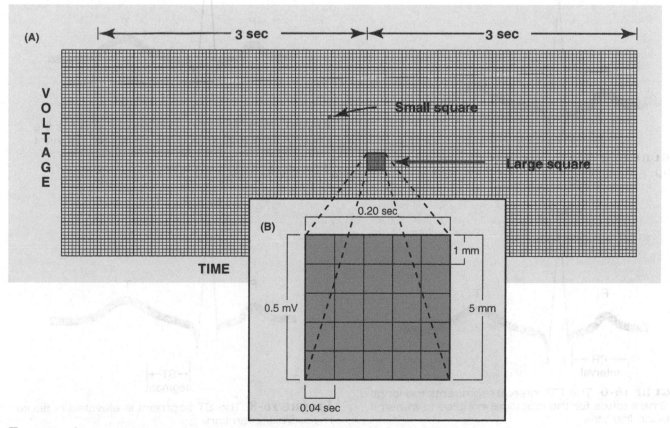

FIGURE 16-4 ECG and monitor graph paper.

When reading the ECG paper vertically, one small block represents 0.04 second. Each large block is five small blocks wide. Each of these represents 0.20 seconds. When reading the ECG paper vertically, each small block represents 1 mm. Each large block represents 5 mm vertically.

Waves on the ECG

Understanding the electrical conduction of the heart is key to understanding the various rhythms you will see on ECG tracings. You must be able to recognize the various waves on the ECG and understand the heart actions they represent. Knowing the normal values for each wave and interval is also important.

P Wave. The P wave (**Figure 16-5**) represents the pacemaker firing and atrial contraction. This wave is usually considered abnormal if it exceeds three small blocks on the ECG paper.

PR Interval. The PR interval (**Figure 16-6**) extends from the beginning of the P wave to the beginning of the Q wave. This interval represents the length of time it takes for the impulse to travel through the atrium and AV node. The normal time value is 0.12 to 0.20 second, or three to five small blocks on the ECG paper.

QRS Complex. The QRS complex (**Figure 16-7**) consists of three separate waves: The Q wave, or the first downward stroke; the R wave, the first upward stroke; and the S wave, the last downward stroke. This impulse begins in the AV node, and represents the electrical impulse traveling through the bundle of His, bundle branches, and Purkinje fibers. The normal time interval is 0.06 to 0.10 second.

ST Segment. The ST segment (**Figure 16-8**) begins at the end of the S wave, and ends at the beginning of the T wave. It becomes elevated during an acute **myocardial infarction,** or heart attack. It is depressed when the heart is not getting enough oxygen.

T Wave. The T wave (**Figure 16-9**) represents the resting and electrical recovery of the ventricles. It is

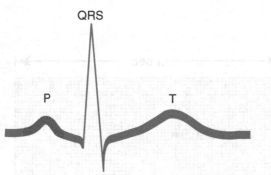

FIGURE 16-5 The P wave indicates the pacemaker firing.

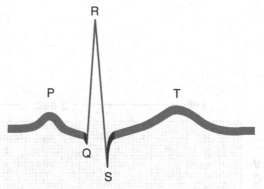

FIGURE 16-7 The QRS complex represents the impulse traveling through the bundle of His, right and left bundle branches, and Purkinje fibers, causing ventricular contraction.

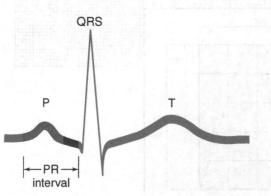

FIGURE 16-6 The PR interval represents the length of time it takes for the electrical impulse to transmit through the atria.

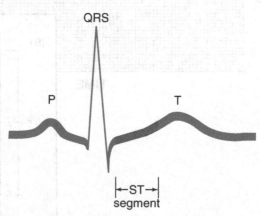

FIGURE 16-8 The ST segment is elevated in acute myocardial infarction.

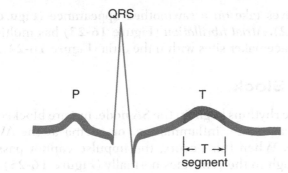

FIGURE 16-9 The T wave represents the resting phase of the heartbeat.

normally no more than 10 small blocks high in the chest leads, and five small blocks high in other leads.

Calculating the Heart Rate

The top of the ECG strip is marked with small vertical lines. Each of these represents 3 seconds. You can estimate the heart rate by counting the number of QRS complexes in 6 seconds, then multiplying by 10. Another method is to find an R wave that falls on a heavy black line (**Figure 16-10**). Begin counting the heart rate at the *next* heavy black line. Count the next heavy line as 300. The next heavy line is 150. Continue to count the heavy black lines as 100, 75, 60, and 50. The line on which the next R wave falls determines the approximate rate. These methods of estimating the rate are accurate only for regular rhythms. If the rhythm appears very irregular (such as atrial fibrillation), do not use this method.

IDENTIFYING CARDIAC RHYTHMS

The ability to identify the various electrical rhythms seen on the ECG and cardiac monitor is very im-

portant. Follow your facility policy for documenting these rhythms and entering them in the medical record. If a patient is being monitored continuously, you may be required to run a strip at the beginning of the shift. You may also be required to print a strip of any abnormal rhythms that occur. To do this, you must recognize what is normal, so you can identify what is abnormal.

Rhythms Originating in the SA Node

You will recall that the SA node is the normal pacemaker for the heart. The conduction pathway for rhythms originating in the SA node is pictured in **Figure 16-11**. Normal sinus rhythm, **Figure 16-12**, is the normal rhythm you expect to see. Sometimes

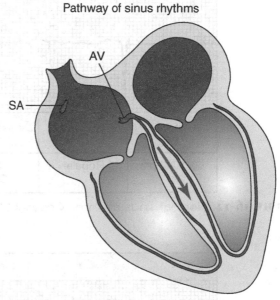

FIGURE 16-11 Normal conduction pathway within the atrium, with the electrical impulse beginning in the SA node.

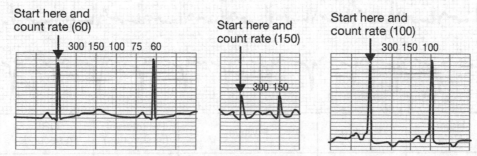

FIGURE 16-10 Count the rate by locating an R wave that falls on a heavy black line. Begin counting at the *next* heavy black line. Count that as line 300. The next heavy line is 150. Continue to count the heavy black lines as 100, 75, 60, and 50. The line on which the next R wave falls determines the approximate rate.

abnormal rhythms begin in the SA node. These are pictured in Figures 16-13, 16-14, 16-15, 16-16, and 16-17.

Rhythms Originating in the Atria

Some rhythms originate in the atria, but outside of the SA node (Figures 16-18, 16-19, and 16-20. The conduction pathway for these rhythms is pictured in Figure 16-21. *Atrial flutter* is a rhythm in which the

P waves take on a sawtoothed appearance (Figure 16-22). *Atrial fibrillation* (Figure 16-23) has multiple pacemaker sites within the atria (Figure 16-24).

AV Block

Some rhythms begin in the SA node, but are blocked by scar tissue, inflammation, or edema at the AV node. When this occurs, the impulse cannot pass through to the ventricles normally (Figure 16-25).

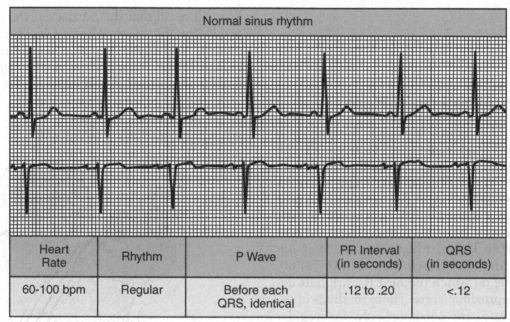

Heart Rate	Rhythm	P Wave	PR Interval (in seconds)	QRS (in seconds)
60-100 bpm	Regular	Before each QRS, identical	.12 to .20	<.12

FIGURE 16-12 Normal sinus rhythm. (Copyright Marquette Electronics, Marquette, WI)

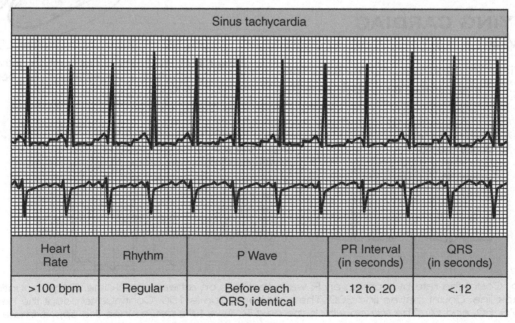

Heart Rate	Rhythm	P Wave	PR Interval (in seconds)	QRS (in seconds)
>100 bpm	Regular	Before each QRS, identical	.12 to .20	<.12

FIGURE 16-13 Sinus tachycardia. (Copyright Marquette Electronics, Marquette, WI)

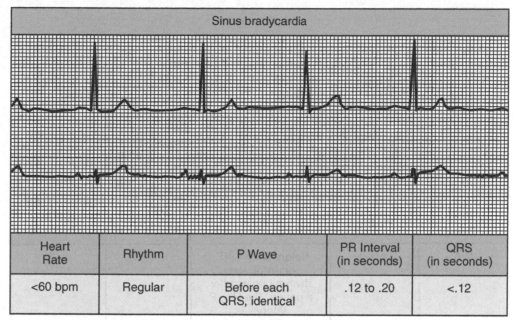

Heart Rate	Rhythm	P Wave	PR Interval (in seconds)	QRS (in seconds)
<60 bpm	Regular	Before each QRS, identical	.12 to .20	<.12

FIGURE 16-14 Sinus bradycardia. (Copyright Marquette Electronics, Marquette, WI)

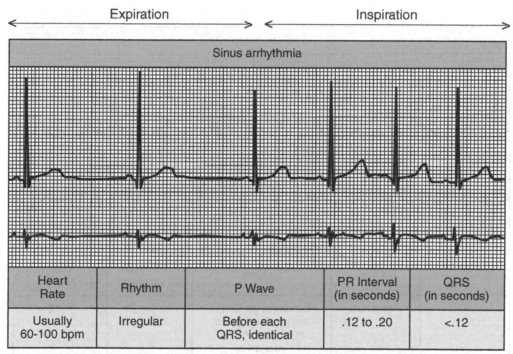

Heart Rate	Rhythm	P Wave	PR Interval (in seconds)	QRS (in seconds)
Usually 60-100 bpm	Irregular	Before each QRS, identical	.12 to .20	<.12

FIGURE 16-15 Sinus arrhythmia. (Copyright Marquette Electronics, Marquette, WI)

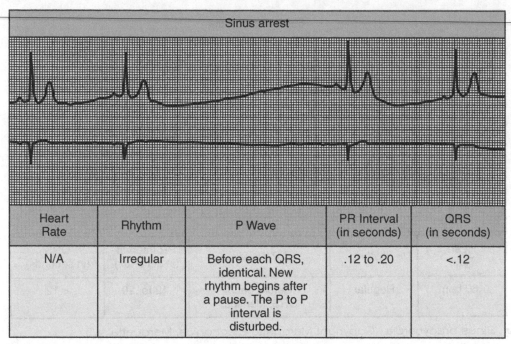

Heart Rate	Rhythm	P Wave	PR Interval (in seconds)	QRS (in seconds)
N/A	Irregular	Before each QRS, identical. New rhythm begins after a pause. The P to P interval is disturbed.	.12 to .20	<.12

FIGURE 16-16 Sinus arrest. (Copyright Marquette Electronics, Marquette, WI)

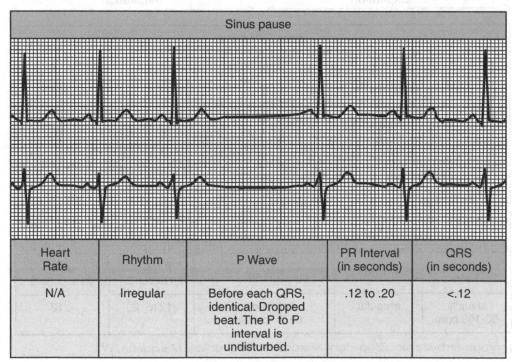

Heart Rate	Rhythm	P Wave	PR Interval (in seconds)	QRS (in seconds)
N/A	Irregular	Before each QRS, identical. Dropped beat. The P to P interval is undisturbed.	.12 to .20	<.12

FIGURE 16-17 Sinus pause. (Copyright Marquette Electronics, Marquette, WI)

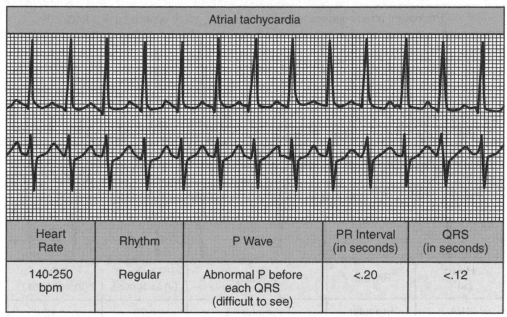

Heart Rate	Rhythm	P Wave	PR Interval (in seconds)	QRS (in seconds)
140-250 bpm	Regular	Abnormal P before each QRS (difficult to see)	<.20	<.12

FIGURE 16-18 Atrial tachycardia. (Copyright Marquette Electronics, Marquette, WI)

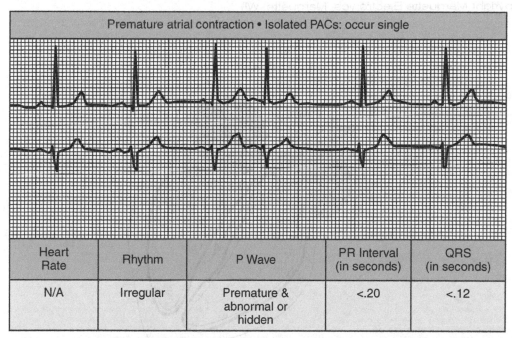

Heart Rate	Rhythm	P Wave	PR Interval (in seconds)	QRS (in seconds)
N/A	Irregular	Premature & abnormal or hidden	<.20	<.12

FIGURE 16-19 Premature atrial contractions. (Copyright Marquette Electronics, Marquette, WI)

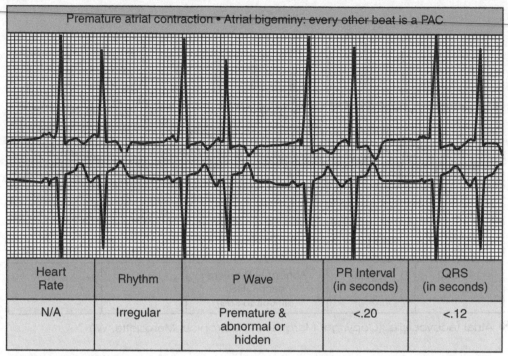

Premature atrial contraction • Atrial bigeminy: every other beat is a PAC

Heart Rate	Rhythm	P Wave	PR Interval (in seconds)	QRS (in seconds)
N/A	Irregular	Premature & abnormal or hidden	<.20	<.12

FIGURE 16-20 Premature atrial contractions occurring every other beat. This may also be called atrial bigeminy. (Copyright Marquette Electronics, Marquette, WI)

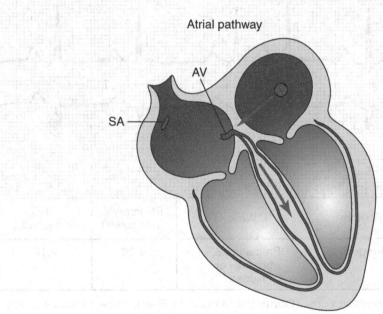

FIGURE 16-21 Example of a conduction pathway when the pacemaker is in the atria, but outside of the SA node. The rhythm produced by this pathway will appear abnormal on the ECG.

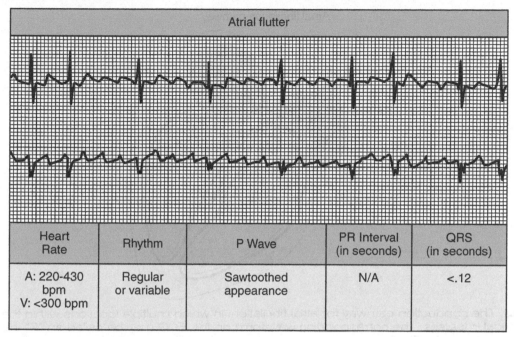

	Atrial flutter			
Heart Rate	Rhythm	P Wave	PR Interval (in seconds)	QRS (in seconds)
A: 220-430 bpm V: <300 bpm	Regular or variable	Sawtoothed appearance	N/A	<.12

FIGURE 16-22 Atrial flutter is distinguished by sawtoothed P waves. (Copyright Marquette Electronics, Marquette, WI)

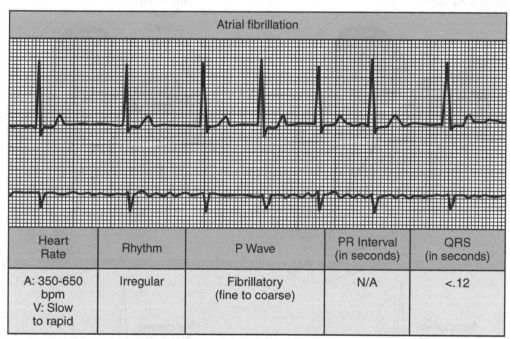

	Atrial fibrillation			
Heart Rate	Rhythm	P Wave	PR Interval (in seconds)	QRS (in seconds)
A: 350-650 bpm V: Slow to rapid	Irregular	Fibrillatory (fine to coarse)	N/A	<.12

FIGURE 16-23 Atrial fibrillation. (Copyright Marquette Electronics, Marquette, WI)

Atrial fibrillation pathway

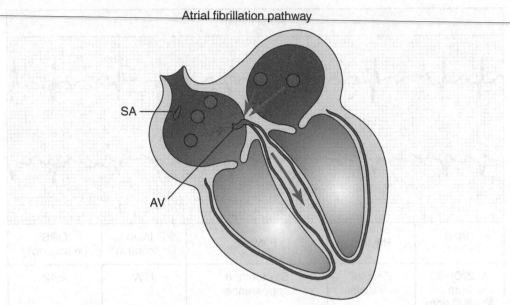

FIGURE 16-24 The conduction pathway for atrial fibrillation, in which multiple locations within the atria generate electrical impulses. The corresponding waveform on the ECG may be called an "F" wave, or fibrillatory wave, instead of a P wave.

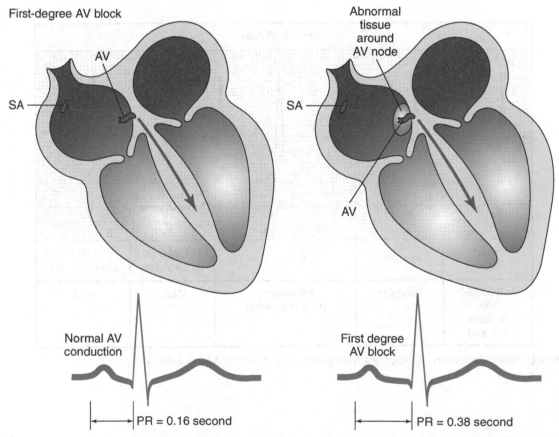

First-degree AV block

Abnormal tissue around AV node

AV

SA

SA

AV

Normal AV conduction

First degree AV block

PR = 0.16 second

PR = 0.38 second

FIGURE 16-25 In an atrioventricular block, scar tissue within the atria prevents the electrical impulse from taking its normal path through the tissue. In first-degree AV block, this is reflected by a prolonged PR interval.

Rhythms Originating in the AV Junction

Rhythms originating in the AV junction are called *junctional rhythms*. In these rhythms, the pacemaker is somewhere between the atria and the ventricles (Figure 16-26). The appearance of the P wave is the key that the SA node is not acting as the pacemaker (Figure 16-27). The rhythm pictured in Figure 16-28 has flattened P waves, indicating that the pacemaker is in the AV junction. The P waves in Figure 16-29 have different configurations, indicating multiple pacemaker sites within the AV junction.

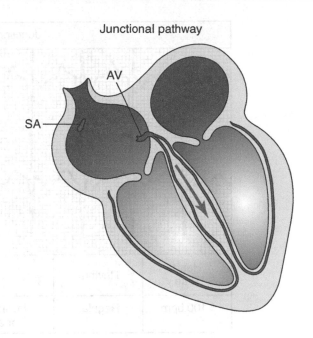

Junctional pathway

AV

SA

FIGURE 16-26 The conduction pathway for junctional rhythms begins in the AV junction.

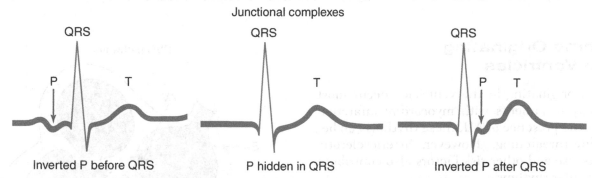

Junctional complexes

QRS   QRS   QRS

P   T   T   P   T

Inverted P before QRS   P hidden in QRS   Inverted P after QRS

FIGURE 16-27 Various P waves generated from different locations in the AV junction.

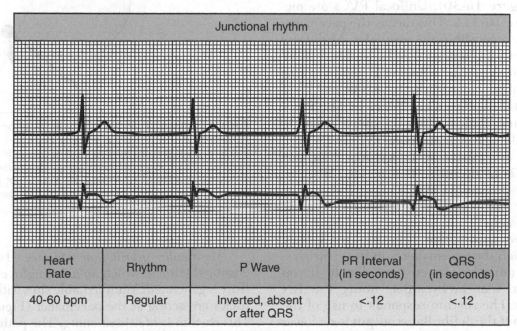

Junctional rhythm

Heart Rate	Rhythm	P Wave	PR Interval (in seconds)	QRS (in seconds)
40-60 bpm	Regular	Inverted, absent or after QRS	<.12	<.12

FIGURE 16-28 Junctional rhythm. (Copyright Marquette Electronics, Marquette, WI)

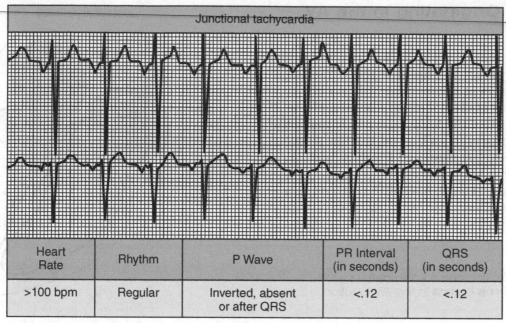

FIGURE 16-29 Junctional tachycardia. (Copyright Marquette Electronics, Marquette, WI)

Heart Rate	Rhythm	P Wave	PR Interval (in seconds)	QRS (in seconds)
>100 bpm	Regular	Inverted, absent or after QRS	<.12	<.12

Rhythms Originating in the Ventricles

Rhythms originating in the ventricles occur most commonly in patients with myocardial infarction (MI). In the presence of MI, these rhythms can become life-threatening. However, arteriosclerotic heart disease and other risk factors also contribute to ventricular rhythms.

Premature ventricular contractions (PVCs) are individual beats in which the pacemaker is in the ventricles (**Figure 16-30**). Unifocal PVCs are pictured in **Figure 16-31A**. This means the pacemaker is one irritable area within the ventricles. Multifocal PVCs are shown in **Figure 16-31B**. In this rhythm, several irritable sites within the ventricles are acting as the pacemaker. Patients who have had an MI are often medicated to eliminate PVCs. In MI, PVCs can quickly cause critical or life-threatening complications. Multifocal PVCs, and more than six PVCs in one minute, are especially dangerous. Bigeminy (**Figure 16-32A**), trigeminy (**Figure 16-32B**), and quadrigeminy (**Figure 16-32C**) mean PVCs every two, three, or four heartbeats. Report PVCs to the nurse immediately.

Ventricular tachycardia (**Figure 16-33**) is a rhythm in which the pacemaker is in the ventricles. This rhythm must be treated immediately. If you identify ventricular tachycardia, notify the RN without delay. The rhythm responds to use of the defibrillator, but the defibrillator output is set lower than would be used for ventricular fibrillation.

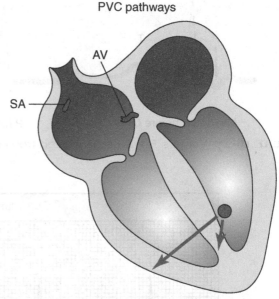

FIGURE 16-30 In PVCs, various locations within the ventricles generate an electrical impulse. Although the impulse is reflected on the ECG, a PVC does not result in a normal heartbeat. Because the heart does not contract normally, blood is not pumped through the system as a result of this beat.

Ventricular fibrillation (**Figure 16-34**) is a chaotic rhythm in which no meaningful electrical activity is generated. Many irritable sites within the ventricles are acting as the pacemaker (**Figure 16-35**). This rhythm is life-threatening. The patient requires immediate CPR and defibrillation.

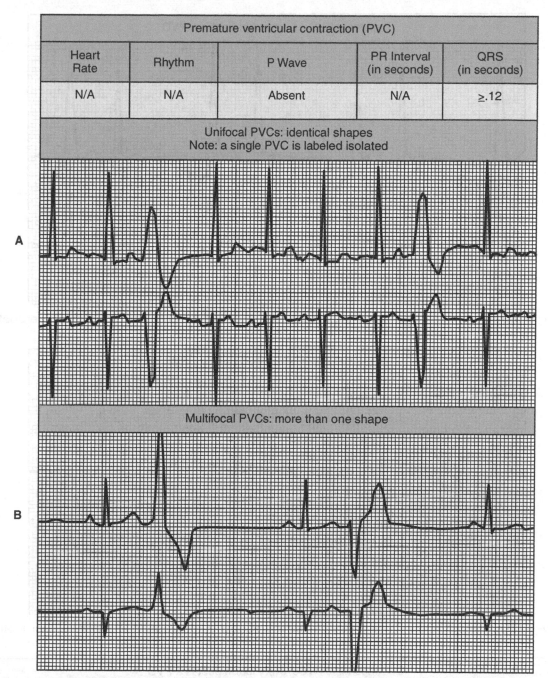

Premature ventricular contraction (PVC)				
Heart Rate	Rhythm	P Wave	PR Interval (in seconds)	QRS (in seconds)
N/A	N/A	Absent	N/A	≥.12

Unifocal PVCs: identical shapes
Note: a single PVC is labeled isolated

A

Multifocal PVCs: more than one shape

B

FIGURE 16-31   (A) Unifocal PVCs are generated by one pacemaker within the ventricles. (Copyright Marquette Electronics, Marquette, WI). (B) Multifocal PVCs are generated by multiple irritable sites within the ventricles. (Copyright Marquette Electronics, Marquette, WI)

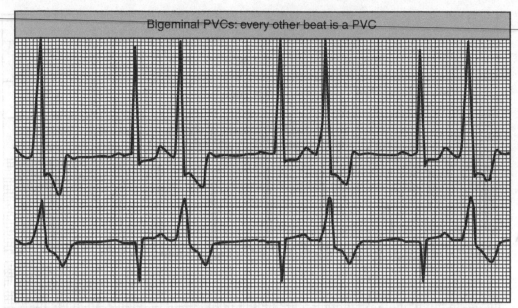

FIGURE 16-32(A) Every other beat is a PVC in bigeminy. (Copyright Marquette Electronics, Marquette, WI)

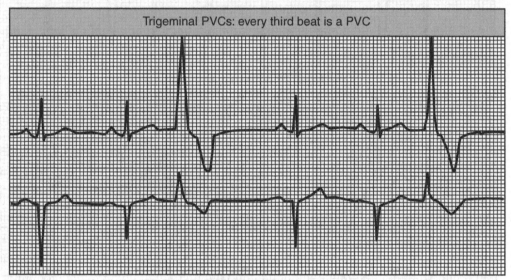

FIGURE 16-32(B) Every third beat is a PVC in trigeminy. (Copyright Marquette Electronics, Marquette, WI)

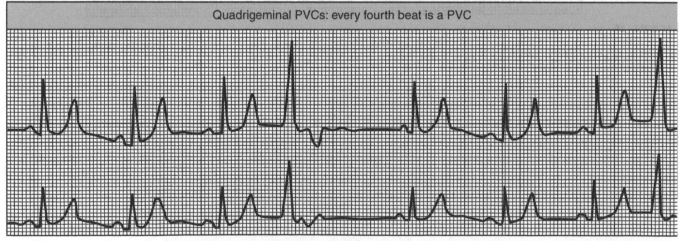

FIGURE 16-32(C) Every fourth beat is a PVC in quadrigeminy. (Copyright Marquette Electronics, Marquette, WI)

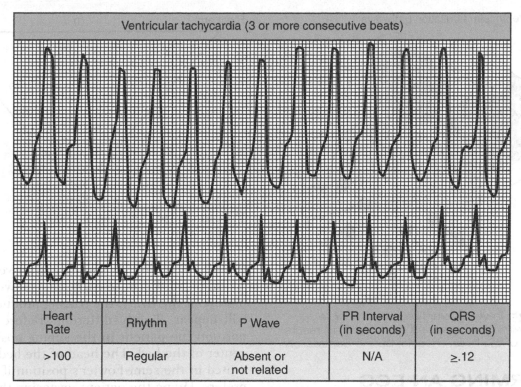

Heart Rate	Rhythm	P Wave	PR Interval (in seconds)	QRS (in seconds)
>100	Regular	Absent or not related	N/A	≥.12

FIGURE 16-33 Three or more consecutive PVCs is ventricular tachycardia. This tracing shows multiple consecutive PVCs; there are no normal beats in between. (Copyright Marquette Electronics, Marquette, WI)

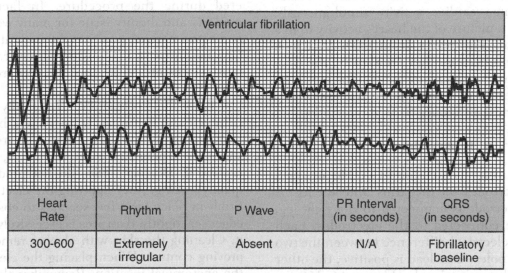

Heart Rate	Rhythm	P Wave	PR Interval (in seconds)	QRS (in seconds)
300-600	Extremely irregular	Absent	N/A	Fibrillatory baseline

FIGURE 16-34 Ventricular fibrillation indicates sudden cardiac death. Lifesaving measures must be initiated immediately. (Copyright Marquette Electronics, Marquette, WI)

Ventricular fibrillation pathways

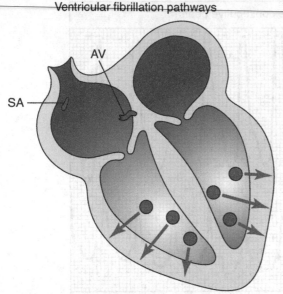

FIGURE 16-35 In ventricular fibrillation, multiple irritable sites within the ventricles are firing. This results in a quivering of the heart muscle, but no contraction.

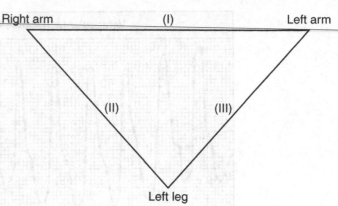

FIGURE 16-36 Einthoven's triangle.

PERFORMING AN ECG

The heart is a three-dimensional muscle. The ECG gives us the ability to look at the heart from different dimensions. The ECG consists of 12 leads. The leads record the same cardiac activity simultaneously. Each provides a picture of the heart's activity from a different angle. The waves from each lead look slightly different because they are viewing the electrical activity from different positions. Each lead has a positive pole and a negative pole. The unit measures the electrical difference between the poles.

Einthoven's Triangle

Willem Einthoven invented the ECG. He arranged recording electrodes on the arms and left leg. A grounding electrode is connected to the right leg. Leadwires are connected to the electrodes. Each measures the electrical difference between the two electrodes, or poles. One lead is positive, the other negative. Einthoven's triangle (**Figure 16-36**) displays the position of the electrodes. Because the heart is three-dimensional, its electrical activity must be viewed in three dimensions. Twelve electrodes must be used for a complete analysis of the heart's electrical activity.

The 12-Lead ECG

Twelve leads are used to record the standard ECG. The placement and location of the electrodes define each lead (**Figure 16-37**). Six leads show the

frontal plane, and six show the transverse or horizontal plane. Because each lead shows a different picture of the heart, the tracing produced by each will appear slightly different. Before beginning, position the patient in the supine position in the center of the bed. The head of the bed may be elevated in the semi-Fowler's position if the patient prefers. Drape the patient, exposing the arms and legs. The patient must be relaxed and not too cold, to reduce muscle trembling; trembling will interfere with the ECG. The chest need not be uncovered during the procedure. In fact, this is a modesty and dignity issue for many women. If the bed is too narrow, position the patient's hands under the buttocks. This will reduce trembling and muscle tension. Make sure the feet are not touching the footboard of the bed.

Place the electrodes on flat, fleshy areas. Avoid bony or muscular areas. If the patient has an amputated extremity, you may place electrodes on the stump. If a pregelled electrode is dry, discard and replace it. Dry electrodes do not produce a high-quality tracing. After applying the electrode, hold it firmly in place for a few seconds to ensure that the edges seal tightly. If an area is excessively hairy, shave it. Cleaning the skin with alcohol removes oil, improving contact. When placing the electrodes, use the anatomical position. Remember that right and left on the patient are opposite to right and left on your body when you are facing the patient.

Two types of electrodes are commonly used. A conductive jelly is necessary to transmit the electrical impulse. Some disposable electrodes are prepackaged with gel. When using disposable pre-gelled electrodes, make sure they are not past the package expiration date. After the expiration date, the gel may be too dry. For other electrodes, a separate bottle of gel is used. Apply the gel to the skin surface, then attach the electrode immediately. Avoid allow-

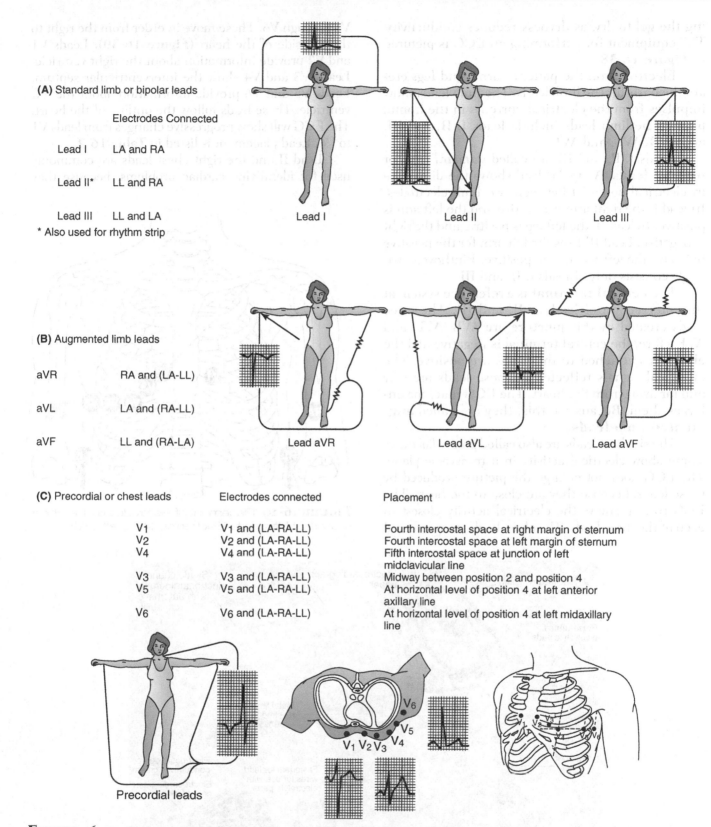

(A) Standard limb or bipolar leads

	Electrodes Connected
Lead I	LA and RA
Lead II*	LL and RA
Lead III	LL and LA

* Also used for rhythm strip

Lead I   Lead II   Lead III

(B) Augmented limb leads

aVR	RA and (LA-LL)
aVL	LA and (RA-LL)
aVF	LL and (RA-LA)

Lead aVR   Lead aVL   Lead aVF

(C) Precordial or chest leads

	Electrodes connected	Placement
V1	V1 and (LA-RA-LL)	Fourth intercostal space at right margin of sternum
V2	V2 and (LA-RA-LL)	Fourth intercostal space at left margin of sternum
V4	V4 and (LA-RA-LL)	Fifth intercostal space at junction of left midclavicular line
V3	V3 and (LA-RA-LL)	Midway between position 2 and position 4
V5	V5 and (LA-RA-LL)	At horizontal level of position 4 at left anterior axillary line
V6	V6 and (LA-RA-LL)	At horizontal level of position 4 at left midaxillary line

Precordial leads

FIGURE 16-37 Standard ECG leads, with corresponding electrode placement.

~~ing the gel to dry, as dryness reduces conductivity.~~ The equipment for performing an ECG is pictured in **Figure 16-38.**

Electrodes on the patient's arms and legs create the basis for the limb leads. The limb leads show impulses from the electrical currents in the frontal plane. The limb leads include leads I, II, and III, and AVR, AVL, and AVF.

Leads I, II, and III are called *standard leads* or **bipolar leads.** A bipolar lead shows the difference in electrical potential between two limb electrodes. In lead I, the right arm is negative and the left arm is positive. In lead II, the left leg is positive and the right is negative. Lead III uses the left arm for the negative pole and the left leg for the positive. Einthoven's triangle consists only of leads I, II, and III.

The **central terminal** is a reference system at the intersection of leads I, II, and III. The three leads created by this juncture are AVR, AVL, and AVF. Here, the central terminal is negative and the electrodes attached to the limbs are positive. The electrical signals reflected in these leads are tiny and far away from the heart. The ECG machine enlarges them. Because of this, they are called **augmented limb leads.**

The six chest leads are also called *precordial leads.* These show electrical activity in a transverse plane. The ECG does not enlarge the picture produced by these leads, because they are close to the heart. The ECG tracing shows the electrical activity closest to each of the three leads. The chest leads are numbered

V1 through V6. These move in order from the right to the left side of the heart (**Figure 16-39**). Leads V1 and V2 provide information about the right ventricle. Leads V3 and V4 show the interventricular septum. Leads V5 and V6 provide information about the left ventricle. These leads follow the outline of the heart. The ECG will show progressive changes from leads V1 to V6. Lead placement is listed in **Table 16-2.**

Lead II and the right chest leads are commonly used for identifying cardiac problems, because they

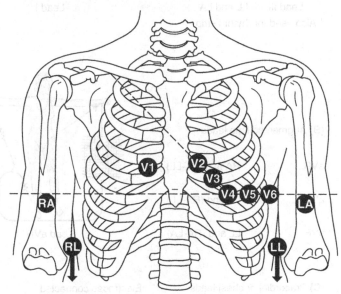

FIGURE 16-39 Placement of electrodes on the chest. (Copyright Marquette Electronics, Marquette, WI)

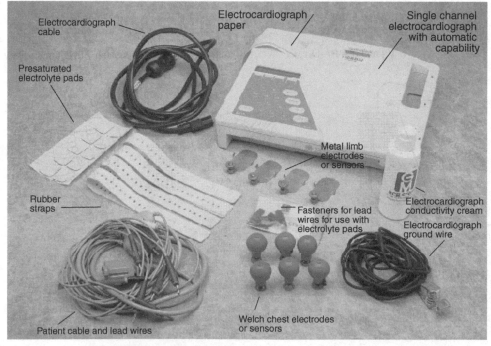

FIGURE 16-38 Equipment and supplies necessary for performing an electrocardiogram.

Table 16-2 Lead Placement

V1—right sternal border, fourth intercostal space

V2—left sternal border, fourth intercostal space

V3—midway between V2 and V4

V4—fifth intercostal space, midclavicular line

V5—horizontal to V4, anterior axillary line

V6—fifth intercostal space at the midaxillary level

RA and LA—anywhere on the arm

RL and LL—a few inches above the ankle

show the P wave best. The P wave is often the key to identifying a **dysrhythmia,** or abnormal heart rhythm. Some health care providers use the term *arrhythmia*. This is an older term that technically means "absence of rhythm." *Dysrhythmia* means abnormal rhythm, which describes the condition more accurately.

Remember to treat the patient, not the monitor. For example, the monitor shows a flat line, suggesting absence of heartbeat. However, the patient is talking and in no distress. Check the monitor and correct the problem.

The deflections on the ECG vary from one lead to another. The tracing may appear upright or positive when the current flows toward a positive electrode. The tracing appears upside down or negative when current is flowing toward a negative pole.

Lead Coding

The ECG must be marked so that the person interpreting it can tell one lead from another. This is important to interpretation of the rhythm, and determination of axis deviation and other factors. Coding of each lead is done by using a series of dots and dashes. Many newer ECG machines mark the rhythm strip automatically. If you are using an older unit, you may have to mark each lead manually by pressing the marker button. **Figure 16-40** shows an example of standardized lead coding.

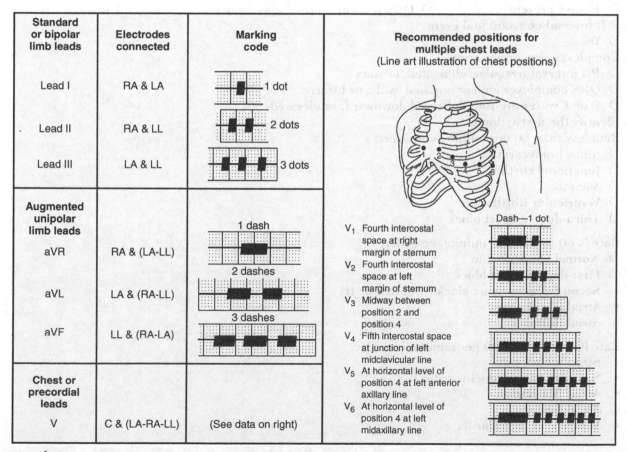

FIGURE 16-40 An example of a manual ECG coding system. (Courtesy of Siemens Burdick, Inc.)

Documentation and Reporting

Label the ECG according to facility policy. This usually includes the date, time, patient name, patient identification number, room number, and physician. Depending on the unit used, this may be done by hand or electronically.

Inform the RN when you have completed the ECG. Identify abnormal or life-threatening dysrhythmias and report these to the RN immediately. The checklist in **Table 16-3** may help you identify common dysrhythmias.

After you have labeled the tracing with the patient's identifying information, roll the rhythm strip up so the V-leads are at the end and lead II is at the beginning of the roll. If a delay in reading the strip is anticipated, a physician or RN can interpret the reading using the rolled strip. Avoid folding the tracing or scratching the surface of the thermal (heat-sensitive) paper, which will permanently mark the strip and may interfere with legibility.

Mounting the ECG

ECG tracings are cut and mounted so that a standard-size copy can be retained in the medical record. Several form styles are available for mounting (**Figure 16-41**). Some have pockets that the leads slide into, and others have self-adhesive tape for mounting the cut portion of the tracing.

Most hospitals use a tool called an *ECG trimmer* (**Figure 16-42**) to cut the tracing, although scissors may be used if necessary. Many physicians prefer that a rhythm strip be mounted first. This is a section that has been run at the beginning or end of the lead II tracing. It is mounted separately from the lead II strip. Cut the leads so the standardization mark is at the beginning of each lead (**Figure 16-43**) for identification purposes.

Table 16-3 Identifying Dysrhythmias		
A. Rate:		
○ 0–60	○ 60–100	○ 100 and over
B. Appearance of QRS complexes:		
○ P wave present	○ QRS present, normal appearance	○ T wave
C. R-R interval constant and even:		
○ Yes	○ No	
D. Complexes appear abnormal:		
○ PR interval irregular, elongated, or wavy		
○ QRS complexes appear notched, wide, or bizarre		
○ P or T waves are flat, deflected downward, or elevated		
E. Identify the dysrhythmia:		
Rate less than 60 per minute, consider:		
○ Sinus bradycardia		
○ Junctional rhythm		
○ Asystole		
○ Ventricular fibrillation		
○ Third-degree heart block		
Rate is 60 to 100 per minute, consider:		
○ Normal sinus rhythm		
○ First-degree heart block		
• Second-degree heart block (Mobitz I or II)		
• Atrial fibrillation		
• Atrial flutter		
Rate is more than 100 per minute, consider:		
• Sinus tachycardia		
• Supraventricular tachycardia		
• Atrial fibrillation		
• Atrial flutter		
• Ventricular tachycardia		

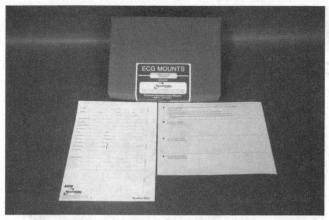

FIGURE 16-41 Various forms for mounting ECGs.

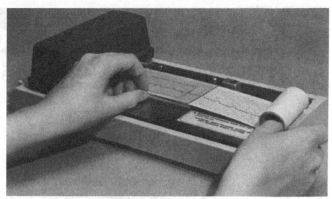

FIGURE 16-42 An ECG trimmer. (Courtesy of Spacelabs Medical, Inc.)

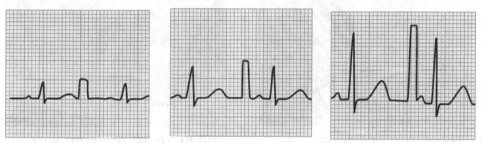

FIGURE 16-43 Standardization markings. (Courtesy of Spacelabs Medical, Inc.)

Procedure **130**

Performing a 12-Lead ECG

Supplies needed:
- ECG unit
- Recording paper
- Electrodes
- Alcohol sponges
- 4 × 4 gauze pads
- Razor
- Plastic bag for used supplies

1. Perform your beginning procedure actions.
2. If necessary, shave excess hair. Shaving is usually not necessary, but excess hair will interfere with electrode adherence to the skin. Remove skin oil with the alcohol sponges. Allow to dry. Rub the area of electrode placement briskly with the 4 × 4 sponge to abrade the area slightly. The area will appear slightly red. This removes dead skin cells, promoting better contact. Never substitute alcohol or acetone pads for electrode paste or gel. The pads impede electrode contact and reduce the recorded quality of electrical impulses.
3. Position the limb electrodes (**Figure 16-44**). Connect the leadwires. For easy visual identification, each is color-coded and lettered.
   - Right arm leadwire is white, and labeled RA
   - Right leg leadwire is green, and labeled RL
   - Left leg leadwire is red, and labeled LL
   - Left arm leadwire is black, and labeled LA
4. Apply electrodes to the chest (**Figure 16-45**). Avoid positioning the electrodes directly on bone, which will cause interference. In the female, position the electrodes below the breast tissue. If the breasts are large, you may have to position the breast laterally.

(continues)

Procedure **130**, *continued*

Performing a 12-Lead ECG

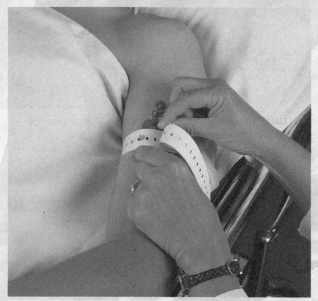

FIGURE 16-44 Attach the limb electrodes so they are snug, but not too tight.

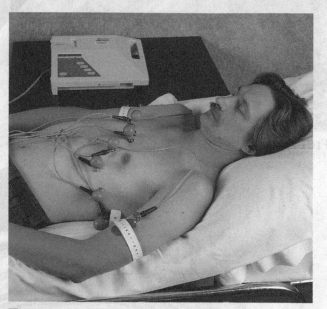

FIGURE 16-45 Attach the suction-cup electrodes to the chest.

a. Palpate the clavicle (collarbone), which is considered the first rib. Continue palpating downward to the fourth rib. Move down slightly to the space between the fourth and fifth ribs. Position lead V1 in the fourth intercostal space, to the right of the sternum.

b. Position lead V2 directly opposite V1 at the left sternal border.

c. Next, position lead V4 in the fifth intercostal space at the midclavicular line.

d. Position lead V3 halfway between V2 and V4.

e. Position leads V5 and V6 laterally to V4. Position V5 in the anterior axillary line. V6 is positioned in the midaxillary line.

5. After applying the electrodes, enter information required by the facility into the ECG cart. Applying electrodes first allows the electrode gel to contact and penetrate the skin surface.

6. Attach the correct leadwire to each electrode. The leadwires are brown.

7. Check the speed on the ECG machine. It should be set to the standard reading of 25 mm/second, unless you are instructed otherwise. Make sure the unit is set to the full voltage. The unit will mark a standardization mark on the paper. Next, enter facility-required patient identification information.

When performing the ECG, if part of a wave extends beyond the paper, reduce the normal standardization to half standardization. Note this adjustment on the ECG strip.

8. Ask the patient to lie still and breathe normally.

9. Press the "AUTO" or "RECORD" button. Check the tracing quality. If artifact is present, try to correct the problem. It may be necessary to use fresh electrodes. The machine will record the ECG (**Figure 16-46**).

10. When the unit finishes recording, remove the leadwires and electrodes. Clean the conductive gel from the patient's skin.

11. Perform your procedure completion actions.

(continues)

Procedure **130**, *continued*

Performing a 12-Lead ECG

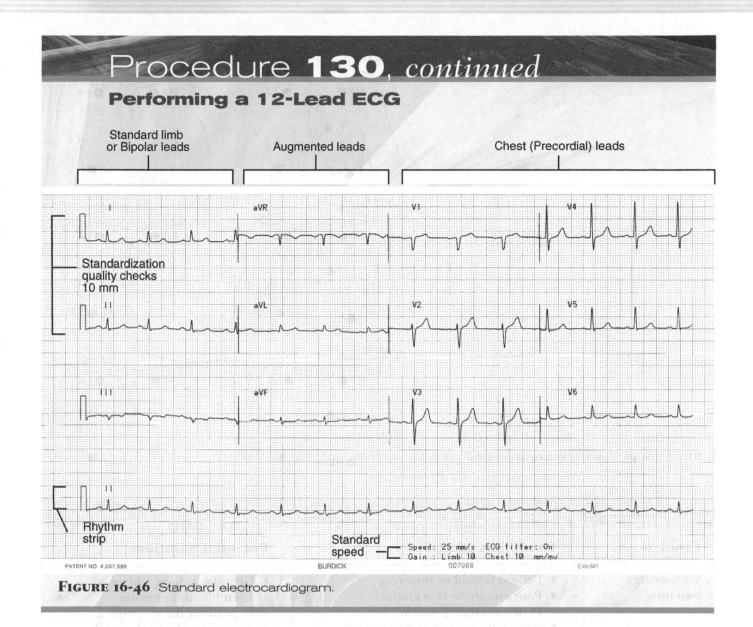

Standard limb or Bipolar leads

Augmented leads

Chest (Precordial) leads

Standardization quality checks 10 mm

Rhythm strip

Standard speed

Speed: 25 mm/s   ECG filter: On
Gain : Limb 10   Chest 10   mm/mv

PATENT NO. 4,207,580   BURDICK   007966   C-00-501

FIGURE 16-46 Standard electrocardiogram.

CONTINUOUS CARDIAC MONITORING

Cardiac monitoring is performed to provide continuous observation of the heart in patients who are at risk of developing dysrhythmias, and those with unstable medical conditions. Two types of monitoring are commonly done. In **hardwire monitoring,** the patient's heart rhythm is displayed on both a monitor at the bedside and at another remote location, usually the nurses' station. A second type of monitoring, called **telemetry,** enables the patient to be ambulatory. A small transmitter sends a signal to a remote location, where the patient's cardiac rhythm is displayed on a monitor screen.

The cardiac monitor displays the patient's heart rate and rhythm. The monitoring unit can produce a printed record of the cardiac rhythm. The monitor can be set to sound an alarm if the heart rate rises above or falls below a certain level. Certain life-threatening dysrhythmias will also cause the alarm to sound.

Setting Up Continuous Cardiac Monitoring

Cardiac monitoring is done using three or five electrodes. Follow the RN's directions and facility policy. The chest leads are most commonly used for monitoring because these appear upright and are easiest to read. However, other leads may also be used, if necessary, to provide a different view of the heart.

Placement of the electrodes on the chest for leads I, II, and III is the same. To change leads, a switch on the monitor is set to correspond with the lead you want to view. **Figure 16-47** shows electrode placement for leads I, II, and III.

Table 16-4 lists cardiac monitoring problems and potential solutions.

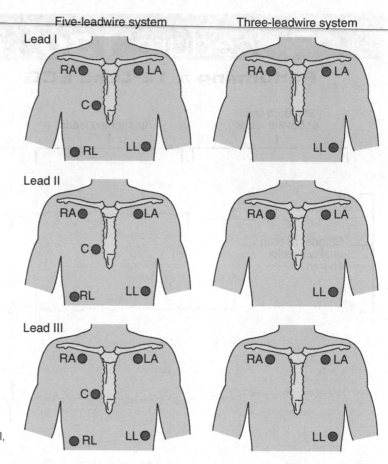

FIGURE 16-47 Electrode placement for leads I, II, and III.

Table 16-4 Troubleshooting for Cardiac Monitoring Problems		
Problem	**Potential Cause**	**Potential Solutions**
Wandering baseline	• Patient is cold or shivering • Poor electrode-skin contact • Poor electrode position • Respirations are interfering with thoracic electrodes	• Give the patient a blanket; keep him or her warm • Reposition the electrodes • Apply new electrodes; make sure they are not too dry
Skin irritation from electrodes	• Electrode has been in the same place too long • Patient is allergic to the adhesive	• Reposition the electrodes • Gently wash adhesive from skin; do not use alcohol • Obtain hypoallergenic electrodes and tape
False alarm—low rate	• Patient movement has shifted the electrical axis • Poor electrode contact • Low-amplitude QRS	• Remove and reapply electrodes. Increase the gain so the QRS is more than one millivolt
False alarm—high rate	• Skeletal muscle activity • Monitor is counting T waves as QRS complexes, which doubles the rate	• Remove and replace electrodes. Ensure that they are positioned so that T waves appear smaller than QRS complexes

(continues)

Table 16-4 Troubleshooting for Cardiac Monitoring Problems (Continued)		
Problem	**Potential Cause**	**Potential Solutions**
		• Move electrodes away from very muscular areas
60-cycle interference (baseline thick and fuzzy)	• The bed is improperly grounded • Interference from other electrical equipment	• Make sure the bed ground is connected to the common ground in the room • Make sure all equipment is attached to the common ground • Check plugs of electrical equipment; make sure they are tight
Artifact	• Patient anxious, chilling, trembling, having a seizure • Patient movement • Patient tapping on or playing with electrode • Static electricity • Electrodes improperly applied • Decreased humidity in room • Short in patient cable or leadwires • Broken leadwires	• Give patient a blanket; keep him or her warm • Reassure the patient; help him or her relax • Monitor the patient to determine if he or she is tapping the electrodes • Check security of electrodes; remove and reapply if needed • Replace broken wires and equipment • Make sure the cables do not have exposed connector wires • Check for sources of static electricity and remove; check the patient's bed; change nylon nightgowns or clothing • Check humidity; increase to 40 percent • Replace and retape leadwires; apply stress loops • Use soap and water to clean leadwires; do not use alcohol. Keep the ends of the connectors dry
Low amplitude	• Monitor malfunction • Loss of QRS amplitude • Poor contact between electrodes and skin • Dried gel • Loose or broken leadwires • Poor connection between patient and monitor • Gain is set too low	• Check all connections to make sure they are secure • Replace electrodes • Increase gain

Procedure 131

Setting Up for Continuous Cardiac Monitoring

Supplies needed:
- Cardiac monitor
- Electrodes
- Leadwires
- Alcohol sponges
- 4 × 4 gauze pad
- Razor (optional)

1. Perform your beginning procedure actions.
2. If necessary, shave excess hair. Shaving is usually not necessary, but excess hair will interfere with electrode adherence to the skin. Remove skin oil with the alcohol sponges. Allow to dry. Rub the area of electrode placement briskly with the 4 × 4 sponge to abrade the area slightly. The area will appear slightly red. This removes dead skin cells, promoting better contact.
3. Position the electrodes. Connect the leadwires.
4. Turn the monitor on, if not done previously.
5. Check the monitor for quality of the tracing, and adjust if necessary.
6. Set the high and low heart rate alarms according to facility policy, or as instructed by the RN.
7. Perform your procedure completion actions

MONITORING THE PULSE TO EVALUATE CIRCULATION

You have learned that counting the pulse enables you to count the number of heartbeats per minute. Pulse points are located throughout the body (**Figure 16-48**). When taking the pulse during routine vital signs, you use the radial pulse. However, other pulses in the body are checked to determine if blood is circulating to various parts of the body.

Apical Pulse

The apical pulse is taken at the apex of the heart. The stethoscope is placed over the lower tip of the heart. Listen for the heart sounds that indicate the closing of valves. These sounds should occur at the same rate as the pulse at the radial artery. The apex of the heart is found:

- On the left side of the front of the chest
- Between the fifth and sixth ribs

HEALTH CARE ALERT

Warm the diaphragm or bell of the stethoscope by rubbing it between your hands. A cold stethoscope may startle the patient and increase the pulse rate. If you are having trouble hearing, reverse the head of the stethoscope. The bell enables you to hear low-pitched sounds more effectively than the diaphragm.

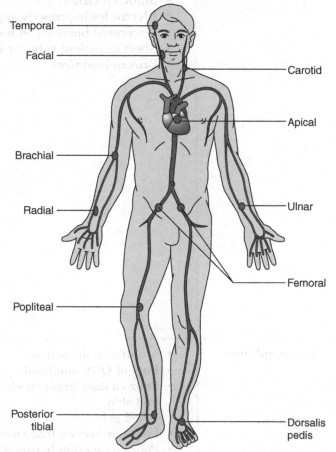

Temporal
Facial
Carotid
Apical
Brachial
Radial
Ulnar
Femoral
Popliteal
Posterior tibial
Dorsalis pedis

FIGURE 16-48 Pulse points.

- Just below the left nipple
- In females, below the left breast

After placing the stethoscope on the chest, listen for two sounds: lub dub. The louder sound (lub) corresponds to the contraction of the ventricles pushing blood forward through the arteries, and closing of the valves to prevent a backflow of blood. This is the sound to be counted. The softer sound (dub) corresponds to the relaxation of the ventricles as they fill with blood. When documenting an apical pulse reading, write "AP" after the value.

Apical-Radial Pulse Rate

The apical-radial pulse rate is a comparison of the apical pulse and the radial pulse. Usually they are the same. Sometimes, though, the contraction of the heart is so weak that it fails to send enough blood to the arteries to expand them. When this happens, no pulse is felt. In this case, the number of loud sounds does not correspond to the number of pulse beats felt at the radial artery.

The difference between the apical pulse and radial pulse is the **pulse deficit.** Pulse deficits are found in some forms of heart disease. Two people will measure the heart rate and radial pulse rate simultaneously. During this procedure, the pulse should be counted for one full minute. The apical or radical pulses may be checked:

- Whenever a pulse deficit exists or is suspected
- Before the RN administers drugs that alter the heart rate or rhythm
- In children whose rapid heart rates are difficult to count at the wrist
- On any child 12 months of age or younger
- Whenever you are unsure of the accuracy of the radial pulse
- In medical conditions in which the radial pulse is imperceptible

Procedure 132

Counting the Apical-Radial Pulse

Supplies needed:
- Stethoscope
- Alcohol sponges or disinfectant

1. Perform your beginning procedure actions.
2. Wipe the stethoscope earpieces and diaphragm with alcohol or disinfectant.
3. Place the stethoscope in your ears with the tips facing slightly forward.
4. Place the stethoscope diaphragm over the apex of the patient's heart.
5. Listen carefully for the heartbeat.
6. After you have located the heartbeat, signal your partner to begin counting the radial pulse.
7. Count the louder (lub) sounds for one full minute while your partner counts the radial pulse.

8. Note results on a pad for comparison. Calculate the pulse deficit, if any.

Example: Apical pulse   =   108
Minus (−) Radial pulse   −82
Pulse Deficit =   26

9. Clean the earpieces and diaphragm of the stethoscope with alcohol or disinfectant.
10. Perform your procedure completion actions.

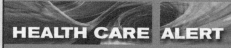

HEALTH CARE ALERT

If the peripheral pulse is weak and hard to palpate, or irregular, check the apical pulse for accuracy. If the pulse is difficult to count, consider using the Doppler ultrasound blood flow detector.

Checking the Femoral Pulse

You may be asked to check the femoral pulse beat. The superficial femoral artery is the main blood vessel responsible for leg circulation. The name of this artery becomes the popliteal artery just above the knee. The artery passes through the knee, and splits into three blood vessels. One of these, the posterior tibial artery, is also used for checking the pulse.

Adjust the bath blanket or draping sheet to expose the patient's groin area. Avoid checking the pulse by reaching down from the abdomen

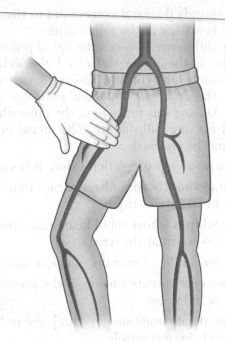

FIGURE 16-49 The femoral pulse is in the crease of the upper leg.

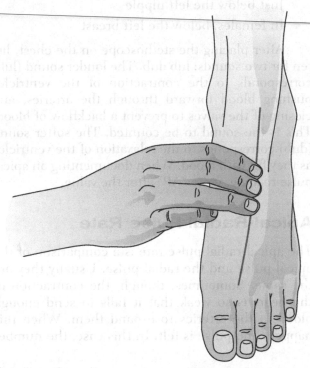

FIGURE 16-50 To locate the dorsalis pedis pulse, draw an imaginary line from the ankle to the area between the great toe and second toe.

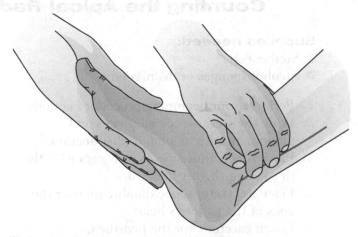

FIGURE 16-51 To locate the posterior tibial pulse, place your fingers in the groove between the Achilles tendon and the tibia. Move your fingers in slightly, toward the tibia.

under the drape. Stand next to the patient's legs when examining the groin area. Move the drape as needed, but avoid unnecessarily exposing the genitals. The femoral pulse is in the center of the crease in the leg, near the groin (**Figure 16-49**). After locating the pulse, count it for one full minute. You may be instructed to mark the pulse with an X in indelible ink. If the pulse is difficult to palpate, you may be instructed to check it using the Doppler instrument.

Dorsalis Pedis and Posterior Tibial Pulses

The posterior tibial and dorsalis pedis pulses are located in the lower extremities. These pulses are checked to determine if blood flow is adequate in the lower legs and feet. In some patients, they may be difficult to palpate. Sometimes a special device, called a *Doppler,* is used to amplify the pulse beat so that you can hear an audible beat. The Doppler is similar to a stethoscope with an amplifier.

To check the dorsalis pedis and posterior tibial pulses, you must first locate the pulse point. The dorsalis pedis artery is located on an imaginary line drawn from the ankle to the area between the great toe and second toe (**Figure 16-50**). It may be easiest to palpate the pulse on the instep. The posterior tibial pulse is located posterior to the inner ankle

(**Figure 16-51**). It may be slightly harder to find. Use two or three fingers.

After locating the pulse, place your fingers or the Doppler device gently over the pulse, and count for one full minute. Avoid pressing too hard, which may obliterate the pulse. If you cannot locate either pulse on a patient, see if you can locate the popliteal artery, behind the knee. This pulse may be easier to locate if you ask the patient to flex the knee. Press deeply into the center of the popliteal space to palpate the pulse. Always notify the RN if you cannot palpate a pulse.

The pulse in the lower extremities may be checked every shift, or more often, in some patients. Because these pulses are often hard to find, the RN may instruct you to mark the location with a pen on the patient's skin, with an X. Absence of pulses in an extremity suggests peripheral arterial disease. The patient may have an obstruction below the lowest palpable pulse. Although the patient's feet and legs may be intact, he or she is at very high risk of injury. A small cut or other injury can result in serious complications because of a lack of blood flow in the extremity.

Procedure 133

Checking the Pulses in the Legs and Feet

Supplies needed:
▶ Disposable exam gloves, if necessary for checking the femoral pulse
▶ Watch with second hand
▶ Note pad and pen

1. Perform your beginning procedure actions.
2. Check the pulse:
   ▶ Femoral pulse:
      ▶ Apply gloves if contact with blood or body fluid is likely.
      ▶ Adjust the bath blanket or draping sheet to expose the patient's groin.
      ▶ Locate and palpate the femoral pulse, in the center of the crease in the leg, near the groin. You may have to press deeply.
      ▶ Count the pulse for one full minute.
   ▶ Dorsalis pedis pulse:
      ▶ Imagine a line between the ankle and the fleshy area between the great toe and second toe. Place two or three fingers on this line, over the instep area.
      ▶ Gently palpate the area to determine the pulse location.
      ▶ Count the pulse for one full minute.
   ▶ Posterior tibial pulse:
      ▶ Place your fingers in the groove between the Achilles tendon and the tibia, slightly above the medial malleolus. Move the fingers in, toward the tibia. You may have to press deeply.
      ▶ Gently palpate the area to determine the pulse location.
      ▶ Count the pulse for one full minute.
3. Mark the pulse location with an X, if instructed to do so.
4. Document the pulse rate on your note pad.
5. Perform your procedure completion actions.

Using the Doppler

A **Doppler** (Figure 16-52) is an instrument that amplifies sounds, similar to a stethoscope. It uses ultrasound to magnify sounds inside the body. It is commonly used for listening to arteries, such as the blood pressure and pulse. Various types of Dopplers are available. Some are handheld units, and some have headsets similar to a stethoscope. This procedure is for a handheld unit, but may be modified for use with other types of Dopplers.

HEALTH CARE ALERT

Use coupling gel or transmission gel, not water-soluble lubricant. Place the probe directly over the artery, then tilt it at a 45-degree angle. Make sure there is sufficient gel between the Doppler and the skin. Turn the Doppler on. Set the volume control to the lowest setting by turning the knob counterclockwise. Move the probe slowly, in a circular motion, to find the center of the artery and Doppler signal. This sounds like a hissing noise at the heartbeat. If the signal sounds distorted, repeat the counterclockwise circle very slowly. Moving the probe too quickly will scramble and garble the signal.

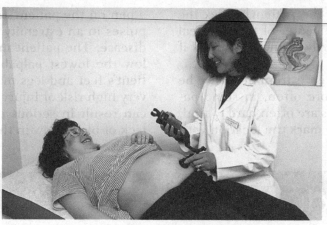

FIGURE 16-52 The Doppler amplifies sounds by using ultrasound to magnify sounds inside the body. The unit pictured here is a handheld unit. Some Dopplers have headsets similar to a stethoscope.

Procedure 134

Using a Doppler to Hear Pulse Sounds

Supplies needed:
▶ Doppler unit
▶ Hibistat®, non-phenol-based disinfectant, or other disinfectant according to facility policy
▶ Conductive jelly
▶ Tissues
▶ Plastic bag for used supplies

1. Perform your beginning procedure actions.
2. Cleanse the Doppler with facility-approved disinfectant.
3. Expose the area to be checked.
4. Apply conductive jelly to the patient's skin or the Doppler unit, depending on the equipment you are using.

5. Hold the tip of the probe at a 45-degree angle over the blood vessel you are examining.
6. Press the "ON" button and adjust the volume so you can hear it clearly.
7. Count the pulse or listen to the blood pressure.
8. Turn the unit off and cover the patient.
9. Wipe the jelly off the patient's skin and the Doppler unit.
10. Cleanse the Doppler with facility-approved disinfectant.
11. Perform your procedure completion actions.

BLOOD PRESSURE

Blood pressure is a measurement of the force of blood against the walls of arteries. Readings vary with illness and activity. A patient has high blood pressure when the blood pressure stays elevated over time. The medical term for high blood pressure is *hypertension*. Hypertension makes the heart work too hard and contributes to hardening of the arteries. High blood pressure increases the risk of several serious diseases. It can also cause complications of conditions such as diabetes. High blood pressure is a serious public health problem. Regular blood pressure monitoring and screening are important.

HEALTH CARE ALERT

The technique you use for measuring the blood pressure affects the accuracy of the reading. The cuff must fit the patient correctly. A cuff that is small will give false high readings. A cuff that is too large or wrapped too loosely will provide false low readings. Cuffs come in many different sizes. Although there is a standard-size adult cuff, obese patients usually require an extra-large cuff. Very small patients require a pediatric cuff. To check the cuff size, compare the length of the rubber bladder with the patient's arm circumference. The bladder should be at least 80 percent of the circumference of the arm. If it is larger or smaller, obtain a different-size cuff.

Table 16-5 Blood Pressure Value (mm Hg)			
Category	**Systolic**	***	**Diastolic**
Normal	120 or less	and	80 or less
Prehypertension	120–139	or	80 to 89
High Blood Pressure			
Stage I hypertension	140–159	or	90–99
Stage II hypertension	160 or greater	or	100 or greater

In 2003, the federal government reviewed and revised the hypertension guidelines. The revised values are listed in **Table 16-5.** Hypertension is a blood pressure value of 140/90 or higher. It is a dangerous condition that may be called a "silent killer" because there are no signs or symptoms. A single elevated reading does not mean you have hypertension. The condition is diagnosed based on various readings at different times of the day, and during different activities.

Prehypertension is a condition that means the person is likely to develop high blood pressure in the future. In this condition, the blood pressure value is between 120/80 mm Hg and 139/89 mm Hg. Health care workers are being encouraged to identify prehypertension, so that patients can decrease their risk.

When systolic and diastolic blood pressures fall into different categories, the higher category should be used to classify blood pressure level. For example, 160/80 mm Hg would be Stage II hypertension (high blood pressure). Both numbers in the blood pressure are important, but for people who are 50 or older, systolic pressure gives the most accurate diagnosis of high blood pressure.

Blood Pressure Monitoring

Vital signs must be taken in a timely manner, and must be accurate. Many hospitals use electronic blood pressure monitoring equipment for routine vital signs. It is commonly used for patients who need frequent blood pressure monitoring, such as every 15 minutes. A memory in the unit retains previous blood pressure values and displays them on demand. Vital signs must be documented promptly,

because many individuals will refer to these values. Report abnormal vital signs to the RN promptly. If a patient is connected to electronic vital sign monitoring equipment (**Figure 16-53**), respond to alarms immediately. Never turn an alarm off.

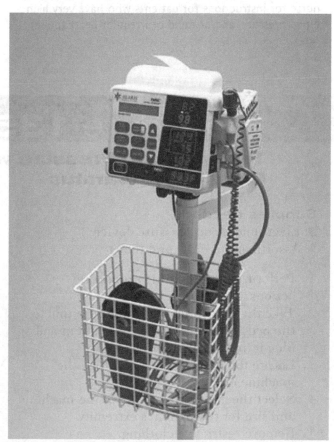

Figure 16-53 All vital signs may be checked with a single instrument. (VitalCheck patient monitor, photo courtesy of Alaris Medical Systems, Inc. San Diego, CA)

Guidelines for Electronic Blood Pressure Monitoring

Patient Selection

● This procedure can be done on patients of all ages and sizes, but appropriately sized cuffs must be used.

● At least one blood pressure reading should be taken using the auscultation method before using the electronic blood pressure device. The auscultation reading is used as a baseline with which to compare electronic values.

Contraindications

Electronic blood pressure monitoring is contraindicated in patients with:

● Extreme hypertension or hypotension

● Very rapid heart rates

● Irregular heart rhythms or atrial dysrhythmias

● Excessive body movement, tremors

Patients for whom electronic blood pressure monitoring is not acceptable should be known to all caregivers and identified on the care plan. If in doubt, check with the nurse for instructions for patients who have very high blood pressure, and/or rapid or irregular heart (pulse) rates.

Application of the Cuff

● Select the proper cuff size. The width should be equal to 80 percent of the arm circumference.

● The upper arm is the preferred location, but the forearm or ankle may also be used.

● Do not place the cuff on an arm with:
  ● Paralysis
  ● An intravenous infusion
  ● A pulse oximeter
  ● Impaired circulation
  ● A dialysis access device
  ● Fracture
  ● Burns
  ● A recent mastectomy or other surgical procedure

Infection Control

● Blood pressure cuffs are a potential source of transmission of infection. Some facilities issue a disposable cuff to each patient. Others require personnel to wipe the cuff with a disinfectant solution after each patient. Follow your facility policies for prevention of infection.

Procedure 135

Taking Blood Pressure with an Electronic Blood Pressure Apparatus

Supplies needed:
▶ Electronic blood pressure device
▶ Assortment of cuffs and tubes

1. Perform your beginning procedure actions.
2. Take the electronic blood pressure unit to the bedside. Place it near the patient and plug it into a source of electricity.
3. Locate the on/off switch and turn the machine on.
4. Select the appropriate cuff for the machine and size for the patient's extremity.
5. Remove restrictive clothing.
6. Squeeze excess air out of the cuff.
7. Connect the cuff to the connector hose.

8. Wrap the cuff snugly around the patient's extremity, verifying that only one finger can fit between the cuff and the patient's skin. Make sure the "artery" arrow marked on the outside of the cuff is correctly placed over the brachial artery.
9. Verify that the connector hose between the cuff and the machine is not kinked.
10. Set the frequency control for automatic or manual.
11. Press the start button.
12. If the cuff will take periodic, automatic measurements, set the designated frequency of measurement.

(continues)

Procedure 135, *continued*

Taking Blood Pressure with an Electronic Blood Pressure Apparatus

13. Set upper and lower alarm limits for systolic, diastolic, and mean blood pressure readings.

14. Remove the cuff at least every 2 hours and alternate sites, if possible. Evaluate the skin

for redness and irritation. Report abnormalities to the nurse.

16. Perform your procedure completion actions.

CARING FOR A PATIENT FOLLOWING AN ANGIOGRAM OR ARTERIOGRAM

An **angiogram** or **arteriogram** is an X-ray study of the blood vessels. It may be done on an inpatient or outpatient basis. Specific vessels are studied by positioning a catheter into the artery. **Contrast medium** is a special dye that is injected through the catheter during the X-ray. It enables the physician to see inside the blood vessel and identify potential problems. The patient is positioned on his or her back on an X-ray table. The groin area is prepped by shaving and scrubbing, then draped with sterile drapes. Local anesthetic is injected into

the skin. Initially, a needle is inserted into the femoral artery. After the skin stick is made, a catheter is inserted into the artery and positioned. The physician views the position of the catheter on a device similar to a television. When the catheter is properly positioned, the contrast medium is injected while the X-ray is being obtained. The catheter is removed upon procedure completion. Pressure must be applied to the puncture site for 10 to 15 minutes thereafter.

The patient will remain on bedrest for 4 to 6 hours after the procedure. He or she will be instructed not to sit up or bend the leg that was used for the study. He or she may be discharged after this, if there are no complications.

Guidelines for Caring for a Patient Post-Arteriogram (or Angiogram)

- Maintain bedrest for 4 to 6 hours, or according to facility policies.
- Keep the head of the bed flat for 3 hours.
- The RN may permit elevation of the head of the bed 10 to 15 degrees after 2 hours.
- After 3 hours, the patient may sit in the high Fowler's position for an hour, if he or she is stable.
- Keep the operative extremity in full extension while the patient is on bedrest.
- Evaluate vital signs and peripheral pulses (in this case, check the pedal pulse) immediately after the procedure.
- Monitor vital signs at the frequency specified by facility policy, or:
  - Monitor vital signs every 15 minutes (4 times) during the first hour.

- Monitor vital signs every 30 minutes (4 times) during the second and third hours.
- Monitor vital signs every hour thereafter until the patient is discharged.
- Monitor the puncture site for bleeding and signs of hematoma immediately on return and each time vital signs are taken. If active bleeding is present, apply firm pressure with your gloved hand for 15 minutes.
- The patient may be on special bleeding precautions if he or she is receiving anticoagulant therapy.
- Assist the patient to eat and drink while in the flat position.
- Encourage fluids. (This will help flush dye from the system.)
- Monitor I&O.
- Verify that the patient has voided before he or she is discharged.

(continued)

Guidelines for Caring for a Patient Post-Arteriogram (or Angiogram) (Continued)

- Inform the RN immediately if the patient develops signs and symptoms of complications:
  - Bleeding or hematoma at puncture site
  - Drainage or swelling at the insertion site
  - Deterioration or loss of distal pulse(s)
  - Temperature or sensory deterioration in operative extremity
  - Cool, mottled, or bluish skin in operative extremity
  - Increasing coldness in one leg compared with the other leg
  - Excessive warmth, numbness, tingling in operative extremity

- Numbness or tingling sensation in either leg
- Change in strength of either leg
- Weakness in either leg
- Unrelieved pain in operative extremity
- Fever
- Chills
- Other abnormal vital signs
- Inability to void after 4 hours
- Capillary refill more than 3 seconds

CARDIAC CATHETERIZATION

Cardiac catheterization is a diagnostic procedure in which a catheter is threaded through the blood vessels into the heart. Depending on the nature of the procedure performed, certain complications are possible during and after the procedure. These include:

- Nausea
- Vomiting
- Low blood pressure
- Slow pulse (bradycardia)
- Internal bleeding (the patient may complain of thigh, back, or groin pain)
- Hematoma formation at the puncture site
- Myocardial infarction

Care after Cardiac Catheterization

Patients undergoing cardiac catheterization require close monitoring after the procedure. The RN will instruct you on special monitoring and things to watch for. When monitoring the patient, communicate regularly with the RN and report changes immediately. Depending on the technique used in the procedure, the patient may be able to go home in as little as three hours. However, the physician may write an order requiring the patient to stay on bedrest until the morning after the procedure. Instruct the patient to move the affected extremity as little as possible. Follow your facility policies and the RN's instructions.

Procedure 136

Monitoring after Cardiac Catheterization

Supplies needed:

- Disposable exam gloves (for checking femoral pulse)
- Stethoscope
- Blood pressure cuff
- Watch with second hand

1. Perform your beginning procedure actions.
2. Check the patient's blood pressure and apical pulse every 15 minutes, or more often

as directed. The RN may increase the interval to 30 or 60 minutes after the patient has stabilized.
3. Check the peripheral pulses in the affected extremity:
   - Radial pulse in the upper extremity
   - Dorsalis pedis and posterior tibial pulses in the lower extremity

(continues)

Procedure **136**, *continued*

Monitoring after Cardiac Catheterization

4. Evaluate the affected extremity for:
   ▶ Color
   ▶ Skin temperature
   ▶ Complaints of pain
   ▶ Complaints of numbness or tingling
5. Monitor the site of the skin puncture for edema, bleeding, and signs of hematoma development. Question the patient about pain in the extremity.
6. Ask the patient if he or she is having chest pain. If present, remain in the room and use the call signal to alert the RN.
7. Question the patient about groin, thigh, or back pain.
8. Monitor for signs and symptoms of other complications.
9. Perform your procedure completion actions.

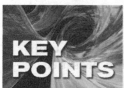
KEY POINTS

▶ Cardiovascular disorders are the leading cause of death in the United States.

▶ Electrical activity within the heart causes the heart to beat.

▶ The cardiac cycle consists of contraction and relaxation.

▶ The sinoatrial node is the primary pacemaker of the heart; this pacemaker fires at 60 to 100 beats per minute.

▶ Any tissue within the heart can act as a pacemaker; the rate may be a key to which area of the heart is acting as the primary pacemaker.

▶ The electrical impulse in a healthy heart begins in the SA node, then travels to the AV node, through the bundle of His, right and left bundle branches, and Purkinje fibers, causing the ventricles to contract.

▶ The working phase of the heart is systole; the resting phase is diastole.

▶ Understanding the normal conduction of the heart is key to identifying various rhythms on an ECG or cardiac monitor.

▶ Each heartbeat shows up as five waves on the ECG; each wave represents an electrical impulse and corresponding heart action.

▶ When reading the ECG paper vertically, one small block represents 0.04 second. Each large block is five small blocks wide. Large blocks represent 0.20 second. When reading the ECG paper vertically, each small block represents 1 mm. Each large block represents 5 mm vertically.

▶ The heart is three-dimensional; the ECG views the heart from various dimensions. The ECG consists of 12 leads recording the same cardiac activity simultaneously.

▶ A dysrhythmia is an abnormal heart rhythm.

▶ In hardwire cardiac monitoring, the patient's heart rhythm is displayed on both a monitor at the bedside and at another remote location, usually the nurses' station.

▶ In telemetry monitoring, the patient can be ambulatory because the monitor is battery-operated and sends a signal to a remote location.

▶ The cardiac monitor displays the patient's heart rate and rhythm; it can produce a printed record of the cardiac rhythm.

(continues)

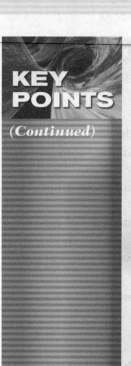

KEY POINTS

(Continued)

▶ The monitor will sound an alarm if the heart rate rises above or falls below a certain level; certain life-threatening dysrhythmias will also cause the alarm to sound.

▶ Cardiac monitoring is commonly done in leads I, II, and III. Electrode placement for these leads is the same; a switch on the monitor is turned to designate the lead.

▶ The apical pulse is taken at the apex of the heart and reflects the sound of valves closing.

▶ The apical-radial pulse rate is a comparison of the apical pulse and the radial pulse.

▶ The difference in value between the apical pulse and radial pulse is the pulse deficit.

▶ A Doppler is an instrument that uses ultrasound to amplify sounds inside the body.

▶ Palpating the dorsalis pedis and posterior tibial pulses provides information about blood flow in the feet and lower legs.

▶ Normal blood pressure is less than 120/80.

▶ Prehypertension is a condition that means the person is likely to develop high blood pressure in the future. In this condition, the blood pressure value is between 120/80 mm Hg and 139/89 mm Hg.

▶ Hypertension is blood pressure of more than 140/90 mm Hg.

▶ At least one blood pressure reading should be taken using the auscultation method before using an electronic blood pressure device. The auscultation reading is used as a baseline with which to compare electronic values.

▶ An angiogram or arteriogram is an X-ray study of the blood vessels. Contrast medium is a special dye that is injected during this procedure, enabling the physician to see inside the blood vessels and identify potential problems.

▶ The patient will remain on bedrest for 4 to 6 hours after an angiogram or arteriogram. He or she will be instructed not to sit up or bend the leg that was used for the study.

▶ Cardiac catheterization is a diagnostic procedure in which a catheter is threaded through the blood vessels to the heart; complications can occur during and after the procedure, and close monitoring is required.

CLINICAL APPLICATIONS

1. Mr. Darien's monitor shows a rate of 50 beats per minute. The P waves appear slightly flat. Based on this information, which area of the heart may be acting as the pacemaker?

2. Mrs. Gonsalves's PR interval is 0.24 second. The rest of her ECG appears normal. Is the problem in the atria or ventricles? Do you think this condition is life-threatening?

3. Mr. Han does not speak English. His daughter is interpreting for him. You are asked to perform an ECG on this patient. The patient and his daughter are not familiar with the ECG procedure. How will you explain it to them?

4. The RN instructs you to change Mrs. Jefferson's monitor from lead III to lead I. Will you move the electrodes? How will you change the lead?

5. Mr. Ferrier had a cardiac catheterization earlier in your shift. He returned to the unit 30 minutes ago. During your routine check, the patient tells you that he has "a little pain and tightness in his chest." What action will you take?

CHAPTER REVIEW

Multiple-Choice Questions

Select the one best answer.

1. The ECG measures the:
   a. blood flow within the heart.
   b. electrical activity within the heart.
   c. blood flow through the large blood vessels.
   d. brain activity.

2. During diastole, the heart is:
   a. working.
   b. sending ventricular impulses.
   c. resting.
   d. conducting atrial impulses.

3. When the pacemaker is in the SA node, the heartbeat is usually:
   a. 10 to 30 beats per minute.
   b. 20 to 60 beats per minute.
   c. 40 to 80 beats per minute.
   d. 60 to 100 beats per minute.

4. When the pacemaker is in the AV node, the heartbeat is usually:
   a. 10 to 20 beats per minute.
   b. 20 to 40 beats per minute.
   c. 40 to 60 beats per minute.
   d. 60 to 100 beats per minute.

5. When the pacemaker is in the ventricles, the heartbeat is usually:
   a. 10 to 50 beats per minute.
   b. 20 to 40 beats per minute.
   c. 40 to 60 beats per minute.
   d. 60 to 100 beats per minute.

6. The heartbeat occurs:
   a. as a result of ventricular contraction.
   b. when the SA node fires.
   c. as the impulse travels through the bundle of His.
   d. when you see the T wave on the ECG.

7. Each small block on the ECG paper represents:
   a. 0.40 second.
   b. 0.04 second.
   c. 0.10 second.
   d. 0.20 second.

8. Each large block on the ECG paper represents:
   a. 0.40 second.
   b. 0.04 second.
   c. 0.20 second.
   d. 0.10 second.

9. The dorsalis pedis pulse is usually found:
   a. over the instep of the foot.
   b. near the inner fibula.
   c. near the medial malleolus.
   d. on the ball of the foot.

10. The patient who has had a cardiac catheterization:
    a. is ambulated immediately upon return to the unit.
    b. is at low risk of myocardial infarction.
    c. has usually had a CVA.
    d. requires monitoring every 15 minutes until stable.

11. The AV junction is:
    a. in the upper left atrium.
    b. in the general area of the AV node.
    c. the regular pacemaker for the heart.
    d. near the bottom of the bundle of His.

12. The pulse deficit is:
    a. normally at least 30 in most people.
    b. a symptom of a heart attack.
    c. the difference between the apical and radial pulses.
    d. an early warning of prehypertension.

13. A Doppler instrument:
    a. amplifies sounds within the body.
    b. automatically takes blood pressure.
    c. is needed during the arteriogram.
    d. should be used routinely for all patients.

14. Prehypertension is a blood pressure value between:
    a. 116/70 and 136/80 mm Hg.
    b. 120/80 mm Hg and 139/89 mm Hg.
    c. 140/90 and 160/80 mm Hg.
    d. 150/90 and 200/100 mm Hg.

15. Electronic blood pressure monitoring is contraindicated in all of the following *except*:
    a. patients with extreme hypertension or hypotension.
    b. patients with very rapid or very slow heart rates.
    c. patients with irregular heart rhythms or atrial dysrhythmias.
    d. patients who weigh less than 100 pounds or under the age of 12.

16. An angiogram or arteriogram is:
    a. a procedure to open blocked arteries.
    b. an X-ray study of the blood vessels.
    c. a study of the conduction system.
    d. contraindicated in patients with pulse deficit.

17. After the arteriogram, you should do all of the following *except*:
    a. force fluids.
    b. keep the operative leg extended.
    c. ambulate the patient early.
    d. make sure the patient voids.

EXPLORING THE WEB

2003 Blood Pressure Guidelines (NIH)	http://www.nhlbi.nih.gov
Alaris Clinical Resources	http://www.alarismed.com
American Heart Association	http://www.americanheart.org
Arteriogram	http://adam.about.com
Cardiovascular Technologists and Technicians	http://www.bls.gov
ECG Learning Center	http://medstat.med.utah.edu
ECG Library	http://www.ecglibrary.com
Examination of Cardiovascular System	http://www.fortunecity.com
Lower Extremity Arterial Reconstruction	http://www.perspectivesinnursing.org
Measure and Monitor a Casualty's Pulse	http://www.medtrng.com
Measuring BP with a Doppler Device	http://www.findarticles.com
Measuring Thigh B/P	http://www.findarticles.com
Medical Patient Simulators and Interactive Tutorials	http://medi-smart.com
Nurse Bob's MICU Survival Guide	http://rnbob.tripod.com
Stroke, CVA, and TIA	http://www.nursingceu.com
Understanding the Heart's Electrical Message	http://www.emergencyekg.com
Yale Heart Book	http://www.med.yale.edu

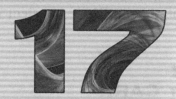

CHAPTER 17

Emergency Procedures

OBJECTIVES:

After reading this chapter, you should be able to:

- Spell and define key terms.
- Define resuscitation.
- List the ABCs of emergency care.
- List signs and symptoms of airway obstruction and describe how to treat this condition.
- Differentiate respiratory failure from respiratory arrest.
- Differentiate the pocket mask from the bag-valve mask and demonstrate how each is used.
- State when CPR is used.
- Explain the purpose of the crash cart.
- Describe postresuscitation care.

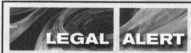

LEGAL ALERT

In some states and facilities, PCTs are not permitted to perform the procedures in this chapter. Your instructor will explain your responsibilities in your state and facility. Perform these procedures only if you are permitted to do so by state law and facility policies. Doing only tasks that you have been instructed to do, and doing things in the way that you were taught, protects patients from injury. It also protects you from injury, legal exposure, and liability.

RESUSCITATION

Emergencies involving the circulatory and respiratory systems are always life-threatening. Emergency procedures are those that are performed to save a patient's life. Without intervention, the patient will die or have lasting injury. If breathing stops, the patient must be treated quickly. After four to six minutes without oxygen, the patient's brain begins to die. **Resuscitation** means saving. Resuscitation is necessary in emergencies in which the breathing stops or the heart stops beating.

When the patient stops breathing, the brain is without oxygen, and the risk of brain damage increases with the passage of time. Although resusci-

tation procedures may be successful, the patient may still suffer brain damage. Resuscitation is most successful if performed immediately. If the patient is without oxygen for a prolonged period, recovery will not be possible.

Hypothermia, or low body temperature due to prolonged cold exposure, preserves the vital organs. Patients with this condition may be able to be resuscitated after a longer period without oxygen and still have a complete recovery. Patients in several well-publicized cases of cold exposure were successfully resuscitated from one to two hours after the event occurred.

Advance Directives

Each patient in a health care facility has the right to execute an **advance directive.** An *advance directive* is a document that designates the patient's wishes if he cannot speak for himself. Advance directives can be in the form of a **living will,** which specifies the patient's wishes if she is in a terminal condition. The patient also has the right to designate a surrogate decision maker, called a **health care proxy.** The document that the patient signs to appoint the health care proxy is called a **durable power of attorney for health care.** This document allows the health care proxy to make decisions on behalf of the patient. State laws vary on how advance directives are implemented, but patients in all states have the right to execute these documents. The health care facility informs the patient of this right upon admission. The facility is obligated to follow the patient's written directions found in these documents.

The person designated as the proxy in the durable power of attorney for health care should be familiar with the patient's wishes. The authority for making decisions takes effect only if the patient becomes physically or mentally unable to speak for himself or herself. If the patient subsequently regains the ability to make decisions, he or she resumes the power of attorney. Your facility will have a procedure for securing another person, usually a relative, to make decisions on the patient's behalf if he or she has not designated a proxy or executed a durable power of attorney for health care. The durable power of attorney for health care covers only health care decisions, and only for the period of time in which the patient is unable to make decisions personally. It does not cover management of finances or other areas of the patient's life.

Health care workers sometimes become confused about the meaning of a living will if the patient specifies that no heroic procedures are to be undertaken if the patient is in a terminal irreversible condition. If the patient is not known to be in a terminal condition, resuscitation will be done (unless otherwise ordered). For example, a 32-year-old patient in good health enters the hospital for a diagnostic procedure that involves the injection of contrast materials into the veins. The patient has an allergic reaction to the contrast material and suffers a cardiac arrest. In this case, *CPR would be done,* because the patient is not known to be in a terminal condition. In contrast, an elderly patient enters the hospital for insertion of a central intravenous catheter to be used for pain management as part of terminal care for cancer. The patient is known to have inoperable cancer, as documented by two or more physicians. The patient experiences a complication during the procedure and has a cardiac arrest. In this case, the provisions of the living will would be honored, and *CPR would not be done.*

Consent

Consent means giving permission for treatment when the person is conscious and alert. All patients have the right to refuse treatment for any reason. They also have the right to have the consequences of the refusal explained to them. Spouses or legal guardians have the right to give consent or refuse treatment for patients who are mentally confused, unless another person has been designated as the health care proxy. Inform the RN if a patient or guardian refuses care.

THE ABCs OF EMERGENCY CARE

ABC is a mnemonic used to remember action to take in an emergency. ABC stands for:

- A = Airway
- B = Breathing
- C = Circulation

In any emergency, the ABCs are always your primary concern. Sometimes bleeding, open fractures, and other conditions distract you from the ABCs. Always evaluate the ABCs before caring for other problems.

The procedures in this chapter provide an overview of information learned in a **cardiopulmonary resuscitation (CPR) class. CPR stands for:**

- C = cardio, or heart
- P = pulmonary, or lungs
- R = resuscitation, or saving

During CPR, the heart is squeezed between the sternum and the spine. This provides only about one-quarter to one-third of the normal blood flow, but it is sufficient to sustain life in many patients. CPR classes may be offered through your employer. Many health care facilities have certified instructors. The American Heart Association (AHA) and American Red Cross (ARC) offer classes providing certification in these procedures. If you will be responsible for performing any of the procedures in this chapter, take a CPR class sponsored by the AHA or ARC. Special courses are available for health care professionals. The class involves hands-on practice in which you will learn to perform emergency procedures using manikins.

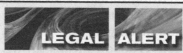

LEGAL ALERT

Your facility may have designations for different levels of emergency care, ranging from comfort care to full advanced life support. Become familiar with the criteria for these levels. Many facilities have ethics committees made up of professionals from many disciplines. The committee meets to review difficult care situations.

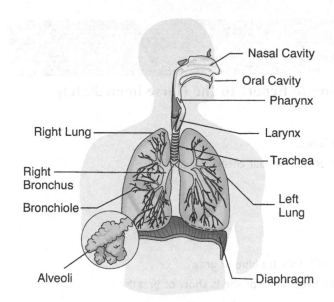

FIGURE 17-1 The respiratory system. A foreign body in the lower airway may cause an obstruction.

Table 17-1 Normal Respiratory Rates

Age	Normal Respiratory Rate per Minute
Infant	30–60
Toddler	24–40
Preschool child	22–34
School-aged child	18–30
Teenager	12–26
Adult	12–20

Table 17-2 Monitoring for Breathing Adequacy

The patient is talking, respirations are between 12 and 20, and there is no apparent distress.

The rhythm is regular.

The patient's color is normal, with no cyanosis or gray coloration.

Look at the patient's chest. It should expand equally with each inspiration.

Listen for breath sounds by placing your ear next to the patient's nose and mouth, if necessary. The sounds should be quiet, without gurgling, wheezing, gasping, or other abnormal sounds.

Feel for breath movement on your cheek and ear.

PROTECTING THE AIRWAY

The **airway** (Figure 17-1) is the structure through which air enters and leaves the body. This passageway must be open to take oxygen into the body. The lower airway extends from the back of the throat into the lungs. The patient may be unable to breathe if there is an obstruction or blockage in the lower airway.

The most common cause of airway obstruction is the tongue falling into the back of the throat. This commonly occurs during unconsciousness. Using an oral or nasal airway (Chapter 14) keeps the tongue from blocking the back of the throat, and allows air to pass. Food and other foreign objects may also block the lower airway.

MAINTAINING THE PATIENT'S BREATHING

The normal respiratory rate is determined by age. Normal respiratory rates for various age groups are listed in **Table 17-1**.

Respiratory failure occurs when breathing is insufficient to sustain life. **Respiratory arrest** occurs when breathing stops. It is caused by many conditions, including heart attack, brain attack (stroke or CVA), overdose, drowning, electrocution, poisoning, and traumatic injuries. Follow the criteria in **Table 17-2** to determine if the patient's breathing is adequate. Abnormal respirations are often a warning of an impending crisis. Stay with the patient and use the call signal to request assistance if the patient is in distress. Report abnormalities to the RN immediately.

Signs and symptoms of abnormalities to report are listed in the Observe & Report box.

Opening the Airway

If you discover a patient who is in respiratory failure, or respiratory arrest, remain in the room and signal for help. You must open the patient's airway if he or she cannot do this independently. Opening

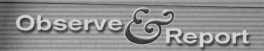

Observe & Report

Signs and Symptoms of Inadequate Breathing to Report to the Nurse Immediately

- Movement in the chest is absent, minimal, or irregular.
- Breathing movement appears to be in the abdomen, not the lungs.
- Air movement cannot be detected by listening and feeling for breath on your cheek and ear.
- Respiratory rate is too slow or rapid.
- Respirations are irregular, gasping, very deep, or shallow.
- Respirations appear labored.
- Patient is short of breath.
- Patient's skin, lips, tongue, earlobes, mucous membranes, or nail beds are blue or gray.
- Patient is unable to speak at all, or cannot speak in sentences because he or she is short of breath.
- Respirations are noisy.
- Nasal flaring is present during inspiration.
- The muscles below the ribs and/or above the clavicles retract inward during respiration.

the airway lifts the tongue from the back of the throat, making breathing easier. This procedure, as well as some other emergency procedures in this chapter, is most effective when the patient is lying in the supine position. Always remove the pillow. Position the patient correctly before beginning.

Because of the nature of the situation, you may not have time to wash your hands or perform other beginning procedure actions. Immediately after the patient is safe, wash your hands thoroughly. Avoid contact with the patient's secretions if you are not wearing gloves or other personal protective equipment.

The **head-tilt, chin-lift maneuver** is the most common method of opening the airway. If the patient has a neck injury, use the jaw-thrust maneuver first. If you cannot successfully open the airway with this procedure, use the head-tilt, chin-lift method.

The **jaw-thrust maneuver** is used to open the airway of patients with known or suspected neck in-

> **SAFETY ALERT**
>
> Do not be distracted by copious bleeding in an unconscious patient. Always check the adequacy of the patient's airway first. If airway, breathing, and circulation are adequate, quickly apply gloves and take measures to stop the bleeding.

juries, and for those whose airway cannot be opened using the head-tilt, chin-lift method. In some facilities, this procedure is used for patients with head and facial injuries. This is because patients with injuries of the head and face often have neck injuries. The purpose of the procedure is to open the airway without moving the head or neck.

After the airway has been opened, it may be necessary to insert an oral airway, or to suction. Follow your facility policy and the RN's directions.

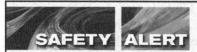

Procedure 137

Head-Tilt, Chin-Lift Maneuver

1. Place one hand on the patient's forehead. Place the fingers of the opposite hand below the center of the jawbone, directly under the chin.

2. Tilt the head back gently.

3. With your fingertips, lift the lower jaw forward (Figure 17-2). The lower teeth

(continues)

Procedure **137**, *continued*

Head-Tilt, Chin-Lift Maneuver

should almost touch the upper teeth. Avoid pressing on the neck, which may worsen the airway obstruction.

4. Keep the patient's mouth open. If necessary, pull the patient's lower lip forward. Avoid inserting your fingers into the mouth.

5. If the patient cannot maintain this position, support the airway manually by holding your hands in place, if necessary.

6. As soon as the patient is safe, and the RN or other professionals have assumed responsibility for care, wash your hands well.

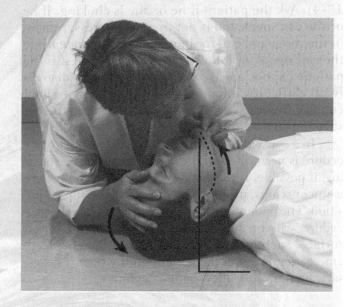

FIGURE 17-2 Use the head-tilt, chin-lift technique to open the airway.

Procedure **138**

Jaw-Thrust Maneuver

1. Move the patient into the supine position as a single unit. Avoid twisting the neck, back, or spine during movement.

2. Pull the head of the bed away from the wall.

3. Position yourself above the patient's head.

4. Position your elbows on the mattress.

5. Using your forearms, stabilize the sides of the head to prevent movement.

6. Place one hand on each side of the lower jaw, just below the ears (**Figure 17-3**).

7. Use the tips of your fingers to push the lower jaw forward.

8. Keep the patient's mouth open. If necessary, pull the patient's lower lip forward. Avoid inserting your fingers into the mouth.

9. If the patient cannot maintain this position, support the airway manually by holding your hands in place, if necessary.

10. As soon as the patient is safe, and the RN or other professionals have assumed responsibility for care, wash your hands well.

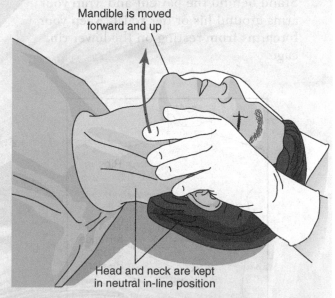

Mandible is moved forward and up

Head and neck are kept in neutral in-line position

FIGURE 17-3 Position your fingers at the angle of the jaw, pushing it forward and upward.

Choking

A patient who is choking will be unable to speak, cough, or breathe. One or both hands at the throat is the universal distress sign for choking (**Figure 17-4**). Ask the patient if he or she is choking. If he or she can speak and is not in great distress, remain in the room and call for immediate assistance using the call signal, or follow your facility policies. If the patient cannot speak, or is in respiratory distress (with difficulty inhaling air, cyanosis, or a silent cough), you must act quickly by performing the obstructed airway procedure.

In a conscious patient, the obstructed airway procedure is performed with the patient sitting or standing, if possible. If this is not possible, or if the patient is unconscious, position the patient in the supine position. The patient must be on a firm surface. The procedure will be ineffective if performed on a soft surface, such as a mattress. This is a life-and-death emergency. Position the patient on the floor if necessary. Remove the pillow before beginning.

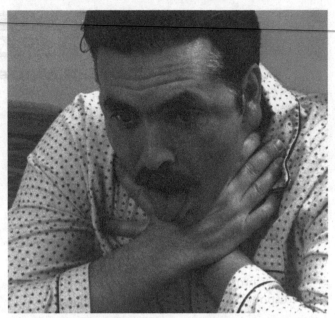

FIGURE 17-4 One or both hands at the throat is the universal distress signal for choking.

Procedure 139

Obstructed Airway Procedure, Conscious Patient

1. Tell the patient you will help.
2. Stand behind the patient and wrap your arms around his or her waist. Keep your forearms from resting on the lower rib cage.

3. Position your hands at the patient's midline, just above the navel and well below the xiphoid process (**Figure 17-5**).
4. Make a fist with one hand. Position the thumb next to the abdomen (**Figure 17-6A**).
5. Grasp your fist with the other hand.
6. Press your fist into the abdomen, using quick, upward thrusts. Deliver each thrust with the intent of freeing the obstruction (**Figure 17-6B**).
7. Repeat the abdominal thrusts until the foreign body is expelled or the patient loses consciousness. Each new thrust is a

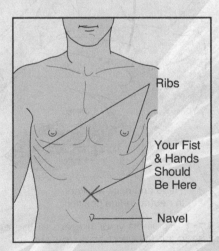

FIGURE 17-5 Position the hands slightly above the navel. Thrust forcefully with the thumb side of the fist against the midline.

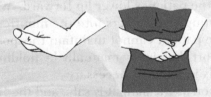

FIGURE 17-6(A) Clench your fist, keeping the thumb straight.

(continues)

Procedure **139**, *continued*

Obstructed Airway Procedure, Conscious Patient

separate, distinct movement. Avoid pressing on the ribs.

8. Continue the procedure until the RN provides further directions or the patient loses consciousness. If the patient loses consciousness, activate the EMS system and begin CPR. Each time you open the airway to give rescue breaths, look for an obstruction in the mouth. If you see something, remove it.

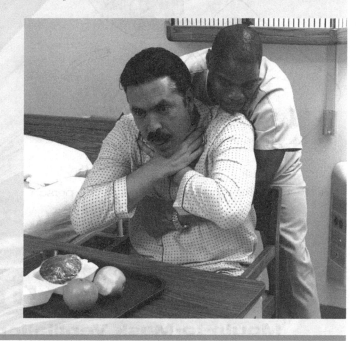

FIGURE 17-6(B) Grasp your clenched fist with the opposite hand. Avoid pressing against the ribs with your forearms.

Mouth-to-Mask Resuscitation

When a patient stops breathing, his or her respirations must be sustained by artificial means to prevent brain damage and other complications. If you have taken a CPR class previously, you may have learned mouth-to-mouth **ventilation.** This is a technique of breathing for the patient. Most health care facilities discourage staff from using this method on patients because of the risk of disease transmission. Various **adjunctive devices** are used instead. An *airway adjunct* is a secondary device used to maintain respirations. Before using an airway adjunct to ventilate the patient, insert an oral airway, if available.

Mouth-to-mask ventilation is performed using a **pocket mask.** The mask has a special valve that prevents the patient's exhaled air and secretions from entering the caregiver's mouth. This infection control feature protects the user. Some pocket masks have an oxygen inlet. This is connected to oxygen extension tubing. The oxygen source is turned up to 15 liters per minute, or as high as possible. The extra oxygen is best for the patient, but both masks are effective. Room air contains approximately 21 percent oxygen. You do not use all the oxygen when you breathe. You exhale extra oxygen, so there is more than enough for the patient to use. He or she must be positioned in the supine position with the airway open for effective ventilation. The mask can be turned upside down for infant resuscitation.

Most pocket masks are clear plastic. This is so you can see the position of the patient's mouth. Monitoring the color of the patient's lips will help you see how well the patient is being oxygenated. Sometimes the patient will vomit during artificial ventilation. You will see this in the mask. If vomiting occurs, quickly turn the patient on his or her side, then clear the mouth and continue ventilation. If suction is available, quickly suction before proceeding with ventilation.

Bag-Valve-Mask Resuscitation

The **bag-valve mask (BVM)** (Figure 17-7) is commonly used in health care facilities to support patients who are in respiratory arrest. Some units are disposable; others are cleaned and sterilized after each use. Bag-valve-mask devices come in various sizes to fit infants, children, and adults. Select the mask that fits the patient's face the best. In addition to being used to support patients who are not breathing, this device may also be used to assist patients whose ventilations are not adequate. An oral airway is inserted before the bag-valve-mask device is used. The respiratory care professional usually performs

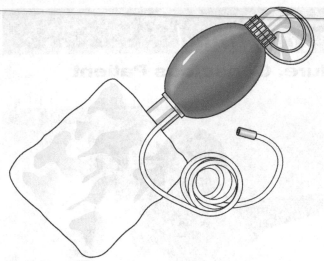

FIGURE 17-7 The bag-valve mask is a two-person device.

this procedure. If the mask is applied directly to the patient's face, he or she is given 1 breath every 5 to 6 seconds or 10 to 12 breaths a minute for adults. If the patient has an endotracheal tube or other advanced airway, he or she is given 1 breath every 6 to 8 seconds, or 8 to 10 breaths per minute.

The bag-valve mask has a bag that refills itself. An oxygen inlet at the end is connected to the oxygen source with connecting tubing. The oxygen flow is set at 15 liters. The bag is connected to a mask that fits the patient's face. A clear mask is also used for the BVM system. As the ventilator squeezes the bag, a valve inside closes the air inlet, forcing oxygen into the patient's lungs. When the bag is released, the patient exhales passively. The BVM device may also be connected to an **endotracheal tube,** a large tube that is inserted into the lungs to maintain breathing. The RCP usually cares for the airway when an endotracheal tube is present.

Procedure **140**

Mouth-to-Mask Ventilation

Supplies needed:
- Disposable exam gloves
- Pocket mask with antireflux (one-way) valve
- Oxygen connecting tubing (if available)
- Oxygen source (if available)

1. Pull the head of the bed away from the wall.
2. Connect the mask to the oxygen connecting tubing and oxygen source. Turn the oxygen on to 15 liters, or the maximum the flow meter will allow. If oxygen is not available immediately, proceed to the next step. Do not delay ventilation.
3. Apply gloves.
4. Open the patient's airway using the head-tilt, chin-lift method.
5. Position yourself at the patient's head.
6. Position the mask on the patient's face, with the small end over the bridge of the nose and the wide end on the patient's chin. The ventilation port should be centered over the patient's mouth.
7. Seal the mask to the patient's face by positioning your thumbs on the top of the mask and your fingers at the sides. Hold the airway in the open position.

8. Take a normal breath, then seal your mouth over the ventilation port, exhaling into the mask (**Figure 17-8**). The ventilation should take 1 second. During the ventilation, look at the patient's chest. It should rise as you blow air in.

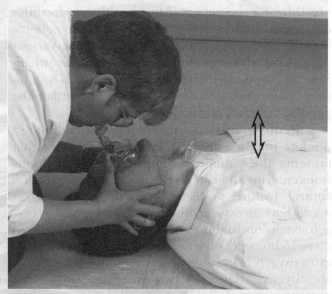

FIGURE 17-8 Give two full ventilations, allowing for exhalation between each. Make sure the chest rises and falls with each ventilation.

(continues)

Procedure **140**, *continued*

Mouth-to-Mask Ventilation

9. Remove your mouth from the mask and allow the patient to exhale passively. Continue to breathe into the mask once every 5 to 6 seconds for adults and 1 breath every 6 to 8 seconds for infants and children. Remember to take a normal breath, not a deep breath, before administering ventilation. Your objective is to avoid overinflating the patient's lungs.

Using the bag-valve mask requires training and practice. Mastering this task is a challenge for many health care workers. The AHA recommends that two rescuers use this device. A single rescuer may have difficulty sealing the mask on the patient's face. This often takes two hands. Having a second person available to squeeze the bag is best. As with the other procedures, the patient's airway must be open, and he or she must be in the supine position.

Procedure **141**

Bag-Valve-Mask Ventilation, Two Rescuers

Supplies needed:
▶ Disposable exam gloves
▶ Bag-valve-mask device, correct size to fit the patient
▶ Oxygen connecting tubing (if available)
▶ Oxygen source (if available)

1. Assemble the bag-valve-mask system. Attach the oxygen connecting tubing and connect it to the oxygen source. Turn the oxygen on to 15 liters, or the maximum the flow meter will allow. If oxygen is not available immediately, proceed to the next step. Do not delay ventilation.
2. Apply gloves.
3. Open the patient's airway using the head-tilt, chin-lift method.
4. Position yourself next to the patient's head.
5. Position the mask on the patient's face, with the small end over the bridge of the nose and the wide end on the patient's chin. The ventilation port should be centered over the patient's mouth.
6. Seal the mask to the patient's face by positioning your thumbs on the top of the mask and your fingers at the sides. Hold the airway in the open position.
7. While one rescuer maintains the face seal, the other squeezes the bag. During the ventilation, look at the patient's chest. It should rise as you squeeze the bag.
8. Release the bag, but keep the mask in contact with the face. This allows the patient to exhale passively. Continue to ventilate once every 5 to 6 seconds, or 1 breath every 6 to 8 seconds if the patient has an endotracheal tube or other advanced airway.

CARDIOPULMONARY RESUSCITATION

Cardiac arrest is a condition in which the heart stops beating. You have learned that cardiopulmonary resuscitation is used as a lifesaving meas-ure in the care of a patient whose heart has stopped beating. For CPR to be effective, the patient's upper torso must be on a firm surface. Health care facilities have emergency backboards for this purpose. If a backboard is not available, do not delay to get it. Any firm object, such as a meal tray, can be used. If the patient has fallen to the floor, perform CPR there. CPR is approximately one-quarter to one-third as effective as the human heart, but this is adequate to circulate oxygen to the body. For maximum effectiveness, CPR should be started immediately after the heart stops. However, if the time of the cardiac arrest is unknown, give the patient the benefit of the doubt and begin CPR.

CPR is practiced on a manikin during an AHA or ARC basic life support program. The information here is presented for your information and understanding. Do not attempt to perform this procedure until you are properly trained.

When a cardiac arrest occurs, health care facilities call a "code." This is paged over the intercom, or the operator sets off the pagers of an emergency

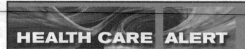

HEALTH CARE ALERT

Always take complaints of chest pain seriously. If a patient complains of chest pain, assist him or her to stop all activity and assume a comfortable position. Notify the RN promptly.

response team. Each agency has a different keyword to page that denotes a code situation. After the code has been called, many individuals will respond to the patient's room, bringing emergency supplies, equipment, and medications to save the patient's life. Learn the procedure and keywords for codes in your health care facility. Learn how to call a code.

Procedure 142

One-Rescuer CPR, Adult

Supplies needed:
- Disposable exam gloves
- Adjunctive ventilation device

1. Gently shake the patient and ask, "Are you OK?"
2. Call for help by following your facility policy for calling a code or getting emergency assistance.
3. Open the patient's airway using the head-tilt, chin-lift procedure.
4. Stand next to the patient's head. Place your ear next to the patient's nose and mouth. Simultaneously look at the patient's chest to see if it is rising and falling. Feel and listen for breathing on your cheek and ear.
5. If the patient is not breathing, give two breaths through a pocket mask or other adjunctive device.
6. Locate the carotid pulse (**Figure 17-9**), and palpate it lightly for 5 to 10 seconds.
7. If the pulse is absent, position the heel of one hand on the center of the chest. Use an imaginary line between the nipples as your landmark. Proper hand placement is very important to prevent injury.
8. Place the heel of your other hand on top of the first hand and interlace your fingers (**Figure 17-10**).

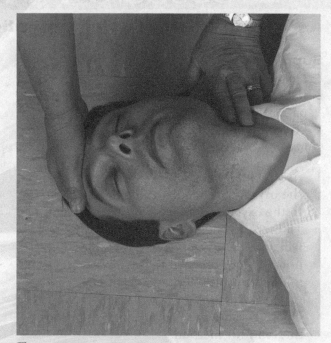

FIGURE 17-9 The carotid pulse is easy to locate, and provides a good indication of heart action.

9. Compress the sternum straight down 1½ to 2 inches at a rate of 100 compressions a minute (**Figure 17-11**). Downward pressure should be on the sternum only. Avoid pressing on the ribs with your fingers. Keep

(continues)

Procedure **142**, *continued*

One-Rescuer CPR, Adult

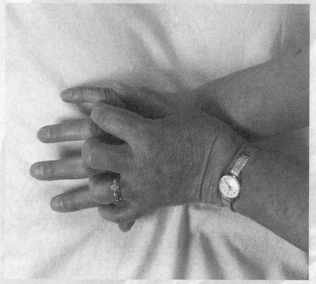

FIGURE 17-10 Interlace your fingers and elevate them slightly during chest compressions to avoid pressure on the rib cage.

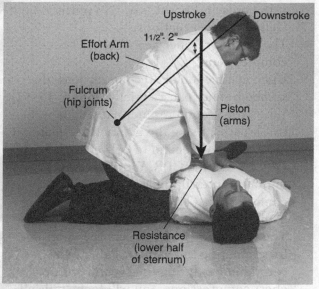

FIGURE 17-11 Position your shoulders directly over the sternum. Keep your back straight and your elbows locked.

your fingers interlaced and slightly elevated from the chest. Compressions should be smooth and rhythmic. Completely release pressure, but maintain hand contact with the chest between each compression. The release in pressure allows the heart to refill with blood.

10. At the end of each 30 compressions, deliver 2 full breaths through the pocket mask or other adjunctive device.
11. Repeat this cycle until help arrives or you are exhausted and unable to continue.
    If a second rescuer joins you while CPR is in progress, see Procedure 143.

Procedure **143**

Two-Rescuer CPR, Adult

Supplies needed:
▶ Disposable exam gloves
▶ Adjunctive ventilation device

1. If the code team or other help has not yet arrived when the second rescuer appears, instruct him or her to repeat the call for help.
2. Upon the second rescuer's return, complete a cycle of 30 compressions and 2 ventilations.

3. Stop CPR and move to the head.
4. Locate the carotid pulse and assess for spontaneous pulse return.
5. During the pulse check, the second rescuer prepares to perform chest compressions. He or she positions himself or herself opposite the first rescuer and locates the landmark. He or she places hands on the chest in preparation for beginning chest compressions.

(continues)

Procedure **143**, *continued*

Two-Rescuer CPR, Adult

6. If the pulse is absent, say, "No pulse."
7. Deliver two ventilations.
8. The second rescuer begins chest compressions.
9. Upon completion of 30 compressions, the second rescuer pauses briefly (**Figure 17-12**).
10. When the second rescuer pauses, deliver two breaths, using the adjunctive device. Take only one second to deliver each breath. Quickly resume CPR. Your goal is to minimize interruptions to chest compressions.(That is, you want to stop compressions for the least possible time.)
11. The ventilator (first rescuer) is responsible for evaluating the patient. Palpate the carotid pulse during the second rescuer's chest compressions. You will feel a pulse if the compressions are effective.
12. CPR is physically demanding. If the compressor is fatigued, his or her compressions may not be as deep or effective. To prevent this, alternate positions every 2 minutes, or after about 5 cycles of 30 compressions and 2 ventilations.
13. Count out loud, substituting the word "switch" or "change" for "one," then continuing with "two, and three, and four, and five," and so forth.

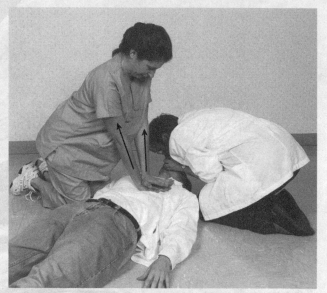

FIGURE 17-12 After 30 compressions, the compressor pauses briefly, while the ventilator gives 2 full breaths.

14. The first rescuer delivers two ventilations.
15. Both rescuers move simultaneously to change places. The first rescuer moves to the chest and locates proper hand placement. The second rescuer moves to the head.
16. The first rescuer begins chest compressions. Repeat the sequence until the code team arrives.

THE RECOVERY POSITION

If the patient is unresponsive, but is breathing and has a pulse, he or she should be positioned in the recovery position to prevent complications (**Figure 17-13**). The recovery position is a modified lateral position. The patient's position must:

- Be stable
- Avoid pressure on the chest
- Avoid pressure on the lower arm
- Allow the airway to remain open

FIGURE 17-13 If the victim is breathing but not conscious, place him in the recovery position.

Continue to monitor the patient according to facility policy to ensure that the pulse and respirations remain adequate. Take vital signs according to the nurse's instructions.

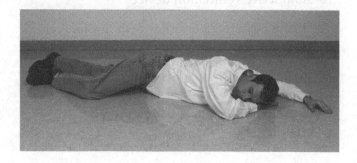

Procedure 144

Positioning the Patient in the Recovery Position

1. Kneel beside the patient and straighten his or her legs.
2. Place the arm nearest you above the patient's head with the palm up and the elbow bent slightly.
3. Position the opposite arm across the chest.
4. Place your lower hand on the patient's thigh on the far side of the body. Pull the thigh up slightly, closer to the center of the patient's body.
5. Place your upper hand on the patient's shoulder on the opposite side of the body.
6. With one hand on the thigh and the other on the shoulder, roll the patient on the side facing you.
7. Move the patient's upper hand close to the cheek, bending the elbow. This hand should be close to the face, but not under the body. Adjust the upper body so that the hip and knee are at right angles.
8. Tilt the patient's head back slightly to keep the airway open. Now place the upper hand, palm facing down, under the cheek to maintain the head position.
9. Continue to monitor the patient closely for adequate breathing.

INTRODUCTION TO THE CRASH CART

The **crash cart** (Figure 17-14) is an emergency supply cart. It typically contains a firm backboard for performing chest compressions, a cardiac monitor with defibrillator, equipment and supplies for ventilation, instruments used in emergency procedures, an assortment of needles and syringes, and emergency drugs. Some facilities keep intravenous solutions and other supplies on the crash cart as well. **Intubation equipment** is also stored in the cart. This equipment is used to insert an endotracheal tube into the lungs.

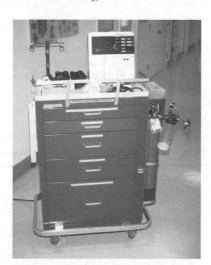

FIGURE 17-14 An emergency resuscitation cart (crash cart).

In many facilities, the crash cart is checked each shift. A checklist is used, and each item in the cart is checked. Checking the crash cart is an important responsibility. The checklist will list each supply in the cart and state how many of each item should be present. The person checking the cart will also check to ensure that the packaging is intact on sterile supplies. He or she may also check the expiration dates for sterile supplies and medications. The cart must be fully stocked and ready to use at all times. It is resupplied immediately after a code. Do not be tempted to remove items from the cart in a nonemergency situation. In addition to ensuring that the cart is fully stocked, checking each shift helps personnel become familiar with the location of items in the cart so they can be reached quickly in an emergency.

DEFIBRILLATION

Defibrillation is a method of treatment that uses an electric shock to reverse disorganized activity in the heart during cardiac arrest. Early defibrillation has proven to be critical to survival in cardiac arrest. Defibrillators are placed in various locations in the community and are used by rescuers who have been taught to use the devices in case of cardiac arrest. Public access to defibrillation has been highly successful. Some studies have shown that the chance of survival doubles when early access to defibrillation is available. The speed with which defibrillation is done is the key to success. Early defibrillation (within 5 minutes) is a high-priority goal in the community. In health care facilities, the goal is to defibrillate within 3 minutes.

Automatic External Defibrillators

Automatic external defibrillators (AEDs) (Figure 17-15) are computerized devices that are simple to learn and operate. The AED is used *only* when a patient is unresponsive, not breathing, and pulseless. When the device is attached to the victim's chest, the unit determines if an electrical shock is necessary to reestablish or regulate the heartbeat. Several different models are available, and the operating instructions are slightly different for each. The four basic steps to using an AED are:

- Turn the power on
- Apply the electrode pads to the patient's chest
- All rescuers stand back to allow the machine to analyze the heart rhythm
- All rescuers continue to stand back; the operator of the unit presses the shock button and/or follows the unit's instructions, which are usually audible through a voice-synthesized message.

Hospitals normally use manual, portable defibrillators for caring for patients who have experienced a cardiac arrest. These defibrillators are operated by qualified licensed personnel. The AED is not routinely used in the hospital. However, some large campuses have AEDs available in strategic locations, such as the cafeteria. Some facilities have defibrillators that can be used as AEDs, or switched to regular defibrillator mode. If your facility purchases an AED (or dual-purpose defibrillator), employees will be taught to use it. Although the AED is simple to operate, only those who are properly trained may use the device. CPR and use of the AED are included in basic life support classes for health care professionals.

Some safety concerns with use of the defibrillator are:

- Remove medication patches and wipe the chest well to remove medication residue. Some topical medications increase the risk of burns or fire.
- Excessive coarse chest hair will interfere with patch use. In an emergency, the fastest way to remove hair is to apply a patch, then pull it off. This will remove hair with it. Use a new patch for analyzing the heart rate and defibrillating.

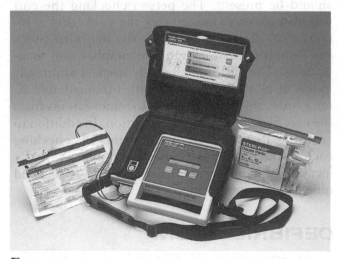

FIGURE 17-15 An automatic external defibrillator will analyze the electrical activity of the heart and deliver a series of shocks to restore organized electrical activity and a normal heart rhythm.

SAFETY ALERT

Before AED use: Do not use the AED on a newborn (from birth to 1 year of age) patient who is in cardiac arrest. Newborns should receive CPR only. Small children, ages 1 to 8, may be defibrillated by using pediatric patches. Children over 8 years of age and 55 pounds should be defibrillated with adult patches. Make sure that the patient and all rescuers are dry, and that no one is in standing water. Follow all manufacturers' recommendations on safety and where the unit can and cannot be used. (Read the owner's manual and facility policy and procedure manual.) If the patient is on or near steel or metal grating, move him or her, if possible. If not, clear all unnecessary personnel from the steel. Do not kneel on steel grating. Essential rescuers should stand with their feet flat on the grating, with legs close together and not touching, before delivering treatment. Remove the patient's shirt, if possible, and place the shirt between the steel and the patient.

Procedure **145**

Managing Cardiac Arrest Using an AED

Supplies needed:
- Disposable exam gloves
- Automatic external defibrillator
- Oropharyngeal airway
- Pocket mask or bag-valve mask
- Nonrebreather mask
- Oxygen tank setup

1. Perform your beginning procedure actions, as appropriate in an emergency. If you witness the person's collapse, and an AED is immediately available, deliver a shock before beginning CPR. If the arrest is unwitnessed, no AED is available, or you arrive on a scene where another rescuer is doing CPR:
2. Briefly question the person doing CPR about the arrest event.
   - How long has the victim been in cardiac arrest?
   - How long has CPR been in progress?
   - Do you know two-rescuer CPR?
3. Determine whether the patient is a candidate for an AED:
   - Unresponsive
   - No respirations
   - Pulseless

NOTE: If the patient has sustained trauma before collapse, do not attach the AED. Continue CPR and transport immediately.

4. Turn the automatic external defibrillator on.
5. Attach the monitoring-defibrillation pads to the cables if the pads are not attached.
6. Attach the AED to the patient.
   - Place the top right pad below the right midclavicular area.
   - Place the lower pad over the lower left ribs.
7. Instruct the rescuer to stop CPR.
8. Ensure that all individuals are standing clear of the patient.
9. Give the order, "ALL CLEAR."
10. Visually check to ensure that no one is in contact with the patient or any electrically conductive material touching the patient.
11. Initiate rhythm analysis by pressing the analysis button.

12. Wait for the machine to analyze the rhythm.
13. Press the button to deliver shock if instructed.

   CAUTION: *Never deliver a shock if anyone is touching the patient or the patient is wet (dry the patient), touching metal (move away from metal), or wearing a nitroglycerin patch. If a patch is present, remove it with a gloved hand.*

14. If no shock is indicated:
    - Check the pulse.
    - If none, perform CPR for 1 minute.
    - Press the "analyze" button.
    - If no shock is indicated, repeat steps 11 and 12.
15. If no shock is still indicated, check the pulse. If no pulse, resume CPR and initiate transport.
16. Repeat steps 11 through 13 until three shocks have been delivered.
17. Check for pulse.
18. If no pulse, direct the assistant and rescuer to resume CPR.
19. Check the pulse during CPR to confirm the effectiveness of CPR.
20. Insert an airway adjunct (Procedures 117 and 118).
21. Ventilate the patient.
22. After one minute of CPR, repeat steps 11 through 13.
23. Check for pulse. If the patient has a pulse:
    - Check for respirations.
    - If breathing is adequate, provide oxygen at high liter flow through a nonrebreather mask.
    - If breathing is inadequate or absent, ventilate the patient using a bag-valve mask.
24. Transport the patient.

NOTE: If a resuscitated patient suffers cardiac arrest during transport, repeat steps 11 through 13 until a total of six shocks have been given or the patient regains a pulse. If the patient is pulseless:

- Continue CPR
- Continue transport

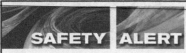

Understanding Manual Defibrillation

PCTs frequently assist with code situations in the health care facility. Follow the RN's instructions. Defibrillation is delivery of an electrical shock. This may be performed during a cardiac arrest. It is also used to treat several other electrical disturbances of the heart.

Two types of electrical rhythms commonly cause cardiac arrest. **Ventricular fibrillation** (Figure 17-16) is a quivering of the heart muscle. In this condition, the monitor shows a great deal of disorganized electrical activity. The quivering action does not circulate blood to the body. This rhythm causes 50 percent to 60 percent of all cardiac arrests. **Asystole** (Figure 17-17) occurs when the heart stops beating; 20 percent to 25 percent of all cardiac arrests are caused by this rhythm. Several other less common rhythm disturbances account for the remaining instances of cardiac arrest.

When a cardiac arrest occurs, the patient's pulse and respirations cease. He or she appears clinically dead. A combination of CPR, drugs, and defibrillation may be used to restore the heart to a normal rhythm. Initially, a licensed health care professional will apply the monitor electrodes to the patient's chest. When the monitor is successfully connected, the RN or other licensed professional instructs others to stop performing CPR. He or she will analyze the rhythm on the monitor, then give the command to resume CPR.

Ventricular fibrillation is a rhythm that responds to defibrillation. Asystole does not respond well to this treatment. If the monitor displays ventricular fibrillation, the licensed person will instruct you to continue CPR until the defibrillator is prepared. The RN or other professional will apply special conductive jelly and defibrillator paddles to the patient's chest. He or she will give the

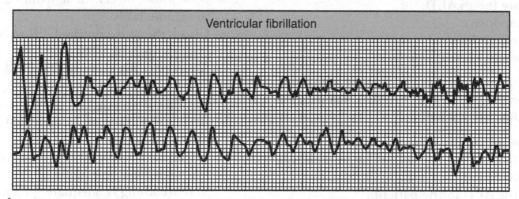

FIGURE 17-16 Ventricular fibrillation is a quivering of the heart. (Copyright Marquette Electronics, Marquette, WI)

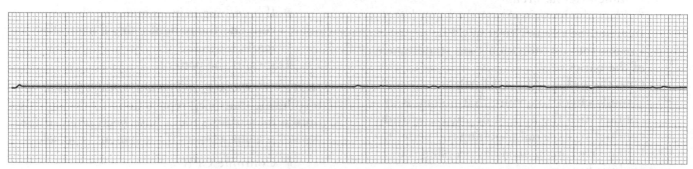

FIGURE 17-17 During asystole, there is no electrical or mechanical activity of the heart. (Copyright Marquette Electronics, Marquette, WI)

command to "Stand back" or "clear" the patient. When this command is given, quickly stop what you are doing. Stand back so that your body and clothing do not touch the patient, the bed, equipment such as intravenous fluids and machinery, or supplies attached to the patient. When the RN gives the command to stand back or stay clear, do so quickly. The electrical impulse used for defibrillation is very strong. The shock is conducted through the patient's body. Those in contact with the patient, bed, or other equipment will also receive a shock. If a healthy heart receives this shock, serious complications can occur. When the RN is certain that all staff are clear, he or she will press the button to defibrillate. The paddles deliver an electrical shock to the patient's chest. Multiple shocks are often necessary. The shocks may convert the disorganized rhythm into a more effective one that will circulate blood to the body. If the shocks are not effective, CPR continues. Medications are administered and the shocks will be repeated.

If the patient is in asystole, CPR will be performed and certain drugs will be given. The objective of the drugs is to irritate the heart muscle into ventricular fibrillation. If this can be accomplished, defibrillation may be used successfully to shock the heart back into a normal rhythm.

A physician directs the code situation. He or she will determine how long resuscitation will continue. Sometimes the patient is resuscitated for a prolonged period. In other situations, resuscitation is brief. This determination must be made by the physician, based on his or her professional judgment and the patient's response to lifesaving measures.

Assisting with a Code

The PCT's responsibilities in a code will be determined by the employer, and are set out in the job description. Your responsibilities may also be outlined in the policy and procedure manual. In general, you must know how to function in a code situation, but your role and responsibility will vary according to facility policy.

Many facilities have "mock code" practices. These are not announced in advance. When personnel respond to the code, a manikin is being used. However, the code is conducted as if it were a real patient. This provides all staff with an opportunity to practice their skills, learn their responsibilities, and become comfortable with and proficient in providing lifesaving care. Always follow the directions of the RN or other licensed health care professional in an emergency situation. You may be asked to perform chest compressions, act as a messenger by transporting blood samples to the laboratory, record the times that CPR was started and stopped, or record the times defibrillation was delivered. A code is a very busy time for everyone. Many tasks must be accomplished in a rapid, orderly manner. Become familiar with your facility policies and your responsibilities so that you are confident in your ability to perform your best in this highly critical situation.

POSTRESUSCITATION CARE

Postresuscitation care is care given to a patient who has been successfully resuscitated. Although the patient's heartbeat has been restored, he or she will continue to be in critical, unstable condition for a period of time. Cardiac arrest may recur. Thus, the patient needs very frequent, careful monitoring. Report your findings to the RN frequently. Report abnormalities immediately.

After a cardiac arrest, the patient is usually transferred to an intensive care unit (ICU), coronary care unit (CCU), or other specialized unit with high staff-to-patient ratios. The location depends on services available in the hospital, as well as availability of bed space. You may monitor the patient before the transfer, or while working in a special care unit after the patient arrives. Once again, your responsibilities are determined by your facility policy and the procedures of the unit on which you are working.

When monitoring and caring for a patient after a code, you will do all or some of these things:

● Check vital signs frequently.

● Monitor the quality of the pulse and respirations.

● Be alert to the breathing and heartbeat at all times; they may stop again at any time.

● Monitor the rhythm on the cardiac monitor.

● Administer oxygen at high liter flows.

● Check capillary refill.

● Monitor the pulse oximeter values.

● Monitor the patient's color.

● Draw blood specimens.

● Insert an indwelling catheter and monitor urinary output carefully.

● Monitor intravenous fluids.

● Monitor level of consciousness.

● Report changes in the patient's condition to the RN immediately.

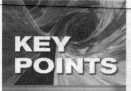

KEY POINTS

▶ Resuscitation is used to treat patients in emergencies in which the breathing stops or the heart stops beating.

▶ Hypothermia and cold temperatures preserve vital organs so that resuscitation may be successful after a prolonged period.

▶ ABC, or A (airway), B (breathing), C (circulation), is a mnemonic used to remember action to take in an emergency.

▶ CPR is a method of squeezing the heart between the sternum and the spine that is used to treat patients who are in cardiac arrest; it is one-quarter to one-third as effective as the normal heartbeat.

▶ CPR certification is available through the American Heart Association and the American Red Cross; the PCT should complete a basic life support class if he or she is performing the procedures in this chapter.

▶ An obstruction in the lower airway may cause the patient to be unable to breathe.

▶ The most common cause of airway obstruction is the tongue falling into the back of the throat.

▶ A patient with a complete airway obstruction cannot speak, cough, or breathe.

▶ The respiratory rate is determined by the patient's age.

▶ Respiratory failure occurs when breathing is insufficient to sustain life.

▶ Respiratory arrest occurs when breathing stops.

▶ The head-tilt, chin-lift maneuver is the most common method of opening the airway.

▶ The jaw-thrust maneuver is used to open the airway if a neck injury is suspected.

▶ Airway adjuncts are secondary devices used to maintain respirations.

▶ Mouth-to-mouth resuscitation is not recommended because of the risk of transmitting infection.

▶ The pocket mask with a one-way valve is used to deliver mouth-to-mask resuscitation; oxygen may be attached to some masks.

▶ The bag-valve mask is a two-person device that is used to ventilate nonbreathing patients.

▶ Cardiac arrest is a condition in which the heart stops beating.

▶ The crash cart is an emergency supply cart that must be checked each shift to ensure that it is fully and correctly stocked.

▶ Intubation is an emergency procedure that is performed to insert an endotracheal tube into the lungs to ventilate the patient.

▶ Defibrillation is performed to reverse certain electrical disturbances in the heart; staff must stand clear of the patient and bed when the shock is delivered.

▶ Patients who have been resuscitated are very unstable after the event.

▶ Postresuscitation care includes checking vital signs frequently, monitoring the quality of the pulse and respirations, being alert to the breathing and heartbeat at all times, monitoring the rhythm on the cardiac monitor, administering oxygen at high liter flows, checking capillary refill, monitoring the patient's color, drawing blood specimens, inserting an indwelling catheter and monitoring urinary output carefully, and monitoring intravenous fluids.

CLINICAL APPLICATIONS

1. Mr. Lieu has fallen on the floor in his room. He apparently hit his head on the nightstand on the way down and is bleeding profusely. You discover this patient on the floor as you pass the doorway. His pulse is 140 and weak, and respirations are shallow, rate of 10. What action will you take first? Second? Third?

2. The RN enters Mr. Lieu's room and hears the patient gurgling. She tells you to quickly open the airway, and picks up the phone to call for additional assistance. Which method will you use?

3. Mr. Lieu gasps, then stops breathing. You hear staff pushing the crash cart toward the room. What action will you take first? Second?

4. Mr. Lieu experienced a respiratory arrest and was successfully resuscitated. The bleeding from the laceration on his head was controlled and the injury was sutured by the emergency physician. During the event, you got a great deal of blood on your uniform that soaked through to your skin. What action will you take?

5. The RN informs you to monitor Mr. Lieu until a bed becomes available in the specialized care unit. What type of monitoring will you perform?

CHAPTER REVIEW

Multiple-Choice Questions

Select the one best answer.

1. Low body temperature caused by prolonged cold exposure is:
   a. hypothermia.
   b. hyperthermia.
   c. thermogenesis.
   d. thermality.

2. You enter a room and find the patient with no pulse or respirations. Your first action is to:
   a. begin chest compressions immediately.
   b. run to get the RN.
   c. call for help.
   d. begin artificial respiration.

3. The normal respiratory rate in an adult is between:
   a. 8 and 20 per minute.
   b. 12 and 20 per minute.
   c. 14 and 24 per minute.
   d. 16 and 30 per minute.

4. Mrs. Gonzales is having difficulty breathing when you enter the room. You should:
   a. check her vital signs.
   b. perform the jaw thrust maneuver.
   c. stay with the patient and call for help.
   d. begin CPR.

5. When connecting an oxygen source to the bag-valve mask, set the liter flow at:
   a. 6 liters per minute.
   b. 8 liters per minute.
   c. 12 liters per minute.
   d. 15 liters per minute.

6. When checking an adult patient to determine if CPR is necessary, check the:
   a. radial pulse.
   b. carotid pulse.
   c. brachial pulse.
   d. femoral pulse.

7. When performing one-person CPR on an adult, compress the sternum at a rate of:
   a. 40 per minute.
   b. 60 per minute.
   c. 100 per minute.
   d. 110 per minute.

8. Defibrillation may be successful in reversing:
   a. ventricular fibrillation.
   b. respiratory arrest.
   c. sinus rhythm.
   b. asystole.

9. When you are delivering an electrical shock with an AED:
   a. instruct another PCT to start an IV.
   b. make sure someone is holding the airway open.
   c. continue chest compressions at a rate of 100 a minute.
   d. tell everyone else to stand back and stay clear.

10. The crash cart is usually checked every:
    a. shift.
    b. day.
    c. week.
    d. month.

EXPLORING THE WEB

American Association of Critical Care Nurses	http://www.aacn.org
American College of Emergency Physicians	http://www.acep.org/webportal
American Heart Association	http://www.americanheart.org
Combined Health Information Database	http://chid.nih.gov
Emergency-nurse	http://www.emergency-nurse.com
Emergency Nurses Organization	http://www.ena.org
Emergency Nursing	http://dmoz.org
Emergency Nursing World	http://ENW.org
EMS Resource	http://www.emsresource.net
EMS Village	http://www.emsvillage.com
Ex-EMT Gets Prison For Fatal Prank	http://www.cbsnews.com/stories
Former Virginia EMT guilty of manslaughter in defibrillator prank death	http://legalsoapbox.freeadvice.com
Futures in Nursing—Emergency Nursing	http://www.futuresinnursing.org
JEMS weigh in on EMT defibrillator prank	http://www.jems.com/products/articles/15693
JEMS Editor-in-Chief A.J. Heightman's analysis of defibrillator prank	http://www.jems.com/products/articles/15693/#A.J.'sTake
MediSmart online emergency tutorials	http://medi-smart.com
MERGINET	http://www.merginet.com/index.cfm
National Association of EMS Educators	http://www.naemse.org
National Center for Emergency Medicine Informatics	http://www.ncemi.org
Neonatal Resuscitation Program	http://www.aap.org
North Carolina College of Emergency Physicians	http://www.nccep.org
Nurse Bob's MICU Survival Guide	http://rnbob.tripod.com
Nurses for a Healthier Tomorrow	http://www.nursesource.org/emergency.html
OHSU Division of Hematology	http://www.ohsu.edu
The Stamford Hospital EMS Institute	http://www.emsinstitute.com
Yale University School of Medicine Heart Book	http://www.med.yale.edu/library/heartbk

Appendix A
Guidelines for Hand Hygiene

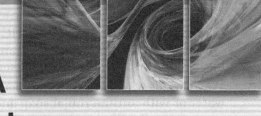

INTRODUCTION

In 2002, the CDC published the results of extensive handwashing studies, as well as new recommendations for cleansing hands. Each recommendation is categorized on the basis of existing scientific data, theoretical rationale, applicability, and economic impact. The CDC system for categorizing recommendations is:

Category IA. Strongly recommended for implementation and strongly supported by well-designed experimental, clinical, or epidemiologic studies

Category IB. Strongly recommended for implementation and supported by certain experimental, clinical, or epidemiologic studies and a strong theoretical rationale

Category IC. Required for implementation, as mandated by federal or state regulation or standard

Category II. Suggested for implementation and supported by suggestive clinical or epidemiologic studies or a theoretical rationale

No recommendation. Unresolved issue. Practices for which insufficient evidence or no consensus regarding efficacy exist

Recommendations

1. Indications for handwashing and hand antisepsis
   - When hands are visibly dirty or contaminated with proteinaceous material or are visibly soiled with blood or other body fluids, wash hands with either a non-antimicrobial soap and water or an antimicrobial soap and water (IA).
   - If hands are not visibly soiled, use an alcohol-based hand rub for routine decontamination of hands in all other clinical situations described in the preceding item (IA).

- Alternatively, wash hands with an antimicrobial soap and water in all clinical situations (IB).
- Decontaminate hands before having direct contact with patients (IB).
- Decontaminate hands before donning sterile gloves when inserting a central intravascular catheter (IB).
- Decontaminate hands before inserting indwelling urinary catheters, peripheral vascular catheters, or other invasive devices that do not require a surgical procedure (IB).
- Decontaminate hands after contact with a patient's intact skin (e.g., when taking a pulse or blood pressure, and lifting a patient) (IB).
- Decontaminate hands after contact with body fluids or excretions, mucous membranes, nonintact skin, and wound dressings if hands are not visibly soiled (IA).
- Decontaminate hands if moving from a contaminated body site to a clean body site during patient care (II).
- Decontaminate hands after contact with inanimate objects (including medical equipment) in the immediate vicinity of the patient (II).
- Decontaminate hands after removing gloves (IB).
- Before eating and after using a restroom, wash hands with a non-antimicrobial soap and water or with an antimicrobial soap and water (IB).
- Antimicrobial-impregnated wipes (i.e., towelettes) may be considered as an alternative to washing hands with non-antimicrobial soap and water. Because they are not as effective as alcohol-based hand rubs or washing hands with an antimicrobial soap and water for reducing bacterial counts on the

hands of health care workers (HCWs) they are not a substitute for using an alcohol-based hand rub or antimicrobial soap (IB).

- Wash hands with non-antimicrobial soap and water or with antimicrobial soap and water if exposure to *Bacillus anthracis* is suspected or proven. The physical action of washing and rinsing hands under such circumstances is recommended because alcohols, chlorhexidine, iodophors, and other antiseptic agents have poor activity against spores (II).

- No recommendation can be made regarding the routine use of non-alcohol-based hand rubs for hand hygiene in health care settings (unresolved issue).

2. Hand-hygiene technique

- When decontaminating hands with an alcohol-based hand rub, apply product to palm of one hand and rub hands together, covering all surfaces of hands and fingers, until hands are dry (IB).

- Follow the manufacturer's recommendations regarding the volume of product to use.

- When washing hands with soap and water, wet hands first with water, apply an amount of product recommended by the manufacturer to hands, and rub hands together vigorously for at least 15 seconds, covering all surfaces of the hands and fingers. Rinse hands with water and dry thoroughly with a disposable towel. Use towel to turn off the faucet (IB).

- Avoid using hot water, because repeated exposure to hot water may increase the risk of dermatitis (IB).

- Liquid, bar, leaflet, or powdered forms of plain soap are acceptable when washing hands with a non-antimicrobial soap and water. When bar soap is used, soap racks that facilitate drainage and small bars of soap should be used (II).

- Multiple-use cloth towels of the hanging or roll type are not recommended for use in health care settings (II).

3. Surgical hand antisepsis

- Remove rings, watches, and bracelets before beginning the surgical hand scrub (II).

- Remove debris from underneath fingernails using a nail cleaner under running water (II).

- Surgical hand antisepsis using either an antimicrobial soap or an alcohol-based hand rub with persistent activity is recommended before donning sterile gloves when performing surgical procedures (IB).

- When performing surgical hand antisepsis using an antimicrobial soap, scrub hands and forearms for the length of time recommended by the manufacturer, usually 2 to 6 minutes. Long scrub times (e.g., 10 minutes) are not necessary (IB).

- When using an alcohol-based surgical hand-scrub product with persistent activity, follow the manufacturer's instructions. Before applying the alcohol solution, prewash hands and forearms with a non-antimicrobial soap and dry hands and forearms completely. After application of the alcohol-based product as recommended, allow hands and forearms to dry thoroughly before donning sterile gloves (IB).

4. Other recommendations

- Do not add soap to a partially empty soap dispenser. This practice of "topping off" dispensers can lead to bacterial contamination of soap (IA).

- Provide workers with hand lotions or creams to minimize the occurrence of irritant contact dermatitis associated with hand antisepsis or handwashing (IA).

- Do not wear artificial fingernails or extenders when having direct contact with patients at high risk (e.g., those in intensive-care units or operating rooms) (IA).

- Keep natural nail tips less than one-quarter inch long (II).

- Wear gloves when contact with blood or other potentially infectious materials, mucous membranes, or nonintact skin could occur (IC).

- Remove gloves after caring for a patient. Do not wear the same pair of gloves for the care of more than one patient, and do not wash gloves between uses with different patients (IB).

- Change gloves during patient care if moving from a contaminated body site to a clean body site (II).

- No recommendation can be made regarding wearing rings in health care settings (unresolved issue).

- Monitor workers' adherence to recommended hand-hygiene practices and provide personnel with information regarding their performance (IA).

- Encourage patients and their families to remind workers to decontaminate their hands (II).

- Store supplies of alcohol-based hand rubs in cabinets or areas approved for flammable materials (IC).

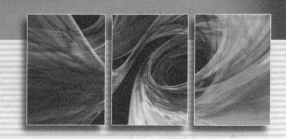

Latex Allergy

Health care workers are at risk for developing latex allergy because they frequently use latex gloves. Many of the products used in patient care contain latex, as do many household and personal items. Persons who have hay fever, hand dermatitis, and food allergies (such as to bananas, avocados, kiwi fruits, and chestnuts) are at increased risk of latex allergy. The amount and type of exposure needed to cause latex sensitivity is not known, although it is believed that wearing latex gloves when a rash is present on the hands increases the risk. A skin rash is often the first sign that a worker is becoming sensitive to latex. Some of the most common items that may contain latex are listed in Table A-1. This list is for example purposes only and may not be all-inclusive. For additional information see http://www.niosh.gov.

Table A-1 Common Items in the Health Care Facility that Contain Latex (This list is not all inclusive.)

Adhesives, skin	Dressings:
Anesthesia circuits, bags, oxygen masks	Action Wrap
	Airstrips (some)
Band-Aids	BDF Elastoplast
	Bioclusive
Blood pressure cuffs and tubing	Butterfly closures (J&J)
	Centurion brief
Catheters	Coban (3M)
cardiac	Comfeel (Coloplast)
condom	Duoderm (Squibb)
Coude	Dyna-flex
feeding	Lyofoam (Acme)
indwelling & systems	Metalline
pulmonary	Montgomery strap (J&J)
straight	Opraflex (Lohmann)
vascular	Opsite
	PinCare (Hollister)
CPR manikins & medical training aids	Reston foam (3M)
	Selopor
Crutch tips, axillary pads, hand grips	Spandage (Medi-tech)
	Venigard
Dental braces with rubber bands	Webril (Kendall)
	Xerofoam (Sherwood)
Diapers, rubber pants	

(continues)

Table A-1 Common Items in the Health Care Facility that Contain Latex (This list is not all inclusive.) (Continued)

Dressings, latex in package only:
  Active Strips (3M)
  CURAD
  Nu-Derm (J&J)
  Steri-strip wound closure system
  Tegaderm
  Tegasorb

Elastic on underwear, socks, clothing

Elastic wrap:
  ACE
  Dyna-flex
  Elastikon (J&J)

Electrode bulbs, pads, grounding

Enemas, ready-to-use (Fleet Pediatric and Mineral oil have latex valve; will soon change)

Foods handled with latex gloves

G-tubes, buttons

Gloves:
  clean
  orthodontic
  sterile
  surgical

Identification bracelets

Incentive deep breathing exerciser

IV access:
  bags
  buretrol ports
  injection ports
  needleless systems
  PRN adapters
  pumps
  Y-sites

IV ports or syringes

Medication training aids

Medication vial stoppers

Penrose drains

Pulse oximeters

Reflex hammers

Respirators

Resuscitators, manual

Shoe covers

Spacer (for metered dose inhalers)

Sphygmomanometer (blood pressure cuff)

Stethoscope tubing

Storage bags, plastic, zippered

Suction tubing

Syringes
  bulb
  disposable

Tapes:
  adhesive felt (Acme)
  cloth
  Moleskin
  pink
  Waterproof (3M)
  Waterproof (J&J)
  Zonas

Theraband (also strip, tube), other OT supplies

Therapeutic mattresses

Thermometer probes

Tourniquets

Vascular stockings (Jobst)

Wheelchair cushions, tires

Three types of reactions can occur in persons using latex products:

1. Irritant contact dermatitis-contact dermatitis—the development of dry, itchy, irritated areas on the skin, usually the hands. However, this problem may have many other causes as well, so one should not assume that a latex sensitivity is present without further diagnostic testing. *Irritant contact dermatitis is not a true allergy.*

2. Allergic contact dermatitis (delayed hypersensitivity)—a sensitivity to the chemicals used during the manufacturing process. The reaction is similar to the symptoms of poison ivy.

3. Latex allergy—a serious reaction to latex. This type of allergy is diagnosed with a blood or skin test. Even low exposure to latex can cause sensitive individuals to react. Reactions usually begin shortly after exposure to latex, but can occur hours later. Mild reactions cause hives, itching, and skin redness. More severe reactions cause respiratory symptoms, including runny nose, sneezing, itchy eyes, difficulty breathing, and wheezing. Anaphylactic shock is the most severe reaction. This type of shock is similar to that experienced by persons who are allergic to bee stings.

Preventing Latex Allergy

Many health care facilities have latex-free carts. Some facilities are becoming latex-free. Health care workers should take the following steps to protect themselves from latex exposure and allergy in the workplace:

- Use nonlatex gloves for activities that are not likely to involve contact with infectious materials (food preparation, routine housekeeping, maintenance, etc.). If latex gloves are used, avoid powdered gloves, which increase sensitivity through inhalation of latex proteins when gloves are removed.

- Use barrier protection as necessary when handling known or potentially infectious materials. If you use latex gloves, use powder-free gloves. Hypoallergenic latex gloves do not reduce the risk of latex allergy. However, they may reduce reactions to chemical additives in the latex (allergic contact dermatitis). *Cloth stethoscope covers provide an excellent barrier against latex exposure, but can be a potential source of contamination to patients.* Make sure your stethoscope cover is laundered regularly to reduce the potential risk of transmission.

- Avoid oil-based hand creams or lotions (which can cause glove deterioration) unless they have been shown to reduce latex-related problems and maintain glove barrier protection.

- After removing latex gloves, wash hands with a mild soap and dry thoroughly.

- Attend educational classes about latex exposure provided by your employer.

- Become familiar with procedures for preventing latex allergy.

- Learn to recognize the symptoms of latex allergy: skin rashes; hives; flushing; itching; nasal, eye, or sinus symptoms; asthma; and shock.

- If you develop symptoms of latex allergy, avoid direct contact with latex gloves and other latex-containing products until you can see a physician experienced in treating latex allergy.

- If you have latex allergy, consult your physician regarding precautions to use, such as:

  - Avoiding contact with latex gloves and other latex-containing products

  - Avoiding areas where you might inhale the powder from latex gloves worn by other workers

  - Informing your employer and your health care providers (physicians, nurses, dentists, etc.) that you have latex allergy

  - Wearing a Medic Alert® bracelet

- Carefully follow your physician's instructions for dealing with allergic reactions to latex.

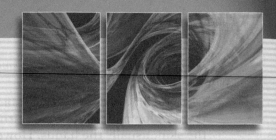

Mercury

Mercury is a neurotoxic, heavy metal that is linked to numerous health problems in wildlife and humans. In the book *Alice in Wonderland* (1865), the author selected a hat maker as the character who hosted a demented tea party. At the time, most hatters were considered mentally unbalanced, giving rise to the expression "mad as a hatter." Slurred speech, tremors, irritability, shyness, depression, and other neurological symptoms were common among those in the hat-making profession. Today, we know that these are all signs of mercury poisoning. In the mid-1800s, hat makers shaped felt and wool hats by using hot solutions of mercuric nitrate. They usually worked in poorly ventilated areas, leading to chronic occupational exposure to mercury and consequent neurological damage.

There is approximately 1 gram of mercury in a thermometer. Although it may not sound like much, this is enough mercury to contaminate a lake with a surface area of about 20 acres, to the degree that fish from the lake would be unsafe to eat. Mercury thermometers have been used for many years. However, in recent years the trend in health care has been to avoid the use of products containing mercury, because they can be very toxic if broken. This is true even if mercury exposure occurs in very small amounts. When mercury vaporizes, it is extremely toxic. However, the vapors are invisible, odorless, and tasteless. If mercury is combined with some other elements, the toxicity may increase. Mercury will conduct electricity.

A *mercury thermometer* is a small glass tube containing liquid mercury, a silvery-white substance that registers body heat. Alternative products are being used in many glass thermometers because of mercury's potential for toxicity. Some thermometers contain a red or blue liquid. These are alcohol thermometers and contain no mercury. Another, less common thermometer contains galin-

stan, a substance that is similar to mercury in appearance. These thermometers are mercury-free, however, and are generally marked as such.

Although most hospitals have eliminated mercury thermometers, many other common equipment items contain mercury, including some sphygmomanometers. No good substitute has been found to replace the mercury in the blood pressure apparatus. The alternative substances are not as sensitive.

Many battery-operated devices are used in the health care facility. The batteries likely contain mercury. It is found in diagnostic equipment and chemicals used in the laboratory, cleaning products, fluorescent light bulbs, switches, relays, thermostats, and many electrical devices. Mercury exposure can be toxic in small amounts, particularly if the mercury vaporizes and is inhaled. Women of childbearing age, pregnant women, and small children are at great risk for the toxic effects of mercury exposure. Mercury enters the body by:

- Inhalation of mercury vapor and/or dust; the threat is significant if mercury is broken or spilled in a small, poorly ventilated room.
- Absorption through skin of vapor, dust, and direct contact.
- Ingestion of metallic inorganic and organic forms, directly or indirectly through the food chain.

Once mercury enters the body, it is not easily excreted. It is fat-soluble, so the toxins accumulate in the tissues. Liver, brain, spinal cord, kidney, nervous, and fetal tissue are especially vulnerable, and mercury tends to accumulate and concentrate in these areas. Once inside the body, mercury:

- Alters cell membrane physiology
- Inhibits production and action of enzymes

- Damages the brain, spinal cord, liver, and kidneys
- Decreases the velocity of nerve impulses. Over time, mercury toxicity may cause shaking or trembling of the hands and loss of fine motor control

The effects of mercury exposure tend to be cumulative and irreversible. Mercury has a half-life of 70 days. After entering the body, it is slowly excreted, but its effects (and damage) are not readily reversed. Signs and symptoms of excessive mercury exposure and toxicity are:

- Headaches, vertigo, nausea, diarrhea
- Restlessness, irritability
- Tremors, loss of fine motor control
- Psychological disturbances, including mood and personality changes
- Blurred vision
- Lesions on skin with prolonged contact
- Increased perinatal mortality

MERCURY SPILLS

Even small mercury spills must be cleaned up properly to prevent contamination and illness. Never dispose of mercury in toilets, drains, sinks, or other wastewater collection systems. It will end up in the water supply, where it poisons wildlife and waterfowl. Because we depend on lakes and streams for our drinking water, over time the mercury may find its way back to humans. Spill kits and products that suppress mercury vapors are available, but these products are quite expensive. If you accidentally break a device containing mercury, inform the RN promptly. Follow facility policies and procedures for picking up mercury. If no procedures are available, apply shoe covers, gloves, face mask, and eye protection. Pick up broken glass and other debris and place it in a puncture-resistant container. Use an index card to consolidate the droplets, then seal them in a plastic bag or covered container. Small droplets can be picked up with adhesive tape or wet paper towels. Seal the container and affix a label identifying the material as "mercury spill debris." Consult the RN for information regarding where to discard this material.

E X P L O R I N G   T H E   W E B

Going Green (resource kit for eliminating mercury in health care)	http://www.noharm.org
Mercury Consumption Advice and Fish Advisories	http://www.epa.gov
Mercury Free at NIH	http://orf.od.nih.gov
Mercury Information	http://www.epa.gov
Mercury Thermometers and Your Family's Health	http://www.noharm.org
Planning and Holding a Mercury Thermometer Exchange	http://www.noharm.org
Ross-EPS Mercury Products and Information	http://www.epsross.com
Sustainable Hospitals	http://www.sustainablehospitals.org
What You Need to Know about Mercury in Fish and Shellfish	http://www.epa.gov

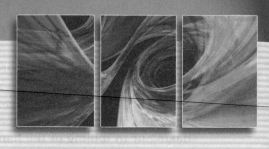

Appendix B
Abbreviations and
Medical Terminology

ABBREVIATION PROBLEMS

Misinterpretation of handwritten abbreviations is a major cause of error in health care facilities. Each facility maintains a list of acceptable abbreviations that may be used in documentation and other communications within the facility. In 2004, the JCAHO began checking for terms on its "listing of dangerous abbreviations" when it conducts facility surveys. These abbreviations must not be used in handwritten clinical documentation. Many of the abbreviations on the JCAHO list are used for medication administration. Facilities are required to expand their "do not use" lists by adding at least three abbreviations, acronyms, or symbols of their own choosing to the list each quarter. The JCAHO lists of dangerous abbreviations appear in Tables B-1 and B-2.

Table B-1 JCAHO "Minimum List" of Dangerous Abbreviations, Acronyms, and Symbols		
Abbreviation	**Potential Problem**	**Preferred Term**
U (unit)	Mistaken as zero, four, or cc.	Write "unit"
IU (international unit)	Mistaken as IV (intravenous) or 10 (ten).	Write "international unit"
Q.D., Q.O.D. (Latin abbreviation for once daily and every other day)	Mistaken for each other. The period after the Q can be mistaken for an "I" and the "O" can be mistaken for "I."	Write "daily" and "every other day"
Trailing zero (X.0 mg), lack of leading zero (.X mg)	Decimal point is missed.	Never write a zero by itself after a decimal point (X mg), and always use a zero before a decimal point (0.X mg)
MS MSO_4 $MgSO_4$	Confused for one another; can mean morphine sulfate or magnesium sulfate.	Write "morphine sulfate" or "magnesium sulfate"

Table B-2 Abbreviations to Omit in Addition to the JCAHO "Minimum Required List"		
μg, μg (for microgram)	Mistaken for mg (milligrams), resulting in thousand-fold dosing overdose.	Write "mcg"
H.S. (for half-strength, or Latin abbreviation for bedtime)	Mistaken for either half-strength or hour of sleep (at bedtime); q.H.S. mistaken for every hour. All can result in dosing error.	Write out "half-strength" or "at bedtime"
T.I.W. (for three times a week)	Mistaken for three times a day or twice weekly, resulting in overdose.	Write "3 times weekly" or "three times weekly"
S.C. or S.Q. (for subcutaneous)	Mistaken as SL for sublingual, or "5 every"	Write "Sub-Q," "subQ," "subcu," or "subcutaneously"
D/C (for discharge)	Interpreted as discontinue whatever medications follow (typically discharge meds).	Write "discharge"
c.c. or cc (for cubic centimeter)	Mistaken for U (units) when poorly written.	Write "mL" for milliliters
A.S., A.D., A.U. (Latin abbreviation for left, right, or both ears) O.S., O.D., O.U. (Latin abbreviation for left, right, or both eyes)	Mistaken for each other (e.g., AS for OS, AD for OD, AU for OU, etc.).	Write "left ear," "right ear," or "both ears"; "left eye," "right eye," or "both eyes"

The Institute for Safe Medication Practices (ISMP) also maintains an extensive listing of potentially unsafe abbreviations. The ISMP list of unacceptable abbreviations appears in Table B-3. Your facility will have a listing of acceptable and unacceptable abbreviations. Become familiar with this list and review it regularly.

Table B-3 ISMP Unacceptable Abbreviations			
Dose Designations and Other Information	**Intended Meaning**	**Misinterpretation**	**Correction**
Drug name and dose run together (especially problematic for drug names that end in "L" such as Inderal40 mg; Tegretol300 mg)	Inderal 40 mg Tegretol 300 mg	Mistaken as Inderal 140 mg Mistaken as Tegretol 1300 mg	Place adequate space between the drug name, dose, and unit of measure

(continues)

Table B-3 ISMP Unacceptable Abbreviations (Continued)

Dose Designations and Other Information	Intended Meaning	Misinterpretation	Correction
Numerical dose and unit of measure run together (e.g., 10mg, 100mL)	10 mg 100 mL	The "m" is sometimes mistaken as a zero or two zeros, risking a 10- to 100-fold overdose	Place adequate space between the dose and unit of measure
Abbreviations such as mg. or mL. with a period following the abbreviation	mg mL	The period is unnecessary and could be mistaken as the number 1 if written poorly	Use mg, mL, etc. without terminal period
Large doses without properly placed commas (e.g., 100000 units; 1000000 units)	100,000 units 1,000,000 units	100000 has been mistaken as 10,000 or 1,000,000; 1000000 has been mistaken as 100,000	Use commas for dosing units at or above 1,000, or use words such as 100 "thousand" or 1 "million" to improve readability

Drug Name Abbreviations	Intended Meaning	Misinterpretation	Correction
ARA A	vidarabine	Mistaken as cytarabine (ARA C)	Use complete drug name
AZT	zidovudine (Retrovir)	Mistaken as azathioprine or aztreonam	Use complete drug name
CPZ	Compazine (prochlorperazine)	Mistaken as chlorpromazine	Use complete drug name
DPT	Demerol-Phenergan-Thorazine	Mistaken as diphtheria-pertussis-tetanus (vaccine)	Use complete drug name
DTO	diluted tincture of opium, or deodorized tincture of opium (Paregoric)	Mistaken as tincture of opium	Use complete drug name
HCl	hydrochloric acid or hydrochloride	Mistaken as potassium chloride (The "H" is misinterpreted as "K")	Use complete drug name unless expressed as a salt of a drug
HCT	hydrocortisone	Mistaken as hydro-chlorothiazide	Use complete drug name
HCTZ	hydrochlorothiazide	Mistaken as hydrocortisone (see as HCT250 mg)	Use complete drug name

(continues)

Table B–3 ISMP Unacceptable Abbreviations (Continued)			
Drug Name Abbreviations	**Intended Meaning**	**Misinterpretation**	**Correction**
MgSO₄**	magnesium sulfate	Mistaken as morphine sulfate	Use complete drug name
MS, MSO₄**	morphine sulfate	Mistaken as magnesium sulfate	Use complete drug name
MTX	methotrexate	Mistaken as mitoxantrone	Use complete drug name
PCA	procainamide	Mistaken as Patient Controlled Analgesia	Use complete drug name
PTU	propylthiouracil	Mistaken as mercaptopurine	Use complete drug name
T3	tylenol with codeine No. 3	Mistaken as liothyronine	Use complete drug name
TAC	triamcinolone	Mistaken as tetracaine, Adrenalin, cocaine	Use complete drug name
TNK	TNKase	Mistaken as "TPA"	Use complete drug name
ZnSO₄	zinc sulfate	Mistaken as morphine sulfate	Use complete drug name
Stemmed Drug Names	**Intended Meaning**	**Misinterpretation**	**Correction**
"Nitro" drip	nitroglycerin infusion	Mistaken as sodium nitroprusside infusion	Use complete drug name
"Norflox"	norfloxacin	Mistaken as Norflex	Use complete drug name
"IV Vanc"	intravenous vancomycin	Mistaken as Invanz	Use complete drug name
Symbols	**Intended Meaning**	**Misinterpretation**	**Correction**
ℨ	Dram	Symbol for dram mistaken for "3"	Use the metric system
ℳ	Minim	Symbol for minim mistaken as "mL"	
x3d	For three days	Mistaken as "3 doses"	Use "for three days"
> and <	Greater than and less than	Mistaken as opposite of intended; mistakenly use incorrect symbol; "< 10" mistaken as "40"	Use "greater than" or "less than"

(continues)

Table B-3 ISMP Unacceptable Abbreviations (Continued)

Symbols	Intended Meaning	Misinterpretation	Correction
/ (slash mark)	Separates two doses or indicates "per"	Mistaken as the number 1 (e.g., "25 units/10 units" misread as "25 units and 110" units)	Use "per" rather than a slash mark to separate doses
@	At	Mistaken as "2"	Use "at"
&	And	Mistaken as "2"	Use "and"
+	Plus or and	Mistaken as "4"	Use "and"
°	Hour	Mistaken as a zero (e.g., q2° seen as q 20)	Use "hr," "h," or "hour"

**Identified abbreviations are also included on the JCAHO's "minimum list" of dangerous abbreviations, acronyms and symbols that must be included on an organization's "Do Not Use" list, effective January 1, 2004. An updated list of frequently asked questions about this JCAHO requirement can be found on their website at www.jcaho.org.

GENERAL ABBREVIATIONS

Table B-4 lists abbreviations that you may encounter in the course of your work. This table is for your learning and understanding only. Do not use the abbreviations listed in this book unless they have been approved for clinical documentation or other communications in your facility.

Table B-4 General Abbreviations

Abbreviation	Meaning	Abbreviation	Meaning
1°	first, primary, first degree	A&P	anatomy and physiology
1×, 2×, etc.**	one time, one person, two times, etc.	AAROM	active assistive (assisted) range of motion
2°	second, secondary, second degree; secondary to	ABCs	airway, breathing, circulation
3°	third, tertiary, third degree	abd.	abdomen, abduction
3P's	pain, pallor, pulselessness	ABT, ABX	antibiotic therapy
4P's	pain, pallor, pulselessness, paralysis	a̅c	before meals
		ACT	active, actively, activities
a̅**	before	AD	activity director, activities director
@**	at		

(continues)

Table B-4 General Abbreviations (Continued)

Abbreviation	Meaning	Abbreviation	Meaning
AD, Alz.	Alzheimer's disease	APIE	assessment, plan, implementation, evaluation
ad lib	as desired		
ADA	American Dietetic Association, American Diabetic Association, Americans with Disabilities Act	AROM	active range of motion
		as tol	as tolerated
		ASAP	as soon as possible
add.	Adduction	ASCVD	arteriosclerotic cardiovascular disease
ADLs	Activities of daily living		
adm	admission, administer, administrator, administration (context-dependent)	ASHD	arteriosclerotic heart disease
		assign	assignment
		assist	assistance
adm, trans, d/c	admission, transfer, discharge	ax	axillary (under the arm)
adv dir	advance directive	B, (B), B̄	bilateral, both
AEB	as evidenced by	B&B ◯	bowel and bladder
AED	automatic external defibrillator	BB	bedbath
		BBP	bloodborne pathogens
AFO	ankle foot orthosis	BEE	basal energy expenditure
AIDS	acquired immune deficiency syndrome	bid	twice a day
aka	above-the-knee amputation, also known as	bil, bilat	bilateral
ALF	assisted living facility	BKA	below-the-knee amputation
alt	alternate, alternating	BLE	both lower extremities
am	morning	BM	bowel movement
AMA	against medical advice	BP	bedpan
amb	ambulate	BP or B/P	blood pressure
amt	amount	BPM	beats per minute
ant	anterior	BR, B/R	bedrest, bathroom

(continues)

Table B-4 General Abbreviations (Continued)

Abbreviation	Meaning	Abbreviation	Meaning
BRP	bathroom privileges	CHF	congestive heart failure
BS	blood sugar	ck or √	check
BSC	bedside commode	ck freq or √ freq	check frequently
BSE	breast self-examination	cl liq	clear liquid
BUE	both upper extremities	CM	care map
c, cm	centimeter	CMA	certified medication aide
C	Celsius, centigrade, cane	CNA	certified nursing assistant, certified nurse aide, certified nurses aide
c̄	with		
C1, C2, C3, etc.	first cervical vertebra, second cervical vertebra, third cervical vertebra, etc.	CNS	Clinical Nurse Specialist
		c/o	complains of
C & S	culture and sensitivity	COLD, COPD	chronic obstructive lung (pulmonary) disease
c. diff	*Clostridium difficile*		
CA	cancer	communic	communicate, communication
CAD	coronary artery disease	confid	confidential, confidentiality
cal, kcal	calorie, kilocalorie		
cath	catheter	consc.	conscious
CB	call bell, call light, call signal	COTA	Certified Occupational Therapy Assistant
CBB	complete bedbath	CP	care plan, clinical pathway, critical pathway, chest pain, cold pack (context-dependent)
CBC	complete blood count		
CBE	charting by exception	CPM	continuous passive motion machine
cc	cubic centimeter		
CC	chief complaint	CPR	cardiopulmonary resuscitation
CDC	Centers for Disease Control and Prevention	CS	central supply, central service, central stores
C/D/I or CDI	clean, dry, and intact	cu	cubic
chem	chemicals, chemistry	CV	cardiovascular

(continues)

Table B-4 General Abbreviations (Continued)

Abbreviation	Meaning	Abbreviation	Meaning
CVA	cerebrovascular accident, stroke	DR, D/R	dining room
CXR	chest x-ray	Dr.	doctor
d	day	DSD	dry sterile dressing
DAR	data, action, response	DSM	dietary services manager
D/C, DC**	discontinue, discharge	DT	dietetic technician
DD	developmental disability	DVT	deep vein thrombosis (blood clot)
DDS	Doctor of Dental Science (dentist)	Dx	diagnosis
decub	pressure ulcer, decubitus ulcer	E	enema
dep	dependent	ECG	electrocardiogram
dept.	department	ED	emergency department, emergency room
diab	diabetes, diabetic	EEG	electroencephalogram
disinfec	disinfectant	EENT	eye, ear, nose, and throat
DJD	degenerative joint disease	EKG	electrocardiogram
DM	diabetes mellitus	EMR	electronic medical record
DNR	do not resuscitate	ENT	ear, nose, and throat
DNS	Director of Nursing Service	EOB	edge of bed
DO	Doctor of Osteopathy	ER	emergency room, emergency department
DOA	dead on arrival	ESRD	end-stage renal disease
DOB	date of birth	et	and
doc	documentation	ETOH	ethanol (often used to refer to alcoholic beverages)
DON	Director of Nursing		
DPOA, DPOA-HC	durable power of attorney, durable power of attorney for health care	ETT	endotracheal tube
		Eval	evaluation
DPM	Doctor of Podiatric Medicine	ex.	exercise

(continues)

Table B-4 General Abbreviations (Continued)

Abbreviation	Meaning	Abbreviation	Meaning
exam	examination	gt	gait
ext.	extension, extremity, external	gtt	drop
F	Fahrenheit, fair (context-dependent)	GU	genitourinary
		Gyn	gynecology
FB	foreign body	h	hour
FBS	fasting blood sugar	H	hydrogen
FC	focus charting, Foley catheter	H & P	history and physical
		H_2O	water
FE	Fleet's enema	H_2O_2	hydrogen peroxide
FF	force fluids	HAV, HBV, HCV, etc.	hepatitis A virus, hepatitis B virus, hepatitis C virus, etc.
flex	flexion		
flu	influenza	HCP	health care professional, health care proxy
freq	frequently		
FS	frozen section, fingerstick	HCW	health care worker
FSBS	fingerstick blood sugar	HD	Huntington's disease
FU or F/U	follow up	hemi	half, hemiplegia
FUO	fever of unknown origin	HEPA	high-efficiency particulate air (respirator or filter)
FWB	full weight bearing		
FWW, fw/w	front-wheeled walker	Hg	mercury
Fx	fracture	HIV	human immunodeficiency virus
G	good	HMO	health maintenance organization
g/c, GC	geriatric chair		
gen'l.	general, generalized	HNP	herniated nucleus pulposis (slipped disc)
GERD	gastroesophageal reflux disease	HOB	head of bed
GI	gastrointestinal	HOH	hard of hearing, hand-over hand
G/T, GT, G-tube	gastrostomy tube	hosp	hospital

(continues)

Table B-4 General Abbreviations (Continued)

Abbreviation	Meaning	Abbreviation	Meaning
hr	hour	irrig	irrigate, irrigation
HR	heart rate	isol	isolation
hs, HS**	bedtime (hour of sleep)	IV	intravenous
ht	height	J-tube	jejunostomy tube
HWB	hot water bottle	K or K+	potassium
Hx	history	KVO	keep vein open
hyper	high, fast, too much	L	liter, left
hypo	low, not enough	L/min or LPM	liters per minute
Ⓘ, ind.	independent, independently	L1, L2, etc.	first lumbar vertebra, second lumbar vertebra, etc.
I & O	intake and output	LA	left arm, left atrium
IC	infection control	lab	laboratory
ID	initial dose, identification	lat	lateral
IDCP	interdisciplinary care plan	lb, #	pound
IDDM	insulin-dependent diabetes mellitus	LBP	low back pain
IDT	interdisciplinary team	LBQC	large-based quad cane
IM	intramuscular	LE	lower extremity, late entry
immob	immobilize, immobility	LL	left leg
inc rept	incident report	LLC	long leg cast
incont	incontinent, incontinence	LLE	left lower extremity
infec	infection	lg	large
info	information	liq	liquid
inj	injury	LLQ	left lower quadrant
int.	internal	LOB	loss of balance
IPPB	intermittent positive pressure breathing	loc	local, localized

(continues)

Table B-4 General Abbreviations (Continued)

Abbreviation	Meaning	Abbreviation	Meaning
LOC	level of consciousness, level of care	min req	minimum required, minimum requirement
LOM	limitation of motion, loss of motion	mL or ml	milliliter
LPM or L/min	liters per minute	mm	millimeter
LPN	licensed practical nurse	mm Hg or mmHg	millimeters of mercury
lt	left	MN, midnoc	midnight
LTC	long-term care	mod	moderate
LTCF	long-term care facility	MR	mental retardation
LTG	long-term goal	MRSA	methicillin-resistant *Staphylococcus aureus*
LUQ	left upper quadrant	MRSE	methicillin-resistant *Staphylococcus epidermis*
LV	left ventricle		
LVN	licensed vocational nurse	MS	multiple sclerosis
M	meter	MS, MSO$_4$	morphine sulfate
MA	medication aide	MSDS	material safety data sheets
max	maximum	mult.	multiple
M'caid	Medicaid	N & V	nausea and vomiting
M'care, Mcr.	Medicare	NA or N/A	not applicable, nursing assistant, nurse aide, nurses aide (context-dependent)
MD	muscular dystrophy, medical doctor		
MDR	main dining room	Na$^+$	sodium
MDS	Minimum Data Set	NACEP	Nurse Aide Competency Evaluation Program
mech soft	mechanical soft	NANDA	North American Nursing Diagnosis Association
med rec	medical record, medical records	NAR	no adverse reaction
meds, med	medication, medications	NAS	no added salt
MI	myocardial infarction (heart attack)	NATCEP	Nurse Aide Training and Competency Evaluation Program
min	minimum, minimal		

(continues)

Table B-4 General Abbreviations (Continued)			
Abbreviation	**Meaning**	**Abbreviation**	**Meaning**
NBQC	narrow-based quad cane	NWB	no weight bearing, non-weight bearing
N/C, no c/o	no complaints	O, os	mouth
neg, or −	negative	O₂	oxygen
NG	nasogastric	OA	osteoarthritis, obstructed airway
NGT	nasogastric tube		
NH	nsg home, nursing home	obj	objective
NIC	Nursing Interventions Classification	OBRA	Omnibus Budget Reconciliation Act
NIDDM	non-insulin-dependent diabetes mellitus	obs	observations
		OBS	organic brain syndrome
NIOSH	National Institutes of Occupational Safety and Health	occ	occasional
NKA	no known allergies	OOB	out of bed
NN	Nurses' Notes	OR	operating room
NNO	no new orders	ORIF	open reduction, internal fixation
NO	new orders		
noc	night	os, O	mouth*
NOC	Nursing Outcomes Classification	OSHA	Occupational Safety and Health Administration
NP	Nurse Practitioner	OT	occupational therapist, occupational therapy
NPO	nothing by mouth	P	poor, pulse (context-dependent)
NREM	nonrapid eye movement sleep		
		p̄	after
N/S, NSS	normal saline, normal saline solution	P&P	policies and procedures
nsg dx., Ndx	nursing diagnosis	PA	physician's assistant, public address system (intercom) (context-dependent)
nsg proc.	nursing process		
NVD	nausea, vomiting, and diarrhea	PACU	postanesthesia care unit
		PB, PBB	partial bath, partial bed bath

(continues)

Table B-4 General Abbreviations (Continued)

Abbreviation	Meaning	Abbreviation	Meaning
$\overline{pc}$	after meals	PU, pu	pressure ulcer, pickup
PCT	patient care technician	PUD	peptic ulcer disease
PE	physical examination	PVD	peripheral vascular disease
peds or pedi	pediatrics	PWB	partial weight bearing
PEG	percutaneous endoscopic gastrostomy	$\overline{q}$	each, every
per	by, through	$\overline{q}2h$, $\overline{q}3h$, $\overline{q}4h$, etc.	every 2 hours, every 3 hours, every 4 hours, etc.
pm	afternoon or evening	$\overline{qd}$* **	every day
PN	progress notes	$\overline{q}h$	every hour
pneu	pneumonia	$\overline{q}hs$**	every night at bedtime
po, per os**	by mouth	qid	4 times a day
POMR	problem-oriented medical record	$\overline{q}m$ or $\overline{q}$ am	every morning
pos or ⊕	positive	$\overline{qod}$* **	every other day
postop	postoperative	$\overline{q}s$	sufficient quantity
PPE	personal protective equipment	qt	quart
		quad	quadrant, four
PPS	postpolio syndrome, prospective payment system	R	rectal, respirations, right
preop	preoperative	RA	rheumatoid arthritis, right arm, right atrium
prep	prepare	RAI	Resident Assessment Instrument
prn	as needed	RC	retention catheter
prog	prognosis	RCP	respiratory care practitioner
PROM	passive range of motion	RD	registered dietitian
pt or Pt	patient	re:	regarding
PT	physical therapist, physical therapy	reg	regular
PTA	physical therapy assistant	regs	regulations

(continues)

Table B-4 General Abbreviations (Continued)

Abbreviation	Meaning	Abbreviation	Meaning
rehab	rehabilitation	$\overline{s}$	without
REM	rapid eye movement sleep	SBA	standby assistance
reps	repetitions	SBQC	small-based quad cane
res or Res	resident (nursing home resident or resident physician)	sc, sq, sub-q**	subcutaneous
		SEC	single-end cane
resp, R	respirations	semi	half, partial
RL	right leg	SLP	speech language pathologist
RLE	right lower extremity		
RLQ	right lower quadrant	sm	small
		SNF	skilled nursing facility
rm	room	SNU	skilled nursing unit
RN	registered nurse	SOAP	subjective, objective, assessment, plan
RNA	restorative nursing assistant		
		SOB	shortness of breath
R/O	rule out	SOC	standards of care
ROM	range of motion	SOMR	source-oriented medical record
rot.	rotation		
rt	right	SOOB	sitting out of bed
RT	respiratory therapy, respiratory therapist	SP, std prec, Std. prec.	standard precautions*
r/t	related to	S/P	status post (after)
RUE	right upper extremity	spec	specimen
RUQ	right upper quadrant	S/R, SR	side rail
RV	right ventricle	SS	social service
RW	rolling walker	S/S, S&S, S & S	signs and symptoms
Rx	prescription, therapy, treatment	SSE	soapsuds enema
Ⓢ	shower	st	sterile

(continues)

Table B-4 General Abbreviations (Continued)

Abbreviation	Meaning	Abbreviation	Meaning
ST	speech therapy	TIAN	toilet in advance of need
S/T	skin tear	TID	three times a day
stat	immediately, at once	TKO	to keep open
std, stds	standard, standards	TLC	tender loving care
STG	short-term goal	TO	telephone order
STNA	state-tested nursing assistant	TPN	total parenteral nutrition
str.	strength	TPR	temperature, pulse, respiration
STR, STRC	straight cane	trach	tracheostomy
subj	subjective	TT	therapeutic touch, tray table (context-dependent)
supp	suppository	TTWB	toe-touch weight bearing
SW	social worker	TWE	tap-water enema
Sx	symptoms	Tx	traction, treatment
T, temp	temperature	UA or U/A	urinalysis
T&R	turn and reposition	UAP	unlicensed assistive personnel
T1, T2, etc.	first thoracic vertebra, second thoracic vertebra, etc.	UE	upper extremity
TB	tuberculosis, tub bath (context-dependent), (TB)	unconsc.	Unconscious
TBP or TrBP	transmission-based precautions	UR, U/R	utility room
TCU	transitional care unit	URI	upper respiratory infection
TDO	telephone doctors' order	UTI	urinary tract infection
TF	tube feeding	vag	vaginal
THA	total hip arthroplasty	vc, VC, v/c	verbal cues
THR	total hip replacement	vent	ventilator
TIA	transient ischemic attack	VRE	vancomycin-resistant *Enterococcus*

(continues)

Table B-4 General Abbreviations (Continued)

Abbreviation	Meaning	Abbreviation	Meaning
VRSA	vancomycin-resistant *Staphylococcus aureus*	XR or X/R	X-ray
VS, v/s, vitals	vital signs	y/o	years old
W	walker	yr	year
WA or W/A	while awake	↑	up, increase
WB	weight bearing	↓	down, decrease
WBAT	weight bearing as tolerated	//	parallel
w/c, WC	wheelchair	±, +/−**	plus or minus
WFL	within functional limits	△ [triangle]	change, change to
WNL	within normal limits	° * *	degrees, hour
WP,W/P	whirlpool	Ø	zero, none, nothing
wt	weight	*	important
x or X	times	♀	female
		♂	male

*On JCAHO list
**On ISMP list

Abbreviations Related to the Heart and Cardiac Care

Table B-5 Abbreviations Related to the Heart and Cardiac Care

Abbreviation	Meaning	Abbreviation	Meaning
1°	first degree	A tach, atrial tach	atrial tachycardia
2°	second degree	ant	anterior
3°	third degree	A&P	anatomy and physiology
A fib	atrial fibrillation	A—P, A→P	anterior to posterior
A flutter	atrial flutter		

(continues)

Table B-5 Abbreviations Related to the Heart and Cardiac Care (Continued)

Abbreviation	Meaning	Abbreviation	Meaning
arrhy	arrhythmia	LLQ	left lower quadrant (of abdomen)
atrial tach, A tach	atrial tachycardia	LUL	left upper lobe (of lung)
AV	atrioventricular (node)	LUQ	left upper quadrant (of abdomen)
BBB	bundle branch block	LV	left ventricle
B/P, BP	blood pressure	med	medial, medium, medication (context-dependent)
BPM	beats per minute		
brady	bradycardia, slow	MI	myocardial infarction (heart attack)
cath	catheter, catheterization		
CHF	congestive heart failure	Mobitz 2	second-degree atrioventricular block, Type 2
circ	circulation		
CV	cardiovascular, cerebrovascular (context-dependent)	node, nodal, junct	refers to the atrioventricular node (atrioventricular junction)
CVA	cerebrovascular accident (stroke)	NSR	normal sinus rhythm
defib	defibrillator, defibrillate, defibrillation	P	pulse
		PAC	premature atrial contraction
dysrhy	dysrhythmia	pacer	pacemaker
ECG, EKG	electrocardiogram	PJC	premature junctional contraction
Fem	femoral		
fem—pop	femoral-popliteal	PNC	premature nodal contraction
HR	heart rate		
LA	left atrium, left apex, left arm (context-dependent)	post	posterior
		post tib	posterior tibial (pulse)
lat	lateral	PP	pedal pulse
LL	left leg, left lung (context-dependent)	PVC	premature ventricular contraction
LLL	left lower lobe (of lung)	QRS	QRS complex

(continues)

Table B-5 Abbreviations Related to the Heart and Cardiac Care (Continued)

Abbreviation	Meaning	Abbreviation	Meaning
R	respirations	SA	sinoatrial (node)
RA	right atrium, right apex, right arm (context-dependent)	sinus tach	sinus tachycardia
		ST	refers to the ST segment
RL	right leg, right lung (context-dependent)	SVT	supraventricular tachycardia
RLL	right lower lobe (of lung)	tach, tachy	tachycardia, fast
RLQ	right lower quadrant (of abdomen)	V fib	ventricular fibrillation
		V flutter	ventricular flutter
RML	right middle lobe (of lung)	V tach	ventricular tachycardia
RP	radial pulse	WAP	wandering atrial pacemaker
RUL	right upper lobe (of lung)		
RUQ	right upper quadrant (of abdomen)	Wenckebach	second-degree atrioventricular block, Type 1, Wenckebach phenomenon
RV	right ventricle		
R—R	refers to the R-to-R interval	WPW	Wolff-Parkinson-White syndrome

Measurements

Table B-6 Measurements and Volume

Abbreviation	Meaning	Abbreviation	Meaning
amt	amount	oz**, z	ounce*
cc***	cubic centimeter	tsp**, z	teaspoon, dram
gtt	drop	>, ≥**	greater than
ml or mL	milliliter	<, ≤**	less than
L	liter	ss**, $\overline{ss}$, $\dot{s}\dot{s}$	one-half

*On JCAHO list
**On ISMP list

Table B-7 Height and Weight

cm	centimeter
ft	feet
in	inches
kg	kilogram
lb, #	pound
oz, z	ounce

Medical Terminology

Table B-8 Word Roots

Root	Meaning	Root	Meaning
abdomin (o)	abdomen	dermat (o)	skin
aden (o)	gland	encephal (o)	brain
angi (o)	vessel	enter (o)	small intestine
arteri (o)	artery	erythr (o)	red
arth (o)	joint	fibr (o)	fiber
bronch (i) (o)	bronchus	gastr (o)	stomach
cardi (o)	heart	geront (o)	elderly
cephal (o)	head	gloss (o)	tongue
cerebr (o)	brain	glyc (o)	sugar
chol (e)	bile	gynec (o)	female
col (o)	colon	hem (o)	blood
crani (o)	skull	hemat (o)	blood
cyst (o)	bladder, cyst	hepat (o)	liver
cyt (o)	cell	hydr (o)	water
dent (i) (o)	tooth	hyster (o)	uterus

(continues)

Table B-8 Word Roots (Continued)

Root	Meaning	Root	Meaning
lapar (o)	abdomen, flank, loin	proct (o)	rectum
laryng (o)	larynx	psych (o)	mind
lith (o)	stone	pulm (o)	lung
mamm (o)	breast	py (o)	pus
mast (o)	breast	rect (o)	rectum
men (o)	menstruation	rhin (o)	nose
my (o)	muscle	splen (o)	spleen
myel (o)	bone marrow, spinal cord	stern (o)	sternum
nephr (o)	kidney	thorac (o)	chest
neur (o)	nerve	thromb (o)	clot
ocul (o)	eye	tox (o)	poison
opthalm (o)	eye	trache (i) (o)	trachea
oste (o)	bone	ur (o)	urine
ped (i) (o)	child	urethr (o)	urethra
pharyng (o)	throat	urin (o)	urine
phleb (o)	vein	uter (i) (o)	uterus
pneum (o)	lung, air	ven (o)	vein

Table B-9 Prefixes

Prefix	Meaning	Prefix	Meaning
a, an	without, not	bi	double, two
ab	away from	bio	life
ad	toward	brady	slow
ante	before	circum	around
anti	against	dys	difficult, abnormal

(continues)

Table B-9 Prefixes (Continued)

Prefix	Meaning	Prefix	Meaning
epi	on, over	per	by, through
hemi	half	peri	around
hyper	high, above, excessive	poly	many
hypo	low, below normal	post	after
inter	between	pre	before
intra	inside, within	pseud	false
leuk	white	retro	backward
micro	small	semi	half, partial
neo	new	septic	infection
non	not	sub	under, below
pan	all	tachy	fast

Table B-10 Suffixes

Suffix	Meaning	Suffix	Meaning
algia	pain	pathy	disease
alysis	analyze	penia	deficiency
ectomy	surgical removal	phasia	speaking
emia	blood	plegia	paralysis
gram	record	pnea	breathing
itis	inflammation of	ptosis	sagging, falling
logy	study of	rrhagia	excessive flow
lysis	destruction of	rrhea	discharge
megaly	enlargement	scope	instrument that examines
meter	instrument that measures	stasis	constant
ostomy	surgical opening	therapy	treatment
otomy	surgical opening	uria	condition of urine

E X P L O R I N G   T H E   W E B

Acronym Finder	http://www.acronymfinder.com
American Medical Writers' Association	http://www.amwa.org
Analysis of PDAs in Nursing	http://www.rnpalm.com
Anat Line	http://anatline.nlm.nih.gov
Assorted Encyclopedias on the Web	http://edis.win.tue.nl
Best Health	http://www.besthealth.com
CareNurse nursing resource directory	http://www.care-nurse.com
Center for Human Simulation (Visible Human Project)	http://www.uchsc.edu/sm/chs/open.html
Combined Health Information Database	http://child.nih.gov/index.html
Diseases Database	http://www.diseasesdatabase.com
Dorland's Medical Dictionary	http://www.mercksource.com
Electronic Discovery Resources	http://www.discoveryresources.org
Free e-books	http://www.e-book.com/au/freebooks.htm
Focus on Medterms.com	http://www.medterms.com
Free-ed.net	http://www.free-ed.net
Gray's Anatomy	http://www.bartleby.com
Guidelines for Medical Record Documentation	http://www.southernhealth.com
Harvey Project	http://harveyproject.org
Health Science Resources	http://library.shu.edu/health.htm
HIPAA	http://www.hhs.gov/ocr/hipaa
Incident Reports Protected from Review	http://echo.forensicpanel.com
Incident Reports-Types, Rates, Injuries, JCAHO, Harvard Study	http://www.riskmanco.com
InfoPlease Health Information	http://www.infoplease.com
ISMP Abbreviations Listing and related information	http://www.ismp.org
JCAHO Abbreviations Information	http://www.jcaho.org
JCAHO abbreviation implementation tips	http://www.jcaho.org
Lawrence's Medical Resources	http://www.vex.net/~lawrence
Med Term Web	http://ec.hku.hk
MT Desk	http://mtdesk.com
National Institutes of Health (NIH)	http://health.nih.gov
Online Medical Dictionary	http://cancerweb.ncl.ac.uk
Online Tutorials	http://medi-smart.com
Patient's Guide to Med Term	http://www3.bc.sympatico.ca
Science Web	http://www.scienceteacherprogram.org
Stedman's Online Medical Dictionary	http://www.stedmans.com

Appendix C
Electronic Communication

About the Internet

The *Internet* is a worldwide network of computers that exchange information very quickly. A connection to the Internet provides you with unlimited information, including electronic mail (e-mail), newsgroups, mailing lists, and the World Wide Web (WWW). Most hospitals have Internet access for employee use. Many also use an *intranet*, a private computer network within an organization. It is used to share company information and other resources among employees. An intranet uses regular Internet protocols and usually works like a private version of the Internet.

E-Mail

Sending and receiving electronic mail on the Internet (or an intranet) is like using a very fast post office. It is one of the most useful functions for sending and receiving messages, subscribing to informational lists, and communicating quickly and directly with others. To send e-mail, you simply type the recipient's address; insert a subject in the next box, which is a general subject line; and type your message in the message area. Click the "send" button and you are done! There are also features that allow you to attach files for the recipient to download. Typing the recipient's e-mail address accurately is important. One wrong space, letter, or character will cause the message to be returned or delivered to the wrong person.

E-mail addresses all follow a basic pattern. The name, which can be the recipient's real name or a self-designated screen name, is listed first. This is followed by the symbol @, followed by the Internet service provider (ISP) or company Internet name and a suffix. The suffix often denotes the type of organization, if the message is not going directly to an individual's computer. For example, the abbreviation ".com" at the end denotes a business, ".gov" indicates a governmental agency, ".org" indicates a nonprofit organization, and ".edu" indicates an educational institution. An example of an e-mail address is PCTnancy@StJohnHospital.org.

E-mail arrives quickly, usually within a few minutes. The recipient can respond to the message; cut, copy, and paste it and send it to someone else; save it in a file; or delete it from the system entirely. The recipient can also click a button and send you a quick response.

Surfing the Web

The World Wide Web, or WWW, is the fastest growing part of the Internet. It contains information, news, articles, photographs and other images, and informational resources. The Web uses *hypertext* to create links to other Web sites. These links appear in color (usually blue) on your screen. When you click on the colored word, you will be connected to other related documents. On some Web sites, you can read abstracts or the full text of nursing- and caregiver-related articles. Many hospitals have their procedure manuals online to be accessed using the Internet or an intranet. Some sites even allow you to view pictures and hear sounds, such as breath sounds! Many of the state nursing boards have Web sites.

To gain access to a specific Web site, you must know the *Uniform Resource Locator (URL)* of that site. Unlike an e-mail address, the URL contacts organizations rather than individuals. An example of a URL is http://www.cdc.gov. This address will take you to the Web site of the Centers for Disease Control and Prevention. In addition to accessing the CDC, there are many hypertext links in this site's pages to connect you to other governmental and private sites containing related subject matter.

Getting Information

You find information on the Internet by doing a search. A number of searching services, called *search engines*, are available. These engines have different names, such as Google, Yahoo!, Gopher, Web Crawler, AltaVista, Metacrawler, and Lycos. Some search engines search for general information, and several are specifically for medical information. Most general search engines will also locate medical information.

Some Internet servers have search engines that can be accessed by clicking with your mouse on the home page or by typing the search terms into a box in the browser. For servers that do not have this feature, you must type in the Web address. After you connect to the Web site of the search engine, you type the information you are looking for into a box on the Web page. If the search is too broad, you can click a "Help" link to obtain instructions and suggestions for narrowing it. For example, a search for information on "Nursing Assistants" will look up both "Nursing" and "Assistants." That is, the search engine will also search for any other material with "Assistants" in the title, such as physical therapy assistants, assistant professors, and so forth, and will return far too many "hits" (results) to be useful. Depending on the search engine, it may help to put one or both terms in parentheses or quotation marks. For example, "nursing+assistant" or ("nursing assistant") may be acceptable forms. The directions for narrowing a search vary with the search engine used, but most are very user-friendly and simple to use.

Listservs

Listservs are mailing lists. You receive messages via email, and can respond to them if you wish. There are a number of nursing-related listservs. Some are specifically for nursing assistants and PCTs, and others are for nurses only. Many welcome subscribers from all health disciplines. There are also listservs for many specific diseases. Using these lists allows you to interact with your colleagues. Many list users share information, policies, and ideas with each other. Some lists are for the purpose of personal and professional support.

HIPAA, Patient Confidentiality, and the Internet

One disadvantage of using the Internet is that you must protect confidential information. You would not want to send a medical record, test results, or other confidential information over the Internet because hackers could get into your system or the receiving system and read the information. You could also click the wrong button and accidentally post sensitive information on a list. Once you click the "Send" button, there is no way to retract the mail.

Encryption services are available to scramble and encode confidential or sensitive information. If your hospital uses an encryption service to e-mail sensitive information, you will be given instructions, a password, and guidelines for when to use it. Always remember that e-mail is not completely secure. Never give out personal or confidential information about yourself or others on the Internet. You never know who is reading it!

Another consideration is that you are being paid to work. If your employer provides Internet access, it expects that you will use it for facility business only. Do not use it for personal communication and e-mail, even if you are connecting to your personal account. Your employer may legally access all information you send and receive over its network. Using your employer's Internet service to communicate with friends and relatives, especially while you are on duty and being paid, is usually considered a form of theft from your employer. Thus, you may be subject to the same penalties as you would face for stealing an item from the facility. Use your employer's computer according to facility policies to conduct facility business only.

Fax Machines

Facsimile (fax) machines transmit printed information from one location to another. Most hospitals do this over telephone lines, but some use the Internet to send and receive faxes. Hospitals frequently use fax machines for transmitting laboratory and X-ray reports, physician orders, and communications with physicians and other health care agencies and facilities. Benefits of using the fax machine include:

- *Speed.* Documents and reports are transmitted immediately. There is no waiting, no being put on hold, and no need to navigate through a voice-mail system.
- *Accuracy.* The receiver of the document receives a hard-copy report, which should be retained in the files. This reduces the risk of errors, and the receiver can make decisions based on information transmitted in the document.
- *Legality.* The hard copy of a faxed document can legally become part of the medical record. Most states and accrediting bodies permit physician orders and other information to be transmitted by fax.

You may be responsible for sending information over a fax machine. This involves placing one or more papers in the machine, dialing the fax number of the receiving party, and pressing the "Start" button. Your facility will teach you how to use the type of machine you will be operating.

Most fax machines now use plain paper, but a few use a thermal paper similar to ECG paper. This paper picks up stray marks and scratches, which may render the original illegible. The fax paper also fades over time. Documents received on thermal paper must be recopied on plain paper, using a photocopier, before being placed in a patient's medical records.

Like all other sensitive medical information, fax transmissions are protected under the HIPAA laws and regulations. Always exercise caution and follow facility policies and procedures for electronic communication.

Sample HIPAA-Compliant Electronic Media Policy

1. Employees have access to various forms of electronic media and services (computers, e-mail, telephones, voice mail, fax machines, external electronic bulletin boards, wire services, online services, and the Internet) (hereinafter referred to as "media").

2. This facility encourages the use of electronic media. However, media are company property and are used to facilitate company business. They are not to be used for personal communication or correspondence. The company server retains copies of all electronic communications. These are subject to random, unannounced monitoring at any time to ensure adherence to facility policies.

3. The following procedures apply to all media that:
   a. are accessed on or from company premises;
   b. are accessed using company computer equipment or via company-paid access methods;
   c. are accessed while the employee is being paid by the company for working;
   d. make reference to the company in any manner; and/or
   e. are used in a manner that identifies the employee with the company.

4. Patient identities and protected health information are not to be indiscriminately disclosed when transmitting messages via electronic media. Always double- and triple-check phone numbers, fax numbers, e-mail addresses, and Web sites before sending confidential or sensitive information. Use encryption whenever possible. Add a disclaimer to fax and e-mail communications, such as:

E-mail Disclaimer

The information in this e-mail message is intended for the confidential use of the addressees only. The information is privileged and confidential. Recipients should not file copies of this e-mail with publicly accessible records or forward this e-mail to others. If you are not an addressee or an authorized agent responsible for delivering this e-mail to a designated addressee, you have received this e-mail in error, and any further review, dissemination, distribution, copying, or forwarding of this e-mail is strictly prohibited. If you received this e-mail in error, please notify us immediately at (xxx) xxx-xxxx. Thank you.

Facsimile Disclaimer

The information contained in this facsimile message is privileged and confidential. It is intended only for the use of the individual named above and the privileges are not waived by virtue of this having been sent by facsimile. If the person actually receiving this facsimile or any other reader of the facsimile is not the named recipient or the employee or agent responsible to deliver it to the named recipient, any use, dissemination, distribution, or copying of the communication is strictly prohibited. If you have received this communication in error, please immediately notify us by telephone and return the original message to us at the above address via U.S. Postal Service. We will reimburse your postage. If you did not receive all of the pages listed above, please call us immediately at (xxx) xxx-xxxx. Thank you.

(continues)

Sample HIPAA-Compliant Electronic Media Policy (Continued)

5. Always transmit the cover sheet last so that it covers the confidential fax information. Reversing the order of the pages before faxing is appreciated by the receiver of the communication. For example, fax pages in this order: page 5, page 4, page 3, page 2, page 1, cover sheet. When you transmit documents in this manner, the information is received in order and protected information is covered after being transmitted through the fax.

6. Company electronic media may not be used for transmitting, retrieving, or storing any communications that are: of a discriminatory or harassing nature; derogatory to any individual or group; obscene; of a defamatory or threatening nature; "chain letters"; for personal use; for sending "spam" mail or virus messages; illegal or against company policy; or contrary to the company's interest.

7. Electronic information created and/or communicated by an employee using media will not generally be monitored by the company. However, the company routinely monitors usage patterns for both voice and data communications (e.g., number called or Web site accessed; call length; times of day called) for cost analysis/allocation and management of the Internet server. The company also reserves the right, in its discretion, to review any employee's electronic files and messages and usage to the extent necessary to ensure that media are being used in compliance with the law and with company policy. Therefore, employees should not assume that electronic communications are private and confidential.

8. Employees must respect other people's electronic communications. Employees may not attempt to read or "hack" into other systems or logins; "crack" passwords; breach computer or network security measures; or monitor electronic filings or communications of other employees or third parties, except by explicit direction of company management.

9. Every employee who uses any security measures on a company-supplied computer must provide the company with a sealed, hard-copy record of all passwords and encryption keys (if any) for company use, if required.

10. No e-mail or other electronic communications may be sent that attempt to hide the identity of the sender or represent the sender as someone else or someone from another company.

11. Media may not be used in a manner that is likely to cause network congestion or significantly hamper other people's ability to access and use the system.

12. Employees may not copy, retrieve, modify, or forward copyrighted materials except as permitted by the copyright owner or as a single copy for reference use only.

13. Any information or messages sent by an employee via an electronic network are statements identifiable with and attributable to the company. All communications sent by employees via a network must comply with company policy, and may not disclose any confidential or proprietary company information.

14. Network services and World Wide Web sites monitor access and usage and can identify at least which company, and often which specific individual, is accessing their services. Accessing a particular bulletin board or Web site leaves company-identifiable electronic "tracks" even if the employee merely reviews or downloads the material and does not post any message.

15. Any employee who violates company policy will be subject to corrective action and/or risk losing the privilege of using media for himself or herself and possibly other employees.

16. Employees are responsible for keeping virus protection up to date by downloading weekly computer updates.

17. Employees must use discretion in opening files. Avoid indiscriminate opening of files attached to e-mail. In general, avoid or delete files with the suffix ".exe." However, you must avoid any files if you are not familiar with the sender or are not expecting the file. Employees may be held responsible for the cost of repairs for damage to computers caused by opening files infected with viruses. Employees will be subject to disciplinary action if data is lost as a result of viral infection of the computer.

MEDICATION AND TREATMENT ORDERS

Comprehensive Medication and Treatment Orders

The following are guidelines for medication and treatment orders. Your state may have additional (or different) rules. Follow your state laws and facility policies if different from guidelines listed here.

Medication and treatment orders should consist of the following:

- Name of medication (do not abbreviate).
- Strength or concentration of medication.
- Dosage (form) of medication.
- Frequency (or time) of administration.
- Length of administration, if applicable (e.g., a cold pack for 20 minutes).
- Route of administration.
- Duration of therapy. (This may be determined by facility stop order. PRN (as needed) medications can be "indefinitely.") For antibi-

otics, narcotic analgesics, anticoagulants, and other time-limited medications, clearly mark the date and time for first and last dose on the medication administration record (MAR).

- Diagnosis or indications for use.
- Date and time of order, including year.
- Full signature and title of person issuing order.

Guidelines for working with comprehensive medication orders include:

- Verify allergies, and advise the physician immediately if the patient is allergic to an ordered medication.
- Inform the physician if the patient has orders for another, similar medication.
- PRN orders should specify the condition for which the medication is administered (reason), and the frequency of administration.
- Avoid dose-range or time-range orders.
- When a physician changes an order that is currently being used, the nurse must first discontinue the current order, then write a new order reflecting the change.
- Avoid statements such as, "Resume previous orders" or other blanket reinstatements.
- Orders for parenteral or enteral nutrition therapy must specify the solution/fluid, amount, flow rate, pump/gravity/bolus use, and so on. For tube feeding, note the number of calories per day, and down time, if any. (For example, note if pump is off for an hour each day for shower and ADL care.)
- Treatment orders should specify the area of the body to be treated.
- Restraint orders must be reviewed every 24 hours. Use the least restrictive restraint possible for the least amount of time to keep the patient safe.

Refer to information on page xv.

Telephone Orders

Orders received by telephone are acceptable, but must be countersigned by the physician (or other authorized health care provider) within the required time frame as defined by facility policy. Only a licensed nurse may accept a telephone order. Verbal, electronic, and telephone orders may not be given for:

- Cytotoxic chemotherapeutic agents
- Do Not Resuscitate orders
- Investigational drugs
- Biological response modifiers

The nurse accepting the telephone order must read the order back to the physician after writing the order. Documentation on the medical record must validate that the order was read back to the physician. For example, the nurse writes the following on the order sheet:

TO/Dr. Mehaffy/S. Romcevich, RN/RB/SR

This means: "Nurse Romcevich received a telephone order ("TO") from Dr. Mehaffy, read it back ("RB") to Dr. Mehaffy, and initialed the documentation ("SR")."

Fax and E-Mail Orders

Fax and e-mail orders may be accepted. When fax is used as a means of communication, the physician's (or other health care provider's) office and facility should retain the fax documents as part of the medical record. All faxed information must be clearly identified with the patient's name. The following conditions must be met:

- The physician (or other health care provider) must sign and retain the original copy of the order in his or her file. Alternatively, the original may be sent to the facility at a later time and substituted for the fax.
- The facility should photocopy the faxed order, because the thermal paper and ink used in some fax machines fade over time. The fax may be discarded after the facility photocopies it.
- The receiving unit must maintain confidentiality of protected health information, and follow all policies, procedures, and safeguards to ensure that the fax ordering system is not subject to abuse.
- Physician orders should not be left on the fax machine where they may be read by unauthorized persons.
- Patient identities and protected health information are not to be indiscriminately disclosed when transmitting messages via electronic media. Always double- and triple-check fax numbers, e-mail addresses, and Web sites before sending confidential or sensitive information. Use encryption whenever possible. Always add a disclaimer to fax and e-mail communications, as shown earlier in this appendix.
- Always transmit the cover sheet last so that it covers the confidential fax information. Reversing the order of the pages before faxing is appreciated by the receiver of the communication. For example, fax pages in this order: page 5, page 4, page 3, page 2, page 1,

cover sheet. When you transmit documents in this manner, the information is received in order and protected information is covered after being transmitted through the fax.

Standing Orders

Standing orders should be used only with great discretion. Prescription drugs should not be included in standing orders. Avoid using standing orders as a means of notifying the physician of a change in patient condition. If used, a standing order must be validated and made a part of the patient's medical record. Follow normal facility policies for obtaining the physician's signature. Previsit tests may not be ordered by staff personnel as part of a general standing order protocol. Instead, the staff may obtain information about a patient, then the physician may order previsit testing (order sheet or verbal order) on a case-by-case basis.

Other Issues with Orders

- All orders must be reviewed when a patient goes to or returns from the operating room, changes level of care (e.g., ICU to medical unit), or is transferred to another clinical service. Note "orders reviewed" in your documentation.
- Preprinted order lists may be used if individualized to the specific patient by the physician's editing. The preprinted order list must have the physician's editing, the patient's name and medical record number in the upper right-hand corner, the date, and the physician's signature.
- DNR orders require a physician's order with each admission and change in level of care. They must be reviewed and renewed while the patient is hospitalized. The state-required forms must be on the chart. *Read the forms.* Do not assume that every advance directive contains a DNR order.
- If an individual states that he or she is the appointee in a durable power of attorney for health care for a patient, request a copy of the verification form.
- A dated, timed, and signed order is required before a patient is discharged.

Validating Orders

All orders must be countersigned as required by state law and facility policy. The physician (or other health care provider) must sign his or her own orders. One health care provider cannot sign an order given by another provider.

Transcribing and Noting Orders

- A licensed nurse is responsible for transcribing orders, such as telephone orders.
- The nurse must verify the accuracy of the transcription, and retains responsibility for accurate transcription.
- Transcribe verbal and telephone orders exactly as given by the physician (or other health care provider).
- Check the list of acceptable abbreviations. Misinterpretation of handwritten abbreviations is a major cause of error in health care facilities. If an unauthorized abbreviation is used, contact the physician for clarification. Do not guess at the meaning.
- Draw a horizontal line down and across the page below the order and the physician's signature in such a manner as to prevent any additional orders from being inserted.
- When transcribing medication orders, order the drug(s) from the pharmacy. List the medication and start time on the MAR.
- Order tests and schedule procedures promptly. Note these on the Kardex. Check to determine whether special preparation (such as NPO or a laxative solution) is needed. If so, order the appropriate preparation, schedule it, and note it on the Kardex and other appropriate location.
- Admission orders and postoperative orders must be transcribed as soon as possible, within a maximum of 60 minutes after receipt.
- All health care professional orders (including verbal, telephone, fax, etc.) must be noted and authenticated by a licensed nurse. The nurse must write "noted," date the order, note the time the order was authenticated, and sign the order with his or her name and title.
- The health unit coordinator or other qualified paraprofessional may assist the RN with order transcription as permitted by state law and the state nurse practice act. If transcription is delegated, the nurse and other paraprofessional both sign off on the order.

Appendix D
Procedures and Other
Useful Information

CARING FOR A PATIENT WITH A T-TUBE

T-tubes are named for their shape. This T-shaped tool is used to drain bile and keep the common bile duct open after cholecystectomy (gallbladder removal surgery). The crossbar of the T is placed in the common bile duct. The other end of the tube exits the skin through an incision in the right upper quadrant. The T-tube is seldom sutured in place, but it usually fits tightly. It may be kept in place for six weeks or more. The tube is normally attached to a sterile closed drainage system that includes a catheter bag. Attaching the T-tube to a sterile leg drainage bag provides the patient with more mobility. You may use the bag to collect the bile. Measure it in a graduated pitcher. The bile drainage is very irritating, so keeping it from contacting the skin is a high priority. Applying dry sterile dressings around the insertion site (Procedure 22) will help protect the skin. Check the T-tube every few hours to make sure it is not kinked or obstructed.

T-Tube Drainage

Observe the patient closely for bile leakage, which will irritate the skin and may indicate obstruction. During the first 24 hours after surgery, the tube will drain approximately 300 mL to 500 mL of blood-tinged bile. Inform the RN promptly if drainage exceeds 500 mL during the first 24 postoperative

hours. Daily drainage usually decreases to 200 mL or less after five days, although it may be as much as 1,000 mL. Bile is normally thick, sticky, and gummy or syrupy, and green-brown in color. To prevent excessive bile loss, secure the T-tube drainage system at abdominal level. If bile drainage is excessive (more than 1,000 mL daily), the RN or physician must return the bile to the patient's digestive system orally or through a nasogastric tube. PCT responsibilities include:

- Check the T-tube for patency and site condition every hour for the first 8 hours.
- After the first 8 hours, check the tube every 4 hours, or as instructed.
- Provide conscientious skin care and frequent dressing changes.
- Keep the skin clean and well protected. Use Montgomery straps to avoid irritating the skin with tape.
- Monitor urine and stools carefully. Promptly report color changes to the RN.
- Monitor the patient for jaundice in the skin and sclera, and notify the RN if jaundice is present.
- Inform the RN if the color or viscosity of the T-tube drainage changes, or if the drainage increases.
- Monitor and document strict intake and output.

Procedure D-1

Caring for a T-Tube or Similar Wound Drain

Supplies needed:
- Graduated collection container
- Disposable exam gloves, 1 pair
- Sterile gloves, 1 pair
- Disposable underpad
- Sterile 4 × 4 gauze pads
- Transparent dressings
- Normal saline solution
- Sterile cleaning solution
- Sterile basins, 2
- Povidone-iodine sponges
- Sterile precut drain dressings
- Tape
- Skin protectant, such as petroleum jelly, zinc oxide, or aluminum-based gel
- Montgomery straps, if used
- Plastic bag for used supplies

1. Perform your beginning procedure actions.
2. Check the expiration date on each sterile item and inspect for tears, cracks, or other packaging problems. If the normal saline or cleansing solution has been opened, check the date. Discard if it has been open longer than 24 hours, or according to facility policies.
3. Open the plastic trash bag and position it at the foot of the bed, or tape it to the side of the table in the open position. Make sure you will not have to reach across the sterile field to discard trash.
4. Clean the overbed table with disinfectant solution and allow it to dry. Cover with a disposable underpad, according to facility policy.
5. Position additional underpads under the patient to contain spills, if needed.
6. Wash your hands or use alcohol-based hand cleaner.
7. Open sterile equipment and establish a sterile field.
8. Using sterile technique, place one sterile 4 × 4 gauze pad in each basin.
9. Pour 50 mL of cleansing solution into one basin.
10. Pour 50 mL of normal saline solution into the second basin.
11. Wash your hands or use alcohol-based hand cleaner.
12. Apply disposable exam gloves. Apply other PPE, if necessary.
13. Carefully remove the soiled dressing and discard it in the plastic bag.
14. Remove soiled gloves and discard them in the plastic bag.
15. Wash your hands or use alcohol-based hand cleaner.
16. Apply sterile gloves and other PPE, if indicated.
17. Inspect the incision and tube for edema, warmth, redness, tenderness, induration, irritation, or other signs and symptoms of infection.
18. Rinse the cleansing solution using a 4 × 4 gauze pad and normal saline solution.
19. Pat dry gently with 4 × 4 pads, or allow to air-dry.
20. Cleanse the skin with a povidone-iodine sponge by working in a circle beginning at the T-tube and moving outward.
21. Allow the area to dry.
22. Lightly apply a skin protectant around the tube.
23. Apply a sterile precut drain dressing on each side of the T-tube.
24. Apply a sterile 4 × 4 gauze pad or transparent film over the T-tube and other dressings. Make sure the tubing is not kinked or blocked. Avoid placing the dressing over the open end of the T-tube where it connects to the drainage system. Fasten the dressings with tape or Montgomery straps.
25. Remove your gloves and discard them in the plastic bag.
26. Perform your procedure completion actions.

Clamping the T-Tube

The T-tube is usually clamped for one hour before and one hour after each meal. Clamping the tube alters the flow of bile so it moves back to the duodenum to aid digestion. Clamping the tube may be an RN procedure in your facility. However, you must understand the purpose of clamping the tube. You will monitor the patient's response to clamping and watch for signs of obstructed bile flow. Check the bile drainage level in the closed-system drain bag regularly. Monitor for and report to the RN promptly:

- Fever
- Chills
- Rapid pulse
- Nausea and/or vomiting
- Complaints of pain or fullness in the right upper quadrant
- Jaundice
- Foamy, dark urine
- Clay-colored stools

USING A CLOSED WOUND DRAINAGE SYSTEM

The Jackson-Pratt and Hemovac drains are commonly used for closed drainage systems. The drains are placed directly in a wound, and drainage goes into an expandable container. A record of the amount and character of drainage is entered in both the output record and the nursing notes. It is your responsibility to:

- Report either heavy or light drainage
- Report a change in the appearance, amount, or character of drainage
- Make sure the flow of drainage is not blocked

Observations to make and report include:

- Drain is not intact or patent
- Drain appears blocked, dislodged, or kinked
- Surrounding skin appears abnormal (erosion, red, hot, swollen, macerated)
- Drainage is eroding surrounding healthy skin
- Drainage is purulent, cloudy, foul- or abnormal-smelling
- Drainage color changes or appears abnormal
- Amount of drainage decreases markedly or stops entirely
- Amount of drainage increases markedly
- Patient has fever, tachycardia, hypotension
- Urinary output decreases

Closed wound drainage promotes healing and prevents swelling of the postoperative wound. Various systems are used to apply gentle suction to the wound. This removes accumulated serosanguineous fluid and reduces tension on the suture line. It also decreases the risk of skin breakdown, eliminates the need for many dressing changes, and helps reduce the risk of infection.

Hemovac® and Jackson-Pratt® closed drainage systems are the most common. These systems use perforated tubing and a vacuum unit to remove wound drainage. The proximal end of the tube is in the wound bed. The tubing usually has its own exit site, and is commonly sutured to the skin to prevent displacement. It seldom extends through the suture line. Thus, the patient will have two surgical wounds. The drain is usually left in place for 7 to 10 days, but the length of time is determined by the wound drainage. Wound drainage must be frequently emptied and measured to maintain suction and prevent pulling and stretching on the suture line. Select the proper PPE needed for the procedure, and use conscientious aseptic technique.

Procedure D-2

Caring for a Closed Wound Drainage System

Supplies needed:
- Graduated collection container
- Sterile basin
- Alcohol sponges
- Povidone-iodine sponges or swabsticks or sterile cleaning solution
- Sterile normal saline solution for rinsing
- Sterile 4 × 4 gauze pads
- Disposable underpad
- Disposable exam gloves (2 pair), or sterile gloves if facility policy
- Protective gown

(continues)

Procedure **D-2**, *continued*

Caring for a Closed Wound Drainage System

▶ Eye protection
▶ Surgical mask
▶ Plastic bag for used supplies

1. Perform your beginning procedure actions.
2. Clean the overbed table with disinfectant solution and allow it to dry. Cover with a disposable underpad, according to facility policy.
3. Position an additional underpad on the edge of the bed where you will be working, to contain spills, if needed.
4. Open the plastic trash bag and position it at the foot of the bed, or tape it to the side of the table in the open position. Make sure you will not have to reach across the sterile field to discard trash.
5. Wash your hands or use alcohol-based hand cleaner.
6. Unclip the drain unit from the patient's bed.
7. Using aseptic technique, carefully open the drain spout to allow the unit to fill with air and expand.
8. Empty the unit into a graduated container or sterile basin by gently squeezing and compressing the plastic.
9. Note the amount and appearance of the drainage.
10. Carefully wipe the spout and plug it with an alcohol sponge.
11. Gently compress the unit fully to reestablish the vacuum. Hold the unit closed with one hand while replacing the plug with the other hand.
12. Fasten the unit to the bed or patient's gown. Make sure the container is below the level

of the wound. Leave the drainage tubing loose. It should not be so tight that it pulls on the wound or dislodges.
13. Remove soiled gloves and discard them in the plastic bag.
14. Wash your hands or use alcohol-based hand cleaner.
15. Apply disposable exam gloves.
16. Using sterile technique, place one sterile 4 × 4 gauze pad in each basin.
17. Pour 50 mL of cleansing solution into one basin.
18. Pour 50 mL of normal saline solution into the second basin.
19. Carefully remove the soiled dressing covering the incision and discard it in the plastic bag.
20. Inspect the incision and tube for edema, warmth, redness, tenderness, induration, irritation, or other signs and symptoms of infection.
21. Cleanse the suture line with a povidone-iodine sponge, swabstick, or designated cleansing solution. Rinse with normal saline, if needed, depending on the product you are using.
22. Pat dry gently with 4 × 4 pads, or allow to air-dry.
23. Apply a dressing to the incision, as instructed.
24. Remove your gloves and discard them in the plastic bag.
25. Perform your procedure completion actions.

Procedure **D-3**

Discontinuing an IV and Switching to a Heparin Lock

Supplies needed:
▶ Disposable exam gloves and other protective equipment (mask, eye protection, gown) as needed and as required by facility policy
▶ Sterile heparin lock kit with extension tubing
▶ 2- or 3-mL syringe with 25-gauge needle
▶ Saline, heparin, or designated solution to maintain lock

(continues)

Procedure **D-3**, *continued*

Discontinuing an IV and Switching to a Heparin Lock

- ▶ Alcohol or designated prep solution pads
- ▶ Sharps container

1. Perform your beginning procedure actions.
2. Open the sterile heparin lock package. Prime the extension tubing with saline, or designated solution, as instructed by the RN.
3. Turn the roller clamp to stop the flow of IV solution.
4. Loosen the IV tubing and carefully remove it.
5. Remove the protective cover from the heparin lock and screw the lock into the hub of the cannula.

6. Cleanse the diaphragm of the heparin lock with alcohol and allow it to dry.
7. Insert a 25-gauge needle (attached to a filled syringe) into the rubber diaphragm.
8. Gently pull back on the plunger to establish blood flow.
9. Check the patency of the lock by slowly injecting saline or designated solution into the protective diaphragm.
10. Remove and discard the needle and syringe.
11. Wipe the diaphragm with alcohol.
12. Check for irritation, leakage, and infiltration.
13. Perform your procedure completion actions.

ADDITIONAL METHODS FOR VERSATILE CARDIAC MONITORING

Versatility is sometimes essential to get an accurate snapshot of the heart. There are times, such as during some diagnostic tests, when you may be instructed to perform a three-lead or five-lead ECG. Monitoring of ambulatory patients may be done by using a Holter monitor. The instruction manual for the ECG machine should show pictures for proper lead placement.

Three-Lead ECG

Leads are placed on the shoulder area, at the right apex (RA) and left apex (LA). The leads on the shoulders may be either anterior or posterior. The third lead is positioned on the patient's side, and may be on either the left lung (LL) or the right lung (RL) (**Figure D-1**).

Five-Lead ECG

Leads are placed on the shoulder area, at the right apex (RA) and left apex (LA). The leads on the shoulders may be either anterior or posterior. The next two leads are positioned on the patient's side, on both the left lung (LL) and the right lung (RL). The fifth lead is the ventricular lead (V). This is positioned to the right of the sternum (**Figure D-2**).

Holter Monitor Application

The Holter monitor is a diagnostic tool that allows continuous monitoring for a 24-hour period. It is used both in the hospital and at home to diagnose intermittent or sporadic dysrhythmias. The Holter monitor is used for the patient with abnormal signs and symptoms whose 12-lead ECG is normal. It may also be used to check pacemaker function, and to determine if cardiac medications are effective. The patient is encouraged to go about his or her usual daily activities when the monitor is being used. However, the patient may not bathe when wearing the monitor. By going about normal daily routines, rhythm abnormalities can be correlated with the patient's signs, symptoms, and precipitating factors.

When a Holter monitor is used, special electrodes and leadwires are attached to the patient's chest. A special, battery-operated, magnetic or computer tape recorder records heart activity for a 24-hour period. The patient wears the tape recorder in a leather pouch. The patient must:

- Keep a written diary listing times, daily activities, symptoms, and emotions.
- Avoid handling the electrodes.
- Not remove the tape recorder from the leather pouch.
- Avoid using an electric blanket or heating pad.
- Depress the button marked "event marker" quickly when experiencing a significant symptom.

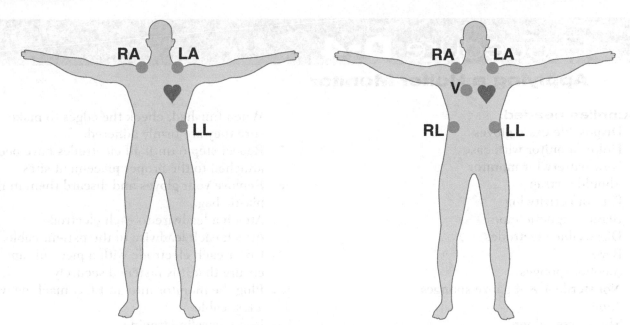

FIGURE D-1 Three-lead ECG.

FIGURE D-2 Five-lead ECG.

Disposable, pre-gelled leads are used for the Holter monitor. Lead placement is different from ECG placement. Four or five leads are used, depending on the device and whether it has an internal ground. Lead placement is listed in Table D–1.

At the end of the 24-hour monitoring period, the patient returns to the physician's office or hospital and the Holter monitor is removed. The rhythm is analyzed by a special scanner or computer, and the physician is provided with a report.

Table D-1 Holter Monitor Electrode Placement		
Electrode	**Lead**	**Location**
A (black)	mV$_1$	Fourth intercostal space at right of sternal edge
B (white)	mV$_5$	Right clavicle, just lateral to sternum
C (brown)	mV$_1$	Left clavicle, just lateral to sternum
D (red)	mV$_5$	Fifth intercostal space at left axillary line
E (green)	ground	Lower right chest wall

Procedure D-4

Applying a Holter Monitor

Supplies needed:
- Disposable exam gloves
- Holter monitor with case
- New battery for monitor
- Shoulder strap
- Patient activity log
- Blank magnetic tape
- Disposable electrodes
- Razor
- Alcohol sponges
- Nonsterile 4 × 4 gauze sponges
- Tape
- Sharps container
- Plastic bag (or wastebasket) for used supplies

1. Perform your beginning procedure actions.
2. Remove the used battery from the monitor and replace it with a new battery.
3. Wash your hands or use alcohol-based hand cleaner.
4. Apply exam gloves.
5. Prepare the skin on the chest in the areas of electrode placement.
   - Dry-shave the hair on electrode placement sites.
   - Rub the shaved areas with alcohol sponges. Allow to air-dry.
   - With a dry 4 × 4 gauze pad, *gently* scrub back and forth on each electrode placement site to abrade the skin. The skin should appear red, but not broken.
   - Discard the razor in the sharps container.
6. Open the package of electrodes and remove the backing paper from one electrode. Apply the electrode to the first placement site by pressing the center of the self-adhesive electrode, then moving out toward the edges. Work in a circle, not side to side.

When finished, check the edges to make sure they are firmly adhered.
7. Repeat step 6 until all electrodes have been attached to the proper placement sites.
8. Remove your gloves and discard them in the plastic bag.
9. Attach a leadwire to each electrode.
10. Attach each leadwire to the patient cable.
11. Cover each electrode with a piece of tape to ensure that it is fastened securely.
12. Plug the monitor into an ECG machine with a test cable.
13. Run a baseline tracing.
14. Validate that the tracing is legible and that the unit is working properly.
15. Have the patient put a shirt on. Assist if necessary.
16. Thread the electrode cable through the buttons of the patient's shirt or below the hem of the shirt.
17. Place the recorder in the carrying case and attach it to the patient's belt or over the shoulder. Make sure there is no tension or pulling on the leadwires.
18. Plug the electrode cable into the monitor.
19. Document the starting time in the patient's activity log.
20. Give the log to the patient and make sure he or she knows how to use it.
21. Demonstrate how to use the "event marker" marker button and ask the patient to do a return demonstration.
22. Inform the patient when to return to have the monitor removed. Remind him or her to bring the activity log.
23. Give the patient a 24-hour phone number in case help is needed.
24. Wash your hands or use alcohol-based hand cleaner.
25. Perform your procedure completion actions.

HEART AND ELECTROCARDIOGRAM STUDY GUIDE

An *electrocardiogram* is a graphic representation of the cardiac cycle.

Anatomy of the Heart

- Four chambers
- Two upper chambers called *atria*
- Two lower chambers called *ventricles*

Circulation

- Deoxygenated blood enters the right atrium and passes into the right ventricle
- Blood travels to the lungs via the pulmonary arteries
- Deoxygenated blood eliminates carbon dioxide and picks up oxygen
- Oxygenated blood travels back to the heart through the pulmonary veins
- Blood enters the left atrium and passes into the left ventricle
- Blood then travels out to the rest of the body

Order of Electrical Conduction (Figure D-3)

- Sinoatrial (SA) node
- Atrioventricular (AV) node
- Bundle of His
- Right and left bundle branches
- Purkinje fibers

Reading an ECG

- Horizontal direction equals time; vertical direction equals voltage
- P wave—positive deflection; atrial depolarization; atrial contraction
- QRS complex—Q/S negative deflections and R positive deflection; ventricular depolarization; ventricular contraction
- T wave—positive deflection; ventricular repolarization; ventricular relaxation

ECG Graph Paper

- Divided into 5 mm and 1 mm squares
- 25 small squares in each large square

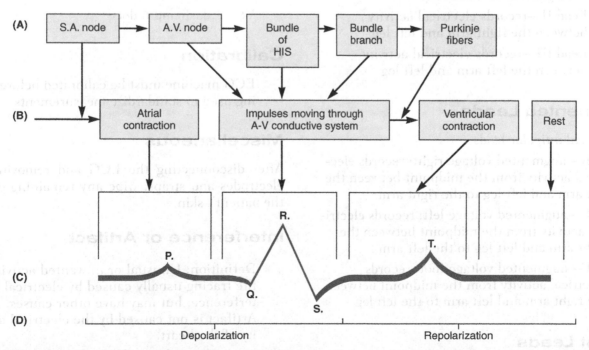

FIGURE D-3 Diagrammatic representations of cardiac impulses on an ECG tracing: (A) course of electrical impulses; (B) cardiac muscle reaction to impulses; (C) ECG tracing of impulse waves; (D) phases of cardiac cycle. (Courtesy of Spacelabs Medical, Inc.)

- Horizontally, one small square represents 0.04 second
- Vertically, one small square represents 1 mm of voltage

Interpretive ECG

Some ECG machines have built-in computer programs to interpret the tracing. However, a physician will manually review and verify each ECG.

Lead Placement

- Four limb leads:
  - Right arm (RA)
  - Left arm (LA)
  - Right leg (RL)—not used as part of the recording; reference point only
  - Left leg (LL)
- Six chest (precordial) leads

Limb Leads

- Called *bipolar* because each uses two limb electrodes that record simultaneously
- The first three leads are recorded
  - Lead I—records electrical activity between the right arm and left arm
  - Lead II—records electrical activity between the right arm and left leg
  - Lead III—records electrical activity between the left arm and left leg

Augmented Leads

- Called *unipolar* leads
- aVR—augmented voltage right; records electrical activity from the midpoint between the left arm and left leg to the right arm
- aVL—augmented voltage left; records electrical activity from the midpoint between the right arm and left leg to the left arm
- aVF—augmented voltage foot; records electrical activity from the midpoint between the right arm and left arm to the left leg

Chest Leads

- Also called *precordial* leads

Remaining Six Leads

- Called unipolar leads
- V1—fourth intercostal space at right margin of sternum
- V2—fourth intercostal space at left margin of sternum
- V4—fifth intercostal space on left midclavicular line
- V3—midway between V2 and V4
- V5—horizontal to V4 at left anterior axillary line
- V6—horizontal to V4 at left midaxillary line

Coding

- Lead I—1 dot
- Lead II—2 dots
- Lead III—3 dots
- aVR—1 dash
- aVL—2 dashes
- aVF—3 dashes
- V1—1 dash and 1 dot
- V2—1 dash and 2 dots
- V3—1 dash and 3 dots
- V4—1 dash and 4 dots
- V5—1 dash and 5 dots
- V6—1 dash and 6 dots

Calibration

- ECG machine must be calibrated before being used to standardize measurements

Miscellaneous

After disconnecting the ECG and removing the electrodes and straps, wipe any remaining gel off the patient's skin.

Interference or Artifact

- Definition: Unusual or unwanted activity in the tracing usually caused by electrical interference, but may have other causes. Artifact is not caused by the electrical activity of the heart.
- Apply electrodes to the fleshy part of a limb to minimize artifact.

- Most common artifacts:
  - Somatic tremor—Occurs when the patient is uncomfortable, moves, talks, coughs, and so on.
  - Alternating current (AC) interference— Electricity present in medical equipment, or wires in the area are leaking a tiny amount of energy into the room
  - Wandering baseline artifact—Occurs when the stylus suddenly moves from the center of the ECG paper, resulting in "wandering" baseline across the ECG paper.
  - Interrupted baseline artifacts—Baseline is interrupted, creating a break between complexes; caused by a broken patient cable or a lead wire that has become detached from an electrode

  Causes of artifact include:
- Electrodes applied too loosely or too tightly
- Corroded or dirty electrodes and/or metal tips of the leadwires
- Inappropriate amount or poor-quality electrode gel or paste
- Lotions, oils, or creams on patient's skin
- Patient is cold

Arrhythmias

- Premature atrial contractions (PAC)
  - Can be experienced by healthy people
  - Seen in patients who use stimulants
  - Cardiac cycle occurs early
  - Usually not life-threatening
- Paroxysmal atrial tachycardia (PAT)
  - Comes on abruptly
  - Heart rate regular at 160–250 bpm
- Atrial fibrillation
  - Rapid, incomplete contractions
  - Irregular irregularity
  - Can be as fast as 400–500 bpm
  - P waves cannot be distinguished
- Premature ventricular contractions (PVCs)
  - May be caused by tobacco, anxiety, alcohol, and epinephrine
  - Ventricles act as pacemaker and fire early in cycle; a pause follows the PVC
- Ventricular tachycardia

  - Seen in patients with cardiac disease
  - Three or more PVCs at 150–250 bpm
  - Life-threatening rhythm

Holter Monitors

Definition: A portable continuous recording of cardiac activity for a 24-hour period, worn by the patient during normal activities of daily living.
- Attach the Holter monitor to the patient.
- Abrade the skin with a dry gauze pad.
- Check the monitor with a test cable.
- Print out a test strip to serve as the patient's baseline and verify that the monitor is working.
- Use four or five electrodes, depending on whether the unit has a built-in ground.
- The patient must keep an activity log or diary listing times, daily activities, symptoms, and emotions.

CALCULATING INTRAVENOUS DRIP RATES

Although intravenous infusions are usually administered through a pump, you must be able to calculate fluid drip rates in the event of pump failure, pump unavailability, power failure, or other reason. Before beginning, you must know:
- The drop factor (information on the tubing package that states how many drops of fluid are in each milliliter)
- The amount of solution to be infused
- The time frame over which the solution is to be infused

Formula for calculating the drip rate:

$$\left(\frac{\text{Total volume to be infused}}{\text{Total hours for infusion}} \right) \times \left(\frac{\text{drop factor}^*}{60 \text{ min/hr}} \right) = \left(\begin{array}{c} \text{drops/min} \\ \text{or mL/hour} \end{array} \right)$$

*Drop factor:
  60 drops/minute, use 1 in the formula
  20 drops/minute, use 1/3 in the formula
  15 drops/minute, use 1/4 in the formula
  10 drops/minute, use 1/6 in the formula

When administering an intermittent infusion, such as antibiotic therapy, use this formula:

$$\frac{\text{Total volume to be infused}}{} \div \frac{\text{minutes to administer}}{60 \text{ minutes/hr}} = \frac{\text{mL}}{\text{hr}}$$

The following estimations may be used:

Prescription	10 drops/mL	15 drops/mL	20 drops/mL	60 drops/mL
10 mL/hr	2	2	4	12
20 mL/hr	3	6	7	21
30 mL/hr	5	7	11	33
40 mL/hr	7	10	15	45
50 mL/hr	8	12	19	57
60 mL/hr	10	15	22	66
70 mL/hr	12	17	26	
80 mL/hr	13	20	29	
90 mL/hr	15	22	33	
100 mL/hr	17	25	36	
110 mL/hr	18	27	38	
120 mL/hr	20	30	40	
130 mL/hr	22	32	43	
140 mL/hr	23	35	46	
150 mL/hr	25	37	52	
160 mL/hr	27	40	55	
170 mL/hr	28	42	59	
180 mL/hr	30	45	62	
190 mL/hr	32	47	65	
200 mL/hr	33	50	68	

Amount per hour	Amount per 8 hours	Amount per 24 hours	Drops per minute
Microdrip (60 drops/mL)			
4	30	90	4
5	40	120	5
6	50	150	6
8	60	180	8
9	70	210	9
10	80	240	10
12	100	300	12
14	110	330	14
18	150	450	18
22	180	540	22
25	200	600	25
30	250	750	30
37	300	900	37
Drop factor 10 drops/mL			
30	240	720	5
40	320	960	6
50	400	1200	8
60	480	1440	10
70	560	1680	11
80	640	1920	13
90	720	2160	15
100	800	2400	16
125	1000	3000	21

Amount per hour	Amount per 8 hours	Amount per 24 hours	Drops per minute
	Drop factor 15 drops/mL		
30	240	720	7
40	320	960	10
50	400	1200	12
60	480	1440	15
70	560	1680	17
80	640	1920	20
90	720	2160	22
100	800	2400	25
125	1000	3000	30

Formula for amount per hour:

$$\frac{\text{Total infusion volume}}{\text{Time of infusion (hours)}} = \text{Milliliters per hour}$$

Formula for infusion time:

$$\frac{\text{Total mL to be infused}}{\text{mL delivered per hour}} = \frac{\text{Infusion time}}{\text{(Hour)}}$$

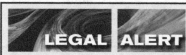

LEGAL ALERT

Always follow your hospital policies and procedures for double-checking the drip rate. For your protection, ask the RN to review your calculations. You should not be ashamed to do this. RNs also check each other's work, especially when giving drugs such as insulin and anticoagulants. This is a routine safeguard that protects you legally and ensures patient safety.

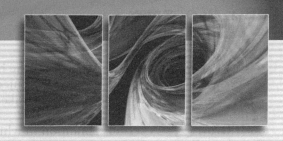

Glossary

NOTE: Numbers in brackets are chapter numbers in which the term first appears.

A

abduction pillow [11]—A special pillow used to keep the legs apart when patients have had hip replacement surgery.

absence seizure [13]—Seizure that begins without warning and consists of a period of unconsciousness, during which the patient blinks rapidly, stares blankly, breathes rapidly, or makes chewing movements. Usually lasts less than a minute, but may occur many times a day.

acupuncture [13]—An ancient practice dating back thousands of years that is used to treat many acute and chronic conditions. Tiny, thin needles are placed in various parts of the body to correct imbalances in energy.

acute pain [13]—Pain that occurs suddenly and without warning that is usually the result of tissue damage, caused by conditions such as injury or surgery. The pain decreases over time, as healing takes place.

adjunctive device [17]—A secondary device used to maintain respirations.

administration set [7]—A flexible, plastic tube through which solution flows; the set is attached to the IV solution on one end and the patient on the other.

advance directive [17]—A document that designates the patient's wishes if he or she cannot speak for himself or herself. Advance directives can be in the form of a living will, which designates the patient's wishes if he or she is in a terminal condition. The patient also has the right to designate a surrogate decision maker, often called a *health care proxy.* The facility is obligated to follow the patient's written directions in these documents.

adverse events [1]—Untoward incidents, events, and injuries associated with patient care and services; may result from commission or omission.

aerobic [6]—Able to live only in the presence of oxygen.

air embolus [7]—A serious complicaton of IV therapy in which air enters the bloodstream, moving freely throughout the body.

air entrainment mask [14]—Also called *Venturi mask, venti mask,* and *high airflow with oxygen enrichment (HAFOE) mask.* An oxygen mask that is similar to a simple mask, but has a large plastic tube at the bottom. It mixes oxygen with room air to obtain the percentage of oxygen ordered by the physician.

airborne [3]—Route of infection whereby very small pathogens suspended in dust and moisture in the air are inhaled by a susceptible host.

airborne precautions [3]—A category of transmission-based precautions that health care workers use to protect themselves from airborne pathogens.

airway [17]—The structure through which air enters and leaves the body.

anaerobic [6]—Able to live without oxygen.

angiogram [16]—*See* arteriogram.

antecubital space [6]—The area in front of the elbow, commonly used for drawing blood or starting an intravenous infusion.

antibodies [7]—Substances produced by the immune system when foreign organisms or materials enter the body; a protective mechanism against foreign materials.

anticoagulants [6]—Medications that thin the blood, preventing clots from forming.

antiembolism stockings [11]—Support hosiery used for patients who have circulation problems or high-risk conditions.

antigens [7]—Foreign substances that cause an allergic reaction, which can be life-threatening; antigens always stimulate an immune response.

appliance [8]—The plastic container into which the contents of the bowel are emptied for patients with ostomies.

aquathermia pad [12]—A plastic pad with coils on the inside used for heating and cooling.

arteriogram [16]—An X-ray study of the blood vessels in which contrast medium is injected through a catheter while an X-ray is taken simultaneously.

aspiration [9]—A serious condition in which food or liquid enters the lungs.

assign [1]—Inform, instruct, or advise another person to complete a task; the person assigning the task must have the authority to do so.

asystole [17]—A lack of rhythm; seen on the cardiac monitor when the heart stops beating.

atelectasis [11]—Inability to expand the lungs due to collapse of the alveolar air sacs.

atrioventricular node [16]—Also known as *AV node;* located on the bottom of the atrium, just above the ventricles; conducts electrical impulses to the ventricles.

audiologist [13]—A person with a degree, license, and certification in audiology (science of hearing) who measures hearing, identifies hearing loss, and participates in rehabilitation of hearing impairment.

augmented limb leads [16]—ECG leads AVR, AVL, and AVF. The electrical signals reflected in these leads are tiny and far away from the heart. The ECG machine enlarges them.

aura [13]—A sensation, smell, taste, or bright light that precedes and may signal the onset of a seizure.

autoclave [4]—Equipment that uses heat and steam to sterilize instruments and other items.

automatic external defibrillator (AED) [17]—A computerized device that uses an electric shock to reverse disorganized activity in the heart during cardiac arrest.

autonomic dysreflexia [13]—A potentially life-threatening complication of spinal cord injury triggered by conditions that would normally cause pain below the level of spinal injury.

B

bag-valve mask (BVM) [17]—*See* bag-valve-mask device.

bag-valve-mask device [15]—Device commonly used in health care facilities to support patients who are in respiratory arrest; consists of a face mask and a ventilation bag.

bandage [5]—Fabric, gauze, net, or elasticized material used to cover dressings to keep the dressings securely in place.

barrier [1]—Something that interferes with communication; can be physical or mental.

battered woman syndrome [13]—A pattern of signs and symptoms, such as fearfulness, hopelessness, and helplessness, commonly seen in women who have experienced physical and emotional abuse over a long period of time.

benchmark [1]—A standard reference point against which performance is measured.

benchmarking [1]—An activity in which an organization establishes best practices by comparing what it is doing with what other, similar organizations are doing, and using this information to improve internal facility work processes.

bevel [6]—The slant or inclination at the end of a needle.

bilevel positive airway pressure (BiPAP) [14]—A ventilatory device that maintains positive airway pressure during both inspiration and expiration.

bioterrorism [3]—The use of biological agents, such as pathogenic organisms or agricultural pests, for terrorist purposes.

bipolar leads [16]—Leads I, II, and III on the ECG; a bipolar lead shows the difference in electrical potential between two limb electrodes.

blood culture [6]—A test done to detect the presence of a systemic infection.

brachytherapy [13]—A form of radiation therapy in which tiny radioactive seeds or pellets are implanted directly inside the body.

bundle of His [16]—Group of fibers in the heart that conducts an electrical impulse after the impulse leaves the AV node; conducts the impulse to the right and left bundle branches and Purkinje fibers. The bundle of His, left and right bundle branches, and Purkinje fibers work together to cause the ventricles to contract.

buried bumper syndrome [9]—An ulceration of the tissue at the feeding tube exit site or the internal mucosal layer of the gastric wall that may occur with a tube that has internal and external retention bumpers holding the tube in place.

butterfly [6]—A winged infusion needle used for drawing blood or starting an intravenous infusion.

C

cannula [15]—An indwelling tube inserted through a tracheostomy stoma to maintain patency.

capillary refill [14]—A test of the patient's peripheral circulation that indicates how well the tissues are being nourished with oxygen.

capillary tube [6]—A slender, short, hollow tube used for collecting a capillary blood specimen.

carbon dioxide (CO_2) [14]—A waste product produced by every cell in the body; transported in the venous blood.

cardiac arrest [17]—A condition in which the heart stops beating.

cardiac cycle [16]—Consists of two phases, contraction and relaxation. During contraction, the heart beats, pumping blood to the body. During the relaxation phase, the heart rests and recovers.

cardiopulmonary resuscitation (CPR) [17]—A lifesaving procedure in which the heart is manually squeezed between the sternum and the spine, to circulate blood throughout the body, while simultaneously providing artificial ventilation to the patient.

carrier [3]—A person who is infected with a disease that can be spread to others; the carrier may not know of the infection.

catheter embolus [7]—A condition in which a sheared piece of an intravenous catheter floats freely in the patient's bloodstream, greatly increasing the risk of complications.

causative agent [3]—The microbe that causes a disease.

Centers for Disease Control and Prevention (CDC) [3]—A federal agency that studies diseases and makes recommendations on protective measures.

central intravenous catheter [7]—A long catheter that is inserted into a vein in the shoulder or neck area; the tip of the catheter is placed in the superior vena cava or right atrium of the heart.

central terminal [16]—A reference system at the intersection of ECG leads I, II, and III; the three leads created by this juncture are AVR, AVL, and AVF.

centrifuge [6]—A device that holds and spins test tubes.

chain of infection [3]—A diagram showing the six factors necessary for an infection to develop.

chart [2]—The binder or notebook containing the patient's medical record.

chemotherapy [13]—Therapy that incorporates the use of medications or drugs to destroy cancer.

chest tubes [15]—Sterile plastic tubes that are inserted through the skin of the chest, between the ribs, and into the space between the pleural membrane that covers the lung and the pleural membrane that lines the chest wall. Chest tubes are used after surgery to drain fluids from the chest.

chronic pain [13]—*See* persistent pain.

CircOlectric bed [11]—An electronic bed that is rotated to reposition the patient between the back and the abdomen. The patient is secured to the inner frame before the bed is moved. The entire inner frame is rotated forward to allow position change without causing stress on the patient.

cleansing enema [8]—An injection of water-based fluid into the anus to remove fecal material from the rectum and lower bowel, stimulate peristalsis, and soften stool.

close call [1]—An event or situation that could have resulted in an adverse event but did not, either by chance or through timely intervention. May also be called a *near miss.*

coagulate [6]—Clot.

coagulation tube [6]—A tube with a blue stopper; used when drawing blood for coagulation (clotting) studies, such as prothrombin time.

colonization [10]—The multiplication of a microbe after it has invaded a wound. Colonization indicates only that the microbe has successfully reproduced; there are no signs or symptoms of infection.

colostomy [8]—The most common type of ostomy; located between the colon and the abdomen.

commercially prepared enema [8]—Small, premeasured container of solution injected into the anus to remove fecal material from the rectum and lower bowel, stimulate peristalsis, and soften stool. Commercially prepared enemas are available with either cleansing or retention enema solutions.

compartment syndrome [11]—Condition that occurs when pressure within the fascia compartment of a muscle builds up, preventing blood and oxygen from reaching the tissues. The primary symptom is severe pain.

competent [1]—Describes someone who knows how to correctly perform the procedures he or she is responsible for.

complementary and alternative medicine (CAM) [13]—A group of diverse systems, practices, and products that are not presently considered part of conventional medicine. Some CAM practices have been proven unsafe or ineffective and are no longer used. Others have proven safe and effective and have become part of mainstream health care.

complex-partial seizure [13]—Temporary change in consciousness that causes abnormal acts, irrational behavior, or loss of judgment; automatic behavior may continue normally. Usually lasts only a few seconds.

congenital disorder [13]—Condition present at birth.

consent [17]—Permission for treatment; given by the patient when he or she is able (conscious and alert), or a health care proxy if the patient is not capable.

constrict [12]—Make smaller.

contact precautions [3]—A category of transmission-based precautions used when caring for patients who have infections spread by skin and wound drainage, secretions, excretions, blood, body fluids, or contact with mucous membranes.

continuous ambulatory peritoneal dialysis (CAPD) [8]—The type of dialysis used at the bedside for patients with end-stage renal disease.

continuous epidural analgesia [13]—Intermittent or continuous infusion of pain medication through a catheter into the epidural space.

continuous passive motion (CPM) [11]—Therapy that prevents stiffness and improves circulation by delivering a form of passive range of motion that moves the joint without using the patient's muscles.

continuous positive airway pressure (CPAP) [14]—Oxygen therapy in which a mask is placed on the patient's face, then connected to a device that creates low levels of pressure.

continuous quality improvement (CQI) [1]—*See* quality assurance.

continuous sutures [5]—A method of closing the skin in which a single thread is used to close an open area.

contraction [16]—One part of the cardiac cycle in which the heart beats, pumping blood to the body.

contrast medium [16]—A special dye that is injected through an intravenous catheter during X-ray procedures. It enables the physician to see inside the blood vessel and identify potential problems.

core body temperature [12]—The normal body operating temperature, deep within the body core.

crash cart [17]—An emergency supply cart containing items needed in cardiac and respiratory arrest and life-threatening emergencies.

critical thinking [1]—Clear, precise, and purposeful mental activities. An essential skill used for solving complex problems, identifying solutions to a problem, drawing inferences, integrating information, distinguishing between fact and opinion, or estimating potential outcomes.

cross-training [1]—*See* multiskilling.

cryotherapy [12]—Cold therapy.

culture and sensitivity testing [10]—A diagnostic test; done to look for the presence of pathogens in exudate in body fluids, secretions, and excretions, and from body cavities and wounds. The culture component of the test determines if a pathogen is present, and, if so, whether the pathogen growth is heavy or light. The culture also identifies the specific pathogen causing the infection. The sensitivity part of the test shows which antibiotics will best eradicate the pathogen.

cytotoxic [5]—Harmful to healing tissue.

D

deep vein thrombosis (DVT) [11]—A blood clot that commonly occurs in the deep veins of the legs.

defibrillation [17]—Delivery of an electrical shock to treat certain types of cardiac arrest and other rhythm disturbances of the heart.

dehiscence [13]—The splitting or gaping open of a suture line.

delegated [1]—Authorized or entrusted to other workers.

delegation [1]—The transfer of responsibility for performance of a nursing activity from a licensed nurse who is authorized to perform the activity to someone who does not already possess that authority.

delirium [13]—An acute confusional state caused by reversible medical problems.

denial [1]—Refusing to admit that something is true.

developmental tasks [1]—Intellectual, social, and emotional tasks and skills that a person must accomplish or acquire at a certain age; are simple in early childhood, but become more complex as a person grows and ages.

dialysis [8]—A treatment done to cleanse the blood of toxins and impurities when the kidneys have failed.

diastole [16]—The resting phase of the cardiac cycle, during which the heart rests and recovers.

diathermy [12]—A heat treatment (may also be called *thermotherapy*).

dilate [12]—Enlarge; make larger.

direct contact [3]—An infection caused by touching an infected person.

distal [4]—Farthest away from the body.

domestic violence [13]—A pattern of forced behaviors perpetrated by a family member that may include repeated battering and injury, psychological abuse, sexual assault, progressive social isolation, deprivation, and intimidation.

Doppler [16]—An instrument that uses ultrasound to amplify sounds, similar to a stethoscope.

dosimeter [13]—A small, personal monitoring instrument that measures the radiation dose received by the individual wearing it.

dressing [5]—Gauze, film, or other synthetic substance that covers a wound, ulcer, or injury.

drop chamber (drip chamber) [7]—A semirigid container at the distal end of intravenous tubing that is filled halfway with fluid; allows easy visualization of the flow rate.

drop orifice [7]—Opening at the distal end of intravenous tubing that controls the size of the drops of fluid.

droplets [3]—Respiratory secretions, such as those produced by sneezing or coughing.

droplet precautions [3]—A category of transmission-based precautions used to prevent the spread of infection for some patients whose infection is spread by droplets in the air.

durable power of attorney for health care [17]—A document that the patient signs to allow the appointed health care proxy to make decisions on behalf of the patient when the patient is unable to do so for himself or herself.

dysrhythmia [16]—Abnormal heart rhythm.

E

ecchymosis [6]—Bruising; dark discoloration caused by bleeding under the skin.

electrocardiogram [16]—A paper tracing, created by an electrocardiograph, that shows heart activity.

electrocardiograph (ECG or EKG) [16]—A diagnostic device that records the activity of the heart.

empathy [1]—Understanding how the patient feels; connecting with and supporting a patient while he or she works through difficult times.

endotracheal intubation [15]—A measure that provides complete control over the airway; commonly called *intubation*.

endotracheal tube (ET tube) [15]—A tube that is passed through the mouth, or less commonly the nose, into the patient's lungs for the purpose of ventilation.

enema [8]—The introduction of fluid into the lower bowel to cleanse the anus, rectum, and lower colon.

enteral tube [9]—A catheter, stoma, or tube (such as a nasogastric or gastrostomy tube) used to provide nutrition and deliver nutrients to the gastrointestinal tract, distal to the oral cavity. The tubes may also be called *enteral access devices*.

ethics [1]—Principles of conduct and moral values.

exacerbate [13]—Escalate, magnify, aggravate, intensify, or worsen.

expectorate [10]—To spit or eject from the mouth.

F

fenestrated drape [9]—A drape with a hole in the center.

filter [7]—A device attached to intravenous tubing that allows fluid to pass, but traps particles; thought by some to help prevent infection.

fingerstick blood sugar (FSBS) [10]—Test to check blood sugar levels; done by collecting a sample of capillary blood with a lancet; the blood is transferred to a reagent strip and read by a handheld meter.

fistula [8]—A connection between an artery and a vein in the arm; used for dialysis access.

flaccid paralysis [13]—Loss of muscle tone and absence of tendon reflexes.

flash sterilization [4]—Quick method of sterilization; units operate rapidly, sterilizing an item within 10 minutes.

flow control clamp [7]—A roller clamp used to regulate the speed or rate of intravenous fluid flow.

fomites [3]—Linen, supplies, equipment, and other items with pathogens on them.

fracture [11]—Broken bone.

G

gastric analysis [10]—A laboratory test done to check for the presence of acid in the stomach.

gastric distention [15]—A condition in which the stomach fills with air, making it difficult for the lungs to expand.

gastrostomy tube (G-tube) [9]—Tube that is surgically inserted through the abdominal wall into the stomach; used for feeding liquid nutritional formula to a patient.

generalized application [12]—A treatment that delivers heat or cold to the entire body.

generalized tonic-clonic seizure [13]—Seizure characterized by loss of consciousness, convulsive activity, stiffening of muscles, and jerking movement of the arms and legs. Usually lasts three to four minutes.

glycated hemoglobin [10]—A measurement of glucose levels in the blood over the past three months; abbreviated %A1C.

graft [8]—A piece of plastic tubing that is surgically inserted to connect an artery to a vein.

grand mal seizure [13]—*See* generalized tonic-clonic seizure.

granulation tissue [5]—A specialized tissue created by the body in response to injury; contains many tiny blood vessels and may appear like a small, red, beadlike mass.

H

hardwire monitoring [16]—Type of cardiac monitoring in which the patient's heart rhythm is displayed on a monitor at the bedside, and at another remote location, usually the nurses' station.

head-tilt, chin-lift maneuver [17]—Most common method of opening the airway; the patient's chin is lifted while gentle pressure is exerted on the forehead to tip the head back.

health care proxy [17]—A surrogate decision maker who authorizes medical care on behalf of the patient if the patient cannot make decisions for himself or herself.

Health Insurance Portability and Accountability Act (HIPAA) [2]—Federal law governing privacy, confidentiality, and medical records. The HIPAA provisions and regulations protect all individually identifiable health information in any form; applies to paper, verbal, and electronic documentation, billing records, and clinical records.

heat exhaustion [12]—Also called *heat prostration*. Condition that develops as a result of overexposure to heat; involves electrolyte imbalance due to heavy perspiration.

heat stroke [12]—Also called *sunstroke*. Condition indicating a profound disruption of the internal temperature-regulating mechanisms in the body; caused by extended exposure to heat.

hematoma [6]—A blood-filled bruise.

hemodialysis [8]—Procedure in which a machine cleans wastes from the blood of a patient whose kidneys have failed.

hemolysis [6]—Breaking of fragile blood cells.

hemothorax [15]—A collection of blood in the chest cavity.

heparin [7]—An anticoagulant solution that prevents blood from clotting.

heparin lock [7]—A cap that covers the end, or hub, of a needle, intravenous catheter, or butterfly that is used to administer intravenous fluids and medications.

high airflow with oxygen enrichment (HAFOE) mask [14]—*See* air entrainment mask.

high-efficiency particulate air (HEPA) respirator [3]—A respirator used to protect employees working in rooms of patients who have diseases spread by the airborne method of transmission.

humidifier [14]—A water bottle attached to an oxygen supply device that moistens the oxygen for comfort and prevents drying of the mucous membranes in the nose, mouth, and lungs; used for liter flows of more than 5.

hydrocollator [12]—A rectangular tank containing very hot water used for heating hot packs.

hydrocolloid dressing [5]—Wound dressing made of a material such as gelatin and pectin; such dressings are self-adhesive and come in various sizes and thicknesses.

hydromassage [12]—The use of agitated water during hydrotherapy to produce the sensation of massage.

hydrotherapy [12]—Water therapy.

hyperpyrexia [12]—Abnormally high body temperature.

hyperthermia [12]—Hyperpyrexia.

hypoallergenic tape [5]—Special tape that reduces the incidence of a skin reaction in patients who are allergic to the adhesive on the back of most bandage tape.

hypothermia [12]—Low body temperature due to prolonged cold exposure; preserves the vital organs for up to several hours in cardiac arrest.

hypothermia-hyperthermia blanket [12]—A full-size aquathermia pad, similar to a K-Pad; used to raise, lower, or maintain the patient's temperature.

hypoxemia [14]—A condition in which there is insufficient oxygen in the blood.

I

immunotherapy [13]—Cancer treatment that uses various biologic agents to alter a patient's immune response and thereby eliminate cancer.

implantable medication pump [13]—Device surgically placed under the abdominal skin, used for long-term medication delivery.

incentive spirometer [11]—Handheld device used for respiratory exercises; used to inflate the lungs, remove mucus, and prevent pneumonia and other complications.

indirect contact [3]—A means of spreading infection by touching contaminated objects and environmental surfaces.

induration [9]—Swelling; enlargement.

infiltration [7]—Condition that occurs when an intravenous needle pierces the vein, allowing the fluid to flow into (*infiltrate*) the surrounding tissue.

Institute for Healthcare Improvement (IHI) [1]—A not-for-profit organization in which membership is voluntary. The IHI advocates safe, effective, efficient, patient-centered care, delivered in a timely manner. Its goals are to reduce or eliminate needless deaths, unnecessary pain, helplessness and dependence, unwanted waiting, and unnecessary waste.

intentionally unsafe acts [1]—Criminal acts, purposefully unsafe acts, acts related to alcohol or substance abuse by health care workers, or any type of patient abuse or neglect.

interdepartmental team [1]—A team made up of workers from two or more different departments.

interdisciplinary team [1]—A team consisting of workers from different disciplines; team members have different training, scopes of responsibility, and levels of expertise.

interpreter [13]—A communication professional who mediates between speakers of different languages.

interrupted sutures [5]—Stitches in which a thread is tied off and knotted separately for each stitch.

intradepartmental team [1]—A team made up of workers from the same department.

intradisciplinary team [1]—A team composed of workers from the same discipline who have similar training, scopes of responsibility, and levels of expertise.

intravenous (IV) therapy [7]—Inserting a needle into a vein for the purpose of administering fluids and medications.

intubation equipment [17]—*See* endotracheal intubation; endotracheal tube.

IV controller [7]—Device that regulates gravity flow of IV fluids by counting drops of solution.

J

Jacksonian seizure [13]—*See* simple-partial seizure.

jaw-thrust maneuver [17]—A method of opening the airway of patients who have known or suspected neck injuries, and in those whose airway cannot be opened using the head-tilt, chin-lift method; opens the airway without moving the neck.

jejunostomy tube (J-tube) [9]—A long, small-bore tube that is threaded through the GI tract until the tip reaches the small intestine. These tubes may be placed through the nose (nasojejunostomy) or surgically through an incision in the abdominal skin. The tubes are used for providing enteral nutrition for patients who do not have a stomach, and patients in whom recurrent formula aspiration is a problem.

junctional fibers [16]—Long, thin fibers in the atrium of the heart that carry electrical impulses.

junctional rhythms [16]—Cardiac rhythms (and beats) originating in the AV node.

K

Kelly (clamp) [6]—A hemostat; a specific type of clamp.

L

lancet [6]—A tiny, sharp, sterile device used to puncture the skin to collect small blood samples.

laryngectomee [15]—A person who has had the voice box (larynx) removed.

laryngectomy [15]—Surgical removal of the larynx, with separation of the airway from the mouth, nose, and esophagus.

laryngoscope [15]—The instrument used to perform the endotracheal intubation procedure; consists of a handle containing batteries, and a blade. The instrument permits the health care professional to visualize the structures in the throat when the tube is inserted.

lethargy [14]—Abnormal sleepiness for no apparent reason.

living will [17]—An advance directive that specifies the patient's wishes if the patient is in a terminal condition.

local [5]—Affecting a single system, area, or body part.

localized application [12]—A treatment that delivers heat or cold to a specific area of the body.

Luer slip [7]—Locking mechanism that makes it difficult to separate needles from their point of attachment on a syringe or intravenous tubing.

lumen [6]—The inside diameter of a needle.

M

maceration [5]—A water-logged appearance of the edges of a wound.

macrodrip [7]—Drop orifice for intravenous infusion that delivers fluid in a larger volume, typically 10 to 15 drops per milliliter of fluid; commonly used for adults.

malpractice [1]—Failure to act in accordance with the acceptable course of conduct, or negligent conduct by a worker that results in damage, harm, or injury to a patient.

massage therapist [13]—A therapist who kneads or manipulates muscles and soft tissue to improve body function, stimulate and improve circulation, promote relaxation and pain relief, and reduce physical and emotional stress.

medical record [2]—A legal document that is a record of the patient's true condition, progress, and care.

medication administration record (MAR)—The flow sheet or other form on which medication administration is documented.

microdraw [6]—A small skin puncture used for collecting blood specimens.

microdrip [7]—Drop orifice for intravenous infusion that delivers fluid in smaller drops, usually 60 drops per milliliter; commonly used for children.

microvette collection device [6]—Closed-system capillary tube that complies with the federal recommendations for capillary tubes.

midstream (clean-catch) urine specimen
[10]—Urine specimen collected to learn if an infection is present; the sample is collected from the middle of the urinary stream and is as sterile as possible.

mode of transmission [3]—The method by which a disease is spread.

modified barium swallow [9]—X-ray study that shows the patient's potential for aspiration.

Montgomery straps [5]—Long strips of adhesive attached to the skin on either side of a wound; after the wound is covered with a dressing, the straps are tied to hold the dressing securely in place.

multiskilling [1]—Teaching a worker to perform expanded skills that were previously the responsibility of other departments or workers.

music therapist [13]—An allied health service that uses music therapeutically to address physical, psychological, cognitive, and/or social functioning, and provide relaxation.

myocardial infarction [16]—Heart attack.

myoclonic seizure [13]—Seizure that consists of one or more myoclonic jerks. The patient remains conscious, but cannot control the muscle movement.

N

N95 respirator [3]—A NIOSH-approved mask with very small pores that may be worn when caring for patients in airborne precautions.

nasogastric tube (NG tube) [9]—Tube inserted through the nose and threaded through the esophagus to the stomach; used for enteral feeding, diagnostic tests, and in some other conditions.

nasopharyngeal airway [14]—A curved, soft, rubber device that is inserted through one nostril; extends from the nostril to the posterior pharynx area, keeping the tongue off the back of the throat.

National Institute of Occupational Safety and Health (NIOSH) [3]—A governmental agency concerned with employee safety; approves masks used in airborne precaution rooms.

nebulizer [14]—An inhalation dispenser that converts liquid medicine into a mist that can be inhaled by the patient.

necrotic tissue [5]—Dead or devitalized tissue that is usually brown or black in appearance; it must be removed for proper wound healing.

negative pressure environment [3]—The ventilation system used in an airborne precaution room; the room air is drawn upward into the ventilation system and is either specially filtered or exhausted directly to the outside of the building.

negligence [1]—Failure to exercise the degree of care considered reasonable in a situation, or failure to act with the prudence that a reasonable person with equal qualifications would exercise in the same circumstances.

nephrostomy tube [8]—A tube that is surgically inserted through the skin and into the kidney to drain urine directly from the kidney to the outside of the body.

nosocomial infection [10]—A hospital-acquired infection, or a new infection that developed in, or is associated with being treated in, a health care facility.

nurse practice act [1]—A document describing the licensed nurse's scope of practice in a particular state.

O

objective [2]—True; factual; not subjective.

occupational therapist (OT) [13]—Therapist who evaluates and treats patients for self-care, work, and ADLs.

open reduction internal fixation (ORIF) [11]—A surgical procedure in which the surgeon manipulates a fractured bone into alignment, then inserts a nail, pin, or rod to hold the bone in place.

oropharyngeal airway [14]—Also called *oral airway*; a curved plastic or rubber device that is inserted into the mouth to the posterior pharynx; used to keep the airway open in unconscious patients by keeping the tongue away from the back of the throat.

orthopedics [11]—Branch of medicine that deals with the prevention or correction of injuries or disorders of the skeletal system and associated structures.

osteoporosis [11]—A decrease in bone mass that leads to fractures with minimal or no trauma.

ostomy [8]—A surgically created opening into the body.

over-the-needle catheter (ONC) [7]—Flexible plastic or Teflon catheter that is threaded into a vein; used for long- or short-term intravenous therapy.

P

paralysis [13]—Loss of voluntary movement and impairment of functions below the level of spinal cord injury; the condition affects sensation and voluntary movement below the level of injury.

paraplegia [13]—Paralysis of the lower half of the body, including both legs; causes loss of bowel and bladder control.

paraprofessionals [1]—Workers who are educated and qualified to act as assistants to licensed personnel.

patient-controlled analgesia (PCA) [11]—A method of enabling patients to self-administer their own pain medications through a pump by intermittent or continuous infusion.

patient-focused care [1]—A method of bringing services to patients, instead of bringing patients to services.

percussion [14]—Clapping against the patient's chest wall to loosen secretions.

percutaneous endoscopic gastrostomy (PEG) [9]—A gastrostomy tube, surgically placed by a physician, that is threaded through the patient's mouth, then out an incision in the abdominal wall over the stomach.

perioperative hypothermia [12]—Hypothermia that develops in the operating room as a result of anesthesia and some other drugs, open body cavities, cold environment, and administration of cold fluids.

perioperative nursing [11]—The care given in hospital surgical department(s), day-surgery units, clinics, and physicians' offices. Perioperative care is provided before, during, and after surgery and other invasive procedures.

peritoneal dialysis [8]—Procedure that filters wastes from the patient's body, using a dialysis solution that is first infused into the abdomen and then drained out after a prescribed period of time.

peritonitis [9]—A very serious inflammation of the peritoneum, the membrane that lines the abdominal cavity; may develop as a complication of intestinal perforation from a tube; has the potential to become life-threatening.

persistent pain [13]—Pain lasting longer than six months; may be intermittent or constant. An older term for this type of pain is *chronic pain*.

personal digital assistant (PDA) [2]—Small handheld computer that operates on battery power; may be used for documentation and storing research information and personal data.

petechiae [6]—Tiny hemorrhagic spots, of pinpoint to pinhead size; caused by escape of blood from the blood vessels into the surrounding skin.

petit mal seizure [13]—*See* absence seizure.

PFR95 respirator [3]—A NIOSH-approved mask with very small pores that may be worn when caring for patients in airborne precautions.

pH [8]—An indication of the acidity or alkalinity of a substance.

phantom pain [13]—Pain that occurs as a result of an amputation. The pain is real, not imaginary.

phlebitis [7]—Irritation of a vein.

phlebotomy [6]—Collection of blood.

physical therapist (PT) [13]—Therapist who prevents physical disability and uses physical methods to evaluate and treat pain, disease, and injury. The PT specializes in muscle development and motor coordination.

piercing pin [7]—A sharp plastic spike that pierces the plastic bag or bottle.

pleural effusion [15]—Fluid that collects around the lungs; often occurs in patients who have cancer.

pneumatic cuffs [11]—Also called *pneumatic hosiery* or *sequential compression device*; a garment that prevents blood clots in surgical patients; promotes blood flow by massaging the legs in a wavelike motion.

pneumothorax [15]—Free air in the chest cavity outside the lung that presses against the lung, preventing the lung from expanding properly.

pocket mask [17]—Clear plastic mask used for ventilation; has a special valve that prevents the patient's exhaled air and secretions from entering the caregiver's mouth.

portal of entry [3]—The place where a pathogen enters the body.

portal of exit [3]—Secretions, excretions, or droplets in which pathogens travel when they leave the body.

postictal [13]—The period of time immediately after a seizure.

postresuscitation care [17]—Monitoring and care given to a patient who has been successfully resuscitated; the patient will be in critical, unstable condition for a period of time and will require very close monitoring.

primary hypothermia [12]—Low body temperature that occurs as a result of overwhelming cold stress.

priorities [1]—Tasks that are the most important. Prioritizing your work means arranging tasks so that they are performed in order of importance. It includes anticipating supply needs and patients' personal needs.

process improvement [1]—Activities designed to evaluate care and facility practices so that staff can identify and correct problems.

professional boundaries [1]—Limits on how a health care worker acts with patients.

proximal [4]—Closest to the body.

psychomotor seizure [13]—*See* complex-partial seizure.

pulse deficit [16]—The difference in value between the apical pulse and the radial pulse.

pulse oximeter [14]—An instrument that measures the level of saturation of hemoglobin with oxygen.

Purkinje fibers [16]—Part of a network of fibers that work together to cause the ventricles to contract; the network includes the bundle of His and left and right bundle branches.

purulent [5]—Pus-filled; pus-like.

Q

quadriplegia [13]—*See* tetraplegia.

quality assurance (QA) [1]—A program designed to conduct internal reviews to identify problems or potential problems and find solutions and methods for improvement. The QA committee meets periodically to evaluate care provided and practices in the facility.

quality improvement (QI) [1]—*See* quality assurance.

quality indicators [1]—Decision-making and research tools used for tracking changes, recognizing potential quality problems, and identifying areas that require further study, investigation, and research. Indicators are measurable items that reflect the level and type of services a facility is delivering. Most can be modified, so if a facility is unhappy with its results, it can change its processes.

R

radiating pain [13]—Pain that moves from the site of origin to other areas.

radiation therapy [13]—The use of high-energy, ionizing beams directed to a cancerous area to destroy cancerous tissue without damaging healthy tissue.

reagents [8]—Chemicals used to perform certain tests on body fluids; they react a certain way when they contact body substances. Reagents come in tablets and strips.

re-engineering [1]—*See* workplace redesign.

refractometer [8]—Instrument used for measuring specific gravity of urine.

rehabilitation [13]—Skilled program(s) designed by a therapist to help patients regain lost skills or to teach new skills.

rehabilitation team [13]—A team of workers from many professions who evaluate and treat patients; design rehabilitation and restorative programs; teach the patient, facility staff, and family members; and serve as consultants when needed.

relaxation [16]—The resting and recovery phase of the heart.

renal calculi [10]—Kidney stones.

renal colic [10]—Flank pain caused by obstruction to the flow of urine, such as from a stone.

reservoir [3]—The place where a disease-causing microbe can grow.

respiratory arrest [17]—Condition that occurs when breathing stops.

respiratory care practitioner (RCP) [13]—A licensed professional who specializes in the care of patients with disorders of the cardiopulmonary system, respirations, and sleep disorders that affect breathing.

respiratory failure [17]—Occurs when breathing is insufficient to sustain life.

respiratory therapist (RT) [13]—*See* respiratory care practitioner.

restorative nursing care [13]—Nursing care designed to assist the patient to attain and maintain the highest possible level of function.

restructuring [1]—*See* workplace redesign.

resuscitation [17]—Saving; reviving.

retention enema [8]—Injection of fluid into the anus to relieve constipation or fecal impaction. An oil-based solution, packaged in a small, commercial container, is used for the retention enema.

root cause analysis (RCA) [1]—A process for identifying the causative or contributing factors associated with adverse events, close calls, or sentinel events. An RCA includes a focused review of the problem or situation. Each facility has specific guidelines for conducting a root cause analysis investigation. The data are used to prevent recurrence of the unsafe situation.

S

secondary hypothermia [12]—Low body temperature that develops as a result of other medical problems, such as shock and sepsis.

seizure [13]—A sudden, spontaneous episode of excessive and scrambled electrical activity caused by interference with impulses in the brain.

seizure precautions [13]—Individualized measures that keep the patient safe during an unexpected seizure.

sentinel events [1]—Type of adverse event that results in patient death or serious physical or psychological injury, or creates a risk of death or serious injury.

septicemia [6]—A generalized infection in the bloodstream.

sequential compression device [11]—*See* pneumatic cuffs.

shunt [8]—A connector that allows blood flow between two locations.

signs [2]—Observations that are seen or made by using the senses.

simple-partial seizure [13]—Seizure that involves only part of the brain; if abnormal muscle activity occurs, muscle spasms may start in one extremity and progressively move upward on that side of the body.

Sims' position [8]—A side-lying position used for giving enemas, rectal examinations, and other rectal treatments. This position promotes evacuation of the bowel.

singultus [11]—Hiccups; intermittent spasms of the diaphragm.

sinoatrial node (SA node) [16]—The normal pacemaker for the heart, located in the right atrium.

skeletal traction [11]—Method of applying traction; ropes and weights are attached to a wire, pin, or tongs that are surgically placed into or through a fractured or surgically repaired bone.

skin traction [11]—Method of applying traction; ropes and weights are attached to a harness or belt worn by the patient; used to keep fractures in alignment and for some other conditions.

sleep apnea [14]—A condition in which patients stop breathing in their sleep. Commonly caused by a blockage or obstruction in the patient's airway that occurs when the patient falls asleep and the muscles relax.

slide clamp [7]—A plastic clamp used to stop or regulate the flow of fluid.

sniffing position [15]—Placement of the head and neck in which the patient appears to be sniffing a flower or other object; the neck is flexed and the head extended.

social worker (LSW) [13]—Therapist who acts as a liaison between hospital and community services; works with both normal and disturbed patients.

source [3]—The pathogen that causes disease.

spastic paralysis [13]—Involuntary movement in which the extremities move in an involuntary pattern, similar to muscle spasms. The patient is aware of the movements, but cannot stop them.

spasticity [2]—Sudden, frequent, violent, intense involuntary muscle contractions that impair function.

speech language pathologist (SLP) [13]—A highly qualified, licensed professional who evaluates patients; plans and directs care for patients who have problems with chewing, swallowing, speech, comprehension, communication, and/or memory loss.

speech therapist (ST) [13]—*See* speech language pathologist.

spores [3]—Microscopic reproductive bodies that are very difficult to eliminate. They can survive in a dormant form until conditions are ideal for reproduction. Active or reactivated spores will multiply and continue to spread infection.

sputum [10]—Secretion from the mucous membranes lining the trachea and lungs.

standard precautions [3]—Measures that health care workers use to prevent the spread of infection to themselves and others.

standards of care [1]—Common health care practices based on laws, facility policies and procedures, information learned in class, job descriptions, and information published in textbooks, journals, literature, and the Internet. Standards may be defined by community, state, and/or national practices. Applying standards of care involves using the degree of care or skill that is expected in a particular circumstance or role.

status epilepticus [13]—A seizure that lasts for a long time, or repeats without recovery.

sterile field [4]—Sterile surface created for use as a work area for sterile procedures.

sterile technique [4]—A microbe-free technique used for performing procedures within body cavities and during certain dressing changes.

stoma [8]—The opening of an ostomy to the outside of the body.

stop order [Appendix C]—A specific time limit on medication administration, as defined by facility policy. If the physician's medication order does not include a specific time limit or a specific number of dosages, the facility will notify the physician that the medication will be stopped on a specific date unless the medication is reordered or continued by the physician.

stylette [15]—A wire inserted through a tube to reduce flexibility of the tube.

subjective [2]—Refers to an opinion that may or may not be true; not objective.

suppositories [8]—Medicine administered into the rectum; usually are given to stimulate bowel elimination, but may also be used for other purposes.

suprapubic catheter [8]—A catheter that is inserted surgically through the abdominal wall directly into the bladder.

surgical asepsis [4]—*See* sterile technique.

susceptible host [3]—The organism in which a disease-causing microbe can grow.

sympathy [1]—Feeling sorry for patients, and taking on their feelings as your own.

symptoms [2]—Things patients notice about their conditions and tell you; cannot be detected by using the senses of a person other than the patient.

systemic [5]—Affecting the entire body.

systemic infection [10]—An infection that spreads throughout the whole body, affecting many systems or organs.

systole [16]—The working phase of the heart.

T

tablet PC (TPC) [2]—*See* personal digital assistant.

tact [1]—The ability to say and do the right things at the right time.

telemetry [16]—Cardiac monitoring in which a small transmitter sends a signal to a remote location, where the patient's cardiac rhythm is displayed on a monitor.

tension pneumothorax [15]—A serious condition in which air trapped between the lung and chest wall cannot escape, leading to a steady buildup of pressure.

tepid [12]—Lukewarm. Tepid water is between 80°F and 93°F.

tetraplegia [13]—Paralysis affecting the arms and legs; complete or incomplete paralysis from the neck downward, affecting all four limbs and the trunk. *Quadriplegia* is an older term for this condition.

therapeutic recreation specialist (TRS) [13]—A therapist who promotes the development of functional independence and facilitates the development, maintenance, and expression of an appropriate leisure lifestyle for persons with mental, physical, emotional, and/or social limitations.

thermotherapy [12]—*See* diathermy.

thrombophlebitis [6]—Inflammation of a vein with clot formation.

total hip arthroplasty (THA) [11]—Removal of a portion of the pelvic bone and femur, and insertion of a prosthesis (artificial body part).

tracheostomy [15]—A surgically created opening into the airway through which a patient breathes.

tracheotomy [15]—The surgical procedure used to create a tracheostomy.

traction [11]—A treatment for fractures of the long bones and some other conditions. The bone ends are pulled into place with ropes and weights. The patient's body weight stabilizes the upper part of the bone; a bag of water or metal disks are attached to pull on the opposite end.

transcutaneous electrical nerve stimulation (TENS) [13]—A nondrug method of managing pain in which mild, harmless electrical current stimulates nerve fibers to block transmission of pain to the brain.

transfusion [7]—Intravenous administration of blood used to treat some medical conditions.

transmission-based precautions [3]—Measures used to prevent the spread of infection when ordinary cleanliness and standard precautions will not avoid the spread of certain pathogens.

transparency [1]—Part of the root cause analysis investigative process that involves keeping people informed. Having transparency in analyses and findings is critical to improving patient safety. Transparency promotes learning and understanding, and enhances trust in the findings and recommendations.

transparent film dressings [5]—Adhesive membranes of various sizes and thicknesses used as a covering for wounds.

transport bag [10]—Sealed plastic bag to which a biohazard label can be affixed; used for transporting laboratory specimens and biohazardous materials.

two-hour postprandial blood sugar (PPBS) [10]—Test in which blood sugar is collected exactly two hours after the patient finishes eating; the blood sugar level should have returned to normal in this period of time.

type and cross-match [7]—Laboratory test that identifies the patient's blood type and Rh factor; the cross-match test determines whether the patient's blood is compatible with the donor blood.

U

unlicensed assistive personnel (UAPs) [1]—Individuals who are trained to assist the licensed nurse in providing direct nursing care to health care consumers; all care is done as delegated by, and under the supervision of, the licensed nurse.

urine specific gravity [8]—Test performed on the nursing unit or in the laboratory that provides a measure of how well the kidneys concentrate urine; provides useful diagnostic information about many different conditions.

urinometer [8]—Instrument used for determining urine specific gravity.

V

vacutainer [6]—A vacuum test tube used for drawing blood.

vector [3]—An insect, rodent, or small animal that spreads disease.

vehicle [3]—Food, water, or other items in which pathogens can live and multiply.

venipuncture [6]—The act of puncturing a vein with a needle.

venti mask [14]—*See* air entrainment mask.

ventilation [17]—Artificial means of providing respiration for a patient using mechanical equipment, adjunctive devices, or mouth-to-mask resuscitation.

ventilator [15]—A mechanical device used to facilitate breathing in patients who have impaired respiratory or diaphragm function.

ventricles [16]—The lower, pumping chambers of the heart.

ventricular fibrillation [17]—Cardiac arrest; a quivering of the heart muscle in which the heart does not pump blood to the rest of the body.

Venturi mask [14]—*See* air entrainment mask.

volumetric intravenous pump [7]—Pump that regulates the flow of IV fluids electronically to ensure accurate flow of IV solutions and drugs.

W

workplace redesign [1]—Combining the services of many different workers and departments, creating larger departments. As part of larger departments, workers provide more services to patients than they did previously.

Y

Yankauer catheter [14]—Rigid suction catheter used to remove secretions and foreign material from the oral cavity; also called a *tonsil tip*.

Y-site [7]—Connection in intravenous tubing for administration of medications.

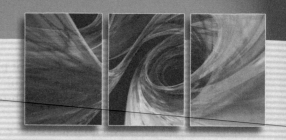

Index

NOTE: Page numbers ending with "f" refer to a figure on the cited page.

A

AAR, 182
ABC, 512
abduction pillow, 322, 323f
ABO system, 182
absence seizure, 385
A1C testing, 290–291
accidental exposure to blood/body fluids, 73
acetest, 190f
acupuncture, 397, 397f
acute pain, 401
adjunctive devices, 517
administration set, 159, 160–161
adolescents, 24–25. *See also* age-appropriate care alert
adulthood, 25–26. *See also* age-appropriate care alert
advance directives, 511–512
advanced respiratory procedures, 448–469. *See also* respiratory procedures
adverse events, 5
AEDs, 524, 525
aerobic microbes, 144
age-appropriate care, 19. *See also* age-appropriate care alert
  adolescents, 24–25
  adulthood, 25–26
  infant, 21
  old age, 26–27
  preschoolers, 22–23
  safety and security, 20
  school-age children, 23–24
  special situations, 20
  toddler, 21–22
age-appropriate care alert
  blood collection, 148, 150
  fingerstick capillary test, 148, 289
  IV administration, 162, 166, 167, 177
  pain, 45

skin, 103
  urine specimen, 198
air embolus, 175
air entrainment mask, 430, 430f
airborne infection, 58
airborne precautions, 73–76
airway, 513
airway adjunct, 517
airway management, 511. *See also* emergency procedures
alcohol-based hand cleaners, 64, 64f
alert. *See* age-appropriate care alert; communication alert; culture alert; difficult patient alert; health care alert; infection alert; legal alert; OSHA alert; procedure alert; safety alert
allergies—hair, 430
alveoli, 416, 416f
anaerobic microbes, 144
anger, 18
angiogram, 505, 506
ankle bandage, 109
antecubital space, 129, 130
Anthrax, 80
antibodies, 182
anticoagulants, 129
antiembolism stockings, 312–315
antigen, 182
antigen-antibody reaction (AAR), 182
anus, 198f
apical pulse, 498–499
apical-radial pulse, 499
appliance, 230, 230f, 231–232
aquathermia pad, 346–347
arm sling, 320
arm whirlpool, 350f
arrhythmia, 491
arteriogram, 505, 506
arteriovenous fistula, 217f
arteriovenous graft, 217f
assignment, 10–12
asystole, 526–527
atelectasis, 309
atrial bigeminy, 480f

atrial fibrillation, 481f, 482f
atrial flutter, 481f
atrial tachycardia, 479f
atrioventricular (AV) block, 476, 482f
atrioventricular (AV) bundle, 471f
atrioventricular (AV) node, 471–472, 471f
audiologist, 398
augmented limb leads, 489f, 490
autoclaving, 88, 89f
automatic external defibrillator (AED), 524, 525
autonomic dysreflexia, 390–391
AV block, 476, 482f
AV bundle, 471f
AV node, 471–472, 471f
aVF (ECG lead), 489f
aVL (ECG lead), 489f
aVR (ECG lead), 489f

B

Bacillus species, 60f
backrub, 31
Bacteroides, 60f
bag valve mask (BVM), 517, 518f
bag valve-mask device, 452
    endotracheal intubation, 453
    tracheostomy, 456
bag valve mask resuscitation, 517–519
bandage, 106. See also Wound care
bandage scissors, 104
bandage-wrapping techniques, 109–111
barrier, 20
barrier equipment, 66. See also Personal protective
    equipment (PPE)
basic IV administration set, 159, 160–161
battered woman syndrome, 376
beginning procedure actions, 81–82
benchmark, 4
benchmarking, 4
bigeminy, 486f
bilevel positive airway pressure (BiPAP), 441
binders, 106, 107
biohazardous waste, 67
bioterrorism, 80
BiPAP, 441
bipolar leads, 489f, 490
bladder irrigation, 213–216
bleeding time, 150–151
blood/body fluid spills, 67
blood collection. See Phlebotomy
blood culture, 144–146
blood culture bottle, 145f
blood glucose equivalent values, 291
blood glucose meters, 287–288
blood glucose testing, 286–289

blood groups/types, 182
blood pressure, 502–505
blood pressure monitoring, 503–505
blood transfer device, 142f, 144
blood transfusion, 182–184
blood tube holders, 139f
body language, 17f
body lice, 100
bolus enteral feeding, 258, 259
bone fracture, 321
bowel elimination, 219–228. See also Urinary and
    bowel elimination
brachial plexus, 389f
brachytherapy, 395–397
breathing adequacy, 417, 513, 514
breathing exercises, 310–311
broken bones (fractures), 318–324
broken glass, 67
Bronchioles, 416, 416f
Buck's traction, 328f
Bundle of His, 471f, 472
buried bumper syndrome, 257
butterfly needle, 126f
butterfly needle and syringe (blood collection),
    126–127, 141–144
butterfly needle (IV therapy), 169–170

C

C. difficile, 60f, 63
CAM, 397
cancer treatment, 392–397
candida, 60f
cannula, 454
CAPD, 218–219
capillary refill, 418
capillary tube, 147
Carbon dioxide (CO_2), 416
cardiac arrest, 519
cardiac care skills, 470–510
    anatomy/basic principles, 470–472
    blood pressure, 502–505
    cardiac catheterization, 506–507
    continuous cardiac monitoring, 495–498
    Doppler, 501, 502
    ECG. See Electrocardiogram (ECG).
    Holter monitor, 570–572, 575
    post-arteriogram care, 505, 506
    pulse, 498–501
cardiac catheterization, 506–507
cardiac cycle, 470
cardiopulmonary resuscitation (CPR), 519–522
cardiovascular system, 41–42
carrier, 58
casts, 319–320

catheter
  cardiac catheterization, 506–507
  central intravenous, 179–181
  epidural, 403–404
  Foley, 197
  Hickman, 180
  indwelling, 196, 197, 202–204, 216–217
  IV, 158, 162, 179–181
  ONC, 158, 158f
  PROTECTIV IV safety system, 165f
  Speci-cath, 205, 205f. *See also* Age-appropriate care
    alert
  straight, 197, 199–201
  suprapubic, 209–210
  urinary elimination, 196–210
catheter breakage/embolus, 175–176
catheter selection considerations, 162
catheterized urine specimen, 278–280
cauda equina, 389f
causative agent, 58
CDC, 73
cell phones, 51–52
Centers for Disease Control and Prevention (CDC), 73
central intravenous catheter, 179–181
central IV dressing change, 181
central terminal, 490
centrifuge, 152–154
cerebellum, 389f
cervical plexus, 389f
cervical traction, 328, 328f
chain of infection, 58, 59
charting, 47–53
chemotherapy, 392–394
chest leads, 489f, 490
chest percussion, 442f
chest tubes, 462–464
children, 21–25. *See also* Age-appropriate care alert
choking, 516–517
CircOlectric bed, 318
claw-type basic frame (traction), 329f, 330
clean-catch urine specimen, 274, 275
cleansing enema, 223, 224–226
close calls, 5
closed bladder irrigation, 215
closed drainage system, opening, 207
clostridium difficile, 60f, 63
CO_2, 416
coagulation tube, 141
coccyx, 389f
code situation, 527
cognitive impairment, 30
cold applications. *See* Heat and cold applications
cold compresses, 360–361
collecting specimens, 266–297. *See also* Specimen
    collection
colloidal oatmeal, 353

colonization, 271
colostomy appliance, 230, 230f, 231–232
colostomy irrigation, 232–234
colostomy stoma, 229, 229f
commercially prepared enema, 223, 226–227
common vehicles, 58
communication, 16–19
communication alert
  cancer, 392
  nonverbal communication, 17
  pain, 402
  patient with limited communication ability, 30
  phlebotomy, 140
  rapport with patient, 20
  reporting observations, 40
compartment syndrome, 326–327
complementary and alternative medicine (CAM), 397
completion procedure actions, 82–83
complex-partial seizure, 385
computerized medical record, 50–53
conduction system of heart, 471f
confidentiality, 38–39, 52
confused mental state, 30
consent, 512
constipation, 402
contact precautions, 76, 77
continuing education, 9–10
continuous ambulatory peritoneal dialysis (CAPD),
    218–219
continuous bladder irrigation, 215–216
continuous cardiac monitoring, 495–498
continuous epidural analgesia, 402
continuous feeding pump, 259–260
continuous passive motion (CPM), 323–326
continuous positive airway pressure (CPAP), 440, 441
continuous quality improvement (CQI), 2
continuous sutures, 117, 117f
contraction (cardiac cycle), 470
contrast medium, 505
conus medullaris, 389f
cool eye compresses, 362, 363
cool soak, 361–362
COPD, 429
core body temperature, 363
coughing and deep breathing exercises, 310–311
CPAP, 440, 441
CPM therapy, 323–326
CPR, 519–522
CQI, 2
crash cart, 523
critical thinking, 4
cross-training, 2
cryotherapy. *See* Heat and cold applications
culture alert
  eye contact, 374
  handshake, 374

Koreans—drinking water, 204
modesty, 196, 219
pain, 45
peri care, 223
personal space, 374
physical distance, 17
post-surgical care, 305
tongue piercings, 432
urinary and bowel elimination, 189, 196, 204, 219, 223
culture and sensitivity testing, 267–269. *See also* Specimen collection
culturette, 268
customer satisfaction/service, 6
cutaneous anthrax, 80
cystostomy tube, 209
cytotoxic products, 105

D

deep breathing exercises, 310–311
deep vein thrombosis (DVT), 308, 313
defibrillation, 523–527
dehiscence, 405
delegation, 10–12
delirium, 382–383
denial, 20
dentures, 300
developmental tasks, 19
diabetic patients, 289–290
dialysis, 217–219
diaphragm, 416f
diastole, 472
diathermy. *See* Heat and cold applications
difficult patient. *See also* Difficult patient alert
language/understanding problems, 29–30. *See also* Communication alert
patients who resist care, 30–31
physically aggressive patients, 31
verbally aggressive patients, 31
yelling/screaming, 31
difficult patient alert
autonomic dysreflexia, 391
backrub, 31
behavior management care plan, 30
chemotherapy, 392, 393
drinking fluids, 204
general information, 17
hair loss, 392
hip surgery, 321
hypoxia, 419
liquid nutritional supplements, 394
nebulizer, 439
NG tube, 240
ostomy, 229
postural drainage, 441, 442

radiation therapy, 395
rewards for positive behavior, 31
suction catheters, 457
wound drainage, 306
direct contact, 57
disabled patient. *See also* Difficult patient alert
cognitive impairment, 30
hearing impairment, 28–29
vision impairment, 28
disaster plan, 80
disposable gloves, 66–68
documentation, 47–53, 538–558, 560–565, 566, 568, 572
domestic violence, 376–381
Doppler, 501, 502
dorsalis pedis pulse, 500–501
double barrel colostomy, 229f
drain (dressing), 112–113, 566–569
drainage, 306–307, 566–569
drainage bag disinfection, 209
dressing, 106, 566–569. *See also* Wound care
drip chamber, 159
drop orifice, 159
droplet infection, 58
droplet precautions, 76
dry heat treatments, 340–343
durable power of attorney for health care, 511–512
DVT, 308, 313
dysrhythmia, 491, 492

E

E. coli, 60f
ECG, 470. *See also* Electrocardiogram (ECG)
ECG coding system, 491, 491f, 574
ECG leads, 488–491, 570–571, 574
ECG paper, 472–474, 573
ECG trimmer, 492, 493f
"Effect of Chronic or Intermittent Hypoxia on Cognition in Childhood: A Review of the Literature, The," 419
Einthoven's triangle, 488, 488f
EKG, 470. *See also* Electrocardiogram (ECG)
elastic bandages, 106
elastic stockings, 312–315
elbow bandage, 110
elderly patients, 26–27. *See also* Age-appropriate care alert
elastic mesh bandages, 106
electrocardiogram (ECG), 472–495, 573–575
atrial bigeminy, 480f
atrial fibrillation, 481f, 482f
atrial flutter, 481f
atrial tachycardia, 479f
AV block, 476, 482f
calculating heart rate, 475

documentation, 492
ECG paper, 472–474
Einthoven's triangle, 488, 488f
junctional rhythms, 483, 483f
junctional tachycardia, 484f
lead coding, 491
leads, 488–491
mounting the ECG, 492–493
normal conduction pathway, 472
normal sinus rhythm, 476f
PR interval, 474, 474f
premature atrial contractions, 479f, 480f
PVCs, 484–487
QRS complex, 472, 474, 474f
reporting, 492
sawtoothed P waves, 481f
sinus arrest, 478f
sinus arrhythmia, 477f
sinus bradycardia, 477f
sinus pause, 478f
sinus tachycardia, 476f
ST segment, 474, 474f
step-by-step procedure, 493–495
T wave, 474–475, 475f
ventricular fibrillation, 484, 487f, 488f
ventricular tachycardia, 484, 487f
electrocardiograph, 470. *See also* Electrocardiogram
(ECG)
electronic blood pressure monitoring, 503–505
emergency procedures, 511–530
ABC, 512
advance directives, 511–512
AEDs, 524, 525
airway, 513
bag-valve mask resuscitation, 517–519
choking, 516–517
code situation, 527
consent, 512
CPR, 519–522
crash cart, 523, 523f
defibrillation, 523–527
head-tilt, chin-lift maneuver, 514–515
jaw-thrust maneuver, 515
mouth-to-mask resuscitation, 517, 518–519
obstructed airway procedure, 516–517
opening the airway, 513–515
postresuscitation care, 527
recovery position, 522, 523
emergency resuscitation cart, 523f
EMLA cream, 163, 163f
empathy, 17
ending procedure actions, 82–83
endotracheal intubation, 449–453
endotracheal tube (ET tube), 448, 448f
enema, 222–227
enteral-feeding formula, 251

enteral nutrition, 239–265
administering the feeding, 251–252
bolus feeding, 258, 259
complications, 253–257
continuous feeding pump, 259–260
equipment alarms, 261
feeding formula, 251
food coloring, 244
G-tube, 248–251
infection control, 257, 258
J-tube, 252–253
NG tube insertion, 240–245
NG tube irrigation, 246, 247
NG tube removal, 247
PEG tube, 248–251
pH testing, 244
reasons for, 240
residual stomach contents, 245–246
enteral tubes, 239
epididymis, 198f
epidural catheter, 403–404
ET tube, 448, 448f
ethics, 14
evacuated blood collection system, 139f
expanded precautions, 77–78
exposure control plan, 73
exposure to blood/body fluids, 73
eye compresses, 362, 363
eye contact, 374
eye protection, 70–72

F

face/eye protection, 70–72. *See also* Respirator;
Surgical mask
FACES pain scale, 46f
fear, 18, 32
fecal impaction, 219, 220f, 228
female Speci-Cath collection device, 278f
femoral plexus, 389f
femoral pulse, 499–500
filters, 159, 160f
filum terminale, 389f
fingernails, 418
fingerstick blood sugar (FSBS), 287, 290
fingerstick capillary test, 148, 289
first dangling and ambulation, 309
first-degree AV block, 482f
fistula, 217
five rights of delegation, 11f
flaccid paralysis, 388
flash sterilization, 96–97
flatus bag, 220–221
flow control clamp, 159
flow meter (oxygen tank), 423, 423f
fluid overload, 177

Foley catheter, 197
food coloring (tube feeding), 244
foot bandage, 109
forearm antisepsis, 299–300
forearm veins, 163f
foreskin, 198f
fractures, 318–324
FSBS, 287, 290

G

G-tube, 248–251
gastric analysis, 274
gastric specimen, 274
gastrointestinal system, 42–43
gastrointestinal system infection, 61
gastrostomy tube (G-tube), 248–251
gauze bandages, 106
gauze sponges, 105
GCS, 312–315
generalized application, 338
generalized tonic-clonic seizure, 384, 384f
genitourinary system, 43
genitourinary system infection, 61
ghb, 290
glans penis, 198f
gloves, 66–68, 94–95
glucose and ketone reagent strips, 191–192
glucose meters, 287–288
glucose testing, 286–289
glycated hemoglobin measurement, 290–291
glycohemoglobin, 290
golden rule, 13
gown, 68–70
graduated compression stocking (GCS), 312–315
graft, 217
gram stain, 268
grand mal seizure, 384, 384f
group A *streptococcus* antigen testing, 270–271
group A *streptococcus pyogenes*, 270
guaiac test, 285
guilt, 18

H

haemophilus, 60f
HAFOE mask, 430
hair loss, 392
hand and forearm veins, 163f
handheld computers, 50–51
handling sharps/needles, 73
handshake, 374
handwashing, 58–63, 88–89
hardwire monitoring, 495
HbA1, 290
HbA1c, 290

head lice, 100
head-tilt, chin-lift maneuver, 514–515
health care alert
    allergies—hair, 430
    aquathermia pad, 346
    bath blanket/towel, 354
    blood pressure measurement, 502
    chest pain, 520
    COPD, 429
    CPM therapy, 326
    Doppler, 501
    gauze sponges, 105
    heat treatments, 341
    ice massage, 360
    phlebotomy, 123
    stethoscope, 498
    tourniquet, 135
    venipuncture, 130, 133, 135
health care proxy, 511
Health Insurance Portability and Accountability Act
    (HIPAA), 38–39
hearing aids, 29
hearing impairment, 28–29
heart, 470, 471f
heart disorders. *See* Cardiac care skills
heat and cold applications, 338–372
    cold compresses, 360–361
    cool soak, 361–362
    dry heat treatments, 340–343
    eye compresses, 362, 363
    general guidelines, 339–340
    heat-related illnesses, 365
    heating pads, 346–347
    hot packs, 341
    hot water bottle, 341–342
    hydrotherapy, 350–358
    hypothermia, 363–365
    hypothermia-hyperthermia blanket, 366–368
    ice packs, 358–360
    moist heat treatments, 343–350
    moist hot packs, 347–350
    sitz bath, 356–358
    tepid sponge bath, 353–356
    therapeutic bath, 353
    warm compresses, 344–346
    warm soak, 343–344
    warmed blankets, 342–343
    whirlpool therapy, 350–353
heat exhaustion, 365
heat prostration, 365
heat-related illnesses, 365
heat stroke, 365
heating pads, 346–347
helplessness, 18
hematoma, 127, 128f, 129, 133, 174
Hemoccult Sensa test, 285

hemodialysis, 217
hemoglobin, 418
hemolysis, 152
hemorrhage, 308
hemothorax, 462
HEPA respirator, 74–75
heparin lock, 168–169, 569–570
hiccups, 307
Hickman central intravenous catheter, 180f
high airflow with oxygen enrichment (HAFOE)
    mask, 430
high efficiency particulate air (HEPA) respirator,
    74–75
hip fracture, 321–323, 324f
hip precautions, 324f
hip prothesis, 322f
HIPAA, 38–39, 561–563
hot packs, 341
hot-syncing, 51
hot water bottle, 341–342
humidifier, 427–428
hydrocollator, 347–350
hydrocolloid dressings, 115, 116
hydromassage, 350
hydrotherapy, 350–358
hyperglycemia, 290
hyperpyrexia, 365
hypertension, 502–503
hyperthermia, 365
hypoglycemia, 290
hypothermia, 363–365
hypothermia-hyperthermia blanket, 366–368
hypoxemia, 309, 417–418, 419

I

ice massage, 360
ice packs, 358–360
IHI, 6
ileostomy, 229f
immunotherapy, 397
implantable medication pumps, 404–405
in-and-out catheterization, 197
in-line filters, 159, 160f
incentive spirometry, 311–312
indirect contact, 57
indwelling catheter, 196, 197, 202–204, 216–217
infant, 21. *See also* Age-appropriate care alert
infant heel stick, 146–150
infection alert
    alcohol-based hand cleaner, 64
    central intravenous catheter, 181
    computers, 50
    dressings, 107, 108
    extra supplies, 88
    general information, 70, 80

hypothermia-hyperthermia blanket, 365
    IV administration, 164
    leukemia, 393
    perineal care, 275
    postpartum patients, 357
    tracheostomy, 456
    urinary leg bag, 208
    whirlpool, 352
    wound culture, 273
infection control, 57–87. *See also* Infection alert
    airborne precautions, 73–76
    beginning procedure actions, 81–82
    bioterrorism, 80
    blood glucose measurement, 288–289
    contact precautions, 76, 77
    droplet precautions, 76
    enteral nutrition, 257, 258
    expanded precautions, 77–78
    exposure to blood/body fluids, 73
    handwashing, 58–63
    isolation measures, 73–80
    needles/sharps, handling, 73
    PPE. *See* Personal protective equipment (PPE).
    procedure completion actions, 82–83
    protective isolation, 78
    respirator, 74–76
    signs/symptoms of infection, 61
    spread of infection, 57–58
    standard precautions, 64–73
    tourniquet, 133
    transmission-based precautions, 73–77
    waste disposal, 67
    waterless hand cleaners, 63, 64
    wound care, 103–104
infiltration, 174–175
initial ambulation, 309
inspection toe, 313
Institute for Healthcare Improvement (IHI), 6
integumentary system, 42
integumentary system infection, 61
intentionally unsafe acts, 5
interdepartmental team, 13
interdisciplinary team, 12
interpreter, 374–375
interrupted sutures, 117, 117f
intradepartmental team, 12–13
intradisciplinary team, 12
intravenous catheters, 158, 162, 179–181
intravenous controllers, 173
intravenous flow rate, 171–172, 575–578
intravenous needles, 158
intravenous pumps, 173
intravenous therapy, 157–188
    air embolus, 175
    basic infusion set, 159, 160–161
    blood transfusion, 182–184

butterfly needle, 169–170
catheter breakage/embolus, 175–176
catheters, 158, 162, 179–181
CDC recommendations, 176–177
central intravenous catheter, 179–181
central IV dressing change, 181
children, 170, 171
complications, 173–177
discontinuing the IV, 179
dressing, 177–178, 181
filters, 159, 160f
fluid overload, 177
hematoma, 174
heparin lock, 168–169
infection, 176
infiltration, 174–175
IV flow rate, 171–172
IV pumps/controllers, 173
IV solution, 158–159
macrodrip/microdrip, 159
marking the container, 160
needles, 158
patient teaching, 162–163
peripheral IV, 161–167, 169–171
phlebitis, 175
precautions, 163–164
site selection, 157–158
special considerations, 159–160
threading a catheter, 164f, 165
troubleshooting, 174
vein, 162, 163f
intubation equipment, 523
irrigation
    bladder, 213–216
    colostomy, 232–234
    NG tube, 246, 247
    wound, 105, 106
isolation measures, 73–80
isolation room, 77–80
IV administration set, 159, 160–161
IV catheters, 158, 162, 179–181
IV controllers, 173
IV flow rate, 171–172
IV heparin lock, 168–169, 569–570
IV needles, 158
IV pumps, 173
IV solution, 158–159
IV therapy, 157–188. *See also* Intravenous therapy
IV-type Balkan frame, 329f
IV-type basic frame, 329f

J

J-tube, 252–253
Jackson, Hughlings, 383
Jackson-Pratt drain, 568–569

Jacksonian seizure, 385
jaw-thrust maneuver, 515
JCAHO accreditation, 9
jejunostomy, 251
jejunostomy tube (J-tube), 252–253
jewelry, 60f
Jobst hose, 312
junction, 472
junctional rhythms, 483, 483f
junctional tachycardia, 484f

K

K-Pad, 346–347
kelly clamp, 127, 127f, 464
ketone reagent strips, 191–192
kidney stones, 280
Klebsiella, 60f
knee bandage, 110
KO, 172
KVO, 172

L

lancet, 146–147
language/understanding problems, 29–30. *See also*
    Communication alert
laryngectomee, 454
laryngectomy, 454
laryngoscope, 449, 450f
larynx, 416f
latex allergy, 533–535
latex tourniquet, 131f
leg exercises, 308–309
leg whirlpool, 350f
legal alert
    child abuse, 376
    documentation, 49, 96
    documenting sterile procedures, 96
    emergency procedures, 511, 512
    platinum rule, 13
    reporting incidents, 5
    reporting observations, 40
    respiratory procedures, 448
    scope of practice, 10
    six rights of medication administration, 158
    standard of care, 9
leukemia, 393
lice, 100
liquid nutritional supplements, 394
liquid oxygen canister, 423f
living will, 511
loboy, 350f
local (localized) condition, 102
localized application, 338
lower leg bandage, 109

lower respiratory tract, 416f
LSW, 399
luer lock, 142f
luer slips, 159
lumbar plexus, 389f
lumen, 124
lungs, 416f

M

Macrodrip, 159
malpractice, 9
massage therapist, 398
mechanical ventilation, 440–441, 464–465
medical record, 47–53, 538–558
mental status, 43
mental status problems, 61
mercury, 536–537
microdraw, 146–150
microdrip, 159
microtainer safety lancets, 147f
microvette collection device, 147
midstream urine specimen, 274, 275
mild hypothermia, 364
mock code practices, 527
mode of transmission, 58
moderate hypothermia, 364
modified barium swallow, 240
moist heat treatments, 343–350
moist hot packs, 347–350
monitoring the heartbeat. See electrocardiogram (ECG)
Montgomery straps, 106, 107
mouth-to-mask resuscitation, 517, 518–519
MRSA, 60f
multifocal PVCs, 485f
multiskilling, 2
multistix reagent strip, 190f
multistix urine testing, 195–196
musculoskeletal system, 43
music therapist, 398
myoclonic seizure, 385

N

N95 respirator, 75f
nail polish, 418
nasal cannula, 428
nasal cavity, 416f
nasogastric tube (NG tube), 240–247
nasojejunostomy, 239
nasopharyngeal airway, 433–434
nasopharyngeal suctioning, 437–438
nausea and vomiting, 307
nebulizer, 438–439
neck breathers, 453–462
needle, 73, 124–125, 138

needle sizes/uses, 138
negative pressure environment, 74
negligence, 9
nephrostomy tube, 210–212
nervous system, 43
NG tube, 240–247
NIOSH-approved respirator, 74–76
nits, 100
noise, 3, 4f
noninvasive mechanical ventilation, 440–441
nonrebreathing mask, 430
normal conduction pathway, 472
normal sinus rhythm, 476f
norovirus, 63–64
nosocomial infection, 288
numeric pain scale, 46f
nun's hat, 276f
nurse practice act, 8–9

O

objective observations, 41
observe & report. *See also* Observe & report (boxes)
  cardiovascular system, 41–42
  dressing/grooming, 44
  drinking, 44
  eating, 44
  gastrointestinal system, 42–43
  genitourinary system, 43
  infection, 41
  integumentary system, 42
  mental status, 44
  musculoskeletal system, 43
  nervous system, 43
  pain, 41
  position, movement, 44
  respiratory system, 42
  sleeping, 44
  walking, 44
observe & report (boxes)
  breathing adequacy, 417, 514
  chest tubes, 464
  diabetic patients, 289–290
  dialysis, 219
  drain observations to report to nurse, 112
  hypothermia-hyperthermia, 368
  infection, 61
  pain observations, 402
  postoperative observation and reporting, 303
  tracheostomy suctioning, 457
  transfusion reaction, 184
  urinary problems, 211
  venipuncture complications to report to nurse, 129
  wound observations to report to nurse, 103
observing the patient, 39–44. *See also* Observe & report

obstructed airway procedure, 516–517
occult blood, stool specimen, 285–286
occupational therapist (OT), 398
old age, 26–27. *See also* Age-appropriate care alert
ONC, 158, 158f
open bladder irrigation, 213–214
open reduction internal fixation (ORIF), 321
opening closed drainage system, 207
opening the airway, 513–515
operating room procedure, 302–303
oral cavity, 416f
ORIF, 321
oropharyngeal airway, 431–433
oropharyngeal suctioning, 436–437
orthopedic beds, 318–319
orthopedic disorders, 318–330
orthopedics, 318
OSHA alert
   exposure control plan, 73
   needle disposal, 125
   needles, razors, etc., 301
   overview of OSHA, 3
   spinal cord injury, 390
   urine sample, 278
   venipuncture, 128
osteoporosis, 321
ostomy, 229–234
ostomy appliance, 230, 230f, 231–232
OT, 398
over-the-needle catheter (ONC), 158, 158f
oxygen administration devices, 428–430
oxygen cannula, 428f
oxygen concentrator, 422f
oxygen cylinder, 426–427
oxygen delivery systems, 422–428
oxygen mask, 429–430, 429f
oxygen safety, 424–425, 431
oxygen therapy, 421–431

P

P. aeruginosa, 60f
pacemaker, 471
PACU, 303–304
pain, 45–47, 401–406
pain management, 305–306
paralysis, 388
paraplegia, 388
patient care technician (PCT)
   continuing education, 9–10
   desirable qualities, 13–15
   job description, 7–8f
   professional boundaries, 15–16
   role/responsibilities, 7–8
   scope of practice, 9, 10
patient-controlled analgesia (PCA), 305–306

patient exercises, 306, 308–309, 310–312
patient-focused care, 6–10
patients who resist care, 30–31
PCA, 305–306
PCT. *See* Patient care technician (PCT)
PCT job description, 7–8f
PDA, 51, 52
pediatric urine specimen collection, 281, 282
PEG tube, 248–251
penis, 198f
percutaneous endoscopic gastrostomy (PEG), 248–251
perineal care, 275
perioperative care, 298–337
   casts, 319–320
   compartment syndrome, 326–327
   complications, 307–308
   CPM therapy, 323–326
   drainage, 306–307
   fractures, 318–324
   hand/forearm antisepsis, 299–300
   hip fracture, 321–323, 324f
   incision care, 309–310
   initial ambulation, 309
   operating room procedure, 302–303
   orthopedic beds, 318–319
   orthopedic disorders, 318–330
   pain management, 305–306
   patient exercises, 306, 308–309, 310–312
   pneumatic cuffs, 316–317
   postoperative care, 303–310
   required skills, 299
   respiratory exercises, 310–312
   shaving operative site, 300–302
   skin care, 300–302
   sling, 320
   support hosiery, 312–315
   traction, 327–330
perioperative hypothermia, 364–365
peripheral IV, 161–167, 169–171
peritoneal dialysis, 218
peritonitis, 249
persistent pain, 401
personal digital assistant (PDA), 51, 52
personal protective equipment (PPE), 66–72
   applying/removing, 78–80
   face/eye protection, 70–72
   gloves, 66–68
   gown, 68–70
personal space, 374
petit mal seizure, 385
PFR95 respirator, 75f
pH, 191, 244
phantom pain, 401
pharynx, 416f
phlebitis, 175

phlebotomy, 123–156
  bleeding time, 150–151
  blood culture, 144–146
  blood transfer device, 144
  butterfly needle and syringe, 126–127, 141–144
  centrifuge, 152–154
  cleansing the skin, 123–124
  complications, 128–129
  infant heel stick, 146–150
  microdraw, 146–150
  needle, 124–125, 138
  precautions, 127–128
  site selection, 130
  syringe method, 126–127, 141–144
  tourniquet, 130–133
  transporting specimen to lab, 152
  vacuum-tube method, 125–126, 136–141
  venipuncture, 130, 133–135
physical disabilities. See Disabled patients
physical distance, 17
physical therapist (PT), 398
physically aggressive patients, 31
piercing pin, 159
pin care, 116–117
platinum rule, 13
pleural effusion, 463
pneumatic cuffs, 316–317
pneumothorax, 462
pocket mask, 517
pointers. See age-appropriate care alert; communica-
    tion alert; culture alert; difficult patient alert;
    health care alert; infection alert; legal alert; OSHA
    alert; procedure alert; safety alert
portable emergency oxygen tank, 422f
portal of entry, 58
portal of exit, 58
post-angiogram care, 505, 506
post-arteriogram care, 505, 506
postanesthesia care unit (PACU), 303–304
posterior tibial pulse, 500–501
postictal, 388
postoperative care, 303–310
postoperative complications, 307–308
postoperative incision care, 309–310
postprandial blood sugar (PPBS), 286
postresuscitation care, 527
postural drainage, 441–443
postural drainage positions, 442f
PPBS, 286
PPE. See Personal protective equipment (PPE)
PR interval, 474, 474f
pre-operative skin care, 300–302
precordial leads, 489f, 490
prehypertension, 503
premature atrial contractions, 479f, 480f
premature ventricular contractions (PVCs), 484–487

preschoolers, 22–23. See also Age-appropriate care
    alert
pressure gauge (oxygen tank), 424
prevention of viral transmission, 289
primary hypothermia, 364
priorities, 14
privacy, 38–39, 53
procedure. See also procedure alert
  AED, 525
  antiembolism stockings, 314–315
  apical-radial pulse, 499
  arm sling, 320
  bag-valve mask ventilation, 519
  bandage-wrapping techniques, 109–111
  bladder irrigation, 213–216
  bleeding time, 150–151
  blood bank, 183
  blood collection, 140–141, 143–144
  blood culture, 145–146
  blood pressure, 504–505
  blood transfer device, 144
  bolus enteral feeding, 259
  butterfly needle & syringe (blood collection),
      140–141
  capillary refill, 418
  cardiac catheterization, 506–507
  catheterization, 199–204, 216–217
  catheterized urine specimen, 278–280
  central IV dressing change, 181
  checking blood products, 183–184
  cold compresses, 361
  colostomy irrigation, 232–234
  continuous cardiac monitoring, 498
  continuous feeding pump, 260
  cool soak, 361–362
  coughing and deep breathing exercises, 310–311
  CPM therapy, 325–326
  CPR, 520–522
  deep breathing exercises, 310–311
  disposable gloves, 67, 68
  Doppler, 502
  dressing—IV infusion site, 178
  dressings, 108, 111–116
  ECG, 493–495
  endotracheal intubation, 452, 453
  enema administration, 224–227
  eye compresses, 363
  fecal impaction, 228
  fingerstick blood sugar, 290
  gastric specimen, 274
  gown, 68–70
  handwashing, 62–63
  head-tilt, chin-lift maneuver, 514–515
  heating pad, 346–347
  heparin lock, 168–169, 569–570
  hot water bottle, 341–342

humidifier, 427
hypothermia-hyperthermia blanket, 367
ice bag, 359–360
incentive spirometry, 312
IV administration set, 160–161
Jackson-Pratt drain, 568–569
jaw-thrust maneuver, 515
microdraw, 149–150
midstream urine sample, 275
mouth-to-mask ventilation, 518–519
nasopharyngeal airway, 433
nasopharyngeal suctioning, 437–438
nephrostomy tube dressing, 212
NG tube, 241–243, 245, 247
obstructed airway, 516–517
oropharyngeal airway, 432–433
oropharyngeal suctioning, 436–437
ostomy appliance, 231–232
oxygen administration, 429, 430
oxygen tank, 425–427
pediatric urine specimen, 282
PEG tube, 249, 250–251
peripheral IV, 166–167, 169–170, 171, 179
pin care, 117
pneumatic compression device, 317
postural drainage, 443
protective eyewear, 72
pulse, 499, 501
pulse oximeter, 420–421
recovery position, 523
rectal suppository, 221–222
rectal swab specimen, 284
rectal tube and flatus bag, 220–221
renal calculi—straining urine, 280–281
residual stomach contents, 246
respirator, 75–76
seizure, 387
shaving operative site, 302
sitz bath, 357–358
small-volume nebulizer treatment, 439
sputum culture, 273
staple removal, 119
sterile field, 92–94
sterile gloves, 94–95
sterile package, 91
sterile tray, 90
sterile urine specimen—indwelling catheter, 277–278
stool specimen, 283–284, 285–286
suctioning a tracheostomy, 457–458
surgical mask, 71–72
suture removal, 118
T-tube, 567
tepid sponge bath, 354–356
throat culture, 270
tracheostomy, 456–462
traction, 330
transfer forceps, 96
24-hour urine specimen, 276–277
urine specific gravity, 194–195
urine specimen collection, 275–282
urine testing, 192, 194–196
vacuum-tube system (blood collection), 140–141
venipuncture, 133–135
warm compresses, 344–346
warm soak, 343–344
wound culture, 272–273
procedure alert
    hemolysis, 152
    phlebotomy, 137, 140
    urine specimen collection, 274, 276
    venipuncture, 131
procedure completion actions, 82–83
professional boundaries, 15–16
prostate gland, 198, 198f
PROTECTIV IV catheter safety system, 165f
protective isolation, 78
proteus, 60f
pseudomonas aeruginosa, 60f
psychomotor seizure, 385
PT, 398
pulmonary embolus, 309
pulse, 498–501
pulse deficit, 499
pulse locations, 316f
pulse oximeter, 418–421
pulse points, 498
purkinje fibers, 471f, 472
PVCs, 484–487

Q

QI, 2
QRS complex, 472, 474, 474f
quadrigeminy, 486f
quadriplegia, 388
quality assurance (QA), 2
quality improvement (QI), 2
quality indicators, 5

R

radiating pain, 401
radiation therapy, 394–397
radio frequency emitting devices, 51–52
RCA, 5–6
RCP, 399
re-engineering, 2
reagent strips, 190–192, 287f
recovery position, 522, 523
rectal suppository, 221–222
rectal swab specimen, 284

rectal tube and flatus bag, 220–221
rectum, 198f
reflex arc, 388, 388f
refractometer, 193, 194f
rehabilitation, 397–401
rehabilitation team, 398–399
reimbursement for health care services, 1–2
relaxation (cardiac cycle), 470
renal calculi, straining urine, 280–281
renal colic, 280
reporting observations, 47–53
reservoir, 58
residual stomach contents, 245–246
resisting care, 30–31
respiration fundamentals, 415–417
respirator, 74–76
respiratory arrest, 513
respiratory care practitioner (RCP), 399
respiratory exercises, 310–312
respiratory failure, 513
respiratory procedures, 415–469
  BiPAP, 441
  capillary refill, 418
  chest tubes, 462–464
  CPAP, 440, 441
  endotracheal intubation, 449–453
  high-risk conditions, 418
  mechanical ventilation, 440–441, 464–465
  nasopharyngeal airway, 433–434
  neck breathers, 453–462
  noninvasive mechanical ventilation, 440–441
  oropharyngeal airway, 431–433
  oxygen therapy, 421–431
  postural drainage, 441–443
  pulse oximeter, 418–421
  respiration fundamentals, 415–417
  respiratory system, 416
  small-volume nebulizer treatment, 438–439
  suctioning, 434–438
  suctioning a tracheostomy, 457–458
  tracheostomy, 454–462
respiratory rates, 513
respiratory system, 42, 416, 513f
respiratory system infection, 61
respiratory therapist (RT), 399
responsible behavior, 14–15
restorative nursing care, 32, 399–401
restructuring, 2
resuscitation, 511. *See also* Emergency procedures
retention enema, 223
retention (Foley) catheter, 197
reverse isolation, 78
Rh factor, 182
rights (dressing changes), 108
root cause analysis (RCA), 5–6
rotavirus, 63–64

RT, 399
rule-out test, 269

S

SA node, 471, 471f
sacral plexus, 389f
sadness, 18
Saf-T-Clik shielded needle adapter, 137f
safety alert
  AED, 524, 526
  arm sling, 320
  bladder irrigation, 213
  clamp, 464
  CPM therapy, 324
  delirium, 383
  dentures, 300
  dialysis, 219
  enteral feeding—food coloring, 244
  fecal impaction, 228
  initial ambulation, 309
  Kelly clamp, 464
  monitoring the patient, 421
  oxygen tank, 423, 431
  perioperative care, 300
  rectal treatment, 228
  removing bed linen, 302
  seizure, 387
  shaving the patient, 301
  shoes, 299
  surgery, 302, 304
  tepid sponge bath, 353
  tourniquet, 133
  unconscious patient, 514
  water temperature, 343
safety blood collection needle, 124f
safety needle, 139f
safety needle and holder, 126f
Sawtoothed P waves, 481f
scabies, 100
school-age children, 23–24. *See also* Age-appropriate
  care alert
sciatic nerve, 389f
scream/yell, patients who, 31
scrotum, 198f
secondary hypothermia, 364
seizure, 383
seizure disorders, 383–388
seizure precautions, 386–387
sentinel events, 5
septicemia, 144
sequential compression device, 316
serious events, 5
severe hypothermia, 364
sharps/needles, handling, 73
shaving operative site, 300–302

Shigella, 60f
shock, 309
shoes, 299
shoulder bandage, 111
shunt, 217
signs, 41
signs (interpreter), 376f
simple-partial seizure, 385
sims' position, 223, 223f
singultus, 307
sinoatrial (SA) node, 471, 471f
sinus arrest, 478f
sinus arrhythmia, 477f
sinus bradycardia, 477f
sinus pause, 478f
sinus tachycardia, 476f
sitz bath, 356–358
six rights of medication administration, 158
skeletal traction, 327, 328f
skin, 100, 101f
skin traction, 327, 328f
sleep apnea, 440
slide clamp, 159
sling, 320
SLP, 399
small-volume nebulizer treatment, 438–439
sniffing position, 451, 451f
social worker (LSW), 399
Sossaman, Marilyn, 16f
source, 58
spastic paralysis, 388
Speci-Cath collection device, 278–280
Speci-Cath insertion kit, 205f
special-needs patients, 373–414
    autonomic dysreflexia, 390–391
    brachytherapy, 395–397
    chemotherapy, 392–394
    delirium, 382–383
    domestic violence, 376–381
    immunotherapy, 397
    interpreter, 374–375
    pain, 401–406
    radiation therapy, 394–397
    rehabilitation, 397–401
    seizure disorders, 383–388
    spinal cord injuries, 388–391
specimen collection, 266–297
    A1C testing, 290–291
    blood glucose testing, 286–289
    culture and sensitivity testing, 267–269
    gastric specimen, 274
    Group A streptococcus antigen testing, 270–271
    guidelines/pointers, 267
    PPE, 267
    preparing the patient, 267
    sputum culture, 273
    stool specimen, 282–286
    swab culture, 268
    throat culture, 269–270
    urine specimen collection, 274–282
    wound culture, 271–273
specimen collection system, 205–206
speech language pathologist (SLP), 399
speech therapist (ST), 399
spinal bed, 318
spinal cord and nerves, 389f
spinal cord injuries, 388–391
spores, 63–64, 80
spouse abuse, 376–381
sputum, 273
sputum culture, 273
ST, 399
ST segment, 474, 474f
stage I pressure ulcer, 101, 101f
stage II pressure ulcer, 101, 101f
stage III pressure ulcer, 101, 102f
stage IV pressure ulcer, 101, 102f
standard leads, 489f, 490
standard precautions, 64–73
standards of care, 9
standards of performance, 9
standards of practice, 9
staphylococcus, 60f
staple removal, 117, 119
status epilepticus, 385
steam sterilization, 96
step-by-step procedure. See Procedure
sterile drape, 92
sterile dressing, 111
sterile field, 91–94
sterile gloves, 94–95
sterile technique, 88. See also surgical asepsis
sterile urine specimen—indwelling catheter, 277–278
sterilization, 96–97
stethoscope, 498
stoma, 229, 229f, 454–462, 454f
stool specimen, 282–286
straight catheter, 197, 199–201
streptococcus, 60f
Stryker frame, 318
subjective observations, 41
suctioning, 434–438
suctioning a tracheostomy, 457–458
sudden cardiac death, 487f
sunstroke, 365
support hosiery, 312–315
suprapubic catheter, 209–210
surgical asepsis, 88–99
    autoclaving, 88, 89f
    documentation, 96
    environmental conditions, 89
    flash sterilization, 96–97

handwashing, 88–89
  opening sterile package, 91
  opening sterile tray, 90
  sterile drape, 92
  sterile field, 91–94
  sterile gloves, 94–95
  tips/pointers, 89–90
  transfer forceps, 96
surgical mask, 71–72
surgicutt bleeding time procedure, 151f
surveyors, 48
susceptible host, 58
suture removal, 117, 118
swab culture, 268
sympathy, 17
symptoms, 41
syringe method of blood collection, 126–127, 141–144
system condition (factor), 102
systemic infection, 271
systole, 472

T

T-tube, 566–568
T wave, 474–475, 475f
table PC (TPC), 51
tact, 13
TED hose, 312, 313f
telemetry, 495
telephone skills, 18–19
TENS, 406
tepid sponge bath, 353–356
testis, 198f
tetraplegia, 388
THA, 322
therapeutic bath, 353
therapeutic recreation specialist (TRS), 399
thermotherapy. *See* heat and cold applications
thirst, 307
threading a catheter, 164f, 165
throat culture, 269–270
tips/pointers. *See* age-appropriate care alert; communication alert; culture alert; difficult patient alert;
  health care alert; infection alert; legal alert; OSHA
  alert; procedure alert; safety alert
titles (multiskilled workers), 2f
TKO, 172
toddler, 21–22. *See also* Age-appropriate care alert
tone of voice, 17f
tongue piercings, 432
total hip arthroplasty (THA), 322
total joint replacement, 321–322
tourniquet, 130–133
TPC, 51
trachea, 416f
tracheostomy, 454–462

tracheostomy dressing, 461–462
tracheostomy oxygen mask, 455f
tracheostomy ties, 461–462
tracheotomy, 453
traction, 327–330
transcutaneous electrical nerve stimulation (TENS), 406
transfer forceps, 96
transfusion reaction, 184
transmission-based precautions, 73–77
transparency, 6
transparent film dressing (IV infusion site), 178
transparent film dressings, 114–115, 115–116
transport bag, 267
trash disposal, 67, 104
trigeminy, 486f
TRS, 399
tube feeding, 239–265. *See also* enteral nutrition
tubular gauze bandages, 106
two-hour postprandial blood sugar (PPBS), 286
12-lead ECG, 488–491
24-hour urine collection, 276–277
type and cross-match, 182

U

UAP, 7
uncertainty, 18
unifocal PVCs, 485f
universal donor, 182
universal recipient, 182
unlicensed assistive personnel (UAP), 7
urethra, 197, 198f
urinary and bowel elimination, 189–238
  bladder irrigation, 213–216
  bowel elimination, 219–228
  catheters, 196–210
  dialysis, 217–219
  drainage bag disinfection, 209
  enema, 222–227
  fecal impaction, 219, 220f, 228
  indwelling catheter, 196, 197, 202–204, 216–217
  nephrostomy tube, 210–212
  opening closed drainage system, 207
  ostomy, 229–234
  rectal suppository, 221–222
  rectal tube and flatus bag, 220–221
  specimen collection system, 205–206
  straight catheter, 197, 199–201
  suprapubic catheter, 209–210
  urinary leg bag, 208, 209
  urine specific gravity, 193–195
  urine testing, 190–196
urinary bladder, 198f
urinary leg bag, 208, 209
urinary retention, 308
urine glucose and ketone reagent strips, 191–192

urine specific gravity, 193–195
urine specimen collection, 274–282
urine testing, 190–196
urinometer, 193, 193f

V

V_1 (ECG lead), 489f
V_2 (ECG lead), 489f
V_3 (ECG lead), 489f
V_4 (ECG lead), 489f
V_5 (ECG lead), 489f
V_6 (ECG lead), 489f
vacutainer, 125
vacuum tube, 136, 136f
vacuum-tube method of blood collection, 125–126,
    136–141
vas deferens, 198f
vector
vein
    arm, 131f
    forearm, 163f
    hand, 163f
venipuncture, 123, 130, 133–135. *See also* Phlebotomy
venti mask, 430
ventilator, 464
ventricles, 472
ventricular fibrillation, 484, 487f, 488f, 526
ventricular tachycardia, 484, 487f
Venturi mask, 430, 430f
verbal pain scale, 46f
verbally aggressive patients, 31
viral transmission, prevention of, 289
vision impairment, 28
VitalCheck patient monitor, 503f
volumetric intravenous pumps, 173
VRE, 60f

W

wall-outlet oxygen, 425–426
warm compresses, 344–346
warm eye compresses, 362, 363

warm soak, 343–344
warmed blankets, 342–343
waste disposal, 67, 104
waterless hand cleaners, 63, 64
wedge bed, 318
wet-to-dry dressings, 113–114
whirlpool therapy, 350–353
wife abuse, 376–381
winged infusion needle, 141f
wireless Internet technology, 51
Wong-Baker FACES pain scale, 46f
workplace redesign, 2
workplace reorganization, 2
worry, 18
wound care, 100–122
    bandage, 106
    bandage-wrapping techniques, 109–111
    changing clean dressing, 108
    cleansing the wound, 105
    dressing, 106
    dressing around a drain, 112–113
    factors to consider, 102–103
    hydrocolloid dressings, 115, 116
    infection control, 103–104
    pin care, 116–117
    removing a dressing, 104
    staple removal, 117, 119
    sterile dressing, 111
    suture removal, 117, 118
    transparent film dressings, 114–115, 115–116
    wet-to-dry dressings, 113–114
    wound irrigation, 105, 106
wound culture, 271–273
wound dehiscence/disruption, 308
wound infection, 271, 309
wound irrigation, 105, 106
wrist bandage, 110

Y

Y-site, 159
Yankauer catheter, 434, 435f
yell/scream, patients who, 31